## THE ULTIMATE CARBOHYDRATE COUNTER

**Low carb products are suddenly everywhere. And yet the body needs carbs to survive. Annette Natow and Jo-Ann Heslin, the nutrition experts you can trust, explain in clear language how carbs got such a bad reputation and how to work them into your diet in a healthy way.**

This revised version of *The Carbohydrate, Sugar, and Fiber Counter* features entirely new introductory information to help health-conscious eaters navigate a carb-obsessed marketplace. Look inside to learn how to count carbs for weight loss and how to sort through the marketing gimmicks in order to make the best carb choices.

In the tradition of the entire bestselling *Counter* series from Natow and Heslin, *The Ultimate Carbohydrate Counter* provides the most up-to-date figures as well as concise, honest guidance on healthy eating.

## THE ULTIMATE CARBOHYDRATE COUNTER

**An essential reference for counting carbs and eating right!**

**Books by Annette B. Natow and Jo-Ann Heslin**

The Antioxidant Vitamin Counter

Calcium Counts

The Calorie Counter (Third Edition)

The Cholesterol Counter (Sixth Edition)

The Complete Food Counter

Count on a Healthy Pregnancy

The Diabetes Carbohydrate and Calorie Counter (Second Edition)

Eating Out Food Counter

The Fat Attack Plan

The Fat Counter (Fifth Edition)

The Food Shopping Counter (Second Edition)

Get Skinny the Smart Way

The Healthy Heart Food Counter

Megadoses: Vitamins as Drugs

The Most Complete Food Counter

No-Nonsense Nutrition for Kids

The Pocket Encyclopedia of Nutrition

The Pocket Fat Counter (Second Edition)

The Pocket Protein Counter

The Pregnancy Nutrition Counter

The Protein Counter (Second Edition)

The Sodium Counter

The Ultimate Carbohydrate Counter

The Vitamin and Mineral Food Counter

Published by POCKET BOOKS

# THE ULTIMATE CARBOHYDRATE COUNTER

Annette B. Natow, Ph.D.
and Jo-Ann Heslin, M.A., R.D.

POCKET BOOKS
New York London Toronto Sydney

POCKET BOOKS, a division of Simon & Schuster, Inc.
1230 Avenue of the Americas, New York, NY 10020



ISBN: 0-7434-6439-7

The previous edition of this book was published as *The Carbohydrate, Fiber, and Sugar Counter.*

First Pocket Books paperback printing of this revised edition January 2005

10 9 8 7 6 5 4 3 2 1



Manufactured in the United States of America

*To our families, who support us through every project:*
*Harry, Allen, Irene, Sarah, Meryl, Laura, Marty,*
*George, Emily, Steven, Rebecca, Joseph, Kristen,*
*Brian, Karen, and John.*

# ACKNOWLEDGMENTS

For graciously sharing her knowledge, Karen J. Nolan, Ph.D.

For all her support and help, our agent, Nancy Trichter.

For her suggestions and editing skills, Sara Clemence.

Without the tireless cooperation of Steven Natow, M.D., and Stephen Llano, *The Ultimate Carbohydrate Counter* would never have been completed.

A special thank you to our editor, Micki Nuding.

*"Since carbohydrates constitute the largest part of an ordinary diet, their withdrawal changes eating habits materially, and people find it difficult to be without the familiar bread, potatoes, cereals, sugars and fruits."*

Mary Swartz Rose, Ph.D.
*Feeding the Family*
The Macmillan Company, 1919

# CONTENTS

# SORTING OUT CARBOHYDRATES

*Carbohydrates, carbs, complex carbs, simple carbs,*
*"good" carbs, "bad" carbs, net carbs,*
*effective carbs, impact carbs—*
***Help!***

As consumers become more carb-conscious, sorting out carbs and selecting nutrient-rich carbohydrate foods becomes increasingly difficult. To shop and eat wisely, you need to understand carbs.

## What are carbohydrates?

Carbohydrates are the starches, fibers, and sugars found in food. All plant foods—fruits, vegetables, beans, and grains—are rich in carbohydrates. Fruits have more sugar. Vegetables, beans, and grains have more starch. Both have fiber.

Sugars and starches are your body's main source of energy. Fiber is not digested or absorbed by the body, but it does help digestion and offer protection against certain diseases. During digestion, sugar molecules move easily into the bloodstream and travel to cells where they are burned for energy. Starches are more complex, made up of many sugar molecules. During digestion, the larger starch molecules are slowly broken apart to yield smaller sugar fragments, which are sent to the cells to be converted into energy. If you eat more carbohydrate than your body needs for energy, the leftover is stored as fat.

### Pounds or energy?

*When you gain weight, your body is actually warehousing energy it doesn't need—as a result, your hips, thighs, and tummy get larger. When you lose weight, you pull that extra energy out of storage and your hips, thighs, and tummy get smaller.*

## What's a simple carbohydrate?

Simple carbohydrates are carbohydrate foods that contain a lot of sugar—like syrups, jelly, honey, soda, and molasses. Complex carbohydrates are foods that contain a lot of starch—like whole grains, cereals, beans, and vegetables. Complex carbs are also rich in fiber, vitamins, and minerals. Most simple carbohydrate foods are poor sources of important nutrients. But there are exceptions. Milk, yogurt, fruits, and some vegetables have a lot of sugar, but they are rich in important vitamins and minerals, too.

**FOODS HIGH IN CARBOHYDRATES**

| Complex Carbs | Simple Carbs |
|---|---|
| Bagels | *Natural Sugar* |
| Beans | Fruits |
| Breads | Fruit juice |
| Cereals | Honey |

| Complex Carbs | Simple Carbs |
|---|---|
| Corn | Milk |
| Crackers | Unsweetened yogurt |
| Grains | |
| Pasta | *Added Sugar* |
| Peas | Cake |
| Popcorn | Candy |
| Potatoes | Cookies |
| Pretzels | Fruit drinks |
| Rice | Jellies/jam |
| Rolls | Gelatin |
| Squash | Soda |
| Tortillas | Sweetened yogurt |
| Vegetables | Sweetened cereal |

> *"Everything you see, I owe to pasta."*
> Sophia Loren

## Which foods have "good" carbs and which have "bad" carbs?

Complex carbs—those foods high in starch—are sometimes called "good carbs." Foods high in sugar or those that are refined, like white flour and pasta, are referred to as "bad carbs." These terms can be misleading and are used more by food marketers than food professionals. There is no question that foods high in sugar—table sugar, candy, cake, cookies, soda—are not the best carb choices. But milk, yogurt, and fruits are also high in natural sugar and they are good choices.

We recommend not worrying about good carbs and bad carbs. Instead, when making choices, pick foods with naturally occurring sugars, like milk and fruit, or those that are less processed, like brown rice and whole wheat bread, more often. Choose foods with added sugars, like fruit drinks, desserts, and sweetened cereal, and those that are highly processed, like white rice and white bread, less often.

## How do you figure the net carbs in foods?

When lowfat foods hit the market in the 1990s, the FDA (Food and Drug Administration) had already legally defined a lowfat food as one that had 3 grams of fat or less in one serving. No similar definition exists for "low carb," "net carbs," or "net impact carbs." These terms were coined by diet doctors to highlight foods that have less impact on blood sugar. More recently, food manufacturers have begun to use these terms to promote new lower carb brands.

"Net carbs" are arrived at by subtracting fiber, glycerin, and sugar alcohols from the total carbohydrates on the nutrition label. To produce new low carb versions of typically higher carb foods, like bread, cereal, cookies, and energy bars, food companies replace some of the carbohydrates with fiber, glycerin, and sugar alcohols. The reasoning behind these substitutions is that your body does not use these carbs effectively.

This is true for fiber. Your body does not digest fiber, so it provides no calories and doesn't have to be counted as part of total carbohydrates. Most experts agree that fiber can be subtracted from the total carbohydrate count for a food. But subtracting glycerin and sugar alcohols to arrive at "net carbs" is more creative math than sound science.

Glycerin, a food additive that helps hold moisture in foods, can also add sweetness. It can be converted to sugar in the body and has the same calories as sugar. But since glycerin is a food additive and not technically a sugar, it's been suggested that it doesn't count as an "effective carb," and therefore can be subtracted from the total carb. Most experts don't agree.

What about sugar alcohols? They appear in the ingredients listing with names that often end in "ol"—mannitol, sorbitol, and xylitol. Sugar alcohols have little or no effect on blood sugar, but they still contain calories. Subtracting them from total carbs is a little like cheating on a math test.

### And the net carb is?

*In many cases, low carb foods do not have fewer carbs or calories. They just have fewer "net carbs."*

*A chocolate chip energy bar has 30 grams of total carbs. The manufacturer subtracts 26 grams of sugar alcohols, advertising the bar as "4 grams net carbs." The nutrition panel still reads 270 calories and 30 grams of total carbs for a 2-ounce bar. So, what's been lost?*

## Is low carb beer healthier?

Classifying beer as "healthy" is a stretch, but advertisements for low carb beer and other low carb alcoholic drinks do make them sound like better choices. The good news is that the federal government has established standards for labeling alcoholic beverages low carb.

Beers or other alcoholic beverages labeled or advertised as "low carb" must have less than 7 grams of carbohydrate in a serving. An alcoholic drink with more than 7 grams of carb, but less carb than the original version, can be labeled or advertised as "reduced carb" or "lower carb."

Low carb or not, don't forget that a bottle of beer or a shot of alcohol has at least 100 calories and some can have much more. Check BEER AND ALE on page 59 and LIQUOR/LIQUEURS, page 313 for a complete listing.

# UNDERSTANDING CARBS

Glucose, a simple sugar, is the only sugar your body will burn for energy, but you won't find it in a package on the supermarket shelves or on a menu at your local restaurant. You have to eat an apple, a roll, or a plate of spaghetti first, so that your body can convert the carbohydrates in those foods into the glucose it needs for energy. Let's take a closer look at how all this happens.

After you chew and swallow carbohydrates, they pass through your stomach into the small intestines, where digestion actually takes place. Sugars are easy to break down because they contain only two molecules of sugar bound together. Once the bond is broken the sugar travels through the intestinal wall and enters the bloodstream quickly. Starches are more complex, made up of many small sugar molecules. It takes time to break the larger starch structures apart. But that's good, because the sugar is released into the body more slowly. Fiber is made up of many sugar molecules, too, but the bonds that hold these sugars together can't be broken down in the human digestive tract. Because fiber can't be digested, it moves down into the large intestine where it adds softness and bulk to stools.

All sugars that are digested and absorbed travel in the bloodstream first to the liver, where they are converted to glucose. That's the only sugar your body burns for energy. The liver is the glucose gatekeeper, sending it into the bloodstream or into storage to maintain a constant blood sugar level.

The process of digestion and absorption changes the carbohydrates in sugar, fruits, vegetables, breads, and milk into glucose. And glucose has only one job—to supply energy for your body.

## Using Glucose

Glucose is the primary fuel for every cell in your body and the most preferred fuel for your brain, red blood cells, and nervous system. Your body keeps close tabs on its glucose levels. When levels rise after a meal, the hormone insulin acts like a key, unlocking cells so glucose can enter them and provide energy. If you have not eaten in a while and your blood sugar begins to fall, another hormone triggers the release of glucose from storage. On a daily basis, your blood sugar goes up and down to meet your energy needs.

If not enough carbohydrates are available to be broken down into glucose, your body can use fat and protein for energy. These are both less efficient forms of fuel. When fat is burned for energy, a small amount of glucose is still needed to completely break down the fat. If no carbohydrate is available, fat can't be broken down completely, and compounds called *ketones* are formed. These compounds can disrupt your body's normal balance and cause dehydration. Your body needs some carbs everyday to prevent *ketosis.*

## Glycemic Index

Decades ago, researcher David Jenkins at the University of Toronto coined the term *glycemic index.* This index ranks a food by how quickly it can be converted to glucose and enter your bloodstream. Foods with a high glycemic index—rice, white bread, potatoes—raise blood sugar levels quickly. Foods with a low glycemic index—beans, whole grains, meat, fat—raise blood sugar levels more slowly, either because they are high in fiber that can't be broken down, or because they don't have any carbohydrates in them. It takes longer for your body to process these foods into glucose to be used for fuel.

In theory, a blast of sugar into your blood stream requires a corresponding blast of insulin to escort the sugar into your cells for energy. When the blood sugar is quickly used up, blood sugar levels drop, and you feel hungry again. Many low carb diet programs hang their hats on this scientific premise.

They claim that eating the wrong carbohydrates makes us ravenous, so we eat more and more. The "bad" carbs—foods high in sugar or highly refined, like white bread—move quickly into the bloodstream and need to be either moved into cells or placed into storage. After this happens, blood sugar drops and your body sends a signal that it needs more glucose. You in turn feel hungry. Low carb diet plans believe cutting carbs will cut hunger. But remember the old caveat: *If something sounds too good to be true, it probably is.*

The theory behind the glycemic index is correct. Some foods do raise blood sugar quickly; others do not. But in practice, it's not that simple.

The glycemic index was devised based on eating one food at a time. Glucose was given a rating of 100 and individual foods were measured against it. White bread has a very high glycemic index. But if you add peanut butter, the glycemic response is lowered because peanut butter, a high fat food, has a low glycemic index. The same goes for a baked potato, another high glycemic food: top it with cheese sauce and broccoli, and the glycemic index plunges.

And it gets even more complicated. Ripe fruits have a lower glycemic index than unripe. That's right, a hard peach will raise your blood sugar faster than a ripe, juicy one. Cooking pasta al dente is fine; overcook it, and its glycemic value goes up. Regular ice cream has a low glycemic index, because the fat in it slows down the absorption of sugar. Even sugars vary: glucose is high on the index, but fructose (fruit sugar) is low.

Most researchers, even those who have extensively studied the glycemic index, feel there is little evidence to support its use in weight control. This is why the concept of net carbs isn't as clear-cut as you are led to believe. Net carbs are based on the assumption that the blood sugar response, or the glycemic index, for a certain food is constant and will be the same for everyone. That simply isn't true.

First, the food would have to be eaten alone, so no other food or cooking condition would affect the blood sugar response. Second, not everyone regulates blood sugar the same. If you exercise regularly, are a normal weight, and eat slowly, you regulate your blood sugar more efficiently. If you are overweight, sedentary, sick, or have diabetes, your ability to regulate blood sugar may be impaired.

*Bottom line:* More research is needed about the health applications of the glycemic index. Eating more foods with a low glycemic index may lower the risk for heart disease and help to control diabetes. But if you are trying to lose weight, the best approach is still to reduce calories and increase activity.

## GLYCEMIC INDEX OF COMMON FOODS

| High (greater than 70) | |
|---|---|
| White rice | 126 |
| Baked potato | 121 |
| Cornflakes | 119 |

## GLYCEMIC INDEX OF COMMON FOODS (continued)

| | |
|---|---|
| **High (greater than 70)** | |
| Rice cakes | 117 |
| Jellybeans | 114 |
| Carrots | 101 |
| White bread | 101 |
| **Glucose** | **100** |
| Wheat bread | 99 |
| Soda | 97 |
| Sucrose | 92 |
| Cheese pizza | 86 |
| Spaghetti | 83 |
| Popcorn | 79 |
| Corn | 78 |
| Banana | 76 |
| Orange juice | 74 |
| **Moderate (between 56 and 69)** | |
| Peas | 68 |
| Orange | 62 |
| Bran cereal | 60 |
| Apple juice | 58 |
| Pumpernickel bread | 58 |
| **Low (55 and below)** | |
| Apple | 52 |
| Nonfat milk | 46 |
| Kidney beans | 42 |
| Fructose (fruit sugar) | 32 |

Source: *Dietary Reference Intakes for Energy, Carbohydrate, Fiber, Fat, Fatty Acids, Cholesterol, Protein and Amino Acids, Part 1,* Institute of Medicine of the National Academies, The National Academies Press, Washington, DC, 2002.

# HOW MUCH SHOULD YOU EAT?

## Carbohydrates

In the last decade, carbohydrates have gone from the dietary penthouse to the dietary doghouse. Not so long ago, you were told to eat all the carbs you wanted. Today, even a little is considered too much. So how much do you really need?

The National Academy of Sciences' Recommended Dietary Allowance (RDA) for carbohydrates is 130 grams a day. The FDA has set 300 grams of carb as the Daily Value (DV), the amount needed by the "typical" consumer. This Daily Value is used on nutrition labels to compare the amount of carbs in one serving of food. For example, if a cup of cereal has 15 grams of carbohydrates, it would provide 5% of your Daily Value of 300 grams. And, it's been estimated that you need at least 50 to 100 grams of carbs a day to prevent ketosis caused by the incomplete breakdown of fat.

That still does not answer the question—*how much carb do you need to eat each day?*

It's not an easy question to answer. Vegetarians, athletes, and many populations throughout the world base their diet on carbohydrates, getting as much as 80% of their daily calories from carbs. Most food professionals believe that eating 40% or less of your daily calories as carb would be considered a low carb diet. On average, Americans get approximately 50% of their daily calories from carbs.

But that still doesn't answer the question—*how much carb do you need each day?*

The truth is, until long-term studies are done, it's impossible to say what amount of carb is right for you. In the meantime, we suggest that you stick with the recommendation of at least 130 grams of carbs a day—choosing more foods high in fiber and fewer foods high in sugar.

If you want to eat a percentage of your daily calories as carbs, that's easy to figure out. If 40% or lower is considered a low carb diet:

40% of 1,500 calories = 600 carb calories
40% of 1,800 calories = 720 carb calories
40% of 2,000 calories = 800 carb calories

To figure out how many grams of carbs to eat a day, you need to know that 1 gram of carb = 4 calories. Using the numbers above:

40% of 1,500 calories = 150 grams carb
(600 carb calories ÷ 4 = 150)
40% of 1,800 calories = 180 grams carb
(720 carb calories ÷ 4 = 180)
40% of 2,000 calories = 200 grams carb
(800 carb calories ÷ 4 = 200)

In every example, you would more than meet the RDA of 130 grams of carb a day and stay well above the minimum needed to prevent ketosis.

Set your own target daily carb intake, using the equation below. Your target may change depending on whether you are trying to lose weight, are on a low carb diet, are an athlete, or are eating a high carb, lowfat diet.

**Your target daily carb intake is:**

*______% of _____ calories a day = _____ carb calories*

*______ carb calories ÷ 4 = _____ carb grams*

## Sugar

Most of us enjoy sweets. Babies are born with a preference for sweets. Both amniotic fluid and breast milk are slightly sweet tasting. Anthropologists believe that our ability to taste the difference between sweet plants and bitter plants may have helped humans to evolve; sweet plants are more often edible and bitter ones are more likely to be poisonous.

Today, however, our passion for sweets is creating a global epidemic of overweight people. Clearly, we are eating too much sugar. Too many sugary foods can crowd out more nutritious choices. We drink more soda than milk in this country, and buy far more sugared drinks than fruit juice.

Cereals, grains, fruits, vegetables, milk, and plain yogurt all contain sugars. These are *natural* sugar choices and contain vitamins, minerals, and fiber, too. Soda, candy, fruit drinks, cakes, cookies, ice cream, jelly, and syrup, in contrast, offer little more than sweetness and calories, and are loaded with *added sugar.*

**We Love Sweets—**

*According to surveys, Americans eat 146 pounds of sugar a year: 45 pounds of regular sugar (about 2 ounces a day), 58 pounds of corn syrup sweeteners (mainly in processed foods), and more than 1 pound of honey and maple syrup.*

*And if that's not enough, on top of that, we eat over 16 pounds of artificial sweeteners.*

You can't rely on the nutrition label to help you sort out the difference between natural sugar and added sugar, but the difference is significant. The nutrition label on a quart of milk tells you that one cup has 14 grams of sugar, all of it from naturally occurring *lactose*, or milk sugar. The label on fruit punch tells you that the same size serving has 30 grams of sugar, almost all of it from added sugar. How can you tell natural sugars from added sugars? Rely on the ingredient listing. Check for the terms below. On food labels, ingredients are listed in descending order by volume, so those ingredients closest to the beginning of the listing will contribute larger amounts to each serving of food.

**SUGAR BY ANY OTHER NAME**

| | |
|---|---|
| Barley Malt | Honey |
| Beet juice | Invert sugar |
| Brown rice syrup | Malt syrup |
| Brown sugar | Maltodextrin |
| Cane syrup | Maple sugar |
| Corn sweetener | Maple syrup |
| Corn syrup | Molasses |

| | |
|---|---|
| Crystalline fructose | Muscavado |
| Dextrose | Raw sugar |
| Evaporated cane juice | Sorghum |
| Fruit juice concentrate | Sucrose |
| Fructose | Sugar in the raw |
| High fructose corn syrup (HFCS) | Turbinado |

Americans currently eat 15% to 21% of their daily calories as sugar, with teenagers eating the most. Studies have shown, over and over, that as sugar intake goes up, vitamin and mineral intake goes down. We should all be eating less sugar, but there is no specific recommendation on how much to eat every day. The National Academy of Sciences' US Dietary Reference Intakes suggest 25% of daily calories from added sugar as the maximum. Obviously, people should eat less. The World Health Organization (WHO) has suggested limiting added sugars to no more than 10% of total calories, though some experts feel this amount is unrealistically low.

Without clear-cut recommendations, you need to decide for yourself how much sugar to eat. We'd suggest attempting to eat closer to the WHO recommendation of 10% total calories as sugar, keeping in mind the 25% recommendation as the healthy upper limit.

## YOUR DAILY TARGET SUGAR INTAKE

| Total Calories | Suggested Intake 10% total calories = grams sugar | | Upper Limit 25% of total calories = grams sugar | |
|---|---|---|---|---|
| | Calories | Sugar | Calories | Sugar |
| 2,400 | 240 | 60 | 600 | 150 |
| 2,300 | 230 | 58 | 575 | 144 |
| 2,200 | 220 | 55 | 550 | 138 |
| 2,100 | 210 | 53 | 525 | 131 |

## YOUR DAILY TARGET SUGAR INTAKE (continued)

| Total Calories | Suggested Intake 10% total calories = grams sugar | | Upper Limit 25% of total calories = grams sugar | |
|---|---|---|---|---|
| | Calories | Sugar | Calories | Sugar |
| 2,000 | 200 | 50 | 500 | 125 |
| 1,900 | 190 | 48 | 475 | 119 |
| 1,800 | 180 | 45 | 450 | 113 |
| 1,700 | 170 | 43 | 425 | 106 |
| 1,600 | 160 | 40 | 400 | 100 |
| 1,500 | 150 | 38 | 375 | 94 |
| 1,400 | 140 | 35 | 350 | 88 |
| 1,300 | 130 | 33 | 325 | 81 |
| 1,200 | 120 | 30 | 300 | 75 |

### WHEN A SUGAR ISN'T A SUGAR

Sugar substitutes have been around for decades. Some, like sugar alcohols, are absorbed slowly by the body, so they have little impact on blood sugar levels. But they do contain calories. Others, called artificial sweeteners, don't raise blood sugar and have no calories. Each has advantages and drawbacks. A high intake of sugar alcohols can cause diarrhea. Some artificial sweeteners lose their sweetness when heated, so they can't be used in cooking.

As more low carb foods are developed and marketed, you'll be eating more foods with sugar substitutes because they will be used to replace regular sugar in foods. Artificial sweeteners are listed in the ingredients, but because they have no calories, they are not listed on the nutrition label. Sugar alcohols do have calories, so they are included under the total carbohydrate value on the nutrition label. As we mentioned earlier, subtracting sugar alcohols from total carbs to arrive at net carbs isn't really a meaningful calculation, because all sugar alcohols still have calories.

**UNDERSTANDING SUGARS**

| Common names | Calories per gram | Found on the Food Label |
|---|---|---|
| ***When a sugar is a sugar:*** | | |
| White sugar | 4 | Under sugar and as part of total carbohydrates on the nutrition facts panel and on the ingredient list. |
| Brown sugar | 4 | |
| Honey | 4 | |
| Molasses | 4 | |
| Raw sugar | 4 | |
| Syrups | 4 | |
| ***When a sugar isn't quite a sugar (sugar alcohols):*** | | |
| Sorbitol | 3 | Under total carbohydrates on the nutrition facts panel and on the ingredient list. |
| Mannitol | 2 | |
| Xylitol | 2 | |
| Isomalt | 2 | |
| Lactitol | 2 | |
| Maltitol | 2 | |
| Trehalose | 4 | |
| ***When a sugar isn't a sugar (artificial sweeteners):*** | | |
| *saccharin:* Sweet and Low, Sweet Twin, Necta Sweet | 0 | On the ingredient list. |
| *aspartame:* Nutrasweet, Equal, Sugar Twin | 4* | |
| *acesulfame-K:* Sunette, Sweet& Safe, Sweet One | 0 | |
| *sucralose:* Splenda | 0 | |
| *neotame* | 0 | |

* This sweetener is almost 200 times as sweet as sugar. Even though it does have calories, so little is used in a serving of food that the calorie amount is negligible.

## Fiber

This is one carbohydrate on which the experts agree: we need to eat more. Fiber isn't digested and provides no calories, yet it's important. Why? Fiber aids in losing weight, managing diabetes, relieving constipation, and protecting against colon cancer. It may even lower the risk for heart disease. All this without calories!

Yet most of us eat too little. We average about 15 grams of fiber, far less than we should be eating each day.

**DAILY FIBER RECOMMENDATIONS**

| | |
|---|---|
| Men | |
| 19–50 years | 38 grams of fiber |
| 50 and older | 30 grams of fiber |
| Women | |
| 19–50 years | 25 grams of fiber |
| 50 and older | 21 grams of fiber |
| pregnant | 28 grams of fiber |

Source: *Dietary Reference Intakes for Energy, Carbohydrate, Fiber, Fat, Fatty Acids, Cholesterol, Protein and Amino Acids, Part 1,* Institute of Medicine of the National Academies, The National Academies Press, 2002.

Slowly start adding foods rich in fiber—beans, berries, bran, fruits, oatmeal, vegetables, and whole grains—to your daily meals. Don't go overboard, because it takes your body a little time to adjust to the extra bulk passing through your digestive tract. And drink plenty of fluids. Fiber soaks up fluids like a sponge. This not only helps you feel fuller longer but also helps form soft, easily passed stools.

## Add a Little Fiber to Your Life

- Eat whole fruits and vegetables instead of drinking juices.
- Eat fruits and vegetables unpeeled.
- Choose whole grains more often—whole wheat, cornmeal, barley, cracked wheat, and rye.
- Use whole grain or high fiber cereals—oatmeal, oat flakes, bran, shredded wheat.
- Eat whole wheat bread, bagels, pasta, pretzels, crackers, and rolls.
- Add beans, lentils, and peas to meals.
- Try soybeans—edemame, soy nuts, tofu, or tempeh.
- Snack on dried fruits, graham crackers, and popcorn.
- Experiment with new versions of old favorites, like brown rice, buckwheat noodles, or baked sweet potatoes.

### Mash It, Smash It, Break It Apart

*Fiber is fiber, no matter what you do in processing or cooking. Canned, pureed pumpkin is a rich source of fiber, as is split pea soup, mashed sweet potatoes, cream of broccoli soup, or a fruit smoothie.*

# CARBOHYDRATES AND WEIGHT LOSS

The doctor of a middle-aged, overweight man who had tried unsuccessfully to lose weight suggested the man cut down on bread and cereals and eat more meat. The pounds began to drop off, and the man was healthier than ever before. He wrote a book detailing his success and it became a huge public success. Sound familiar? That's surprising because none of us were alive when William Banting wrote the first low carbohydrate diet book, *Letter on Corpulence Addressed to the Public,* in 1863. Banting was so excited by his success that he gave away the first printing of the book and sold the second printing for a penny a book.

Today, the bookstores and libraries are overflowing with the latest low carb, high carb, no carb diet scheme. There is no question we all eat too many carbs. In the last 30 years, men have increased their carbohydrate intake from 42% of their total calories to 49%; women went from 45% to 52%. This trend was probably set in motion during the no fat, low-fat decades when everyone was urged to eat as much carbohydrate as they wanted. Between this eat-to-abandon attitude and super-sizing, where bagels grew to the size of salad plates, we've carbed ourselves right out of last season's wardrobe.

Are carbs truly the evil diet temptresses you are led to believe? Can you lose weight on a low carb diet? Should you be eating less carb? No. Yes. And maybe.

Research has shown that you can lose weight on a low carb diet, but it has also shown you can lose weight on a high carb diet. Any diet works that makes you pay attention to what you eat and eat less of it. Low carb diets eliminate or cut down on many foods—candy, cake, cookies, breads, pasta, cereal, fruit, and even some vegetable in the initial stages. When food choices are limited, you eat less, and you lose weight. Many people find they are less hungry when they eat more moderate amounts of carbs. So, yes, low carb diets do work.

If the low carb eating trend makes us all focus on how much sugar and refined carbohydrates we eat and gets us to eat less sugar and more fiber, that's great. Those simple changes will impact positively on our health and help us lose weight.

**For Moms-to-be:**

*Go easy on low carbs if you are pregnant or planning a pregnancy. Bread, pasta, breakfast cereals, and orange juice are key sources of folic acid, a B vitamin that's essential for an unborn baby's neurological development.*

If you are on a low carb diet or are considering trying one, here are some things to consider. First, make sure the carbs you eat are the healthy ones—fruits, vegetables, and whole grains. Second, don't fall for all the "must have" low carb foods popping up on the grocer's shelf. Many of these are high in calories and some aren't even low in carb. Remember the creative net carb math we discussed earlier? (See page 16.) More importantly, many aren't the most nutritious choices for someone trying to lose weight and eat healthy. Think about it—is low carb cake a sensible diet food? And third, don't repeat history. In the not-so-distant past, when people were told to reduce fat, they ate huge amounts of lowfat and no fat foods, without considering the calories they were consuming. If you've decided to cut back on carbs, fine. But that doesn't give you license to eat a half gallon of low carb ice cream. A calorie is a calorie, whether its wrapped up as carbohydrate, protein, or fat.

# COUNTING CARBS

You don't have to be on a diet to count carbs. People with diabetes regularly keep track of the carbs they eat. Those with high triglycerides may have been told by their doctors to eat more moderate amounts of carbohydrates. There is even evidence that high carb intake may increase the level of LDL, or "bad" cholesterol. Athletes routinely eat large amounts of carbs to fuel muscles—"carb loading"—before a major event. Remember the famous pasta dinners the evening before the New York and Boston Marathons?

*The Ultimate Carbohydrate Counter* is the best source you can use to count carbs. With over 15,000 foods listed, values for everything you eat are at your fingertips. The easiest way to determine how many carbs you should be eating each day is to go through the following steps.

### Setting Your Daily Target Carb Intake

1. Find your target calorie zone.
2. Calculate your daily carb calories.
3. Calculate your daily carb grams.
4. Aim to eat less added sugar.
5. Aim to eat more fiber.

## 1. Find your target calorie zone

If you know how many calories you want to eat each day, this step is simple. Just write down the amount. If you are unsure of how many calories you should be eating, think about the target weight you'd like to be. If you want to be 130 pounds, that's your target weight. Next, based on your current activity level, select the activity factor below that best suits you. Last, multiply your target weight by your activity factor to find out how many calories you need each day.

**Activity factor:**

20 = Very active men
15 = Moderately active men or very active women
13 = Inactive men, moderately active women, and people over 55
10 = Inactive women, repeat dieters, seriously overweight people

**Calorie equation:**

**target weight X activity factor**
**= calories needed each day**

your target weight ______ X your activity factor ______

= ______ calories needed each day

For example, if your target weight is 130 and you are a moderately active woman (factor 13) aged 43, you should be eating between 1,600 and 1,700 calories a day.

130 pounds X 13 (moderately active woman)
= 1,690 calories per day

## 2. Calculate your daily carb calories.

In the section "How Much Should You Eat?" we discussed how to calculate your daily carb calories (see page 11). First, you need to decide what percentage of carb you want to eat each day; 40% or lower is considered a low carb eating plan. Let's say you decide to eat 30% of your daily calories as carbs. You have already determined that as a 130-pound woman you need about 1,700 calories a day.

Use the following equation to determine your daily carb calories.

**______% of ______ calories a day**

**= ______ carb calories**

example: *30% of 1,700 calories a day*
*= 510 daily carb calories*

## 3. Calculate your daily carb grams.

In the section "How Much Should You Eat?" we discussed how to calculate your daily carb calories (see page 11). You already know that as a 130-pound woman eating 1,700 calories a day, you can eat 510 carb calories.

Use the following equation to determine your daily carb grams.

**______ daily carb calories ÷ 4**

**= ______ daily carb grams**

example: *510 daily carb calories ÷ 4*
*= 128 daily carb grams*

## 4. Aim to eat less added sugar.

The current recommendation suggests eating approximately 10% of your daily calories as added sugar. As a 130-pound women eating 1,700 calories a day, you should aim for about 170 sugar calories or 43 grams of sugar (see table, page 15–16).

## 5. Aim to eat more fiber.

See the table "Daily Fiber Recommendations" on page 18 to find out how many grams of fiber you should eat each day. For our example, a 43-year-old woman should eat 25 grams, the daily recommendation for women 19 to 50.

Use "Your Daily Carb Diary" on page 29 to keep track of the carbs and calories you eat. You don't have to track your fiber and sugar intakes daily, but it's a good idea to do it once in a while to see if you're meeting the recommendations.

"Your Daily Carb Diary" will tell you a lot about how you eat, why you eat, and what you eat. Research has shown that men are more likely to omit items than women, both sexes are more likely to omit snack items, and meat items are more likely to be underestimated. No one will ever see what you write down, so be honest.

We suggest you note the day and date, because you may eat differently on different days of the week. Some eat more on weekends or days off, others eat more at work. If you keep track, you may begin to see a pattern.

We appreciate that many people eat on a crazy schedule, so the day is broken into 3 periods. That will help you figure out when you do the most eating.

A.M. is from midnight till noon. Many people eat in the middle of the night, so A.M. includes middle-of-the-night noshing, breakfast, coffee break, or morning snack.

Midday is from noon until dinner. It includes lunch and any afternoon or pre-dinner snack, like a drink after work.

P.M. is dinnertime through midnight. It includes your evening meal and after-dinner, TV, and bedtime snacks.

By subtotaling your carbs and calories 3 times during the day, you can make adjustments for unexpected situations. For example, if a client comes in for lunch, you can skip your afternoon snack and eat a lighter dinner to compensate for the extra calories eaten at lunch.

## YOUR DAILY CARB DIARY

Your Target Calorie Zone ___ Your Daily Carb grams ____

Aim for ___ grams sugar daily Aim for ___ grams fiber daily

Day ______________________ Date ______________________

| Food | Portion | Cals. | Carbs | Sugar | Fiber |
|---|---|---|---|---|---|
| AM | | | | | |
| AM Totals | | _____ | _____ | _____ | _____ |
| MIDDAY | | | | | |
| Midday Totals | | _____ | _____ | _____ | _____ |
| PM | | | | | |
| PM Totals | | _____ | _____ | _____ | _____ |
| Daily Totals | | | | | |

# USING YOUR ULTIMATE CARBOHYDRATE COUNTER

*The Ultimate Carbohydrate Counter* lists the portion size, calories, carbohydrate, fiber, and sugar values for more than 15,000 foods. Now you can compare the values in your favorite foods and, when necessary, choose substitutes before you go out to shop or eat. This will save you time and help you decide what to buy.

The counter section of the book is divided into two parts: Part One: Brand Name, Nonbranded (Generic), and Take-Out Foods; and Part Two: Restaurant Chains. Each part lists foods or restaurant chains alphabetically.

In Part One, for each category you will find nonbranded (generic) foods listed first, in alphabetical order, followed by an alphabetical listing of brand name foods. The nonbranded listings will help you estimate calorie values when you don't see your favorite. They can also help you to evaluate store brands. Large categories are divided into subcategories, such as canned, fresh, frozen, and ready-to-eat to make it easier to find what you're looking for. Some categories have "see" and "see also" footnotes, to help you find related items.

Because we eat out so often, we listed more than 500 take-out foods in Part One. These are found in the take-out subcategory in many categories throughout this section. Look there for foods you take-out or order in, because these foods are not nutrition labeled.

Most foods are listed alphabetically. But in some cases, foods are grouped by category. For example, a tuna sandwich is found in the SANDWICH category. Other group categories include:

**ASIAN FOOD** Page 42
includes all types of Asian foods except egg rolls and sushi, which are found in separate categories

**DELI MEATS/COLD CUTS** Page 219
includes all sandwich meats except chicken, ham, and turkey, which are found in separate categories

**DINNER** Page 221
includes all by brand name, except pasta dinners, which are found in a separate category

**LIQUOR/LIQUEUR** Page 313
includes all alcoholic beverages and mixed drinks except beer, champagne, and wine, which are found in separate categories

**NUTRITION SUPPLEMENTS** Page 338
includes all dieting aids, meal replacements, and drinks, except energy bars and energy drinks, which are found in separate categories

In Part Two, Restaurant Chains, 59 national and regional restaurants are listed, including candy, coffee, doughnut, ice cream, pizza, burger, seafood, sandwich, and ethnic food chains. Brand name foods are required by law to have nutrition information on labels. Restaurants, however, provide this information voluntarily.

With *The Ultimate Carbohydrate Counter* as your guide, you will never again wonder how many carbs and calories are in the foods you eat.

# DEFINITIONS

**as prep (as prepared)**—refers to food that has been prepared according to package directions

**lean and fat**—describes meat with some fat on its edges that is not cut away before cooking, or poultry prepared with skin and fat as purchased

**lean only**—refers to lean meat that is trimmed of all visible fat, or poultry without skin

**shelf stable**—refers to prepared products found on the supermarket shelf that are ready-to-eat or are ready to be heated and do not require refrigeration

**take-out**—describes prepared dishes that you purchase ready-to-eat; those included serve as a guide to the calories, carbohydrates, fiber and sugar in products you may purchase.

# ABBREVIATIONS

| | | |
|---|---|---|
| avg | = | average |
| diam | = | diameter |
| fl | = | fluid |
| frzn | = | frozen |
| g | = | gram |
| in | = | inch |
| lb | = | pound |
| lg | = | large |
| med | = | medium |
| mg | = | milligram |
| oz | = | ounce |
| pkg | = | package |
| pt | = | pint |
| prep | = | prepared |
| qt | = | quart |
| reg | = | regular |
| sec | = | second |
| serv | = | serving |
| sm | = | small |
| sq | = | square |
| tbsp | = | tablespoon |
| tr | = | trace |
| tsp | = | teaspoon |
| w/ | = | with |
| w/o | = | without |
| < | = | less than |

# NOTES

Cals = Calories

Carb = Carbohydrates

All carbohydrate, fiber, and sugar values are given in grams.

— (dash) indicates that values are not available

tr (trace) = less than 1 gram of carbohydrate, fiber, or sugar

0 (zero) indicates there are no calories, carbohydrate, fiber, or sugar in that food

Discrepancies in figures are due to rounding, product reformulation, and reevaluation. Labeling law allows rounding of values. Some of the data listed is analysis data, obtained directly from manufacturers, not from labels. Therefore, some values may differ from labels because they have not been rounded.

## PART ONE

# Brand Name, Nonbranded (Generic) and Take-Out Foods

| FOOD | PORTION | CALS | CARB | SUGAR | FIBER |
|---|---|---|---|---|---|
| **ABALONE** | | | | | |
| fresh fried | 3 oz | 161 | 9 | – | – |
| **ACEROLA** | | | | | |
| fresh | 1 | 2 | tr | – | – |
| **ACEROLA JUICE** | | | | | |
| juice | 1 cup | 51 | 12 | – | 1 |
| **ADZUKI BEANS** | | | | | |
| canned sweetened | 1 cup | 702 | 163 | – | – |
| dried cooked | 1 cup | 294 | 57 | – | 17 |
| **AKEE** | | | | | |
| fresh | 3.5 oz | 223 | 5 | – | – |
| **ALCOHOL** *(see* BEER AND ALE, CHAMPAGNE, LIQUOR/LIQUEUR, MALT, WINE*)* | | | | | |
| **ALE** *(see* BEER AND ALE*)* | | | | | |
| **ALFALFA** | | | | | |
| sprouts | 1 tbsp | 1 | tr | – | tr |
| **ALLIGATOR** | | | | | |
| cooked | 3 oz | 126 | 0 | 0 | 0 |
| **ALLSPICE** | | | | | |
| ground | 1 tsp | 5 | 1 | – | – |
| **ALMONDS** | | | | | |
| almond meal | 1 oz | 116 | 8 | – | – |
| almond paste | 1 oz | 127 | 12 | – | – |
| dry roasted w/ salt | 24 nuts (1 oz) | 170 | 6 | 1 | 3 |
| jordan almonds | 10 (1.4 oz) | 190 | 28 | 24 | 1 |
| oil roasted blanched | 1 oz | 174 | 5 | – | 3 |
| oil roasted blanched salted | 1 oz | 174 | 5 | – | – |
| praline | 17 pieces (1.4 oz) | 210 | 21 | 17 | 3 |
| ***Judy's*** | | | | | |
| Sugar Free Coconut Almond Brittle | ¼ piece (1 oz) | 90 | 2 | 0 | 1 |
| ***Keto*** | | | | | |
| Chocolatey Covered | 1 oz | 169 | 7 | 0 | 5 |
| ***Lance*** | | | | | |
| Smoked | 1 pkg (0.8 oz) | 130 | 4 | 0 | 3 |

| FOOD | PORTION | CALS | CARB | SUGAR | FIBER |
|---|---|---|---|---|---|
| ***Low Carb Creations*** | | | | | |
| Soft Almond Brittle | 2 pieces (1 oz) | 170 | 17 | 2 | 2 |
| ***Mama Mellace's*** | | | | | |
| Butter Rum | 1 oz | 150 | 13 | 11 | 2 |
| Cinnamon Roasted | 1 oz | 140 | 14 | 11 | 2 |
| ***Maranatha*** | | | | | |
| Almond Butter | 2 tbsp | 220 | 6 | 2 | 3 |
| Raw Almond Butter | 2 tbsp | 190 | 7 | 2 | 4 |
| Tamari Almonds | ¼ cup | 160 | 6 | 2 | 3 |
| ***Sweet Delights*** | | | | | |
| Almond Roasters | ⅓ pkg (1 oz) | 190 | 6 | 3 | 3 |
| **AMARANTH** | | | | | |
| leaves cooked | 1 cup | 28 | 5 | – | – |
| uncooked | 1 cup (6.8 oz) | 729 | 129 | – | 30 |
| **ANCHOVY** | | | | | |
| canned in oil | 1 can (1.6 oz) | 95 | 0 | 0 | 0 |
| canned in oil | 5 | 42 | 0 | 0 | 0 |
| fresh fillets | 3 (0.4 oz) | 21 | tr | – | – |
| **ANISE** | | | | | |
| seed | 1 tsp | 7 | 1 | – | – |
| **ANTELOPE** | | | | | |
| roasted | 3 oz | 127 | 0 | 0 | 0 |
| **APPLE** | | | | | |
| **CANNED** | | | | | |
| ***Del Monte*** | | | | | |
| Fruit Pleasures Pie Spiced Apples | ½ cup (4.1 oz) | 70 | 18 | 17 | 1 |
| ***Luck's*** | | | | | |
| Fried Apples | ½ cup (4.7 oz) | 130 | 33 | 20 | 2 |
| **DRIED** | | | | | |
| cooked w/o sugar | 1 cup | 145 | 39 | – | 5 |
| rings | 10 | 155 | 42 | – | 6 |
| **FRESH** | | | | | |
| apple | 1 lg | 125 | 32 | – | 6 |
| apple | 1 sm | 63 | 16 | – | 3 |
| apple | 1 med | 81 | 21 | – | 4 |
| w/o skin sliced | 1 cup | 63 | 16 | – | 2 |

| FOOD | PORTION | CALS | CARB | SUGAR | FIBER |
|---|---|---|---|---|---|
| ***Chiquita*** | | | | | |
| Apple | 1 med (5.4 oz) | 80 | 22 | 16 | 5 |
| ***Cool Cut*** | | | | | |
| Apples & Caramel Dip | 1 pkg (4.25 oz) | 180 | 32 | 26 | 3 |
| **TAKE-OUT** | | | | | |
| baked | 1 (5.3 oz) | 126 | 33 | 29 | 3 |
| baked no sugar | 1 (5.9 oz) | 82 | 21 | 18 | 3 |
| **APPLE JUICE** | | | | | |
| mulled cider | 1 serv | 265 | 42 | – | 6 |
| ***Apple & Eve*** | | | | | |
| 100% Juice | 8 fl oz | 110 | 26 | 22 | – |
| Cider | 8 fl oz | 110 | 27 | 24 | – |
| ***Eden*** | | | | | |
| Organic Juice | 8 oz | 80 | 23 | 12 | 0 |
| ***Hansen's*** | | | | | |
| Junior Juice 100% | 1 box (4.23 oz) | 60 | 15 | 14 | 1 |
| ***Langers*** | | | | | |
| 100% Cider | 8 oz | 120 | 28 | 26 | – |
| 100% Juice | 8 oz | 120 | 28 | 26 | – |
| Diet Cocktail | 8 oz | 60 | 14 | 13 | – |
| ***Mott's*** | | | | | |
| 100% Juice | 1 box (8 oz) | 120 | 29 | – | – |
| 100% Juice | 8 fl oz | 120 | 29 | 23 | 0 |
| 100% Natural | 8 fl oz | 120 | 29 | 28 | 0 |
| ***Nantucket Nectars*** | | | | | |
| 100% Pressed | 8 oz | 100 | 25 | 22 | – |
| ***NutraBalance*** | | | | | |
| Plus Fibre | 1 pkg (8 oz) | 120 | 29 | 24 | 10 |
| ***Ocean Spray*** | | | | | |
| 100% Juice | 8 oz | 110 | 28 | 28 | 0 |
| ***Odwalla*** | | | | | |
| Spiced Harvest Cider | 8 fl oz | 130 | 30 | 28 | 0 |
| ***Snapple*** | | | | | |
| Snapple Apple | 8 fl oz | 120 | 30 | 28 | – |
| ***Squeezit*** | | | | | |
| Green Apple | 1 bottle (7 oz) | 110 | 27 | 25 | 0 |
| ***Swiss Miss*** | | | | | |
| Hot Apple Cider Mix | 1 serv | 84 | 20 | 19 | 1 |

| FOOD | PORTION | CALS | CARB | SUGAR | FIBER |
|---|---|---|---|---|---|
| Hot Apple Cider Mix Low Calorie | 1 serv | 14 | 3 | tr | 0 |
| ***Tropicana*** | | | | | |
| Season's Best | 8 oz | 110 | 28 | – | – |
| ***Turkey Hill*** | | | | | |
| Herbal Cider w/ Chamomile & Lemongrass | 1 cup | 100 | 24 | 24 | – |
| ***White House*** | | | | | |
| Juice | 8 oz | 120 | 30 | 26 | – |
| **APPLESAUCE** | | | | | |
| sweetened | ½ cup | 97 | 25 | – | 2 |
| unsweetened | ½ cup | 52 | 14 | – | 2 |
| ***Eden*** | | | | | |
| Organic | ½ cup | 50 | 15 | 11 | 2 |
| Organic Sweet Cinnamon | ½ cup | 50 | 19 | 15 | 4 |
| ***Jok'n'Al*** | | | | | |
| Low Carb | 1 tbsp | 10 | 2 | 1 | – |
| ***Mott's*** | | | | | |
| Single-Serve Cinnamon | 1 pkg (4 oz) | 100 | 26 | – | – |
| Single-Serve Natural | 1 pkg (4 oz) | 50 | 12 | – | – |
| Single-Serve Original | 1 pkg (4 oz) | 100 | 24 | – | – |
| ***White House*** | | | | | |
| Applesauce | ½ cup (4.4 oz) | 90 | 23 | 18 | 2 |
| Chunky | ½ cup (4.4 oz) | 90 | 23 | 18 | 2 |
| Cinnamon | ½ cup (4.5 oz) | 100 | 25 | 21 | 2 |
| Natural Plus | ½ cup (4.4 oz) | 70 | 15 | 13 | 2 |
| **APRICOT JUICE** | | | | | |
| nectar | 1 cup | 141 | 36 | – | 2 |
| **APRICOTS** | | | | | |
| **CANNED** | | | | | |
| ***Del Monte*** | | | | | |
| Halves Unpeeled Lite | ½ cup (4.3 oz) | 60 | 16 | 15 | 1 |
| Orchard Select Halves Unpeeled | ½ cup (4.4 oz) | 80 | 21 | 20 | 1 |
| **DRIED** | | | | | |
| halves | 4 | 32 | 9 | – | 1 |

| FOOD | PORTION | CALS | CARB | SUGAR | FIBER |
|---|---|---|---|---|---|
| **FRESH** | | | | | |
| apricots | 1 | 17 | 4 | – | 1 |
| ***Chiquita*** | | | | | |
| Apricots | 3 med (4 oz) | 60 | 11 | 11 | 1 |
| **FROZEN** | | | | | |
| sweetened | ½ cup | 119 | 30 | – | 3 |
| **ARROWHEAD** | | | | | |
| fresh boiled | 1 med | 9 | 2 | – | – |
| flour | 1 cup | 457 | 113 | – | 4 |
| **ARTICHOKE** | | | | | |
| **CANNED** | | | | | |
| ***Progresso*** | | | | | |
| Hearts | 2 pieces (2.9 oz) | 30 | 6 | 1 | 1 |
| Hearts Marinated | 2 pieces (1.1 oz) | 170 | 2 | 0 | 0 |
| ***S&W*** | | | | | |
| Marinated Hearts | 2 pieces (1 oz) | 20 | 2 | 0 | 1 |
| **FRESH** | | | | | |
| cooked | 1 med | 60 | 13 | – | 7 |
| hearts cooked | ½ cup | 42 | 9 | – | 5 |
| **FROZEN** | | | | | |
| cooked | 1 pkg (9 oz) | 108 | 22 | – | 11 |
| **ARUGULA** | | | | | |
| fresh | ½ cup | 3 | tr | – | tr |
| **ASIAN FOOD** *(see also* DINNER, EGG ROLLS, SUSHI*)* | | | | | |
| **CANNED** | | | | | |
| chow mein chicken | 1 cup | 95 | 18 | – | – |
| ***Chun King*** | | | | | |
| Beef Pepper Oriental BiPack | 1 cup (8.8 oz) | 98 | 13 | 0 | 3 |
| Chow Mein Beef BiPack | 1 cup (8.6 oz) | 78 | 11 | 3 | 3 |
| Chow Mein BiPack Chicken | 1 cup (8.8 oz) | 98 | 11 | 2 | 3 |
| Chow Mein Pork BiPack | 1 cup (8.6 oz) | 78 | 9 | 0 | 2 |
| Hot & Spicy Chicken BiPack | 1 cup (8.6 oz) | 98 | 11 | 0 | 1 |
| Sweet & Sour Chicken BiPack | 1 cup (8.9 oz) | 161 | 29 | 26 | 3 |
| ***La Choy*** | | | | | |
| Beef Pepper Oriental BiPack | 1 cup (8.8 oz) | 98 | 13 | 0 | 3 |

| FOOD | PORTION | CALS | CARB | SUGAR | FIBER |
|---|---|---|---|---|---|
| Chow Mein Beef BiPack | 1 cup (8.6 oz) | 78 | 11 | 3 | 3 |
| Chow Mein Chicken PiBack | 1 cup (8.9 oz) | 98 | 11 | 2 | 3 |
| Chow Mein Shrimp BiPack | 1 cup (8.6 oz) | 52 | 9 | 0 | 3 |
| Main Entree Chow Mein Chicken | 1 cup (9.3 oz) | 80 | 6 | 2 | 3 |
| Oriental Beef w/ Noodles BiPack | 1 cup (8.8 oz) | 156 | 18 | 2 | 4 |
| Oriental Chicken w/ Noodles BiPack | 1 cup (8.7 oz) | 154 | 18 | 3 | 2 |
| Sweet & Sour Chicken BiPack | 1 cup (8.9 oz) | 161 | 29 | 26 | 3 |
| Teriyaki Chicken BiPack | 1 cup (8.6 oz) | 109 | 15 | 5 | 3 |
| **FRESH** | | | | | |
| wonton wrappers | 1 | 23 | 5 | – | – |
| ***Azumaya*** | | | | | |
| Round Wraps | 10 | 160 | 31 | 1 | 1 |
| Square Wraps | 6 | 160 | 31 | 1 | 1 |
| Wrappers Large Square | 3 | 170 | 35 | 1 | 1 |
| ***Nasoya*** | | | | | |
| Egg Roll Wrapper | 3 | 170 | 35 | 1 | 1 |
| Won Ton Wrappers | 8 | 160 | 31 | 1 | 1 |
| **FROZEN** | | | | | |
| ***Amy's*** | | | | | |
| Bowls Teriyaki | 1 pkg (10 oz) | 300 | 59 | 12 | 3 |
| Skillet Meals Teriyaki Stir Fry | 1 cup | 320 | 64 | 9 | 4 |
| Stir Fry Asian Noodle | 1 pkg (10 oz) | 240 | 41 | 6 | 6 |
| Stir Fry Thai | 1 pkg (9.5 oz) | 270 | 36 | 4 | 2 |
| ***Banquet*** | | | | | |
| Fried Rice w/ Chicken & Egg Rolls | 1 meal (8.5 oz) | 330 | 51 | 3 | 5 |
| ***Birds Eye*** | | | | | |
| Easy Recipe Creations Oriental Lo Mein | 2¼ cups | 230 | 40 | 11 | 2 |
| Easy Recipe Creations Sesame Ginger Teriyaki | 2¼ cups | 140 | 24 | 15 | 4 |
| Easy Recipe Creations Spicy Szechuan Cashews | 2¼ cups | 180 | 29 | 18 | 4 |
| ***La Choy*** | | | | | |
| Beef Pepper Oriental | 1 cup (7.1 oz) | 151 | 30 | 7 | 2 |
| Chow Mein Vegetable | 1 cup (8.9 oz) | 108 | 20 | 3 | 5 |

| FOOD | PORTION | CALS | CARB | SUGAR | FIBER |
|---|---|---|---|---|---|
| ***Lean Cuisine*** | | | | | |
| Everyday Favorites Oriental Style Dumplings | 1 pkg (9 oz) | 300 | 51 | 14 | 2 |
| Everyday Favorites Teriyaki Stir Fry | 1 pkg (10 oz) | 290 | 45 | 9 | 4 |
| ***Tyson*** | | | | | |
| Chicken Fried Rice Kit w/ Sauce | 1 pkg (14 oz) | 440 | 69 | 15 | 5 |
| ***Weight Watchers*** | | | | | |
| Smart Ones Chicken Chow Mein | 1 pkg (9 oz) | 200 | 34 | 5 | 3 |
| Smart Ones Hunan Style Rice & Vegetables | 1 pkg (10.34 oz) | 280 | 45 | 4 | 5 |
| Smart Ones King Pao Noodles & Vegetables | 1 pkg (10 oz) | 250 | 37 | 12 | 5 |
| Smart Ones Spicy Szechaun Style Vegetables & Chicken | 1 pkg (9 oz) | 220 | 39 | 1 | 3 |
| **MIX** | | | | | |
| ***Annie Chun's*** | | | | | |
| Chow Mein Noodles w/ Garlic Scallion Sauce | 1 serv | 250 | 39 | 6 | 2 |
| **TAKE-OUT** | | | | | |
| buddha's delight w/ cellophane noodles fat choi jai | 1 serv (7.6 oz) | 211 | 44 | 3 | 2 |
| cha siu bao steamed buns w/ chicken filling | 1 (2.3 oz) | 160 | 26 | 4 | tr |
| chop suey w/ beef & pork | 1 cup | 300 | 13 | – | – |
| chop suey w/ pork | 1 cup | 375 | 29 | – | 2 |
| chow mein chicken | 1 cup | 255 | 10 | – | – |
| chow mein pork | 1 cup | 425 | 21 | – | 3 |
| chow mein shrimp | 1 cup | 221 | 21 | – | 3 |
| chow mein vegetable | 1 serv (8 oz) | 90 | 15 | 2 | 4 |
| filipino chicken adobo | 1 serv (15 oz) | 555 | 45 | tr | 1 |
| fried rice vegetable | 1 cup | 210 | 30 | 3 | 1 |
| fried rice w/ egg | 6.7 oz | 395 | 49 | – | 2 |
| phad thai | 1 serv (9.2 oz) | 232 | 30 | 2 | 1 |
| sesame seed paste bun | 1 (2.5 oz) | 220 | 39 | 12 | 2 |
| shrimp chips | 1¼ cups (1 oz) | 140 | 19 | 1 | 0 |
| shu mai chicken & vegetable dumplings | 6 (3.6 oz) | 160 | 18 | 6 | 1 |

| FOOD | PORTION | CALS | CARB | SUGAR | FIBER |
|---|---|---|---|---|---|
| spring roll | 1 (3.5 oz) | 112 | 37 | – | 5 |
| sweet & sour pork | 1 serv (8 oz) | 250 | 37 | 30 | 2 |
| sweet red bean bun | 1 (2.5 oz) | 130 | 38 | 17 | 2 |
| szechuan chicken w/ lo mein | 1 cup (5.3 oz) | 190 | 35 | 3 | 0 |
| tempura vegetables | 5 pieces (4 oz) | 270 | 31 | 3 | 2 |
| teriyaki chicken plain | ¾ cup | 399 | 7 | – | – |
| teriyaki chicken w/ rice | 1 serv (11 oz) | 430 | 77 | 10 | 1 |
| wonton fried | ½ cup (1 oz) | 111 | 8 | – | 1 |
| **ASPARAGUS** | | | | | |
| **CANNED** | | | | | |
| spears | ½ cup | 23 | 3 | – | 2 |
| ***Del Monte*** | | | | | |
| Cuts & Tips | ½ cup (4.4 oz) | 20 | 3 | 0 | 1 |
| Spears Extra Long | ½ cup (4.4 oz) | 20 | 3 | 0 | 1 |
| Spears Tender Young | ½ cup (4.4 oz) | 20 | 3 | 0 | 1 |
| Tips Hand Selected | ½ cup (4.4 oz) | 20 | 3 | 0 | 1 |
| ***S&W*** | | | | | |
| Green | 6 pieces (4.5 oz) | 15 | 4 | 1 | 1 |
| **FRESH** | | | | | |
| cooked | ½ cup | 22 | 4 | – | 1 |
| cooked | 4 spears | 14 | 3 | – | 1 |
| raw | 4 spears | 15 | 1 | – | tr |
| **FROZEN** | | | | | |
| cooked | 4 spears | 17 | 3 | – | 1 |
| cooked | 1 pkg (10 oz) | 82 | 14 | – | 5 |
| **ATEMOYA** | | | | | |
| fresh | ½ cup | 94 | 24 | – | – |
| **AVOCADO** | | | | | |
| fresh mashed | 1 cup | 407 | 16 | – | 11 |
| fresh peeled california | 1 | 306 | 12 | – | 9 |
| fresh peeled florida | 1 | 340 | 27 | – | 16 |
| ***Chiquita*** | | | | | |
| Fresh | ⅓ med (1 oz) | 55 | 3 | 0 | 3 |
| **TAKE-OUT** | | | | | |
| guacamole | 1 serv (2.2 oz) | 105 | 5 | 1 | 2 |
| **BACON** | | | | | |
| breakfast strips cooked | 3 strips | 156 | tr | – | 0 |

| FOOD | PORTION | CALS | CARB | SUGAR | FIBER |
|---|---|---|---|---|---|
| gammon lean & fat grilled | 4.2 oz | 274 | 0 | 0 | 0 |
| pan fried | 3 strips | 109 | tr | – | 0 |
| ***Health Is Wealth*** | | | | | |
| Uncured Sliced | 2 slices (0.5 oz) | 70 | 0 | – | – |
| ***Ready Crisp*** | | | | | |
| Fully Cooked | 3 slices (0.5 oz) | 70 | 0 | – | – |
| **BACON SUBSTITUTES** | | | | | |
| meatless | 1 strip | 16 | tr | – | tr |
| ***Bac-Os*** | | | | | |
| Chips or Bits | 1½ tbsp (7 g) | 30 | 2 | 0 | 0 |
| ***Lightlife*** | | | | | |
| Fakin' Bacon Bits | 1 tsp | 45 | 1 | 0 | 0 |
| Smart Bacon | 2 strips (0.8 oz) | 45 | 2 | 0 | 0 |
| ***Morningstar Farms*** | | | | | |
| Breakfast Strips | 2 (0.5 oz) | 60 | 2 | 0 | tr |
| **BAGEL** | | | | | |
| cinnamon raisin | 1 lg | 359 | 72 | – | 3 |
| cinnamon raisin toasted | 1 lg | 363 | 73 | – | 3 |
| egg | 1 mini | 72 | 14 | – | 1 |
| egg | 1 lg | 364 | 69 | – | 3 |
| mini onion | 1 (1.4 oz) | 100 | 20 | 1 | 1 |
| oat bran | 1 lg | 334 | 70 | – | 5 |
| onion | 1 lg | 363 | 71 | – | 3 |
| plain | 1 lg | 360 | 70 | – | 3 |
| plain | 1 mini | 72 | 14 | – | 1 |
| poppy seed | 1 lg | 360 | 70 | – | 3 |
| ***Atkins*** | | | | | |
| Cinnamon Raisin | 1 | 200 | 20 | 1 | 11 |
| Onion | 1 | 190 | 19 | 3 | 11 |
| Plain | 1 | 190 | 18 | 0 | 11 |
| ***Otis Spunkmeyer*** | | | | | |
| Barnstormin' Blueberry | 1 (3.6 oz) | 250 | 50 | 6 | 3 |
| Barnstormin' Cinnamon Raisin | 1 (3.6 oz) | 230 | 47 | 6 | 3 |
| Barnstormin' Onion | 1 (3.6 oz) | 230 | 47 | 6 | 3 |
| Barnstormin' Plain | 1 (3.6 oz) | 240 | 49 | 5 | 3 |
| ***Pepperidge Farm*** | | | | | |
| Mini | 1 (1.4 oz) | 120 | 24 | 2 | tr |
| Plain | 1 (3.5 oz) | 290 | 60 | 6 | 2 |

| FOOD | PORTION | CALS | CARB | SUGAR | FIBER |
|---|---|---|---|---|---|
| ***Sara Lee*** | | | | | |
| Blueberry | 1 (2.8 oz) | 210 | 41 | 5 | 2 |
| Cinnamon Raisin | 1 (2.8 oz) | 220 | 45 | 12 | 3 |
| Egg | 1 (2.8 oz) | 210 | 44 | 7 | 2 |
| Oat Bran | 1 (2.8 oz) | 210 | 42 | 7 | 3 |
| Onion | 1 (2.8 oz) | 210 | 44 | 6 | 2 |
| Plain | 1 (2.8 oz) | 210 | 43 | 3 | 2 |
| Poppy Seed | 1 (2.8 oz) | 210 | 41 | 5 | 2 |
| Sesame Seed | 1 (2.8 oz) | 210 | 42 | 5 | 2 |
| ***Thomas'*** | | | | | |
| Everything | 1 (3.6 oz) | 300 | 56 | 7 | 3 |
| Multi-Grain | 1 (3.6 oz) | 280 | 55 | 7 | 4 |
| Plain | 1 (3.6 oz) | 280 | 56 | 7 | 2 |
| ***Uncle B's*** | | | | | |
| Plain | 1 (2.8 oz) | 210 | 41 | 4 | 2 |
| ***Wonder*** | | | | | |
| Blueberry | 1 (3 oz) | 210 | 43 | 9 | 1 |
| Cinnamon Raisin | 1 (3 oz) | 210 | 42 | 9 | 2 |
| Onion | 1 (3 oz) | 210 | 43 | 5 | 1 |
| Plain | 1 (3 oz) | 210 | 43 | 5 | 2 |
| Rye | 1 (3 oz) | 220 | 42 | 1 | 2 |
| Wheat | 1 (3 oz) | 210 | 43 | 5 | 2 |
| **BAKING POWDER** | | | | | |
| baking powder | 1 tsp | 2 | 1 | – | – |
| low sodium | 1 tsp | 5 | 2 | – | – |
| ***Clabber Girl*** | | | | | |
| Baking Powder | 1 tsp | 0 | 1 | – | – |
| ***Davis*** | | | | | |
| Baking Powder | 1 tsp | 0 | 0 | 0 | – |
| ***Rumford*** | | | | | |
| Aluminum Free | ⅛ tsp | 0 | tr | – | – |
| **BAKING SODA** | | | | | |
| baking soda | 1 tsp | 0 | 0 | 0 | 0 |
| **BALSAM PEAR (BITTER GOURD)** | | | | | |
| leafy tips cooked | ½ cup | 10 | 2 | – | 1 |
| leafy tips raw | ½ cup | 7 | 1 | – | – |
| pods cooked | ½ cup | 12 | 3 | – | 1 |

| FOOD | PORTION | CALS | CARB | SUGAR | FIBER |
|---|---|---|---|---|---|
| **BAMBOO SHOOTS** | | | | | |
| canned sliced | 1 cup | 25 | 4 | – | 2 |
| fresh | ½ cup | 21 | 1 | – | 2 |
| fresh cooked | ½ cup | 12 | 2 | – | – |
| ***Chun King*** | | | | | |
| Bamboo Shoots | 2 tbsp (0.8 oz) | 3 | 1 | tr | tr |
| ***La Choy*** | | | | | |
| Bamboo Shoots | 2 tbsp (0.8 oz) | 3 | 1 | tr | tr |
| **BANANA** | | | | | |
| banana chips | 1 oz | 147 | 17 | – | 2 |
| fresh | 1 med | 109 | 28 | – | 3 |
| fresh mashed | 1 cup | 207 | 53 | – | 5 |
| fresh sliced | 1 cup | 138 | 35 | – | 4 |
| powder | 1 tbsp | 21 | 5 | – | 1 |
| whole dried | 1 piece (1.2 oz) | 130 | 33 | 22 | 2 |
| ***Chiquita*** | | | | | |
| Fresh | 1 med (4.4 oz) | 110 | 29 | 21 | 4 |
| **BARBECUE SAUCE** | | | | | |
| barbecue | 1 cup | 188 | 32 | – | – |
| ***Atkins*** | | | | | |
| Barbecue Sauce | 1 tbsp | 15 | tr | 0 | 0 |
| ***Carb Options*** | | | | | |
| Original | 2 tbsp | 10 | 3 | 0 | 0 |
| ***Hunt's*** | | | | | |
| Bold Hickory | 2 tbsp (1.2 oz) | 47 | 11 | 9 | 1 |
| Bold Original | 2 tbsp (1.2 oz) | 46 | 11 | 10 | 1 |
| Hickory & Brown Sugar | 2 tbsp (1.3 oz) | 75 | 18 | 16 | 1 |
| Honey Hickory | 2 tbsp (1.2 oz) | 54 | 12 | 12 | 1 |
| Honey Mustard | 2 tbsp (1.2 oz) | 48 | 12 | 4 | 1 |
| Hot & Spicy | 2 tbsp (1.2 oz) | 48 | 12 | 4 | 1 |
| Light Original | 2 tbsp (1.2 oz) | 23 | 6 | 5 | 1 |
| Mesquite | 2 tbsp (1.2 oz) | 40 | 9 | 8 | 1 |
| Mild | 2 tbsp (1.2 oz) | 41 | 10 | 7 | 1 |
| Mild Dijon | 2 tbsp (1.2 oz) | 39 | 9 | 7 | tr |
| Open Range Original | 2 tbsp (1.2 oz) | 39 | 9 | 8 | 1 |
| Open Range Premier | 2 tbsp (1.3 oz) | 56 | 13 | 12 | 1 |
| Open Range Smokey | 2 tbsp (1.2 oz) | 37 | 9 | 7 | 1 |
| Original | 2 tbsp (1.2 oz) | 40 | 9 | 8 | 1 |
| Teriyaki | 2 tbsp (1.2 oz) | 46 | 11 | 10 | 1 |

| FOOD | PORTION | CALS | CARB | SUGAR | FIBER |
|---|---|---|---|---|---|
| ***Muir Glen*** | | | | | |
| Garlic Mesquite | 2 tbsp (1.3 oz) | 40 | 6 | 6 | tr |
| Hot & Smoky | 2 tbsp (1.2 oz) | 40 | 6 | 6 | tr |
| Original | 2 tbsp (1.2 oz) | 40 | 6 | 6 | tr |
| ***Steel's*** | | | | | |
| Sugar Free | 2 tbsp | 15 | 2 | 0 | 0 |
| **BARLEY** | | | | | |
| flour | 1 cup | 511 | 110 | – | 15 |
| malt flour | 1 cup | 585 | 127 | – | 12 |
| pearled cooked | 1 cup (5.5 oz) | 193 | 44 | – | 6 |
| pearled uncooked | 1 cup | 704 | 155 | – | 31 |
| **BARRACUDA** | | | | | |
| fresh | 3 oz | 122 | 0 | 0 | 0 |
| **BASIL** | | | | | |
| fresh chopped | 2 tbsp | 1 | tr | – | tr |
| ground | 1 tsp | 4 | 1 | – | – |
| leaves fresh | 5 | 1 | tr | – | tr |
| **BASS** | | | | | |
| freshwater raw | 3 oz | 97 | 0 | 0 | 0 |
| sea cooked | 3 oz | 105 | 0 | 0 | 0 |
| sea raw | 3 oz | 82 | 0 | 0 | 0 |
| striped baked | 3 oz | 105 | 0 | 0 | 0 |
| striped bass farm raised | 4 oz | 110 | 0 | 0 | 0 |
| **BAY LEAF** | | | | | |
| crumbled | 1 tsp | 2 | tr | – | – |
| **BEAN SPROUTS** *(see ALFALFA, SPROUTS)* | | | | | |
| **BEANS** *(see also individual names)* | | | | | |
| **CANNED** | | | | | |
| baked beans plain | ½ cup | 118 | 26 | – | 6 |
| baked beans vegetarian | ½ cup | 118 | 26 | – | 6 |
| baked beans w/ beef | ½ cup | 161 | 22 | – | – |
| baked beans w/ franks | ½ cup | 184 | 20 | – | 9 |
| baked beans w/ pork | ½ cup | 134 | 25 | – | 7 |
| baked beans w/ pork & sweet sauce | ½ cup | 140 | 26 | – | 7 |

| FOOD | PORTION | CALS | CARB | SUGAR | FIBER |
|---|---|---|---|---|---|
| baked beans w/ pork & tomato sauce | ½ cup | 124 | 24 | – | 7 |
| refried beans | ½ cup | 134 | 23 | – | – |
| ***Amy's*** | | | | | |
| Vegetarian Baked | ½ cup | 120 | 24 | 9 | 6 |
| ***B&M*** | | | | | |
| Barbeque Baked Beans | ½ cup (4.6 oz) | 210 | 42 | 19 | 9 |
| Maple Baked | ½ cup | 150 | 28 | 12 | 6 |
| Vegetarian 99% Fat Free | ½ cup | 150 | 28 | 12 | 6 |
| ***Bush's*** | | | | | |
| Barbecue | ½ cup (4.6 oz) | 160 | 32 | 13 | 6 |
| Maple Cured Bacon | ½ cup (4.6 oz) | 150 | 28 | 11 | 7 |
| Original | ½ cup (4.6 oz) | 150 | 29 | 5 | 7 |
| Vegetarian | ½ cup (4.6 oz) | 130 | 24 | 4 | 6 |
| ***Eden*** | | | | | |
| Organic Baked w/ Sorghum & Mustard | ½ cup (4.6 oz) | 150 | 27 | 6 | 7 |
| ***Gebhardt*** | | | | | |
| Chili | ½ cup (4.6 oz) | 134 | 31 | 1 | 7 |
| Refried Jalapeno | ½ cup (4.5 oz) | 105 | 19 | 3 | 6 |
| Refried No Fat | ½ cup (4.5 oz) | 92 | 20 | 2 | 6 |
| Refried Traditional | ½ cup (4.5 oz) | 109 | 20 | 2 | 6 |
| Refried Vegetarian | ½ cup (4.5 oz) | 118 | 21 | 3 | 7 |
| ***Health Valley*** | | | | | |
| Honey Baked | ½ cup | 110 | 25 | 11 | 7 |
| Honey Baked No Salt | ½ cup | 110 | 25 | 11 | 7 |
| ***Hunt's*** | | | | | |
| Big John's Beans & Fixin's | ½ cup (4.7 oz) | 127 | 23 | 11 | 6 |
| Homestyle Country Kettle | ½ cup (4.6 oz) | 152 | 31 | 11 | 7 |
| Homestyle Special Recipe | ½ cup (4.7 oz) | 185 | 36 | 22 | 8 |
| Mix & Serve | ½ cup (4.7 oz) | 125 | 30 | 16 | 8 |
| Pork & Beans | ½ cup (4.6 oz) | 157 | 27 | 11 | 7 |
| Pork & Beans | ½ cup (4.5 oz) | 130 | 28 | 16 | 4 |
| ***Open Range*** | | | | | |
| Ranch | ½ cup (4.4 oz) | 124 | 23 | 5 | 8 |
| ***Pringles*** | | | | | |
| Vegetarian | 1 cup (7.9 oz) | 250 | 48 | 24 | 9 |
| ***Rosarita*** | | | | | |
| 3 Bean Recipe Bacon & Jalapeno | ½ cup (4.6 oz) | 117 | 22 | 1 | 5 |

| FOOD | PORTION | CALS | CARB | SUGAR | FIBER |
|---|---|---|---|---|---|
| 3 Bean Recipe Chiles & Chicken | ½ cup (4.6 oz) | 115 | 22 | 3 | 4 |
| 3 Bean Recipe Chilies & Chorizo | ½ cup (4.6 oz) | 111 | 19 | 3 | 4 |
| 3 Bean Recipe Onions & Peppers | ½ cup (4.6 oz) | 104 | 20 | 2 | 5 |
| Fiesta Beans Bacon & Jalapenos | ½ cup (4.6 oz) | 117 | 22 | 1 | 5 |
| Fiesta Beans Chicken & Chilies | ½ cup (4.6 oz) | 115 | 22 | 3 | 4 |
| Fiesta Beans Chilies & Chorizo | ½ cup (4.6 oz) | 110 | 19 | 3 | 4 |
| Fiesta Beans Onions & Peppers | ½ cup (4.6 oz) | 104 | 20 | 2 | 5 |
| Refried Bacon | ½ cup (4.5 oz) | 116 | 19 | 2 | 8 |
| Refried Green Chile | ½ cup (4.5 oz) | 110 | 20 | 2 | 7 |
| Refried Low Fat Black | ½ cup (4.5 oz) | 107 | 23 | tr | 7 |
| Refried Nacho Cheese | ½ cup (4.5 oz) | 108 | 19 | 1 | 6 |
| Refried No Fat | ½ cup (4.5 oz) | 120 | 28 | 1 | 6 |
| Refried No Fat Green Chiles & Lime | ½ cup (4.5 oz) | 101 | 22 | 1 | 8 |
| Refried No Fat w/ Zesty Salsa | ½ cup (4.5 oz) | 105 | 24 | 1 | 6 |
| Refried Onion | ½ cup (4.5 oz) | 114 | 21 | 2 | 6 |
| Refried Spicy | ½ cup (4.5 oz) | 118 | 22 | 2 | 6 |
| Refried Traditional | ½ cup (4.5 oz) | 108 | 19 | 1 | 5 |
| Refried Vegetarian | ½ cup (4.5 oz) | 237 | 42 | 6 | 13 |
| ***S&W*** | | | | | |
| Barbecue Beans Ranch Recipe | ½ cup (4.5 oz) | 100 | 25 | 9 | 8 |
| ***Van Camp*** | | | | | |
| Baked Fat Free | ½ cup (4.6 oz) | 132 | 29 | 11 | 5 |
| Baked Original | ½ cup (4.7 oz) | 143 | 29 | 11 | 6 |
| Baked Southern Style Sauteed Onion | ½ cup (4.8 oz) | 145 | 35 | 18 | 8 |
| Baked Sweet Hickory & Bacon | 1 can (4.8 oz) | 143 | 32 | 14 | 6 |
| Beanee Weenee BBQ | 1 cup (7.7 oz) | 290 | 36 | 12 | 7 |
| Beanee Weenee Baked | 1 cup (9.1 oz) | 410 | 58 | 25 | 10 |
| Beanee Weenee Microwave | 1 cup (7.5 oz) | 260 | 29 | 8 | 6 |
| Beanee Weenee Original | 1 cup (9.1 oz) | 320 | 35 | 10 | 8 |
| Beanee Weenee Zestful | 1 cup (7.7 oz) | 300 | 40 | 16 | 7 |
| Brown Sugar | ½ cup (4.6 oz) | 170 | 31 | 13 | 6 |
| Pork And Beans | ½ cup (4.6 oz) | 110 | 23 | 7 | 6 |
| Vegetarian | ½ cup (4.6 oz) | 110 | 23 | 7 | 5 |

| FOOD | PORTION | CALS | CARB | SUGAR | FIBER |
|---|---|---|---|---|---|
| **FROZEN** | | | | | |
| ***Natural Touch*** | | | | | |
| Nine Bean Loaf | 1 in slice (3 oz) | 160 | 13 | tr | 5 |
| **TAKE-OUT** | | | | | |
| baked beans | ½ cup | 161 | 22 | – | – |
| barbecue beans | 3.5 oz | 120 | 26 | – | – |
| four bean salad | 3.5 oz | 100 | 20 | – | – |
| refried beans | ½ cup | 43 | 5 | – | – |
| three bean salad | ¾ cup | 230 | 31 | – | 1 |
| **BEAR** | | | | | |
| simmered | 3 oz | 220 | 0 | 0 | 0 |
| **BEAVER** | | | | | |
| roasted | 3 oz | 140 | 0 | 0 | 0 |
| simmered | 3 oz | 141 | 0 | 0 | 0 |
| **BEECHNUTS** | | | | | |
| dried | 1 oz | 164 | 10 | – | – |
| **BEEF** *(see also* BEEF DISHES, VEAL*)* | | | | | |
| **CANNED** | | | | | |
| corned beef | 3 oz | 85 | 0 | 0 | 0 |
| ***Armour*** | | | | | |
| Chopped Beef | 2 oz | 170 | 2 | 2 | 0 |
| Corned Beef | 2 oz | 120 | 1 | 1 | 0 |
| Potted Meat | 1 can (3 oz) | 120 | 0 | 0 | 0 |
| Tripe | 3 oz | 90 | 0 | 0 | 0 |
| ***Treet*** | | | | | |
| Luncheon Loaf | 2 oz | 130 | 3 | 3 | 0 |
| Luncheon Loaf 50% Less Fat | 2 oz | 110 | 4 | 2 | 0 |
| **DRIED** | | | | | |
| ***Armour*** | | | | | |
| Sliced | 7 slices (1 oz) | 60 | 2 | 2 | 0 |
| **FRESH** | | | | | |
| bottom round lean & fat trim 0 in Choice roasted | 3 oz | 172 | 0 | 0 | 0 |
| bottom round lean & fat trim 0 in braised | 3 oz | 193 | 0 | 0 | 0 |
| bottom round lean & fat trim ¼ in Choice braised | 3 oz | 241 | 0 | 0 | 0 |

| FOOD | PORTION | CALS | CARB | SUGAR | FIBER |
|---|---|---|---|---|---|
| bottom round lean & fat trim ¼ in Choice roasted | 3 oz | 221 | 0 | 0 | 0 |
| brisket flat half lean & fat trim 0 in braised | 3 oz | 183 | 0 | 0 | 0 |
| brisket flat half lean & fat trim ¼ in braised | 3 oz | 309 | 0 | 0 | 0 |
| brisket point half lean & fat trim 0 in braised | 3 oz | 304 | 0 | 0 | 0 |
| brisket point half lean & fat trim ¼ in braised | 3 oz | 343 | 0 | 0 | 0 |
| brisket whole lean & fat trim 0 in braised | 3 oz | 247 | 0 | 0 | 0 |
| brisket whole lean & fat trim ¼ in braised | 3 oz | 327 | 0 | 0 | 0 |
| chuck arm pot roast lean & fat trim 0 in braised | 3 oz | 238 | 0 | 0 | 0 |
| chuck arm pot roast lean & fat trim ¼ in braised | 3 oz | 282 | 0 | 0 | 0 |
| chuck blade roast lean & fat trim 0 in braised | 3 oz | 284 | 0 | 0 | 0 |
| chuck blade roast lean & fat trim ¼ in braised | 3 oz | 293 | 0 | 0 | 0 |
| corned beef brisket cooked | 3 oz | 213 | tr | – | – |
| eye of round lean & fat trim 0 in Choice roasted | 3 oz | 153 | 0 | 0 | 0 |
| eye of round lean & fat trim ¼ in Choice roasted | 3 oz | 205 | 0 | 0 | 0 |
| flank lean & fat trim 0 in braised | 3 oz | 224 | 0 | 0 | 0 |
| flank lean & fat trim 0 in broiled | 3 oz | 192 | 0 | 0 | 0 |
| ground extra lean broiled medium | 3 oz | 217 | 0 | 0 | 0 |
| ground extra lean broiled well done | 3 oz | 225 | 0 | 0 | 0 |
| ground extra lean fried medium | 3 oz | 216 | 0 | 0 | 0 |
| ground extra lean fried well done | 3 oz | 224 | 0 | 0 | 0 |

| FOOD | PORTION | CALS | CARB | SUGAR | FIBER |
|---|---|---|---|---|---|
| ground extra lean raw | 4 oz | 265 | 0 | 0 | 0 |
| ground lean broiled medium | 3 oz | 231 | 0 | 0 | 0 |
| ground lean broiled well done | 3 oz | 238 | 0 | 0 | 0 |
| ground regular broiled medium | 3 oz | 246 | 0 | 0 | 0 |
| ground regular broiled well done | 3 oz | 248 | 0 | 0 | 0 |
| ground 97% fat free irradiated | 4 oz | 160 | 0 | 0 | 0 |
| ground low-fat w/ carrageenan raw | 4 oz | 160 | tr | – | – |
| porterhouse steak lean & fat trim ¼ in Choice broiled | 3 oz | 260 | 0 | 0 | 0 |
| porterhouse steak lean only trim ¼ in Prime broiled | 3 oz | 185 | 0 | 0 | 0 |
| rib eye small end lean & fat trim 0 in Choice broiled | 3 oz | 261 | 0 | 0 | 0 |
| rib large end lean & fat trim 0 in roasted | 3 oz | 300 | 0 | 0 | 0 |
| rib large end lean & fat trim ¼ in broiled | 3 oz | 295 | 0 | 0 | 0 |
| rib large end lean & fat trim ¼ in roasted | 3 oz | 310 | 0 | 0 | 0 |
| rib small end lean & fat trim 0 in broiled | 3 oz | 252 | 0 | 0 | 0 |
| rib small end lean & fat trim ¼ in broiled | 3 oz | 285 | 0 | 0 | 0 |
| rib small end lean & fat trim ¼ in roasted | 3 oz | 295 | 0 | 0 | 0 |
| rib whole lean & fat trim ¼ in Choice broiled | 3 oz | 306 | 0 | 0 | 0 |
| rib whole lean & fat trim ¼ in Choice roasted | 3 oz | 320 | 0 | 0 | 0 |
| rib whole lean & fat trim ¼ in Prime roasted | 3 oz | 348 | 0 | 0 | 0 |
| shank crosscut lean & fat trim ¼ in Choice simmered | 3 oz | 224 | 0 | 0 | 0 |
| short loin top loin lean & fat trim 0 in Choice broiled | 3 oz | 193 | 0 | 0 | 0 |
| short loin top loin lean & fat trim 0 in Choice broiled | 1 steak (5.4 oz) | 353 | 0 | 0 | 0 |

| FOOD | PORTION | CALS | CARB | SUGAR | FIBER |
|---|---|---|---|---|---|
| short loin top loin lean & fat trim ¼ in Choice braised | 3 oz | 253 | 0 | 0 | 0 |
| short loin top loin lean & fat trim ¼ in Choice broiled | 1 steak (6.3 oz) | 536 | 0 | 0 | 0 |
| short loin top loin lean & fat trim ¼ in Prime broiled | 1 steak (6.3 oz) | 582 | 0 | 0 | 0 |
| short loin top loin lean only trim 0 in Choice broiled | 1 steak (5.2 oz) | 311 | 0 | 0 | 0 |
| short loin top loin lean only trim ¼ in Choice broiled | 1 steak (5.2 oz) | 314 | 0 | 0 | 0 |
| shortribs lean & fat Choice braised | 3 oz | 400 | 0 | 0 | 0 |
| t-bone steak lean & fat trim ¼ in Choice broiled | 3 oz | 253 | 0 | 0 | 0 |
| t-bone steak lean only trim ¼ in Choice broiled | 3 oz | 182 | 0 | 0 | 0 |
| tenderloin lean & fat trim ¼ in Choice broiled | 3 oz | 259 | 0 | 0 | 0 |
| tenderloin lean & fat trim ¼ in Choice roasted | 3 oz | 288 | 0 | 0 | 0 |
| tenderloin lean & fat trim ¼ in Choice broiled | 3 oz | 208 | 0 | 0 | 0 |
| tenderloin lean & fat trim ¼ in Prime broiled | 3 oz | 270 | 0 | 0 | 0 |
| tenderloin lean only trim ¼ in Choice broiled | 3 oz | 188 | 0 | 0 | 0 |
| tenderloin lean only trim ¼ in Select broiled | 3 oz | 169 | 0 | 0 | 0 |
| tip round lean & fat trim 0 in Choice roasted | 3 oz | 170 | 0 | 0 | 0 |
| tip round lean & fat trim ¼ in Choice roasted | 3 oz | 210 | 0 | 0 | 0 |
| tip round lean & fat trim ¼ in Prime roasted | 3 oz | 233 | 0 | 0 | 0 |
| top round lean & fat trim 0 in Choice braised | 3 oz | 184 | 0 | 0 | 0 |
| top round lean & fat trim ¼ in Choice braised | 3 oz | 221 | 0 | 0 | 0 |
| top round lean & fat trim ¼ in Choice broiled | 3 oz | 190 | 0 | 0 | 0 |

| FOOD | PORTION | CALS | CARB | SUGAR | FIBER |
|---|---|---|---|---|---|
| top round lean & fat trim ¼ in Choice fried | 3 oz | 235 | 0 | 0 | 0 |
| top round lean & fat trim ¼ in Prime broiled | 3 oz | 195 | 0 | 0 | 0 |
| top sirloin lean & fat trim 0 in Choice broiled | 3 oz | 194 | 0 | 0 | 0 |
| top sirloin lean & fat trim ¼ in Choice broiled | 3 oz | 228 | 0 | 0 | 0 |
| top sirloin lean & fat trim ¼ in Choice fried | 3 oz | 277 | 0 | 0 | 0 |
| tripe raw | 4 oz | 111 | 0 | 0 | 0 |
| ***Maverick Ranch*** | | | | | |
| Filet Mignon | 4 oz | 120 | 0 | 0 | 0 |
| Ground | 4 oz | 130 | 0 | 0 | 0 |
| Ground Round | 4 oz | 130 | 0 | 0 | 0 |
| Ground Sirloin & Chuck | 4 oz | 130 | 0 | 0 | 0 |
| NY Strip Steak | 4 oz | 150 | 0 | 0 | 0 |
| Rib Eye Steak | 4 oz | 170 | 0 | 0 | 0 |
| Top Round Steak & Roast | 4 oz | 110 | 0 | 0 | 0 |
| Top Sirloin | 4 oz | 160 | 0 | 0 | 0 |
| ***Organic Valley*** | | | | | |
| Extra Lean Ground | 3 oz | 130 | 0 | 0 | 0 |
| Extra Lean Patties | 1 (3.2 oz) | 130 | 0 | 0 | 0 |
| **FROZEN** | | | | | |
| patties broiled medium | 3 oz | 240 | 0 | 0 | 0 |
| **READY-TO-EAT** | | | | | |
| dried beef | 5 slices (21 g) | 35 | tr | – | – |
| ***Alpine Lace*** | | | | | |
| Roast Beef 97% Fat Free | 2 oz | 70 | 1 | 0 | 0 |
| ***Boar's Head*** | | | | | |
| Corned Beef Brisket | 2 oz | 80 | 0 | 0 | 0 |
| Eye Round Pepper Seasoned | 2 oz | 90 | 0 | 0 | 0 |
| Italian Style Oven Roasted Top Round | 2 oz | 80 | 2 | 0 | 0 |
| Roast Beef Cajun | 2 oz | 80 | 0 | 0 | 0 |
| Top Round Deluxe | 2 oz | 90 | 0 | 0 | 0 |
| Top Round Oven Roasted No Salt Added | 2 oz | 90 | 0 | 0 | 0 |

| FOOD | PORTION | CALS | CARB | SUGAR | FIBER |
|---|---|---|---|---|---|
| ***Tyson*** | | | | | |
| Beef Strips Seasoned | 1 serv (3 oz) | 140 | 1 | 1 | 0 |
| **TAKE-OUT** | | | | | |
| roast beef medium | 2 oz | 70 | 0 | 0 | 0 |
| roast beef rare | 2 oz | 70 | 0 | 0 | 0 |

## BEEF DISHES

| FOOD | PORTION | CALS | CARB | SUGAR | FIBER |
|---|---|---|---|---|---|
| **CANNED** | | | | | |
| corned beef hash | 3 oz | 155 | 9 | – | – |
| ***Armour*** | | | | | |
| Corned Beef Hash | 1 cup (8.3 oz) | 440 | 23 | 1 | 2 |
| Corned Beef Hash w/ Peppers & Onions | 1 cup (8.3 oz) | 270 | 23 | 2 | 3 |
| Roast Beef Hash | 1 cup (8.4 oz) | 400 | 23 | 0 | 3 |
| Roast Beef in Gravy | ½ cup (4.6 oz) | 150 | 3 | 0 | 0 |
| Stew | 1 cup (8.6 oz) | 220 | 21 | 0 | 2 |
| ***Mary Kitchen*** | | | | | |
| Corned Beef Hash 50% Reduced Fat | 1 cup (8.3 oz) | 280 | 25 | 1 | 3 |
| **FROZEN** | | | | | |
| ***Banquet*** | | | | | |
| Sandwich Toppers Creamed Chipped Beef | 1 pkg (4 oz) | 120 | 8 | 4 | 0 |
| Sandwich Toppers Gravy & Salisbury Steak | 1 pkg (5 oz) | 210 | 8 | 5 | 2 |
| Sandwich Toppers Gravy & Sliced Beef | 1 pkg (4 oz) | 70 | 5 | 1 | 0 |
| **MIX** | | | | | |
| ***Hamburger Helper*** | | | | | |
| BBQ Beef as prep | 1 cup | 320 | 37 | 8 | 1 |
| Beef Pasta as prep | 1 cup | 270 | 26 | 2 | 1 |
| Beef Romanoff as prep | 1 cup | 280 | 27 | 5 | 0 |
| Beef Stew as prep | 1 cup | 260 | 26 | 6 | 2 |
| Beef Taco as prep | 1 cup | 280 | 31 | 6 | 2 |
| Beef Teriyaki as prep | 1 cup | 290 | 34 | 5 | 2 |
| Cheddar & Broccoli as prep | 1 cup | 350 | 33 | 4 | 0 |
| Cheddar Melt as prep | 1 cup | 310 | 31 | 8 | 1 |
| Cheddar'n Bacon as prep | 1 cup | 330 | 27 | 7 | 2 |
| Cheeseburger Macaroni as prep | 1 cup | 360 | 33 | 9 | 1 |

| FOOD | PORTION | CALS | CARB | SUGAR | FIBER |
|---|---|---|---|---|---|
| Cheesy Hashbrowns as prep | 1 cup | 400 | 39 | 5 | 2 |
| Cheesy Italian as prep | 1 cup | 320 | 28 | 7 | 1 |
| Cheesy Shells as prep | 1 cup | 330 | 30 | 6 | tr |
| Chili Macaroni as prep | 1 cup | 290 | 30 | 5 | 2 |
| Fettuccine Alfredo as prep | 1 cup | 300 | 26 | 5 | 0 |
| Four Cheese Lasagne as prep | 1 cup | 330 | 31 | 6 | 0 |
| Italian Parmesan w/ Rigatoni as prep | 1 cup | 300 | 31 | 6 | tr |
| Lasagne as prep | 1 cup | 270 | 29 | 7 | 2 |
| Meat Loaf as prep | ⅙ loaf | 270 | 11 | 3 | 0 |
| Meaty Spaghetti & Cheese as prep | 1 cup | 290 | 30 | 5 | 1 |
| Mushroom & Wild Rice as prep | 1 cup | 310 | 30 | 4 | 2 |
| Nacho Cheese as prep | 1 cup | 320 | 30 | 5 | tr |
| Pizza Pasta w/ Cheese Topping as pre | 1 cup | 280 | 31 | 9 | 2 |
| Pizzabake as prep | ⅙ pie | 270 | 28 | 4 | tr |
| Potatoes Au Gratin as prep | 1 cup | 280 | 25 | 5 | 2 |
| Potatoes Stroganoff as prep | 1 cup | 250 | 23 | 5 | 2 |
| Reduced Sodium Cheddar Spirals as prep | 1 cup | 300 | 27 | 6 | 0 |
| Reduced Sodium Italian Herby as prep | 1 cup | 270 | 29 | 6 | 2 |
| Reduced Sodium Southwestern Beef as prep | 1 cup | 300 | 32 | 6 | 2 |
| Rice Oriental as prep | 1 cup | 280 | 32 | 2 | 0 |
| Salisbury as prep | 1 cup | 270 | 26 | 4 | 1 |
| Spaghetti as prep | 1 cup | 270 | 27 | 6 | 1 |
| Stroganoff as prep | 1 cup | 320 | 30 | 7 | 0 |
| Swedish Meatballs as prep | 1 cup | 290 | 25 | 3 | 2 |
| Three Cheeses as prep | 1 cup | 340 | 32 | 5 | tr |
| Zesty Italian as prep | 1 cup | 300 | 32 | 8 | 2 |
| Zesty Mexican as prep | 1 cup | 280 | 31 | 8 | 2 |
| **REFRIGERATED** | | | | | |
| ***Morton's Of Omaha*** | | | | | |
| Beef Pot Roast w/ Gravy | 1 serv (3 oz) | 160 | 2 | 0 | 0 |

| FOOD | PORTION | CALS | CARB | SUGAR | FIBER |
|---|---|---|---|---|---|
| ***Smithfield*** | | | | | |
| Beef Tips w/ Gravy | ½ cup | 170 | 6 | – | tr |
| ***Tyson*** | | | | | |
| Roast Beef in Brown Gravy | 1 serv + (3.5 oz) | 160 | 3 | 1 | 0 |
| **SHELF-STABLE** | | | | | |
| ***Lunch Bucket*** | | | | | |
| Beef Stew | 1 pkg (7.5 oz) | 170 | 17 | 0 | 2 |
| ***TastyBite*** | | | | | |
| Beef Roganjosh | 1 pkg (9.5 oz) | 270 | 19 | 6 | 3 |
| Meatballs Vindaloo | 1 pkg (9.5 oz) | 270 | 17 | 6 | 4 |
| **TAKE-OUT** | | | | | |
| beef bourguignon | 1 serv (7 oz) | 254 | 3 | – | 1 |
| bubble & squeak | 5 oz | 186 | 16 | – | 3 |
| bulgoghi korean grilled beef | 1 serv (5.2 oz) | 256 | 5 | 3 | tr |
| cornish pasty | 1 (8 oz) | 847 | 79 | – | 3 |
| greek moussaka | 1 serv (8.5 oz) | 450 | 12 | 4 | 1 |
| irish stew | 1 cup (7 oz) | 280 | 10 | – | – |
| kebab indian | 1 (5.4 oz) | 553 | 2 | – | – |
| kheena | 6.7 oz | 781 | 1 | – | tr |
| koftas | 5 | 280 | 3 | – | tr |
| pot roast w/ gravy | 1 serv (6 oz) | 320 | 4 | 0 | 0 |
| samosa | 2 (4 oz) | 652 | 20 | – | 2 |
| shepherds pie | 1 serv (7 oz) | 282 | 20 | – | 2 |
| steak & kidney pie w/ top crust | 1 slice (5 oz) | 400 | 23 | – | 1 |
| stew | 6 oz | 208 | 6 | – | 1 |
| stew w/ vegetables | 1 cup | 220 | 15 | – | – |
| stroganoff | ¾ cup | 260 | 43 | – | – |
| swiss steak | 4.6 oz | 214 | 10 | – | 2 |
| toad in the hole | 1 (4.7 oz) | 383 | 23 | – | 1 |

## BEEFALO

| | | | | | |
|---|---|---|---|---|---|
| roasted | 3 oz | 160 | 0 | 0 | 0 |

## BEER AND ALE

| | | | | | |
|---|---|---|---|---|---|
| alcohol free beer | 7 fl oz | 50 | 11 | 5 | – |
| ale brown | 10 oz | 77 | 8 | – | 0 |
| ale pale | 10 oz | 88 | 12 | – | 0 |

| FOOD | PORTION | CALS | CARB | SUGAR | FIBER |
|---|---|---|---|---|---|
| beer light | 12 oz can | 100 | 5 | – | 0 |
| beer regular | 12 oz can | 146 | 13 | – | tr |
| black & tan | 1 serv (12 oz) | 146 | 13 | – | 1 |
| boilermaker | 1 serv | 216 | 13 | – | 1 |
| lager | 10 oz | 80 | 4 | – | 0 |
| mead | 1 serv | 250 | 13 | – | 1 |
| pilsener lager beer | 7 fl oz | 85 | 13 | 2 | – |
| shandy | 1 serv | 125 | 12 | – | 1 |
| stout | 10 oz | 102 | 6 | – | 0 |
| ***Amstel*** | | | | | |
| Light | 1 bottle (12 oz) | 95 | 5 | – | – |
| ***Blue Moon*** | | | | | |
| White | 1 bottle (12 oz) | 171 | 13 | – | – |
| ***Bud*** | | | | | |
| Ice Light | 1 bottle (12 oz) | 110 | 7 | – | – |
| ***Budweiser*** | | | | | |
| Beer | 1 bottle (12 oz) | 143 | 11 | – | – |
| Ice | 1 bottle (12 oz) | 148 | 9 | – | – |
| Light | 1 bottle (12 oz) | 110 | 7 | – | – |
| ***Busch*** | | | | | |
| Beer | 1 bottle (12 oz) | 133 | 10 | – | – |
| Ice | 1 bottle (12 oz) | 173 | 13 | – | – |
| Light | 1 bottle (12 oz) | 110 | 7 | – | – |
| ***Clausthaler*** | | | | | |
| Beer | 1 bottle (12 oz) | 96 | 6 | – | – |
| ***Coors*** | | | | | |
| Extra Gold | 1 bottle (12 oz) | 147 | 11 | – | – |
| Light | 1 bottle (12 oz) | 102 | 5 | – | – |
| Nonalcoholic | 1 bottle (12 oz) | 73 | 14 | – | – |
| Original | 1 bottle (12 oz) | 148 | 11 | – | – |
| ***Corona*** | | | | | |
| Light | 1 bottle (12 oz) | 109 | 7 | – | – |
| ***Edison*** | | | | | |
| Light | 1 bottle | 109 | 7 | – | – |
| ***Genessee*** | | | | | |
| 12 Horse | 1 bottle (12 oz) | 152 | 14 | – | – |
| Genny Light | 1 bottle (12 oz) | 96 | 6 | – | – |

| FOOD | PORTION | CALS | CARB | SUGAR | FIBER |
|---|---|---|---|---|---|
| ***Guiness*** | | | | | |
| Draught | 1 bottle (12 oz) | 125 | 10 | – | – |
| ***Hamm's*** | | | | | |
| Beer | 1 bottle (12 oz) | 144 | 12 | – | – |
| ***Heineken*** | | | | | |
| Beer | 1 bottle (12 oz) | 166 | 10 | – | – |
| ***I.C.*** | | | | | |
| Light | 1 bottle (12 oz) | 96 | 3 | – | – |
| ***Icehouse*** | | | | | |
| 5.0 | 1 bottle (12 oz) | 132 | 9 | – | – |
| 5.5 | 1 bottle (12 oz) | 149 | 10 | – | – |
| ***J.W. Dundee*** | | | | | |
| Honey Brown | 1 bottle (12 oz) | 150 | 14 | – | – |
| ***Keystone*** | | | | | |
| Light | 1 bottle (12 oz) | 100 | 5 | – | – |
| ***Kilarney's*** | | | | | |
| Red Lager | 1 bottle (12 oz) | 197 | 23 | – | – |
| ***Killian's*** | | | | | |
| Beer | 1 bottle (12 oz) | 163 | 14 | – | – |
| ***Michelob*** | | | | | |
| Ultra Low Carbohydrate | 1 bottle (12 oz) | 95 | 3 | – | – |
| ***Weinhard's*** | | | | | |
| Amber Ale | 1 bottle (12 oz) | 169 | 14 | – | – |
| Dark | 1 bottle (12 oz) | 150 | 13 | – | – |
| Hefeweizen | 1 bottle (12 oz) | 128 | 9 | – | – |
| **BEET JUICE** | | | | | |
| juice | 7 oz | 72 | 16 | – | – |
| **BEETS** | | | | | |
| **CANNED** | | | | | |
| harvard | ½ cup | 89 | 22 | – | – |
| pickled | ½ cup | 75 | 19 | – | – |
| sliced | ½ cup | 27 | 6 | – | – |
| ***Del Monte*** | | | | | |
| Pickled Crinkle Style Sliced | ½ cup (4.5 oz) | 80 | 19 | 16 | 2 |
| Sliced | ½ cup (4.3 oz) | 35 | 8 | 5 | 2 |
| Whole | ½ cup (4.3 oz) | 35 | 8 | 5 | 2 |

| FOOD | PORTION | CALS | CARB | SUGAR | FIBER |
|---|---|---|---|---|---|
| ***Greenwood*** | | | | | |
| Harvard | 1 serv (4.4 oz) | 100 | 27 | 19 | 1 |
| Pickled | 1 oz | 25 | 6 | 5 | 0 |
| ***S&W*** | | | | | |
| Julienne | ½ cup (4.3 oz) | 30 | 7 | 6 | 1 |
| Pickled Sliced | 1 oz | 15 | 4 | 4 | 1 |
| Pickled Whole | 1 oz | 15 | 4 | 4 | 1 |
| Sliced | ½ cup (4.3 oz) | 30 | 7 | 6 | 1 |
| Whole Small | ½ cup (4.3 oz) | 30 | 7 | 6 | 1 |
| ***Veg-All*** | | | | | |
| Small Sliced | ½ cup | 40 | 8 | 6 | 1 |
| **FRESH** | | | | | |
| greens cooked | ½ cup | 20 | 4 | – | – |
| greens raw | ½ cup | 4 | 1 | – | – |
| greens raw chopped | ½ cup | 4 | 1 | – | – |
| sliced cooked | ½ cup (3 oz) | 38 | 9 | – | – |
| whole cooked | 2 (3.5 oz) | 44 | 10 | – | – |
| whole raw | 2 (5.7 oz) | 70 | 16 | – | – |

**BEVERAGES** *(see* BEER AND ALE, CHAMPAGNE, COFFEE, DRINK MIXERS, ENERGY DRINKS, FRUIT DRINKS, ICED TEA, LIQUOR/LIQUEUR, MALT, MILKSHAKE, SODA, TEA/HERBAL TEA, WATER, WINE*)*

## BISCUIT

| FOOD | PORTION | CALS | CARB | SUGAR | FIBER |
|---|---|---|---|---|---|
| buttermilk | 1 (2 oz) | 191 | 28 | – | 1 |
| plain | 1 (2 oz) | 191 | 28 | – | 1 |
| ***Bisquick*** | | | | | |
| Buttermilk | ½ cup | 150 | 21 | 1 | – |
| Cheese Garlic | ½ cup | 160 | 22 | 2 | – |
| Cinnamon Swirl | ½ cup | 150 | 30 | 6 | – |
| Mix | ⅓ cup (1.4 oz) | 160 | 25 | 1 | – |
| Reduced Fat | ⅓ cup | 140 | 27 | 3 | tr |
| ***Kentucky Kernel*** | | | | | |
| Biscuit | ¼ cup (1 oz) | 171 | 28 | 1 | 1 |
| ***MiniCarb*** | | | | | |
| Buttery as prep | 1 | 255 | 3 | 0 | 2 |
| **REFRIGERATED** | | | | | |
| buttermilk | 1 (1 oz) | 98 | 14 | – | – |
| plain | 1 (1 oz) | 98 | 14 | – | tr |

| FOOD | PORTION | CALS | CARB | SUGAR | FIBER |
|---|---|---|---|---|---|
| ***1869 Brand*** | | | | | |
| Buttermilk | 1 (1.1 oz) | 100 | 12 | 1 | 0 |
| ***Hungry Jack*** | | | | | |
| Butter Tastin' Flaky | 1 (1.2 oz) | 100 | 14 | 2 | 0 |
| Cinnamon & Sugar | 1 (1.2 oz) | 110 | 17 | 5 | tr |
| Flaky | 1 (1.2 oz) | 100 | 14 | 2 | 0 |
| Flaky Buttermilk | 1 (1.2 oz) | 100 | 14 | 2 | 0 |
| ***Pillsbury*** | | | | | |
| Big Country Butter Tastin' | 1 (1.2 oz) | 100 | 13 | 2 | 0 |
| Big Country Buttermilk | 1 (1.2 oz) | 100 | 14 | 2 | 0 |
| Big Country Southern Style | 1 (1.2 oz) | 100 | 14 | 2 | 0 |
| Buttermilk | 1 (2.2 oz) | 150 | 29 | 3 | tr |
| Country | 1 (2.2 oz) | 150 | 29 | 3 | tr |
| Grands Blueberry | 1 (2.1 oz) | 210 | 29 | 10 | tr |
| Grands Butter Tastin' | 1 (2.1 oz) | 200 | 24 | 5 | tr |
| Grands Buttermilk | 1 (2.1 oz) | 200 | 24 | 5 | tr |
| Grands Buttermilk Reduced Fat | 1 (2.1 oz) | 190 | 27 | 5 | tr |
| Grands Extra Rich | 1 (2.1 oz) | 220 | 25 | 6 | tr |
| Grands Flaky | 1 (2.1 oz) | 200 | 25 | 3 | tr |
| Grands Golden Corn | 1 (1.2 oz) | 210 | 26 | 6 | tr |
| Grands HomeStyle | 1 (2.1 oz) | 210 | 25 | 5 | tr |
| Grands Southern Style | 1 (2.1 oz) | 200 | 24 | 5 | tr |
| Southern Style Flakey | 1 (1.2 oz) | 100 | 14 | 2 | 0 |
| Tender Layer Buttermilk | 1 (2.2 oz) | 160 | 27 | 3 | tr |
| **TAKE-OUT** | | | | | |
| buttermilk | 1 (2 oz) | 212 | 27 | – | – |
| oatcakes | 2 (4 oz) | 115 | 16 | – | 1 |
| plain | 1 (35 g) | 276 | 13 | – | – |
| tea biscuit | 1 (3 oz) | 210 | 30 | 12 | 1 |
| w/ egg | 1 (4.8 oz) | 316 | 24 | – | – |
| w/ egg & bacon | 1 (5.2 oz) | 458 | 29 | – | 1 |
| w/ egg & ham | 1 (6.7 oz) | 442 | 30 | – | 4 |
| w/ egg & sausage | 1 (6.3 oz) | 581 | 41 | – | 1 |
| w/ egg & steak | 1 (5.2 oz) | 410 | 21 | – | – |
| w/ egg cheese & bacon | 1 (5.1 oz) | 477 | 33 | – | – |
| w/ ham | 1 (4 oz) | 386 | 44 | – | 1 |
| w/ sausage | 1 (4.4 oz) | 485 | 40 | – | 1 |
| w/ steak | 1 (4.9 oz) | 455 | 44 | – | – |

| FOOD | PORTION | CALS | CARB | SUGAR | FIBER |
|---|---|---|---|---|---|
| **BISON** | | | | | |
| roasted | 3 oz | 122 | 0 | 0 | 0 |
| **BLACK BEANS** | | | | | |
| dried cooked | 1 cup | 227 | 41 | – | 15 |
| ***Bean Cuisine*** | | | | | |
| Pasta & Beans Mediterranean Black Beans & Fusilli | 1 serv | 210 | 30 | 2 | 4 |
| ***Eden*** | | | | | |
| Organic | ½ cup (4.6 oz) | 100 | 18 | 0 | 6 |
| ***Progresso*** | | | | | |
| Black Beans | ½ cup (4.6 oz) | 110 | 17 | 0 | 7 |
| **BLACKBERRIES** | | | | | |
| canned in heavy syrup | ½ cup | 118 | 30 | – | – |
| fresh | ½ cup | 37 | 9 | – | 3 |
| unsweetened frzn | 1 cup | 97 | 24 | – | – |
| **BLACKBERRY JUICE** | | | | | |
| ***Clear Fruit*** | | | | | |
| Blackberry Rush | 8 oz | 90 | 23 | 23 | – |
| ***Everfresh*** | | | | | |
| Clear Fruit Blackberry Rush | 8 oz | 90 | 23 | 23 | – |
| **BLACKEYE PEAS** | | | | | |
| **CANNED** | | | | | |
| w/pork | ½ cup | 199 | 40 | – | – |
| ***Eden*** | | | | | |
| Organic | ½ cup (4.6 oz) | 90 | 16 | 1 | 4 |
| **DRIED** | | | | | |
| cooked | 1 cup | 198 | 36 | – | 16 |
| **FROZEN** | | | | | |
| ***Birds Eye*** | | | | | |
| Blackeye Peas | ½ cup | 110 | 21 | 1 | 4 |
| **BLINTZE** | | | | | |
| ***Cohen's & Wilton*** | | | | | |
| Cheese | 1 | 80 | 10 | 5 | 0 |
| ***Golden*** | | | | | |
| Cheese | 1 (2.1 oz) | 80 | 13 | 5 | 2 |
| Potato | 1 | 90 | 15 | 2 | 2 |

| FOOD | PORTION | CALS | CARB | SUGAR | FIBER |
|---|---|---|---|---|---|
| ***Ratner's*** | | | | | |
| Cheese | 1 (2.1 oz) | 90 | 15 | 3 | tr |
| **TAKE-OUT** | | | | | |
| cheese | 1 (2.7 oz) | 160 | 15 | 4 | tr |
| **BLUEBERRIES** | | | | | |
| canned in heavy syrup | 1 cup | 225 | 56 | – | – |
| fresh | 1 cup | 82 | 20 | – | – |
| unsweetened frzn | 1 cup | 78 | 19 | – | – |
| ***Tree Of Life*** | | | | | |
| Organic | 1 cup (5 oz) | 80 | 20 | 16 | 2 |
| **BLUEFIN** | | | | | |
| fillet baked | 4.1 oz | 186 | 0 | 0 | 0 |
| **BLUEFISH** | | | | | |
| fresh baked | 3 oz | 135 | 0 | 0 | 0 |
| **BOAR** | | | | | |
| wild roasted | 3 oz | 136 | 0 | 0 | 0 |
| **BOK CHOY** *(see* CABBAGE*)* | | | | | |
| **BONITO** | | | | | |
| fresh | 3 oz | 117 | 0 | 0 | 0 |
| **BORAGE** | | | | | |
| fresh chopped | ½ cup | 9 | 1 | – | – |
| fresh chopped cooked | 3½ oz | 25 | 4 | – | – |
| **BOTTLED WATER** *(see* WATER*)* | | | | | |
| **BOYSENBERRIES** | | | | | |
| in heavy syrup | 1 cup | 226 | 57 | – | – |
| unsweetened frzn | 1 cup | 66 | 16 | – | – |
| **BRAINS** | | | | | |
| beef pan-fried | 3 oz | 167 | 0 | 0 | 0 |
| beef simmered | 3 oz | 136 | 0 | 0 | 0 |
| lamb braised | 3 oz | 124 | 0 | 0 | 0 |
| lamb fried | 3 oz | 232 | 0 | 0 | 0 |
| pork braised | 3 oz | 117 | 0 | 0 | 0 |
| veal braised | 3 oz | 115 | 0 | 0 | 0 |
| veal fried | 3 oz | 181 | 0 | 0 | 0 |

| FOOD | PORTION | CALS | CARB | SUGAR | FIBER |
|---|---|---|---|---|---|
| ***Armour*** | | | | | |
| Pork Brains in Milk Gravy | ⅔ cup (5.5 oz) | 150 | 10 | 0 | 0 |
| **BRAN** | | | | | |
| corn | 1 cup (2.7 oz) | 170 | 65 | – | 65 |
| oat | ½ cup (1.6 oz) | 116 | 31 | – | 7 |
| oat cooked | ½ cup (3.8 oz) | 44 | 13 | – | 3 |
| rice | ½ cup (2.1 oz) | 187 | 29 | – | 12 |
| wheat | ½ cup (2 oz) | 63 | 19 | – | 12 |
| ***Hodgson Mill*** | | | | | |
| Oat | ¼ cup | 120 | 23 | 0 | 6 |
| Wheat Unprocessed | ¼ cup | 30 | 10 | 0 | 7 |
| **BRAZIL NUTS** | | | | | |
| dried unblanched | 1 oz | 186 | 4 | – | – |
| **BREAD** | | | | | |
| **CANNED** | | | | | |
| boston brown | 1 slice (1.6 oz) | 88 | 20 | – | 2 |
| **FROZEN** | | | | | |
| ***Marie Callender's*** | | | | | |
| Cornbread & Honey Butter | 1 piece + butter | 210 | 28 | 2 | 1 |
| Original Garlic | 1 piece | 190 | 23 | 5 | 2 |
| Parmesan & Romano Garlic | 1 piece | 200 | 23 | 2 | 2 |
| ***Pepperidge Farm*** | | | | | |
| Garlic | 1 slice (1.8 oz) | 170 | 15 | 2 | 1 |
| Garlic Sourdough 30% Reduced Fat | 1 slice (1.8 oz) | 170 | 22 | 2 | 2 |
| Mozzarella Garlic Cheese | 1 slice (2 oz) | 201 | 21 | 2 | 1 |
| **MIX** | | | | | |
| cornbread | 1 piece (2 oz) | 189 | 29 | – | 1 |
| ***Atkins*** | | | | | |
| Caraway Rye as prep | 1 slice | 150 | 8 | 0 | 5 |
| Country White as prep | 1 slice | 70 | 8 | 0 | 5 |
| Sourdough as prep | 1 slice | 70 | 8 | 0 | 5 |
| ***Buitoni*** | | | | | |
| Focaccia Rosemary & Garlic | 1 piece (1 oz) | 110 | 22 | 2 | 1 |
| ***Carbolite*** | | | | | |
| Bread Mix as prep | 1 slice | 45 | 4 | – | – |

| FOOD | PORTION | CALS | CARB | SUGAR | FIBER |
|---|---|---|---|---|---|
| ***Hodgson Mill*** | | | | | |
| European Cheese & Herb | ¼ cup (1.2 oz) | 130 | 21 | 3 | tr |
| Honey Whole Wheat | ¼ cup (1.2 oz) | 120 | 22 | 2 | 2 |
| ***Keto*** | | | | | |
| Quick Bread All Flavors as prep | 1 slice | 55 | 3 | – | – |
| ***MiniCarb*** | | | | | |
| Country White as prep | 1 slice | 80 | 7 | 0 | 4 |
| **READY-TO-EAT** | | | | | |
| baguette parisian | 2 oz | 120 | 26 | 0 | tr |
| baguette whole wheat | 2 oz | 140 | 29 | tr | 1 |
| challah | 1 slice (2 oz) | 160 | 29 | 5 | 1 |
| cracked wheat | 1 slice | 65 | 12 | – | 1 |
| egg | 1 slice (1.4 oz) | 115 | 19 | – | – |
| french | 1 slice (1 oz) | 78 | 15 | – | 1 |
| french | 1 loaf (1 lb) | 1270 | 230 | – | – |
| gluten | 1 slice | 47 | 8 | – | – |
| italian | 1 slice (1 oz) | 81 | 15 | – | 1 |
| italian | 1 loaf (1 lb) | 1255 | 256 | – | – |
| navajo fry | 1 (5 in diam) | 296 | 48 | – | – |
| navajo fry | 1 (10.5 in diam) | 527 | 85 | – | – |
| oat bran | 1 slice | 71 | 12 | – | 1 |
| oat bran reduced calorie | 1 slice | 46 | 10 | – | – |
| oatmeal | 1 slice | 73 | 13 | – | 1 |
| oatmeal reduced calorie | 1 slice | 48 | 10 | – | – |
| pita | 1 reg (2 oz) | 165 | 33 | – | 1 |
| pita | 1 sm (1 oz) | 78 | 16 | – | 1 |
| pita whole wheat | 1 reg (2 oz) | 170 | 35 | – | 5 |
| pita whole wheat | 1 sm (1 oz) | 76 | 16 | – | 2 |
| protein | 1 slice | 47 | 8 | – | – |
| pumpernickel | 1 slice | 80 | 15 | – | 2 |
| raisin | 1 slice | 71 | 14 | – | – |
| rice bran | 1 slice | 66 | 12 | – | – |
| rye | 1 slice | 83 | 16 | – | 2 |
| rye reduced calorie | 1 slice | 47 | 9 | – | – |
| seven grain | 1 slice | 65 | 12 | – | 2 |
| sourdough | 1 slice (1 oz) | 78 | 15 | – | 1 |
| vienna | 1 slice (1 oz) | 78 | 15 | – | 1 |
| wheat reduced calorie | 1 slice | 46 | 10 | – | 3 |

| FOOD | PORTION | CALS | CARB | SUGAR | FIBER |
|---|---|---|---|---|---|
| wheat berry | 1 slice | 65 | 12 | – | 1 |
| wheat bran | 1 slice | 89 | 17 | – | 3 |
| wheat germ | 1 slice | 74 | 14 | – | – |
| white | 1 slice | 67 | 12 | – | 1 |
| white reduced calorie | 1 slice | 48 | 10 | – | 2 |
| white toasted | 1 slice | 67 | 13 | – | – |
| white cubed | 1 cup | 80 | 15 | – | – |
| whole wheat | 1 slice | 70 | 13 | – | 2 |
| ***Arnold*** | | | | | |
| Bran'nola Country Oat | 1 slice (1.3 oz) | 110 | 20 | 3 | 3 |
| Carb Counting Multigrain | 1 slice | 60 | 9 | – | 3 |
| Country Buttermilk | 1 slice (1.3 oz) | 110 | 20 | 4 | 1 |
| Country Wheat | 1 slice (1.3 oz) | 100 | 19 | 4 | 1 |
| Country White | 1 slice (1.3 oz) | 110 | 21 | 4 | tr |
| Natural 100% Whole Wheat | 1 slice (1.3 oz) | 90 | 16 | 2 | 3 |
| Raisin Cinnamon | 1 slice (1 oz) | 80 | 15 | 7 | 1 |
| ***Atkins*** | | | | | |
| Rye | 1 slice | 60 | 8 | 0 | 5 |
| White | 1 slice | 60 | 8 | 0 | 5 |
| ***Bread Du Jour*** | | | | | |
| French | 3 in slice (2 oz) | 140 | 26 | 3 | 1 |
| ***Damascus*** | | | | | |
| Pita | 1 (2 oz) | 130 | 29 | 0 | 2 |
| Pita Whole Wheat | 1 (2 oz) | 160 | 32 | 0 | 3 |
| Wraps Honey Wheat | ½ wrap (2 oz) | 130 | 28 | 3 | 1 |
| Wraps Plain | ½ wrap (2 oz) | 130 | 29 | tr | 1 |
| Wraps Spinach | 1 (4 oz) | 280 | 52 | tr | 2 |
| Wraps Tomato | 1 12-inch (4 oz) | 240 | 58 | 1 | 2 |
| ***Ecce Panis*** | | | | | |
| Country Wheat | 1 slice (2 oz) | 150 | 32 | tr | 2 |
| ***Freihofer's*** | | | | | |
| Whole Wheat Light | 2 slices | 80 | 19 | 3 | 5 |
| ***Gold Medal*** | | | | | |
| 100% Whole Wheat | 1 slice | 70 | 13 | 1 | 2 |
| ***Home Pride*** | | | | | |
| Carb Action Multigrain | 1 slice | 60 | 8 | – | 1 |
| Carb Action White Fiber | 1 slice | 60 | 10 | – | 4 |
| Wheat | 1 slice (1 oz) | 80 | 14 | 2 | 1 |

| FOOD | PORTION | CALS | CARB | SUGAR | FIBER |
|---|---|---|---|---|---|
| ***La Mexicana*** | | | | | |
| Wraps Chocolate | 1 (1.3 oz) | 120 | 18 | 1 | 1 |
| Wraps Southwestern Mild Chili | 1 (1.3 oz) | 120 | 18 | 1 | 1 |
| Wraps Spinach | 1 (1.3 oz) | 120 | 18 | 1 | 1 |
| Wraps Tomato Basil | 1 (1.3 oz) | 120 | 18 | 1 | 1 |
| ***Milton's*** | | | | | |
| Healthy Multi-Grain | 1 slice (1.4 oz) | 110 | 24 | 6 | 3 |
| ***Pepperidge Farm*** | | | | | |
| Apple Cinammon | 1 slice (1 oz) | 80 | 15 | 4 | 1 |
| Deli Swirl Rye & Pump | 1 slice | 80 | 15 | tr | 1 |
| Farmhouse Butter Topped Wheat | 1 slice | 110 | 21 | 3 | 2 |
| Farmhouse Country Wheat | 1 slice | 110 | 21 | 3 | 2 |
| Farmhouse Hearty White | 1 slice (1.5 oz) | 110 | 20 | 5 | tr |
| Farmhouse Sesame Wheat | 1 slice | 110 | 19 | 2 | 2 |
| Farmhouse Sourdough | 1 slice (1.5 oz) | 110 | 20 | 2 | 1 |
| Natural Whole Grain Whole Wheat | 1 slice (1.2 oz) | 90 | 16 | 2 | 2 |
| Natural Whole Grain Honey Oat | 1 slice (1.2 oz) | 90 | 15 | 2 | 2 |
| Sandwich Pocket Wheat | 1 (2 oz) | 160 | 30 | 2 | 3 |
| Sandwich Pocket White | 1 (2 oz) | 150 | 30 | 2 | 2 |
| Swirl Cinnamon | 1 slice (1 oz) | 90 | 15 | tr | 1 |
| Swirl Raisin Cinnamon | 1 slice (1 oz) | 80 | 14 | 6 | 1 |
| ***Stroehmann*** | | | | | |
| 100% Whole Wheat | 1 slice (1.3 oz) | 90 | 17 | 3 | 2 |
| D'Italiano Italian No Seeds | 1 slice (1 oz) | 80 | 15 | tr | tr |
| D'Italiano Italian Seeded | 1 slice (1 oz) | 80 | 15 | tr | tr |
| Family White | 1 slice (0.8 oz) | 65 | 13 | 1 | 0 |
| Homestyle Split Top Wheat | 1 slices (0.8 oz) | 60 | 13 | 2 | tr |
| Homestyle Split Top White | 1 slice (0.8 oz) | 65 | 12 | 1 | 1 |
| Honey Cracked Wheat | 1 slice (1.2 oz) | 80 | 16 | 2 | 1 |
| King White | 1 slice (0.8 oz) | 65 | 13 | 1 | 0 |
| New York Rye | 1 slice (1 oz) | 80 | 15 | 1 | 1 |

| FOOD | PORTION | CALS | CARB | SUGAR | FIBER |
|---|---|---|---|---|---|
| Potato | 1 slice (1.2 oz) | 100 | 19 | 3 | tr |
| Ranch White | 1 slice (0.8 oz) | 65 | 13 | 1 | 0 |
| Rye | 1 slice (1.1 oz) | 80 | 15 | tr | tr |
| Twelve Grain | 1 slice (1.2 oz) | 90 | 17 | 3 | 1 |
| ***TastyBite*** | | | | | |
| Nan Kontos Massala | ½ loaf (1.4 oz) | 120 | 15 | 1 | 1 |
| Nan Kontos Onion | ½ loaf (1.4 oz) | 120 | 15 | 1 | 1 |
| Nan Kontos Roghani | ½ loaf (1.4 oz) | 125 | 19 | 3 | 1 |
| Nan Kontos Tandoori | ½ loaf (1.4 oz) | 120 | 19 | 3 | 1 |
| Roti Kontos Missy | ½ loaf (1.4 oz) | 125 | 18 | 2 | 2 |
| ***Toufayan*** | | | | | |
| Wraps Sundried Tomato Basil | 1 (2 oz) | 183 | 30 | 1 | 2 |
| **REFRIGERATED** | | | | | |
| ***Pillsbury*** | | | | | |
| Crusty French Loaf | ⅕ loaf (2.2 oz) | 150 | 27 | 3 | tr |
| Grands Wheat | 1 (2.1 oz) | 200 | 27 | 6 | 2 |
| **TAKE-OUT** | | | | | |
| chapatis as prep w/ fat | 1 bread (1.6 oz) | 95 | 18 | 1 | 3 |
| chapatis as prep w/o fat | 1 (2½ oz) | 141 | 31 | – | 5 |
| cornbread | 2 in x 2 in (1.4 oz) | 107 | 18 | – | – |
| cornstick | 1 (1.3 oz) | 101 | 13 | – | tr |
| focaccia | 1 piece (2 oz) | 130 | 23 | 03 | 1 |
| focaccia onion | 1 piece (4.6 oz) | 282 | 43 | 2 | 2 |
| focaccia rosemary | 1 piece (3.5 oz) | 251 | 40 | 1 | 2 |
| focaccia tomato olive | 1 piece (4.7 oz) | 270 | 42 | 1 | 2 |
| garlic bread | 2 slices (2 oz) | 190 | 27 | 1 | 1 |
| irish soda bread | 1 slice (2 oz) | 174 | 34 | – | – |
| naan | 1 bread (3.5 oz) | 286 | 43 | 3 | 2 |
| papadums fried | 2 (1.5 oz) | 81 | 9 | – | 2 |
| paratha | 1 bread (2.1 oz) | 201 | 23 | 1 | 2 |

| FOOD | PORTION | CALS | CARB | SUGAR | FIBER |
|---|---|---|---|---|---|
| **BREAD COATING** | | | | | |
| ***Don's Chuck Wagon*** | | | | | |
| Chicken Baking Mix | ¼ cup (1 oz) | 95 | 21 | 0 | 1 |
| Fish & Chips Mix | ¼ cup (1 oz) | 100 | 21 | 0 | 1 |
| Fish Mix | ¼ cup (1 oz) | 95 | 21 | 0 | 1 |
| Mushroom Batter Mix | ¼ cup (1 oz) | 95 | 21 | 0 | 1 |
| Onion Ring Mix | ¼ cup (1 oz) | 100 | 21 | 0 | 1 |
| Seafood Bake & Fry Mix | ¼ cup (1 oz) | 95 | 21 | 0 | 1 |
| ***Luzianne*** | | | | | |
| Cajun Chicken Coating Mix | 2 tbsp (1 oz) | 100 | 20 | 2 | 1 |
| **BREAD MACHINE MIX** | | | | | |
| ***Betty Crocker*** | | | | | |
| Harvest Wheat | 1/11 loaf | 140 | 25 | 3 | 2 |
| Home-Style White | 1/11 loaf | 130 | 25 | 2 | 0 |
| ***Carbsense*** | | | | | |
| Harvest Wheat as prep | 1 slice | 60 | 4 | 0 | 1 |
| ***Fleischmann's*** | | | | | |
| Apple Cinnamon | ⅛ loaf | 160 | 32 | 12 | 2 |
| Cinnamon Raisin | ⅛ loaf | 160 | 33 | 4 | 2 |
| Country White | ⅛ loaf (1.6 oz) | 170 | 31 | 4 | 2 |
| Cranberry Orange | ⅛ loaf | 150 | 33 | 4 | 2 |
| Honey Oatmeal | ⅛ loaf | 160 | 33 | 5 | 3 |
| Italian Herb | ⅛ loaf | 160 | 29 | 2 | 2 |
| Sourdough | ⅛ loaf | 150 | 29 | 3 | 2 |
| Stoneground Wheat | ⅛ loaf | 160 | 32 | 4 | 3 |
| ***Keto*** | | | | | |
| Cinnamon Raisin as prep | 1 slice | 79 | 6 | tr | 3 |
| French Loaf as prep | 1 slice | 79 | 5 | tr | 3 |
| Sourdough Rye as prep | 1 slice | 79 | 5 | tr | 3 |
| ***Ketogenics*** | | | | | |
| Low Carb Honey Wheat as prep | 1 slice | 80 | 7 | 1 | 5 |
| Low Carb Original White as prep | 1 slice | 62 | 2 | – | – |
| Low Carb Pumpernickel Rye as prep | 1 slice | 80 | 7 | 1 | 5 |
| **BREADCRUMBS** | | | | | |
| dry | 1 cup | 426 | 78 | – | 5 |
| dry seasoned | 1 cup (4 oz) | 441 | 85 | – | 5 |

| FOOD | PORTION | CALS | CARB | SUGAR | FIBER |
|---|---|---|---|---|---|
| fresh | ⅔ cup | 76 | 14 | – | 1 |
| ***Keto*** | | | | | |
| Low Carb Cajun | ½ cup | 185 | 13 | – | 9 |
| Low Carb Italian | ½ cup | 185 | 13 | – | 9 |
| Low Carb Original | ½ cup | 185 | 13 | – | 9 |
| ***Progresso*** | | | | | |
| Garlic & Herb | ¼ cup (1 oz) | 100 | 18 | 1 | 1 |
| Italian Style | ¼ cup (1 oz) | 110 | 20 | 1 | 1 |
| Parmesan | ¼ cup (1 oz) | 100 | 17 | 1 | 1 |
| Plain | ¼ cup (1 oz) | 110 | 19 | 1 | 1 |
| ***Ronzoni*** | | | | | |
| Italian Flavored | ¼ cup | 120 | 21 | 2 | 2 |
| **BREADFRUIT** | | | | | |
| fresh | ¼ small | 99 | 26 | – | – |
| seeds cooked | 1 oz | 48 | 9 | – | – |
| seeds raw | 1 oz | 54 | 8 | – | – |
| seeds roasted | 1 oz | 59 | 11 | – | – |
| **BREADNUTTREE SEEDS** | | | | | |
| dried | 1 oz | 104 | 23 | – | – |
| **BREADSTICKS** | | | | | |
| onion poppyseed | 1 | 64 | 11 | – | – |
| plain | 1 | 41 | 7 | – | – |
| plain | 1 sm | 25 | 4 | – | – |
| ***Bread Du Jour*** | | | | | |
| Original | 1 (1.9 oz) | 130 | 25 | 3 | 1 |
| Sourdough | 1 (1.9 oz) | 130 | 25 | 1 | 1 |
| ***Pepperidge Farm*** | | | | | |
| Snack Sticks Wheat | 9 (1 oz) | 130 | 22 | 4 | 1 |
| ***Pillsbury*** | | | | | |
| Soft | 1 (1.4 oz) | 110 | 19 | 2 | tr |
| Soft Garlic & Herb | 1 (2.1 oz) | 180 | 25 | 3 | tr |
| ***Stella D'Oro*** | | | | | |
| Grissini Style Fat Free | 3 (0.5 oz) | 60 | 12 | 1 | 0 |
| Original | 1 (0.4 oz) | 45 | 7 | 0 | 0 |
| Potato 'N Onion | 1 (0.4 oz) | 45 | 8 | tr | 0 |
| Roasted Garlic | 1 (0.4 oz) | 45 | 8 | tr | tr |
| Sesame | 1 (0.4 oz) | 50 | 7 | tr | tr |

| FOOD | PORTION | CALS | CARB | SUGAR | FIBER |
|---|---|---|---|---|---|
| Snack Stix Cracked Pepper | 4 (0.5 oz) | 70 | 11 | tr | 0 |
| Snack Stix Salted | 4 (0.5 oz) | 70 | 11 | tr | 0 |
| Sodium Free | 1 (0.4 oz) | 45 | 7 | tr | 0 |
| Wheat | 1 (0.3 oz) | 40 | 6 | tr | 0 |
| **BREAKFAST BARS** *(see* CEREAL BARS, ENERGY BARS*)* | | | | | |
| **BREAKFAST DRINKS** | | | | | |
| orange drink powder | 3 rounded tsp | 93 | 24 | – | – |
| orange drink powder as prep w/water | 6 oz | 86 | 22 | – | – |
| ***Carnation*** | | | | | |
| Instant Breakfast French Vanilla as prep w/ 2% milk | 1 serv | 250 | 40 | – | – |
| Instant Breakfast French Vanilla as prep w/ fat free milk | 1 serv | 220 | 40 | – | – |
| Instant Breakfast French Vanilla as prep w/ whole milk | 1 serv | 280 | 39 | – | – |
| **BROAD BEANS** | | | | | |
| canned | 1 cup | 183 | 32 | – | – |
| dried cooked | 1 cup | 186 | 33 | – | – |
| fresh cooked | 3½ oz | 56 | 10 | – | – |
| **BROCCOFLOWER** | | | | | |
| fresh raw | ½ cup (1.8 oz) | 16 | 3 | – | – |
| **BROCCOLI** | | | | | |
| **FRESH** | | | | | |
| chinese broccoli (gai lan) cooked | 1 cup (3.1 oz) | 19 | 3 | – | 2 |
| chopped cooked | ½ cup | 22 | 4 | – | 2 |
| **FROZEN** | | | | | |
| chopped cooked | ½ cup | 25 | 5 | – | – |
| spears cooked | 10 oz pkg | 69 | 13 | – | 4 |
| spears cooked | ½ cup | 25 | 5 | – | 3 |
| ***Birds Eye*** | | | | | |
| Florets | 1 cup | 25 | 4 | 1 | 2 |
| in Cheese Sauce | ½ cup | 70 | 7 | 3 | 2 |
| ***Fresh Like*** | | | | | |
| Spear | 3.5 oz | 26 | 5 | – | 1 |

| FOOD | PORTION | CALS | CARB | SUGAR | FIBER |
|---|---|---|---|---|---|
| ***Health Is Wealth*** | | | | | |
| Broccoli Munchees | 2 (1 oz) | 60 | 10 | 0 | 1 |
| ***Tree Of Life*** | | | | | |
| Cuts | 1 cup (3.1 oz) | 25 | 4 | 1 | 2 |
| **BROWNIE** | | | | | |
| **FROZEN** | | | | | |
| ***Greenfield*** | | | | | |
| Fat Free Homestyle | 1 (1.3 oz) | 110 | 27 | 19 | 0 |
| ***Otis Spunkmeyer*** | | | | | |
| Blue Yonder w/ Walnuts | 1 (2 oz) | 230 | 34 | 22 | 2 |
| ***Weight Watchers*** | | | | | |
| Brownie A La Mode | 1 (3.14 oz) | 190 | 33 | 15 | 2 |
| Double Fudge Brownie Parfait | 1 (5.3 oz) | 190 | 39 | 20 | 2 |
| **MIX** | | | | | |
| plain | 1 (1.2 oz) | 139 | 20 | – | 1 |
| plain low calorie | 1 (0.8 oz) | 84 | 16 | – | 1 |
| ***Atkins*** | | | | | |
| Kitchen Fudge as prep | 1 (2 inch) | 60 | 17 | 0 | 4 |
| ***Aunt Paula's*** | | | | | |
| Low Carb Chef Fudge Brownie as prep | 1 (2.5 inch) | 89 | 9 | 0 | 2 |
| ***Betty Crocker*** | | | | | |
| Chocolate Chunk as prep | 1 | 180 | 25 | 18 | – |
| Dark Chocolate Fudge as prep | 1 | 170 | 24 | 17 | – |
| Dark Chocolate w/ Syrup as prep | 1 | 170 | 25 | 16 | – |
| Fudge as prep | 1 | 170 | 23 | 17 | – |
| German Chocolate Coconut Pecan Filling as prep | 1 | 200 | 29 | 21 | 1 |
| Hot Fudge as prep | 1 | 170 | 23 | 16 | – |
| Original as prep | 1 | 180 | 27 | 19 | – |
| Peanut Butter as prep | 1 | 180 | 23 | 17 | – |
| Stir'n Bake w/ Mini Kisses as prep | 1 serv | 220 | 38 | 27 | 1 |
| Turtle w/ Caramel & Pecans as prep | 1 | 170 | 25 | 16 | – |
| Walnut as prep | 1 | 180 | 23 | 15 | – |

| FOOD | PORTION | CALS | CARB | SUGAR | FIBER |
|---|---|---|---|---|---|
| ***Estee*** | | | | | |
| Brownie Mix as prep | 2 | 100 | 23 | 10 | 1 |
| ***Keto*** | | | | | |
| Chocolate Fudge as prep | 1 | 59 | 2 | 0 | 1 |
| ***MiniCarb*** | | | | | |
| Chocolate Brownie as prep | 1 | 220 | 10 | 1 | 8 |
| ***No Pudge!*** | | | | | |
| All Flavors | 1 | 100 | 21 | 13 | tr |
| ***Sweet Rewards*** | | | | | |
| Low Fat Fudge as prep | 1 | 130 | 27 | 18 | 1 |
| Reduced Fat Supreme as prep | 1 | 140 | 27 | 19 | – |
| **READY-TO-EAT** | | | | | |
| plain | 1 lg (2 oz) | 227 | 36 | – | 1 |
| plain | 1 sm (1 oz) | 115 | 18 | – | 1 |
| w/ nuts | 1 (1 oz) | 100 | 16 | – | – |
| ***Dolly Madison*** | | | | | |
| Fudge | 1 (3 oz) | 330 | 54 | 11 | 1 |
| ***Entenmann's*** | | | | | |
| Little Bites | 3 (2.2 oz) | 290 | 37 | 26 | 1 |
| Ultimate Fudge | 1 (1.6 oz) | 220 | 27 | 18 | 2 |
| ***Greenfield*** | | | | | |
| Blondie Fat Free Apple Spice | 1 (1.3 oz) | 110 | 26 | 19 | 0 |
| ***Health Valley*** | | | | | |
| Bar w/ Fudge Filling | 1 bar | 110 | 26 | 17 | 4 |
| ***Hostess*** | | | | | |
| Brownie Bites | 3 (1.3 oz) | 170 | 21 | 17 | 1 |
| Fudge | 1 (3 oz) | 330 | 54 | 11 | 1 |
| Light | 1 (1.4 oz) | 140 | 28 | 19 | 1 |
| ***Lance*** | | | | | |
| Fudge Nut | 1 (2.25 oz) | 340 | 56 | 26 | 2 |
| ***Little Debbie*** | | | | | |
| Brownie Lights | 1 (2 oz) | 190 | 39 | 27 | 1 |
| Brownie Loaves | 1 (2.1 oz) | 260 | 31 | 21 | 1 |
| Fudge | 1 pkg (2.1 oz) | 270 | 39 | 24 | tr |
| ***Tastykake*** | | | | | |
| Fudge Walnut | 1 (3 oz) | 370 | 52 | 37 | 1 |
| ***Tom's*** | | | | | |
| Fudge Nut | 1 pkg (2.5 oz) | 300 | 45 | 19 | 0 |

| FOOD | PORTION | CALS | CARB | SUGAR | FIBER |
|---|---|---|---|---|---|
| **REFRIGERATED** | | | | | |
| ***Toll House*** | | | | | |
| Brownie Dough | 1/12 pkg (1.5 oz) | 180 | 26 | 18 | 2 |
| **TAKE-OUT** | | | | | |
| plain | 1–2 in sq (2.1 oz) | 243 | 39 | – | – |
| **BRUSSELS SPROUTS** | | | | | |
| **FRESH** | | | | | |
| cooked | ½ cup | 30 | 7 | – | 3 |
| cooked | 1 sprout | 8 | 2 | – | – |
| **FROZEN** | | | | | |
| cooked | ½ cup | 33 | 6 | – | – |
| ***Birds Eye*** | | | | | |
| Brussels Sprouts | 11 sprouts | 35 | 7 | 2 | 3 |
| **BUCKWHEAT** | | | | | |
| groats roasted cooked | 1 cup (5.9 oz) | 647 | 34 | – | 5 |
| groats roasted uncooked | 1 cup (5.7 oz) | 567 | 123 | – | 17 |
| **BUFFALO** | | | | | |
| burger | 4 oz | 150 | 1 | 0 | 0 |
| water buffalo roasted | 3 oz | 111 | 0 | 0 | 0 |
| **BULGUR** | | | | | |
| cooked | 1 cup (6.3 oz) | 151 | 34 | – | 8 |
| uncooked | 1 cup (4.9 oz) | 479 | 106 | – | 26 |
| **BURBOT (FISH)** | | | | | |
| fresh baked | 3 oz | 98 | 0 | 0 | 0 |
| **BURDOCK ROOT** | | | | | |
| cooked | 1 cup | 110 | 26 | – | – |
| fresh | 1 cup | 85 | 20 | – | – |
| **BUTTER** | | | | | |
| clarified butter | 3½ oz | 876 | 0 | 0 | 0 |
| stick | 1 stick (4 oz) | 813 | tr | – | – |
| stick | 1 pat (5 g) | 36 | tr | – | – |
| whipped | 4 oz | 542 | tr | – | – |
| whipped | 1 pat (4 g) | 27 | tr | – | – |
| whipped | 1 tbsp | 70 | 0 | 0 | 0 |

| FOOD | PORTION | CALS | CARB | SUGAR | FIBER |
|---|---|---|---|---|---|
| ***Breakstone's*** | | | | | |
| Salted | 1 tbsp (0.5 oz) | 100 | 0 | 0 | 0 |
| ***Cabot*** | | | | | |
| Butter | 1 tbsp | 100 | 0 | 0 | 0 |
| ***Corman*** | | | | | |
| Light | 1 tbsp | 55 | 0 | 0 | 0 |
| ***Hotel Bar*** | | | | | |
| Stick | 1 tbsp (0.5 oz) | 100 | 0 | – | – |
| ***Keller's*** | | | | | |
| European | 1 tbsp (0.5 oz) | 100 | 0 | 0 | 0 |
| ***Land O Lakes*** | | | | | |
| Salted | 1 tbsp (0.5 oz) | 100 | 0 | – | – |
| Ultra Creamy Salted | 1 tbsp (0.5 oz) | 110 | 0 | – | – |
| ***Organic Valley*** | | | | | |
| Butter | 1 tbsp (0.5 oz) | 100 | 0 | 0 | 0 |
| Unsalted | 1 tbsp (0.5 oz) | 110 | 0 | 0 | 0 |
| **BUTTER BEANS** | | | | | |
| **CANNED** | | | | | |
| ***Van Camp*** | | | | | |
| Butter Beans | ½ cup (4.6 oz) | 110 | 22 | 0 | 7 |
| **FROZEN** | | | | | |
| ***Birds Eye*** | | | | | |
| Speckled | ½ cup | 100 | 20 | 1 | 4 |
| **BUTTER SUBSTITUTES** | | | | | |
| stick | 1 stick | 811 | 1 | – | – |
| ***Keto*** | | | | | |
| Butta | 1 tsp | 43 | 0 | 0 | 0 |
| ***Molly McButter*** | | | | | |
| Natural Butter | 1 tsp | 5 | 1 | – | – |
| Natural Cheese | 1 tsp | 5 | 1 | – | – |
| Roasted Garlic | 1 tsp | 5 | 1 | – | – |
| ***Olivio*** | | | | | |
| Spread | 1 tbsp | 80 | 0 | 0 | 0 |
| **BUTTERBUR** | | | | | |
| canned fuki chopped | 1 cup | 3 | tr | – | – |
| fresh fuki | 1 cup | 13 | 3 | – | – |

| FOOD | PORTION | CALS | CARB | SUGAR | FIBER |
|---|---|---|---|---|---|
| **BUTTERFISH** | | | | | |
| baked | 3 oz | 159 | 0 | 0 | 0 |
| fillet baked | 1 oz | 47 | 0 | 0 | 0 |
| **BUTTERNUTS** | | | | | |
| dried | 1 oz | 174 | 3 | – | – |
| **BUTTERSCOTCH** *(see also* CANDY*)* | | | | | |
| ***Hershey*** | | | | | |
| Chips | 1 tbsp (0.5 oz) | 80 | 10 | – | – |
| ***Nestle*** | | | | | |
| Morsels | 1 tbsp | 80 | 9 | 9 | 0 |
| **CABBAGE** *(see also* COLESLAW*)* | | | | | |
| chinese bok choy shredded cooked | ½ cup | 10 | 2 | – | – |
| chinese pak-choi raw shredded | ½ cup | 5 | 1 | – | – |
| chinese pe-tsai raw shredded | 1 cup | 12 | 2 | – | – |
| chinese pe-tsai shredded cooked | 1 cup | 16 | 3 | – | – |
| danish raw | 1 head (2 lbs) | 228 | 49 | – | 18 |
| danish raw shredded | ½ cup (1.2 oz) | 9 | 2 | – | tr |
| danish shredded cooked | ½ cup (2.6 oz) | 17 | 3 | – | 1 |
| green raw | 1 head (2 lbs) | 228 | 49 | – | 18 |
| green raw shredded | ½ cup (1.2 oz) | 9 | 2 | – | tr |
| green shredded cooked | ½ cup (2.6 oz) | 17 | 3 | – | 1 |
| napa cooked | 1 cup (3.8 oz) | 13 | 2 | – | 0 |
| red raw shredded | ½ cup | 10 | 2 | – | 1 |
| red shredded cooked | ½ cup | 16 | 3 | – | – |
| savoy raw shredded | ½ cup | 10 | 2 | – | – |
| savoy shredded cooked | ½ cup | 18 | 4 | – | – |
| ***Greenwood*** | | | | | |
| Sweet & Sour Red | ½ cup | 100 | 24 | 14 | 0 |
| **TAKE-OUT** | | | | | |
| korean kimchee | ½ cup | 22 | 4 | – | 4 |
| stuffed cabbage | 1 (6 oz) | 373 | 18 | – | – |
| sweet & sour red cabbage | 4 oz | 61 | 8 | – | 3 |

| FOOD | PORTION | CALS | CARB | SUGAR | FIBER |
|---|---|---|---|---|---|
| **CACTUS** | | | | | |
| napoles fresh sliced | ½ cup (1.5 oz) | 7 | 1 | – | – |
| pricklypear fresh | 1 cup (5.3 oz) | 56 | 13 | – | 4 |
| **CAKE** *(see also* CAKE MIX*)* | | | | | |
| angelfood | 1 cake (11.9 oz) | 876 | 197 | – | 5 |
| battenburg cake | 1 slice (2 oz) | 204 | 28 | – | 1 |
| boston cream pie frzn | ⅙ cake (3.2 oz) | 232 | 40 | – | 1 |
| carrot w/ cream cheese icing home recipe | 1 cake 10 in diam | 6175 | 775 | – | – |
| cheesecake | 1 cake 9 in diam | 3350 | 317 | – | – |
| cheesecake | ⅙ cake (2.8 oz) | 256 | 20 | – | 2 |
| cherry fudge w/ chocolate frosting | ⅛ cake (2.5 oz) | 187 | 27 | – | – |
| coffeecake fruit | ⅛ cake (1.8 oz) | 156 | 26 | – | – |
| cream puff shell | 1 (2.3 oz) | 239 | 15 | – | – |
| crumpet | 1 (2.3 oz) | 131 | 31 | – | 2 |
| devil's food cupcake w/ chocolate frosting | 1 | 120 | 20 | – | – |
| devil's food w/ creme filling | 1 (1 oz) | 105 | 17 | – | – |
| eccles cake | 1 slice (2 oz) | 285 | 36 | – | 1 |
| eclair | 1 (1.4 oz) | 149 | 15 | – | tr |
| fruitcake | 1 piece (1.5 oz) | 139 | 27 | – | – |
| fruitcake dark home recipe | 1 cake 7½ in x 2¼ in | 5185 | 738 | – | – |
| jelly roll lemon filled | 1 slice (3 oz) | 210 | 48 | 29 | tr |
| madeira cake | 1 slice (1 oz) | 98 | 15 | – | 1 |
| pound | 1 cake 8½ x 3½ x 3 in | 1935 | 257 | – | – |
| pound | ⅒ cake (1 oz) | 117 | 15 | – | – |
| pound fat free | 1 cake (12 oz) | 961 | 208 | – | – |
| pound cake home recipe | 1 loaf 8½ in x 3½ in | 1935 | 265 | – | – |

| FOOD | PORTION | CALS | CARB | SUGAR | FIBER |
|---|---|---|---|---|---|
| sheet cake w/ white frosting home recipe | 1 cake 9 in sq | 4020 | 694 | – | – |
| sheet cake w/o frosting home recipe | 1 cake 9 in sq | 2830 | 434 | – | – |
| sheet cake w/o frosting home recipe | 1/9 cake | 315 | 48 | – | – |
| sour cream pound | 1/10 cake (1 oz) | 117 | 16 | – | tr |
| sponge | 1/12 cake (1.3 oz) | 110 | 23 | – | – |
| sponge cake dessert shell | 1 (0.8 oz) | 70 | 12 | 7 | 0 |
| sponge w/ creme filling | 1 (1.5 oz) | 155 | 27 | – | – |
| tiramisu | 1 cake (4.4 lbs) | 5732 | 439 | 234 | 3 |
| toaster pastry apple | 1 (1¾ oz) | 204 | 37 | – | – |
| toaster pastry blueberry | 1 (1¾ oz) | 204 | 37 | – | – |
| toaster pastry brown sugar cinnamon | 1 (1¾ oz) | 206 | 34 | – | – |
| toaster pastry cherry | 1 (1¾ oz) | 204 | 37 | – | – |
| toaster pastry strawberry | 1 (1¾ oz) | 204 | 37 | – | – |
| treacle tart | 1 slice (2.5 oz) | 258 | 42 | – | 1 |
| vanilla slice | 1 slice (2½ oz) | 248 | 30 | – | 1 |
| white w/ white frosting | 1/16 cake | 260 | 42 | – | – |
| white w/ white frosting | 1 cake 9 in diam | 4170 | 670 | – | – |
| yellow w/ chocolate frosting | 1/8 cake (2.2 oz) | 242 | 36 | – | 1 |
| yellow w/ chocolate frosting | 1 cake 9 diam | 3895 | 620 | – | – |
| ***Amy's*** | | | | | |
| Toaster Pops Apple | 1 | 140 | 26 | 6 | tr |
| Toaster Pops Strawberry | 1 | 140 | 26 | 6 | tr |
| ***Baby Watson*** | | | | | |
| Cheesecake | 1 slice (3 oz) | 260 | 19 | 15 | tr |
| ***Dolly Madison*** | | | | | |
| Angel Food | 1 slice (2.1 oz) | 160 | 34 | 30 | 1 |
| Apple Crumb | 1 (1.6 oz) | 160 | 28 | 19 | 0 |
| Banana Dream Flip | 1 (3.5 oz) | 390 | 59 | 26 | 1 |
| Bear Claw | 1 (2.75 oz) | 270 | 40 | 16 | 1 |
| Carrot | 1 (4 oz) | 360 | 67 | 46 | 1 |

| FOOD | PORTION | CALS | CARB | SUGAR | FIBER |
|---|---|---|---|---|---|
| Chocolate Snack Squares | 1 (1.6 oz) | 210 | 28 | 22 | 0 |
| Cinnamon Buttercrumb | 1 (1.6 oz) | 170 | 28 | 20 | 0 |
| Cinnamon Buttercrumb Low Fat | 1 (1.5 oz) | 140 | 29 | 24 | 0 |
| Cinnamon Stix | 1 (1.3 oz) | 170 | 21 | 14 | 0 |
| Creme Cakes | 2 (1.9 oz) | 210 | 32 | 21 | 0 |
| Cupcakes Chocolate | 1 (2 oz) | 210 | 35 | 20 | 1 |
| Cupcakes Spice | 1 (2 oz) | 230 | 33 | 25 | 0 |
| Dunkin' Stix | 1 (1.3 oz) | 170 | 20 | 14 | 0 |
| Frosty Angel | 1 (3.5 oz) | 330 | 65 | 50 | 1 |
| Holiday Cupcakes | 1 (1.9 oz) | 180 | 35 | 22 | 0 |
| Honey Bun | 1 (3.7 oz) | 440 | 49 | 22 | 1 |
| Koo Koos | 1 (1.8 oz) | 200 | 29 | 23 | 0 |
| Mini Coconut Loaf | 1 (3.5 oz) | 350 | 62 | 35 | 1 |
| Mini Pound Cake | 1 (3.2 oz) | 310 | 48 | 28 | 1 |
| Raspberry Square | 1 (1.8 oz) | 190 | 28 | 23 | 0 |
| Sweet Roll Apple | 1 (2.2 oz) | 200 | 33 | 16 | 0 |
| Sweet Roll Cherry | 1 (2.2 oz) | 210 | 34 | 19 | 1 |
| Sweet Roll Cinnamon | 1 (2.2 oz) | 230 | 36 | 15 | 1 |
| Texas Cinnamon Bun | 1 (4.2 oz) | 440 | 69 | 33 | 1 |
| Zingers Devil's Food | 2 (2.6 oz) | 270 | 46 | 26 | 1 |
| Zingers Lemon | 1 (1.4 oz) | 150 | 22 | 18 | 0 |
| Zingers Raspberry | 1 (1.4 oz) | 150 | 22 | 18 | 0 |
| Zingers Yellow | 2 (2.5 oz) | 280 | 50 | 29 | 1 |
| ***Drake's*** | | | | | |
| Coffee Cake Low Fat | 1 (1.1 oz) | 110 | 21 | 12 | 0 |
| Yodel's | 1 (1 oz) | 150 | 16 | – | – |
| ***Dutch Mill*** | | | | | |
| Dessert Shells Chocolate Covered | 1 (0.5 oz) | 80 | 8 | 6 | 0 |
| ***Entenmann's*** | | | | | |
| Apple Puffs | 1 (3 oz) | 270 | 37 | 20 | 1 |
| Coffee Cake Cheese Filled Crumb | 1 serv (1.9 oz) | 200 | 25 | 12 | tr |
| Coffee Cake Crumb | 1 serv (2 oz) | 250 | 33 | 13 | 1 |
| Cupcakes Light Chocolate Creme Filled | 1 (2 oz) | 160 | 39 | 33 | 1 |
| Hot Cross Buns | 1 (2.3 oz) | 230 | 37 | 20 | 2 |
| Stollen Fruit | ⅛ cake (2 oz) | 210 | 34 | 17 | 1 |
| Ultimate Crumb Cake | 1/10 cake | 250 | 32 | 15 | tr |

| FOOD | PORTION | CALS | CARB | SUGAR | FIBER |
|---|---|---|---|---|---|
| ***Fillo Factory*** | | | | | |
| Apple Turnovers Vegan | 5 (5 oz) | 270 | 53 | 4 | 2 |
| ***Goody Man*** | | | | | |
| Happy Birthday Cupcake Chocolate | 1 (1.75 oz) | 200 | 34 | 24 | tr |
| Happy Birthday Cupcake White | 1 (1.75 oz) | 190 | 36 | 26 | 0 |
| ***Greenfield*** | | | | | |
| Blondie Fat Free Chocolate Chip | 1 (1.3 oz) | 110 | 27 | 19 | 0 |
| ***Hostess*** | | | | | |
| Angel Food | ⅛ cake (2 oz) | 160 | 33 | 29 | 1 |
| Chocodiles | 1 (1.6 oz) | 240 | 33 | 22 | 1 |
| Chocolicious | 1 (1.6 oz) | 190 | 30 | 19 | 1 |
| Coffee Crumb | 1 (1.1 oz) | 130 | 19 | 10 | 0 |
| Crumb Cake Light | 1 (1 oz) | 100 | 18 | 11 | 0 |
| Cupcakes Chocolate | 1 (1.8 oz) | 180 | 30 | 17 | 1 |
| Cupcakes Orange | 1 (1.5 oz) | 160 | 27 | 20 | 0 |
| Cupcakes Light Chocolate | 1 (1.6 oz) | 140 | 29 | 19 | 1 |
| Ding Dongs | 2 (2.7 oz) | 360 | 44 | 32 | 2 |
| Ho Ho's | 2 (2 oz) | 250 | 34 | 23 | 1 |
| Honey Bun Glazed | 1 (2.7 oz) | 320 | 34 | 25 | 1 |
| Honey Bun Iced | 1 (3.4 oz) | 410 | 42 | 31 | 1 |
| Shortcake Dessert Cups | 1 (1 oz) | 100 | 17 | 10 | 0 |
| Sno Balls | 1 (1.8 oz) | 180 | 31 | 19 | 1 |
| Suzy Q's | 1 (2 oz) | 230 | 35 | 22 | 1 |
| Sweet Roll Cherry | 1 (2.2 oz) | 210 | 34 | 19 | 1 |
| Sweet Roll Cinnamon | 1 (2.2 oz) | 230 | 36 | 15 | 1 |
| Twinkies | 1 (1.5 oz) | 150 | 25 | 14 | 0 |
| Twinkies Light | 1 (1.5 oz) | 130 | 27 | 16 | 0 |
| ***Jell-O*** | | | | | |
| Dessert Delights Cheesecake | 1 bar (1.4 oz) | 160 | 20 | 13 | tr |
| Dessert Delights Chocolate Fudge Pudding | 1 bar (1.4 oz) | 150 | 23 | 15 | 1 |
| ***Lance*** | | | | | |
| Dunking Sticks | 1 (2.75 oz) | 180 | 22 | 15 | tr |
| Fig Cake | ½ piece (2.1 oz) | 110 | 21 | 14 | 1 |

| FOOD | PORTION | CALS | CARB | SUGAR | FIBER |
|---|---|---|---|---|---|
| Fig Cake Fat Free | ½ piece (2.1 oz) | 100 | 22 | 13 | 1 |
| Honey Bun | 1 (3 oz) | 330 | 47 | 13 | 4 |
| Pecan Twirls | 1 pkg (2 oz) | 220 | 32 | 17 | 1 |
| Swiss Rolls | 1 (2.5 oz) | 170 | 23 | 13 | tr |
| ***Little Debbie*** | | | | | |
| Angel Cakes Lemon | 1 (1.6 oz) | 130 | 29 | 22 | 0 |
| Angel Cakes Raspberry | 1 (1.6 oz) | 130 | 29 | 23 | 0 |
| Banana Nut Loaves | 1 (1.9 oz) | 220 | 31 | 19 | tr |
| Banana Twins | 1 (2.2 oz) | 250 | 39 | 29 | 0 |
| Be My Valentine Chocolate | 1 (2.2 oz) | 280 | 38 | 25 | 1 |
| Be My Valentine Vanilla | 1 (2.2 oz) | 290 | 38 | 26 | 0 |
| Blueberry Loaves | 1 (2 oz) | 220 | 29 | 16 | tr |
| Chocolate Chip | 1 (2.4 oz) | 310 | 41 | 32 | tr |
| Christmas Tree Cake | 1 pkg (1.5 oz) | 190 | 26 | 19 | 0 |
| Coconut Creme | 1 (1.7 oz) | 210 | 30 | 24 | 0 |
| Coffee Cake Apple | 1 (2.1 oz) | 230 | 39 | 23 | 0 |
| Cupcake Creme Filled Chocolate | 1 (1.6 oz) | 180 | 26 | 18 | tr |
| Cupcake Creme Filled Orange | 1 (1.7 oz) | 210 | 29 | 22 | 0 |
| Cupcake Creme Filled Strawberry | 1 (1.7 oz) | 210 | 29 | 22 | tr |
| Devil Cremes | 1 (1.6 oz) | 190 | 29 | 20 | 0 |
| Devil Squares | 1 (2.2 oz) | 270 | 39 | 31 | 1 |
| Easter Basket Cake Chocolate | 1 (2.4 oz) | 300 | 40 | 29 | tr |
| Easter Basket Cake Vanilla | 1 (2.5 oz) | 320 | 43 | 32 | 0 |
| Fall Party Cake Chocolate | 1 (2.4 oz) | 290 | 42 | 29 | tr |
| Fall Party Cake Vanilla | 1 (2.5 oz) | 310 | 44 | 31 | 0 |
| Fancy Cakes | 1 (2.4 oz) | 300 | 42 | 33 | 0 |
| Frosted Fudge | 1 (1.5 oz) | 200 | 25 | 18 | tr |
| Golden Cremes | 1 (1.5 oz) | 150 | 26 | 18 | 0 |
| Holiday Cake Roll Cherry Creme | 1 (2.1 oz) | 260 | 37 | 24 | tr |
| Holiday Snack Cake Chocolate | 1 (2.4 oz) | 300 | 41 | 29 | 1 |
| Holiday Snack Cake Vanilla | 1 (2.5 oz) | 320 | 41 | 29 | 0 |
| Honey Bun | 1 (1.8 oz) | 220 | 24 | 13 | tr |
| Pecan Spinwheels | 1 (1 oz) | 110 | 16 | 7 | 0 |
| Snack Cake Chocolate | 1 (2.5 oz) | 310 | 44 | 30 | 1 |
| Strawberry Shortcake Roll | 1 (2.1 oz) | 230 | 41 | 29 | 0 |

| FOOD | PORTION | CALS | CARB | SUGAR | FIBER |
|---|---|---|---|---|---|
| Swiss Rolls | 1 (2.1 oz) | 270 | 38 | 25 | 1 |
| Zebra Cakes | 1 (2.6 oz) | 330 | 45 | 33 | 0 |
| ***Marie Callender's*** | | | | | |
| Cobbler Apple | 1 serv (4.25 oz) | 370 | 45 | 31 | 2 |
| Cobbler Berry | 1 serv (4.25 oz) | 370 | 41 | 29 | 1 |
| Cobbler Cherry | 1 serv (4.25 oz) | 380 | 50 | 32 | 0 |
| Cobbler Peach | 1 serv (4.25 oz) | 380 | 47 | 24 | 0 |
| ***Natural Touch*** | | | | | |
| Toaster Square Blueberry | 1 (2.8 oz) | 180 | 33 | 12 | 6 |
| Toaster Squares Date Walnut | 1 (2.8 oz) | 200 | 36 | 9 | 8 |
| ***Pepperidge Farm*** | | | | | |
| Apple Turnover | 1 (3.1 oz) | 330 | 48 | 5 | 6 |
| Blueberry Turnovers | 1 (3.1 oz) | 340 | 45 | 5 | 6 |
| Cherry Turnover | 1 (3.1 oz) | 320 | 46 | 6 | 6 |
| Large Layer Chocolate Fudge | ⅛ cake (2.4 oz) | 260 | 31 | 20 | 1 |
| Large Layer Coconut | ⅛ cake (2.4 oz) | 260 | 35 | 24 | 0 |
| Large Layer Vanilla | ⅛ cake (2.4 oz) | 250 | 35 | 25 | 0 |
| Mini Turnover Apple | 1 (1.4 oz) | 140 | 15 | 10 | 1 |
| Mini Turnover Cherry | 1 (1.4 oz) | 140 | 16 | 7 | 1 |
| Mini Turnover Strawberry | 1 (1.4 oz) | 140 | 18 | 10 | 0 |
| Peach Turnover | 1 (3.1 oz) | 340 | 47 | 5 | 6 |
| Raspberry Turnovers | 1 (3.1 oz) | 330 | 47 | 6 | 6 |
| ***Philadelphia*** | | | | | |
| Snack Bars Classic Cheesecake | 1 (1.5 oz) | 200 | 17 | 12 | 0 |
| ***Pillsbury*** | | | | | |
| Apple Turnovers | 1 (2 oz) | 170 | 23 | 11 | tr |
| Cherry Turnovers | 1 (2 oz) | 180 | 24 | 12 | 0 |
| ***Sara Lee*** | | | | | |
| Cheesecake 25% Reduced Fat | ¼ cake (4.2 oz) | 310 | 40 | 28 | 2 |
| Cheesecake Cherry Cream | ¼ cake (4.7 oz) | 350 | 55 | 35 | 2 |

| FOOD | PORTION | CALS | CARB | SUGAR | FIBER |
|---|---|---|---|---|---|
| Cheesecake Chocolate Chip | ¼ cake (4.2 oz) | 410 | 47 | 43 | 2 |
| Cheesecake French | ⅙ cake (3.9 oz) | 350 | 24 | 22 | 1 |
| Cheesecake French Strawberry | ⅙ cake (4.3 oz) | 320 | 43 | 26 | 1 |
| Cheesecake Strawberry Cream | ¼ cake (4.7 oz) | 330 | 49 | 36 | 2 |
| Coffee Cake Butter Streusel | ⅙ cake (1.9 oz) | 220 | 25 | 11 | 1 |
| Coffee Cake Crumb | ⅛ cake (2 oz) | 220 | 32 | 17 | 1 |
| Coffee Cake Pecan | ⅙ cake (1.9 oz) | 230 | 24 | 9 | 1 |
| Coffee Cake Raspberry | ⅙ cake (1.9 oz) | 220 | 27 | 13 | 1 |
| Coffee Cake Reduced Fat Cheese | ⅙ cake (1.9 oz) | 180 | 28 | 11 | 0 |
| Layer Cake Coconut | ⅛ cake (2.8 oz) | 260 | 33 | 25 | 1 |
| Layer Cake Double Chocolate | ⅛ cake (2.8 oz) | 260 | 33 | 24 | 2 |
| Layer Cake Fudge Golden | ⅛ cake (2.8 oz) | 260 | 34 | 23 | 1 |
| Layer Cake German Chocolate | ⅛ cake (2.9 oz) | 280 | 35 | 26 | 1 |
| Layer Cake Vanilla | ⅛ cake (2.8 oz) | 260 | 32 | 22 | 0 |
| Original Cheesecake | ¼ cake (4.2 oz) | 350 | 39 | 30 | 1 |
| Pound Cake All Butter | ¼ cake (2.7 oz) | 320 | 38 | 21 | 1 |
| Pound Cake Chocolate Swirl | ¼ cake (2.9 oz) | 330 | 42 | 31 | tr |
| Pound Cake Family Size | ⅙ cake (2.7 oz) | 310 | 36 | 15 | 1 |
| Pound Cake Reduced Fat | ¼ cake (2.7 oz) | 280 | 42 | 26 | tr |
| Pound Cake Strawberry Swirl | ¼ cake (2.9 oz) | 290 | 44 | 25 | tr |

| FOOD | PORTION | CALS | CARB | SUGAR | FIBER |
|---|---|---|---|---|---|
| Strawberry Shortcake | ⅛ cake (2.5 oz) | 180 | 27 | 15 | 1 |
| ***Snack & Smile*** | | | | | |
| Mini Loaf Apple Cinnamon | 1 loaf (2 oz) | 190 | 29 | 16 | 0 |
| Mini Loaf Banana | 1 loaf (2 oz) | 200 | 30 | 17 | 0 |
| Mini Loaf Blueberry | 1 loaf (2 oz) | 190 | 29 | 16 | tr |
| Mini Loaf Carrot | 1 loaf (2 oz) | 200 | 30 | 16 | 0 |
| ***SnackWell's*** | | | | | |
| Streusal Squares Apple Cinnamon | 1 (1.5 oz) | 150 | 31 | 17 | tr |
| Streusal Squares Cherry | 1 (1.5 oz) | 150 | 31 | 16 | tr |
| ***Super*** | | | | | |
| Bun | 1 (2.5 oz) | 270 | 24 | 9 | tr |
| ***Tastykake*** | | | | | |
| Banana Creamie | 1 (1.5 oz) | 170 | 25 | 18 | 0 |
| Bear Claw Apple | 1 (3 oz) | 280 | 50 | 24 | 0 |
| Bear Claw Cinnamon | 1 (3 oz) | 300 | 53 | 27 | tr |
| Big Texas | 1 (3 oz) | 300 | 51 | 21 | tr |
| Breakfast Bun Chocolate Raisin | 1 (3.2 oz) | 330 | 59 | 32 | 1 |
| Bunny Trail Treats | 1 (1.3 oz) | 150 | 25 | 16 | 0 |
| Chocolate Creamie | 1 (1.5 oz) | 180 | 25 | 17 | 0 |
| Chocolate Krimpies | 2 (2.2 oz) | 240 | 38 | 24 | 1 |
| Coffee Roll Glazed | 1 (3 oz) | 300 | 51 | 22 | tr |
| Coffee Roll Vanilla | 1 (3.2 oz) | 320 | 56 | 27 | tr |
| Cupcakes | 2 (2.1 oz) | 200 | 37 | 22 | 1 |
| Cupcakes Butter Cream Cream Filled Iced | 2 (2.2 oz) | 240 | 40 | 26 | 1 |
| Cupcakes Chocolate Cream Filled Iced | 2 (2.2 oz) | 230 | 39 | 25 | 1 |
| Cupcakes Low Fat Vanilla Cream Filled | 2 (2.2 oz) | 190 | 42 | 28 | 0 |
| Cupid Kake | 1 (1.3 oz) | 150 | 25 | 16 | 0 |
| Honey Bun Glazed | 1 (3.2 oz) | 350 | 47 | 22 | 0 |
| Honey Bun Iced | 1 (3.2 oz) | 350 | 47 | 22 | 0 |
| Junior Chocolate | 1 (3.3 oz) | 330 | 54 | 34 | 1 |
| Junior Coconut | 1 (3.3 oz) | 310 | 54 | 35 | 0 |
| Junior Koffee Kake | 1 (2.5 oz) | 270 | 42 | 22 | 1 |
| Junior Pound Kake | 1 (3 oz) | 320 | 45 | 28 | 1 |
| Kandy Kakes Chocolate | 3 (2 oz) | 250 | 35 | 24 | 2 |
| Kandy Kakes Coconut | 2 (2.7 oz) | 330 | 43 | 30 | 2 |

| FOOD | PORTION | CALS | CARB | SUGAR | FIBER |
|---|---|---|---|---|---|
| Kandy Kakes Peanut Butter | 2 (1.3 oz) | 190 | 21 | 14 | 1 |
| Koffee Kake Cream Filled | 2 (2 oz) | 240 | 35 | 20 | 0 |
| Koffee Kake Low Fat Apple | 2 (2 oz) | 170 | 34 | 20 | 1 |
| Koffee Kake Low Fat Lemon | 2 (2 oz) | 180 | 36 | 21 | 0 |
| Koffee Kake Low Fat Raspberry | 2 (2 oz) | 170 | 36 | 16 | 1 |
| Koffee Kakes | 1 (2 oz) | 210 | 34 | 18 | tr |
| Kreepy Kakes | 2 (2.2 oz) | 240 | 38 | 27 | 0 |
| Kreme Krimpies | 2 (2 oz) | 230 | 34 | 21 | 0 |
| Krimpets Butterscotch Iced | 2 (2 oz) | 210 | 38 | 24 | 0 |
| Krimpets Jelly Fillled | 2 (2 oz) | 190 | 38 | 23 | 1 |
| Krimpets Strawberry | 2 (2 oz) | 210 | 37 | 22 | 0 |
| Kringle Kake | 1 (1.3 oz) | 150 | 25 | 16 | 0 |
| Santa Snacks | 2 (2.2 oz) | 240 | 38 | 27 | 0 |
| Sparkle Kake | 1 (1.3 oz) | 150 | 25 | 16 | 0 |
| Tasty Tweets | 2 (2.2 oz) | 240 | 38 | 27 | 0 |
| Tropical Delight Coconut | 2 (2 oz) | 190 | 26 | 16 | 0 |
| Tropical Delight Guava | 2 (2 oz) | 190 | 30 | 20 | 0 |
| Tropical Delight Papaya | 2 (2 oz) | 200 | 32 | 22 | 0 |
| Tropical Delight Pineapple | 2 (2 oz) | 200 | 32 | 22 | 0 |
| Vanilla Creamie | 1 (1.5 oz) | 190 | 25 | 18 | 0 |
| Witchy Treat | 1 (1.3 oz) | 150 | 24 | 15 | 0 |
| ***Tom's*** | | | | | |
| Honey Bun | 1 pkg (3 oz) | 360 | 41 | 15 | 2 |
| Honey Bun Jelly Filled | 1 pkg (4 oz) | 490 | 52 | 20 | 2 |
| Marble Pound | 1 pkg (2.5 oz) | 300 | 35 | 24 | 1 |
| Texas Cinnamon Roll | 1 pkg (4 oz) | 360 | 71 | 56 | 0 |
| ***Weight Watchers*** | | | | | |
| Chocolate Raspberry Royale | 1 (3.5 oz) | 190 | 38 | 22 | 2 |
| Chocolate Eclair | 1 (2.1 oz) | 150 | 25 | 13 | 1 |
| Danish Coffee Cake Apple Cinnamon | 1 piece (1.9 oz) | 160 | 30 | 13 | 1 |
| Danish Coffee Cake Cheese | 1 piece (1.9 oz) | 160 | 29 | 11 | 1 |
| Danish Coffee Cake Raspberry | 1 piece (1.9 oz) | 160 | 30 | 13 | 1 |
| Double Fudge | 1 piece (2.75 oz) | 190 | 36 | 19 | 2 |
| French Style Cheesecake | 1 piece (3.9 oz) | 170 | 28 | 19 | 2 |

| FOOD | PORTION | CALS | CARB | SUGAR | FIBER |
|---|---|---|---|---|---|
| New York Style Cheesecake | 1 piece (2.5 oz) | 150 | 21 | 18 | 1 |
| Strawberry Parfait Royale | 1 (5.24 oz) | 180 | 35 | 22 | 0 |
| Triple Chocolate Eclair | 1 (2.14 oz) | 160 | 25 | 13 | 1 |
| **TAKE-OUT** | | | | | |
| angelfood | 1/12 cake (1 oz) | 73 | 16 | – | 1 |
| apple crisp | ½ cup (5 oz) | 230 | 46 | – | – |
| baklava | 1 oz | 126 | 10 | – | 1 |
| boston cream pie | 1/6 cake (3.3 oz) | 293 | 43 | – | 1 |
| cannoli w/ cannoli cream | 1 | 369 | 42 | 28 | – |
| carrot w/ cream cheese icing | 1/12 cake (3.9 oz) | 484 | 52 | – | – |
| cheesecake w/ cherry topping | 1/12 cake (5 oz) | 359 | 33 | – | – |
| chocolate w/ chocolate frosting | 1/8 cake (2.2 oz) | 235 | 35 | – | 2 |
| coffeecake cheese | 1/6 cake (2.7 oz) | 258 | 38 | – | 1 |
| coffeecake crumb topped cheese | 1/6 cake (2.7 oz) | 258 | 38 | – | 1 |
| coffeecake crumb topped cinnamon | 1/9 cake (2.2 oz) | 263 | 29 | – | 2 |
| cream puff w/ custard filling | 1 (4.6 oz) | 336 | 30 | – | – |
| dutch honey cake | 1 slice (0.8 oz) | 70 | 17 | 8 | 0 |
| french apple tart | 1 (3.5 oz) | 302 | 37 | 15 | 2 |
| fruitcake | 1/36 cake (2.9 oz) | 302 | 54 | – | 3 |
| gingerbread | 1/9 cake (2.6 oz) | 264 | 36 | – | 2 |
| panettone | 1/12 cake (2.9 oz) | 300 | 43 | 21 | 2 |
| petit fours | 2 (0.9 oz) | 120 | 15 | 12 | 0 |
| pineapple upside down | 1/9 cake (4 oz) | 367 | 58 | – | – |
| pound fat free | 1 oz | 80 | 17 | – | – |
| pound cake | 1 slice (1 oz) | 120 | 15 | – | – |
| sacher torte | 1 slice (2.2 oz) | 240 | 30 | 11 | 4 |
| sheet cake w/ white frosting | 1/9 cake | 445 | 77 | – | – |

| FOOD | PORTION | CALS | CARB | SUGAR | FIBER |
|---|---|---|---|---|---|
| strudel apple | 1 piece (2½ oz) | 195 | 29 | – | 2 |
| tiramisu | 1 piece (5.1 oz) | 409 | 31 | 17 | tr |
| trifle w/ cream | 6 oz | 291 | 34 | – | 1 |
| yellow w/ vanilla frosting | ⅛ cake (2.2 oz) | 239 | 38 | – | – |
| **CAKE ICING** | | | | | |
| chocolate ready-to-use | 1/12 pkg (1.3 oz) | 151 | 24 | 21 | – |
| glaze home recipe | 1/12 recipe (1 oz) | 97 | 20 | – | – |
| vanilla ready-to-use | 1/12 pkg (1.3 oz) | 159 | 26 | 26 | – |
| ***Betty Crocker*** | | | | | |
| HomeStyle Mix Coconut Pecan as prep | 2 tbsp | 160 | 21 | 17 | tr |
| HomeStyle Mix White Fluffy as prep | 6 tbsp | 100 | 24 | 23 | – |
| Party Frosting Chocolate w/ Stars | 2 tbsp (1.2 oz) | 140 | 22 | 20 | – |
| Rich & Creamy Butter Cream | 2 tbsp (1.3 oz) | 140 | 23 | 20 | – |
| Rich & Creamy Cherry | 2 tbsp (1.2 oz) | 140 | 23 | 20 | – |
| Rich & Creamy Chocolate | 2 tbsp (1.2 oz) | 130 | 21 | 17 | – |
| Rich & Creamy Cream Cheese | 2 tbsp (1.2 oz) | 140 | 23 | 20 | – |
| Rich & Creamy Dark Chocolate | 2 tbsp (1.3 oz) | 130 | 23 | 16 | 1 |
| Rich & Creamy French Vanilla | 2 tbsp (1.2 oz) | 140 | 23 | 20 | – |
| Rich & Creamy Milk Chocolate | 2 tbsp (1.3 oz) | 130 | 21 | 18 | – |
| Rich & Creamy Rainbow Chip | 2 tbsp (1.2 oz) | 140 | 23 | 20 | – |
| Rich & Creamy Vanilla | 2 tbsp (1.2 oz) | 140 | 23 | 20 | – |

| FOOD | PORTION | CALS | CARB | SUGAR | FIBER |
|---|---|---|---|---|---|
| Toppers Milk Chocolate | 2 tbsp (1.2 oz) | 130 | 22 | 18 | – |
| Toppers Vanilla | 2 tbsp (1.2 oz) | 140 | 24 | 20 | – |
| ***Estee*** | | | | | |
| Frosting as prep | 1/5 pkg | 100 | 20 | 0 | 0 |
| ***Sweet Rewards*** | | | | | |
| Ready-To-Spread Reduced Fat Chocolate | 2 tbsp (1.2 oz) | 120 | 24 | 22 | – |
| Ready-To-Spread Reduced Fat Vanilla | 2 tbsp (1.2 oz) | 130 | 27 | 25 | – |
| **CAKE MIX** | | | | | |
| angelfood | 1/12 cake (1.8 oz) | 129 | 29 | – | 1 |
| angelfood | 10 in cake (20.9 oz) | 1535 | 350 | – | 9 |
| carrot w/o frosting | 1/12 cake (2.5 oz) | 239 | 33 | – | – |
| carrot w/o frosting | 2 layers (29.6 oz) | 2886 | 395 | – | – |
| chocolate pudding type w/o frosting | 2 layers (32.4 oz) | 3234 | 409 | – | – |
| chocolate pudding type w/o frosting | 1/12 cake (2.7 oz) | 270 | 34 | – | – |
| chocolate w/o frosting | 1/12 cake (2.3 oz) | 198 | 32 | – | – |
| chocolate w/o frosting | 2 layers (26.8 oz) | 2393 | 384 | – | – |
| coffeecake crumb topped cinnamon | 1/8 cake (2 oz) | 178 | 30 | – | 2 |
| devil's food w/o frosting | 1/12 cake (2.3 oz) | 198 | 32 | – | – |
| devil's food w/ chocolate frosting | 1 cake 9 in diam | 3755 | 645 | – | – |
| devil's food w/ chocolate frosting | 1/16 cake | 235 | 40 | – | – |
| fudge w/o frosting | 1/12 cake (2.3 oz) | 198 | 32 | – | – |
| gingerbread | 1 cake 8 in sq | 1575 | 291 | – | – |

| FOOD | PORTION | CALS | CARB | SUGAR | FIBER |
|---|---|---|---|---|---|
| gingerbread | 1/9 cake (2.4 oz) | 207 | 34 | – | 2 |
| white w/o frosting | 1/12 cake (2.2 oz) | 190 | 34 | – | – |
| white w/o frosting | 2 layer cake (26 oz) | 2265 | 410 | – | – |
| yellow w/ chocolate frosting | 1/16 cake | 235 | 40 | – | – |
| yellow w/o frosting | 1/12 cake (2.2 oz) | 202 | 34 | – | – |
| yellow w/o frosting | 2 layers (26.5 oz) | 2415 | 411 | – | – |
| yellow w/ chocolate frosting | 1 cake 9 in diam | 3895 | 620 | – | – |
| ***Betty Crocker*** | | | | | |
| Angel Food Fat Free | 1/12 cake | 140 | 32 | 24 | – |
| Angel Food Fat Free Confetti as prep | 1/12 cake | 150 | 34 | 24 | – |
| Cheesecake Chocolate Chip as prep | 1/8 cake | 410 | 32 | 23 | 1 |
| Cheesecake Original as prep | 1/8 cake | 400 | 30 | 20 | – |
| Cheesecake Strawberry Swirl as prep | 1/8 cake | 380 | 32 | 21 | – |
| Pineapple Upside Down as prep | 1/6 cake | 420 | 64 | 43 | – |
| Quick Bread Banana | 1/12 cake | 170 | 25 | 13 | – |
| Quick Bread Cinnamon Streusel as prep | 1/14 cake | 180 | 26 | 15 | – |
| Quick Bread Cranberry Orange as prep | 1/12 cake | 170 | 29 | 16 | – |
| Quick Bread Lemon Poppy Seed as prep | 1/12 cake | 170 | 25 | 12 | – |
| Stir'n Bake Carrot Cake w/ Cream Cheese Frosting as prep | 1/6 cake | 260 | 46 | 32 | – |
| Stir'n Bake Coffee Cake w/ Cinnamon Streusel as prep | 1/6 cake | 230 | 36 | 20 | – |
| Stir'n Bake Devils Food w/ Chocolate Frosting as prep | 1/6 cake | 240 | 42 | 27 | 1 |
| Stir'n Bake Yellow w/ Chocolate Frosting as prep | 1/8 cake | 240 | 43 | 26 | 1 |

| FOOD | PORTION | CALS | CARB | SUGAR | FIBER |
|---|---|---|---|---|---|
| SuperMoist Butter Pecan as prep | 1/12 cake | 240 | 35 | 20 | – |
| SuperMoist Butter Yellow as prep | 1/12 cake | 260 | 36 | 20 | – |
| SuperMoist Carrot as prep | 1/10 cake | 320 | 42 | 24 | – |
| SuperMoist Cherry Chip | 1/10 cake | 300 | 41 | 23 | – |
| SuperMoist Chocolate Fudge as prep | 1/12 cake | 270 | 35 | 21 | 1 |
| SuperMoist Golden Vanilla as prep | 1/12 cake | 240 | 35 | 20 | – |
| SuperMoist Lemon as prep | 1/12 cake | 240 | 35 | 20 | – |
| SuperMoist Milk Chocolate as prep | 1/12 cake | 240 | 34 | 20 | 1 |
| SuperMoist Pineapple as prep | 1/12 cake | 250 | 25 | 20 | – |
| SuperMoist Spice as prep | 1/12 cake | 240 | 36 | 20 | – |
| SuperMoist Strawberry as prep | 1/12 cake | 250 | 35 | 21 | – |
| SuperMoist White as prep | 1/12 cake | 230 | 34 | 18 | – |
| SuperMoist White Light as prep | 1/10 cake | 210 | 43 | 24 | – |
| ***Bisquick*** | | | | | |
| Mix | 1/3 cup (1.4 oz) | 160 | 25 | 1 | – |
| Reduced Fat | 1/3 cup (1.4 oz) | 140 | 27 | 3 | tr |
| ***Carbolite*** | | | | | |
| Cheesecake Chocolate as prep | 1/8 cake | 260 | 2 | – | – |
| ***Carbsense*** | | | | | |
| Zero Carb Baking Mix | 1 oz | 110 | 4 | 0 | 4 |
| ***Dromedary*** | | | | | |
| Date Bread | 1/11 cake (2 oz) | 190 | 29 | 16 | 1 |
| Date Nut Roll | 1/2 in slice | 80 | 13 | – | – |
| Gingerbread | 1 piece (2 in x 2 in) | 100 | 19 | – | – |
| Pound | 1/2 in slice | 150 | 21 | – | – |
| ***Estee*** | | | | | |
| Chocolate as prep | 1/5 cake | 190 | 36 | 25 | 1 |
| White as prep | 1/5 cake | 200 | 38 | 24 | tr |

| FOOD | PORTION | CALS | CARB | SUGAR | FIBER |
|---|---|---|---|---|---|
| ***Hodgson Mill*** | | | | | |
| Gingerbread Whole Wheat | ¼ cup (1 oz) | 110 | 24 | 10 | 2 |
| ***MiniCarb*** | | | | | |
| Carrot as prep | 1 slice | 280 | 10 | 0 | 6 |
| Chocolate as prep | 1 slice | 230 | 16 | 0 | 12 |
| Zero Carb Baking Mix not prep | ½ cup | 55 | 2 | 2 | 2 |
| ***Sweet Rewards*** | | | | | |
| Reduced Fat White as prep | 1/12 cake | 180 | 36 | 20 | – |
| Reduced Fat Yellow as prep | 1/12 cake | 200 | 37 | 21 | – |
| **CALABAZA** | | | | | |
| fresh | ½ cup | 32 | 8 | – | – |
| **CALZONE** | | | | | |
| **TAKE-OUT** | | | | | |
| cheese | 1 (12 oz) | 1020 | 86 | 26 | 8 |
| **CANADIAN BACON** | | | | | |
| grilled | 1 pkg (6 oz) | 257 | 2 | – | 0 |
| ***Boar's Head*** | | | | | |
| Canadian Bacon | 2 oz | 70 | 1 | 1 | 0 |
| ***Hormel*** | | | | | |
| Sandwich Style | 3 slices (2 oz) | 70 | 0 | 0 | 0 |
| ***Jones*** | | | | | |
| Slices | 3 | 70 | 0 | 0 | 0 |
| ***Yorkshire Farms*** | | | | | |
| Uncured | 3 oz | 100 | 9 | – | – |
| **CANADIAN BACON SUBSTITUTES** | | | | | |
| ***Yves*** | | | | | |
| Canadian Veggie Bacon | 1 serv (2 oz) | 80 | 1 | 1 | 1 |
| **CANDY** | | | | | |
| boiled sweets | ¼ lb | 327 | 87 | – | 0 |
| butterscotch | 1 oz | 112 | 27 | – | – |
| butterscotch | 1 piece (6 g) | 24 | 6 | – | – |
| candied cherries | 1 (4 g) | 12 | 3 | – | – |
| candied citron | 1 oz | 89 | 23 | – | – |
| candied lemon peel | 1 oz | 90 | 23 | – | – |
| candied orange peel | 1 oz | 90 | 23 | – | – |
| candied pineapple slice | 1 slice (2 oz) | 179 | 45 | – | – |
| candy corn | 1 oz | 105 | 27 | – | – |

| FOOD | PORTION | CALS | CARB | SUGAR | FIBER |
|---|---|---|---|---|---|
| caramels | 1 piece (8 g) | 31 | 6 | – | – |
| caramels | 1 pkg (2.5 oz) | 271 | 55 | – | – |
| caramels chocolate | 1 piece (6 g) | 22 | 6 | – | – |
| caramels chocolate | 1 bar (2.3 oz) | 231 | 56 | – | – |
| carob bar | 1 (3.1 oz) | 453 | 42 | – | – |
| crisped rice bar almond | 1 bar (1 oz) | 130 | 18 | – | 1 |
| crisped rice bar chocolate chip | 1 bar (1 oz) | 115 | 21 | 9 | 1 |
| dark chocolate | 1 oz | 150 | 16 | – | – |
| fondant chocolate coated | 1 lg (1.2 oz) | 128 | 28 | – | – |
| fondant chocolate coated | 1 sm (0.4 oz) | 40 | 9 | – | – |
| fondant mint | 1 oz | 105 | 27 | – | – |
| fruit pastilles | 1 tube (1.4 oz) | 101 | 25 | – | – |
| gumdrops | 10 sm (0.4 oz) | 135 | 35 | – | – |
| gumdrops | 10 lg (3.8 oz) | 420 | 108 | – | – |
| hard candy | 1 oz | 106 | 28 | – | – |
| jelly beans | 10 sm (0.4 oz) | 40 | 10 | – | – |
| jelly beans | 10 lg (1 oz) | 104 | 26 | – | – |
| lollipop | 1 (6 g) | 22 | 6 | – | – |
| marzipan | 1 oz | 128 | 15 | – | 2 |
| milk chocolate | 1 bar (1.55 oz) | 226 | 26 | – | – |
| milk chocolate crisp | 1 bar (1.45 oz) | 203 | 28 | – | – |
| milk chocolate w/ almonds | 1 bar (1.45 oz) | 215 | 22 | 20 | – |
| nougat nut cream | 0.5 oz | 49 | 8 | – | – |
| peanut bar | 1 (1.4 oz) | 209 | 19 | – | – |
| peanuts chocolate covered | 10 (1.4 oz) | 208 | 20 | – | – |
| peanuts chocolate covered | 1 cup (5.2 oz) | 773 | 74 | – | – |
| pretzels chocolate covered | 1 (0.4 oz) | 50 | 8 | – | – |
| pretzels chocolate covered | 1 oz | 130 | 20 | – | – |
| sesame crunch | 20 pieces (1.2 oz) | 181 | 18 | – | – |
| sesame crunch | 1 oz | 146 | 14 | – | – |
| sweet chocolate | 1 bar (1.45 oz) | 201 | 25 | – | – |
| sweet chocolate | 1 oz | 143 | 17 | – | – |
| truffles | 4 pieces (1.1 oz) | 190 | 14 | 12 | 1 |
| ***100 Grand*** | | | | | |
| Bar | 1 bar (1.5 oz) | 200 | 30 | 27 | tr |
| ***5th Avenue*** | | | | | |
| Snack Size | 1 bar (0.58) | 80 | 10 | – | – |

| FOOD | PORTION | CALS | CARB | SUGAR | FIBER |
|---|---|---|---|---|---|
| ***Almond Joy*** | | | | | |
| Snack Size | 1 (0.6 oz) | 90 | 11 | 9 | – |
| ***Altoids*** | | | | | |
| All Flavors | 3 pieces | 10 | 2 | 2 | – |
| ***At Last!*** | | | | | |
| Chocolate Almond | 1 bar | 120 | 13 | 0 | 6 |
| Chocolate Crisp | 1 bar | 110 | 14 | 0 | 6 |
| Chocolate Mint | 1 bar | 110 | 15 | 0 | 7 |
| Chocolate Peanut Butter | 1 bar | 100 | 15 | 0 | 5 |
| Chocolate Peanut Butter | 1 bar | 120 | 14 | 0 | 5 |
| ***Atkins*** | | | | | |
| Endulge Caramel Nut Chew | 1 bar (1.23 oz) | 140 | 17 | 1 | tr |
| Endulge Chocolate Bar | 1 bar (1.1 oz) | 150 | 2 | 0 | 3 |
| Endulge Chocolate Crunch | 1 bar (1 oz) | 150 | 15 | 0 | 3 |
| Endulge Peanut Butter Cups | 3 pieces | 160 | 17 | 0 | 0 |
| ***Baby Ruth*** | | | | | |
| Bar | 1 bar (2.1 oz) | 270 | 36 | 27 | 2 |
| Fun Size | 1 bar (1 oz) | 130 | 17 | 13 | tr |
| ***Bittyfinger*** | | | | | |
| Bars | 2 | 170 | 27 | 18 | tr |
| ***Body Smarts*** | | | | | |
| Chocolate Peanut Crunch | 2 bars (1.8 oz) | 210 | 34 | 20 | 2 |
| ***Butterfinger*** | | | | | |
| BB's | 1 pkg (1.7 oz) | 230 | 33 | 25 | 1 |
| Bar | 1 (2.1 oz) | 270 | 42 | 29 | 1 |
| Fun Size | 1 bar | 100 | 15 | 10 | 0 |
| ***Cadbury*** | | | | | |
| Milk Chocolate Roast Almond | 10 blocks (1.4 oz) | 220 | 21 | 18 | 1 |
| ***Cape Cod Provisions*** | | | | | |
| Cranberry Bog Frogs | 3 pieces (1.9 oz) | 250 | 34 | 27 | tr |

| FOOD | PORTION | CALS | CARB | SUGAR | FIBER |
|---|---|---|---|---|---|
| ***CarbSlim*** | | | | | |
| Crunch Bites Chocolate Caramel | 1 pkg | 122 | 21 | 0 | 9 |
| Crunch Bites Peanut Butter | 1 pkg | 171 | 21 | 0 | 9 |
| ***Carbolite*** | | | | | |
| Caramel | 1 bar | 100 | 18 | 0 | 0 |
| CarbAway | 1 bar | 100 | 17 | 0 | 0 |
| CarboSnack | 1 bar | 110 | 20 | 0 | 1 |
| Chocolate Truffle | 1 bar (1 oz) | 122 | 17 | 0 | 1 |
| Chocolate Almond | 1 bar (1.75 oz) | 298 | 3 | tr | 2 |
| Chocolate Crisp | 1 bar (1.75 oz) | 256 | 3 | 0 | 1 |
| Chocolate Peanut Butter | 1 bar (1.75 oz) | 256 | 3 | 0 | 0 |
| Crispy Caramel | 1 bar (1 oz) | 130 | 17 | 0 | 0 |
| Milk Chocolate | 1 bar (1.75 oz) | 263 | 1 | 0 | 1 |
| Peanut Butter Cup | 1 | 170 | 17 | 0 | 1 |
| Pecan Cluster | 1 bar | 120 | 15 | 0 | 1 |
| ***Carmello*** | | | | | |
| Snack Size | 1 (0.66 oz) | 90 | 12 | – | – |
| ***Cary's Of Oregon*** | | | | | |
| English Toffee Milk Chocolate Almond | 1 piece (0.75 oz) | 110 | 12 | 10 | tr |
| ***Chunky*** | | | | | |
| Bar | 1 (1.4 oz) | 210 | 24 | 21 | 1 |
| ***Cloud Nine*** | | | | | |
| Australian Orange Peel | ½ bar (1.5 oz) | 220 | 25 | 19 | 2 |
| Butter Nut Toffee | ½ bar (1.5 oz) | 230 | 25 | 21 | 1 |
| Cool Mint Crisp | ½ bar (⅕ oz) | 220 | 26 | 22 | 2 |
| Espresso Bean Crunch | ½ bar (1.5 oz) | 220 | 23 | 19 | 2 |
| Malted Milk Crunch | ½ bar (1.5 oz) | 230 | 26 | 23 | 1 |
| Milk Chocolate | ½ bar (1.5 oz) | 230 | 25 | 23 | 1 |
| Oregon Red Raspberry | ½ bar (1.5 oz) | 230 | 25 | 20 | 2 |
| Peanut Butter Brittle | ½ bar (1.5 oz) | 230 | 24 | 21 | 1 |
| Sundried Cherry | ½ bar (1.5 oz) | 230 | 26 | 22 | 1 |
| Toasted Coconut Crisp | ½ bar (1.5 oz) | 230 | 25 | 22 | 2 |
| Vanilla Dark | ½ bar (1.5 oz) | 230 | 25 | 20 | 2 |

| FOOD | PORTION | CALS | CARB | SUGAR | FIBER |
|---|---|---|---|---|---|
| ***Crunch*** | | | | | |
| Fun Size | 4 bars | 210 | 26 | 22 | tr |
| ***Daboga*** | | | | | |
| Organic Milk Chocolate | 1 bar (2 oz) | 318 | 30 | 28 | 6 |
| ***Del Monte*** | | | | | |
| Radical Raizins Cinnamon | 1 pkg (0.7 oz) | 70 | 18 | 16 | 0 |
| Radical Raizins Rainbow | 1 pkg (0.7 oz) | 70 | 18 | 16 | 0 |
| ***Doctor's CarbRite*** | | | | | |
| Sugar Free Dark Chocolate | 1 oz | 124 | 2 | 0 | 2 |
| Sugar Free Dark Chocolate With Almonds | 4 sq (1 oz) | 132 | 16 | 0 | 4 |
| Sugar Free Milk Chocolate | 1 oz | 128 | 0 | 0 | 0 |
| Sugar Free Milk Chocolate With Peanuts | 4 sq (1 oz) | 132 | 12 | 0 | 0 |
| Sugar Free Milk Chocolate With Soy Crisps | 4 sq (1 oz) | 120 | 12 | 0 | 2 |
| Sugar Free Mint Chocolate | 1 oz | 128 | 0 | 0 | 0 |
| ***Estee*** | | | | | |
| Caramels Vanilla & Chocolate | 5 | 115 | 26 | 3 | 0 |
| Dark Chocolate | ½ bar (1.4 oz) | 200 | 23 | 15 | 0 |
| Milk Chocolate | ½ bar (1.4 oz) | 230 | 17 | 15 | 0 |
| Milk Chocolate w/ Almonds | ½ bar (1.4 oz) | 230 | 16 | 14 | 0 |
| Milk Chocolate w/ Crisp Rice | ½ bar (1.2 oz) | 370 | 29 | 24 | 0 |
| Milk Chocolate w/ Fruit & Nuts | ½ bar (1.4 oz) | 220 | 18 | 15 | 0 |
| Mint Chocolate | ½ bar (1.4 oz) | 200 | 23 | 15 | 0 |
| Peanut Brittle | ⅓ box (1.3 oz) | 160 | 28 | 1 | 1 |
| Peanut Butter Cups | 5 | 200 | 19 | 13 | 1 |
| Sugar Free Assorted Fruit | 5 | 30 | 16 | 0 | 0 |
| Sugar Free Assorted Mint | 5 | 30 | 16 | 0 | 0 |
| Sugar Free Butterscotch | 2 | 25 | 12 | 0 | 0 |
| Sugar Free Fruit Gum Drops | 23 | 80 | 36 | 0 | 0 |
| Sugar Free Gourmet Jelly Beans | 26 | 70 | 24 | 0 | 0 |
| Sugar Free Gummy Apple Rings | 5 | 70 | 28 | 0 | 0 |
| Sugar Free Gummy Bears Assorted Fruit | 17 | 100 | 30 | 0 | 0 |
| Sugar Free Licorice Gum Drops | 11 | 90 | 36 | 0 | 0 |
| Sugar Free Peppermint Swirl | 3 | 30 | 14 | 0 | 0 |
| Sugar Free Sour Citrus Slices | 9 | 60 | 30 | 0 | 0 |
| Sugar Free Toffee | 5 | 30 | 16 | 0 | 0 |
| Sugar Free Tropical Fruit | 5 | 30 | 16 | 0 | 0 |

| FOOD | PORTION | CALS | CARB | SUGAR | FIBER |
|---|---|---|---|---|---|
| ***Fauchon*** | | | | | |
| Assorted | 3 pieces (1.1 oz) | 170 | 16 | 12 | 3 |
| ***Ferrero Rocher*** | | | | | |
| Candy | 1 piece (0.4 oz) | 73 | 6 | 5 | tr |
| ***Godiva*** | | | | | |
| Chocolatier Dark Chocolate w/ Raspberry | 1 bar (1.5 oz) | 220 | 28 | 22 | 0 |
| Chocolatier Milk Chocolate | 1 bar (1.5 oz) | 230 | 26 | 25 | 0 |
| Milk Chocolate w/ Whole Almonds | 1 bar (⅕ oz) | 230 | 20 | 18 | 0 |
| Mochaccino Mousse | 2 pieces (1.25 oz) | 210 | 17 | 14 | 0 |
| Truffles Assorted | 2 pieces (1.5 oz) | 220 | 24 | 20 | 0 |
| ***Goetze's*** | | | | | |
| Cow Tales | 1 pkg (1 oz) | 110 | 20 | 11 | tr |
| ***Gol D Lite*** | | | | | |
| Milk Chocolate Crisp | 1 bar | 125 | 15 | 0 | 0 |
| Seashell Truffle | 1 piece | 54 | 6 | 0 | 1 |
| ***Goobers*** | | | | | |
| Peanuts | 1 pkg (1.38 oz) | 210 | 20 | 17 | 1 |
| ***Hershey*** | | | | | |
| Amazin'Fruit Gummy Candy | 1 snack pkg (0.7 oz) | 60 | 15 | 10 | – |
| Bar | 1 (0.6 oz) | 100 | 9 | – | – |
| Candy-Coated Milk Chocolate Eggs | 4 pieces | 90 | 12 | – | – |
| Cookies 'n' Mint | 1 bar (0.6 oz) | 90 | 11 | – | – |
| Hugs | 1 piece | 25 | 3 | – | – |
| Hugs w/ Almonds | 1 piece | 25 | 3 | – | – |
| Kisses | 1 | 25 | 3 | – | – |
| Kisses w/ Almond | 1 | 25 | 3 | – | – |
| Milk Chocolate | 1 bar (0.6 oz) | 90 | 10 | – | – |
| Milk Chocolate w/ Almonds | 1 bar (0.6 oz) | 100 | 9 | – | – |
| Miniature Milk Chocolate | 1 (0.3 oz) | 45 | 5 | – | – |
| Nuggets Cookies 'n' Creme | 1 (0.35 oz) | 50 | 5 | – | – |
| Nuggets Cookies 'n' Mint | 1 (0.35 oz) | 50 | 6 | – | – |
| Nuggets Milk Chocolate | 1 (0.35 oz) | 50 | 6 | – | – |

| FOOD | PORTION | CALS | CARB | SUGAR | FIBER |
|---|---|---|---|---|---|
| Nuggets Milk Chocolate w/ Almonds | 1 (0.35 oz) | 50 | 5 | – | – |
| PayDay Snack Size | 1 (0.66 oz) | 90 | 11 | 8 | – |
| Pot Of Gold Solitaires | 5 pieces | 90 | 8 | – | – |
| ReeseSticks Snack Size | 2 pieces (1.2 oz) | 190 | 19 | 14 | 1 |
| S'mores | 1 bar | 240 | 31 | 20 | tr |
| Special Dark Miniature | 1 (0.3 oz) | 45 | 5 | – | – |
| Sweet Escapes Chocolate Toffee Crisp | 1 bar (0.66 oz) | 80 | 12 | – | – |
| Sweet Escapes Peanut Butter Crispy | 1 bar (0.7 oz) | 70 | 12 | – | – |
| Sweet Escapes Triple Chocolate Wafer | 1 bar (0.7 oz) | 80 | 14 | 12 | – |
| Tastetations Butterscotch | 3 pieces (0.6 oz) | 60 | 12 | – | – |
| Tastetations Caramel | 3 pieces (0.6 oz) | 60 | 12 | – | – |
| Tastetations Chocolate | 3 pieces (0.6 oz) | 60 | 12 | – | – |
| Tastetations Chocolate Mint | 3 pieces (0.6 oz) | 60 | 12 | – | – |
| Tastetations Peppermint | 3 pieces (0.6 oz) | 60 | 15 | – | – |
| ***Hint Mint*** | | | | | |
| All Flavors | 2 pieces | 10 | 2 | 2 | – |
| ***Jolly Rancher*** | | | | | |
| Lollipops All Flavors | 1 (0.6 oz) | 60 | 16 | 12 | – |
| ***Joyva*** | | | | | |
| Halvah Chocolate Covered | 1 serv (2 oz) | 380 | 20 | 19 | 3 |
| Halvah Marble | 1 serv (2 oz) | 390 | 18 | 10 | 2 |
| ***Judy's*** | | | | | |
| Sugar Free Almond Caramel Cluster | 1 piece (1.5 oz) | 200 | 10 | 0 | 2 |
| Sugar Free Cashew Caramel Cluster | 1 pieces (1.5 oz) | 190 | 12 | 1 | 1 |
| Sugar Free English Toffee | 1 piece (1.5 oz) | 220 | 9 | 0 | 3 |

| FOOD | PORTION | CALS | CARB | SUGAR | FIBER |
|---|---|---|---|---|---|
| Sugar Free Macadamia Caramel Cluster | 1 piece (1.5 oz) | 220 | 9 | tr | 2 |
| Sugar Free Peanut Brittle | ¾ cup | 100 | 2 | 0 | tr |
| Sugar Free Pecan Almond Cluster | 1 piece (1.5 oz) | 220 | 9 | 0 | 2 |
| ***Junior Mints*** | | | | | |
| Snack Size | 1 box (0.7 oz) | 75 | 16 | 16 | tr |
| ***Kit Kat*** | | | | | |
| Bar | 1 (0.5 oz) | 80 | 10 | 8 | – |
| ***Klein*** | | | | | |
| Sugar Free Hard Candy All Flavors | 3 pieces | 12 | 5 | 0 | 0 |
| ***Krackel*** | | | | | |
| Bar | 1 (0.6 oz) | 90 | 11 | – | – |
| Miniature | 1 (0.3 oz) | 45 | 5 | – | – |
| ***Lambertz*** | | | | | |
| Petits Soleils Chocolate Coated Gingerbread | 1 piece (0.4 oz) | 47 | 7 | 5 | tr |
| ***Lance*** | | | | | |
| Chocolaty Peanut Bar | 1 (2 oz) | 290 | 32 | 23 | 2 |
| Cinnamon Chews | 1 pkg (1.06 oz) | 120 | 28 | 22 | 0 |
| Fruit Chews | 1 pkg (1.06 oz) | 120 | 28 | 22 | 0 |
| Gum Ball Pops | 1 (0.45 oz) | 45 | 12 | 12 | tr |
| K-Nuts | 4 pieces (1.5 oz) | 240 | 23 | 17 | 0 |
| Mint Chews | 1 pkg (1.06 oz) | 120 | 28 | 22 | 0 |
| Peanut Bar | 1 (1.75 oz) | 270 | 23 | 15 | 2 |
| Pop-A-Lance | 1 piece (0.42 oz) | 45 | 11 | 10 | 0 |
| Popcorn'n'Carmel | 1 bar (0.75 oz) | 90 | 20 | 14 | 0 |
| Starlight Mints | 3 pieces (1 oz) | 60 | 15 | 11 | 0 |
| Strawberry Chews | 1 pkg (1.06 oz) | 120 | 28 | 22 | 0 |
| Suckers | 3 pieces (0.5 oz) | 50 | 13 | 10 | 0 |

| FOOD | PORTION | CALS | CARB | SUGAR | FIBER |
|---|---|---|---|---|---|
| Whistle Pop | 1 (0.67 oz) | 70 | 19 | 17 | tr |
| ***Landies Candies*** | | | | | |
| Sugar Free Almond Clusters | 2 pieces (1.5 oz) | 240 | 17 | tr | 2 |
| Sugar Free Bon Bons Peanut Butter | 2 (1.5 oz) | 240 | 17 | 0 | tr |
| Sugar Free Coconut Clusters | 2 pieces (1.5 oz) | 250 | 18 | tr | 1 |
| Sugar Free Cookies & Cream | 2 pieces (1.5 oz) | 240 | 23 | 0 | tr |
| Sugar Free Dark Almond Bark | 1 piece (1.5 oz) | 230 | 23 | 0 | 2 |
| Sugar Free Dark Miniature Bars | 7 pieces (1.5 oz) | 230 | 26 | 0 | 2 |
| Sugar Free Milk Minature Bars | 7 pieces (1.5 oz) | 240 | 21 | 0 | tr |
| Sugar Free Mint Discs | 7 pieces (1.5 oz) | 240 | 21 | 0 | tr |
| Sugar Free Peanut Clusters | 2 (1.5 oz) | 240 | 17 | 0 | 2 |
| Sugar Free White Almond Bark | 1 piece (1.5 oz) | 230 | 21 | 0 | tr |
| Sugar Free White Caps | 6 pieces (1.5 oz) | 230 | 24 | 0 | 0 |
| ***Lean Protein Bites*** | | | | | |
| Milk Chocolate | 1 pkg (1 oz) | 120 | 1 | 0 | 0 |
| Peanut Butter | 1 pkg (1 oz) | 120 | 1 | 1 | 0 |
| White Chocolate | 1 pkg (1 oz) | 120 | 2 | 2 | 0 |
| ***Lifesavers*** | | | | | |
| Gummi Shapes Barnum's Animals | 1 pkg (0.8 oz) | 70 | 18 | 13 | – |
| ***Lindt*** | | | | | |
| Dark Chocolate 70% Cocoa | 4 blocks (1.4 oz) | 220 | 13 | 11 | 2 |
| Lindor Truffles | 3 pieces | 220 | 16 | 15 | 0 |
| ***Low Carb Chef*** | | | | | |
| Gummi Bears | 14 pieces | 138 | 30 | 0 | 0 |
| Jelly Beans | 37 pieces | 120 | 36 | 0 | 0 |
| Sugar Free Caramel Marshmallow Treats | 3 pieces | 140 | 28 | 0 | 0 |
| Sugar Free Cherry Cordials | 3 pieces | 250 | 28 | 0 | tr |

| FOOD | PORTION | CALS | CARB | SUGAR | FIBER |
|---|---|---|---|---|---|
| Sugar Free Coconut Clusters | 4 pieces | 210 | 19 | 0 | 3 |
| Sugar Free Milk Chocolate Covered Vanilla Caramels | 3 pieces | 160 | 27 | 0 | 0 |
| Sugar Free Peanut Butter Cups | 1 piece | 200 | 19 | 0 | 1 |
| Sugar Free Peanut Butter Truffes | 2 pieces | 200 | 19 | 0 | 1 |
| Sugar Free Peanut Clusters | 4 pieces | 210 | 16 | 0 | 2 |
| Sugar Free Pecan Turtles | 1 pieces | 120 | 20 | 0 | 1 |
| Sugar Free Peppermint Patties | 3 pieces | 150 | 28 | 0 | 3 |
| ***M&M's*** | | | | | |
| Plain | 1 pkg (1.7 oz) | 240 | 34 | 31 | 1 |
| ***Milk Duds*** | | | | | |
| Snack Size | 4 boxes (1.3 oz) | 160 | 26 | 18 | 0 |
| ***Mon Cheri*** | | | | | |
| With Hazelnuts | 2 pieces | 120 | 10 | 10 | 1 |
| ***Mounds*** | | | | | |
| Bar | 1 (0.68 oz) | 90 | 11 | – | – |
| ***Mr. Goodbar*** | | | | | |
| Miniature | 1 (0.3 oz) | 45 | 4 | – | – |
| ***Necco*** | | | | | |
| Bridge Mix | ¼ cup (1.5 oz) | 180 | 27 | 23 | tr |
| Chocolate Covered Raisins | 30 pieces (1.5 oz) | 170 | 30 | 27 | 1 |
| Malted Milk Balls | 11 pieces (1.5 oz) | 180 | 28 | 25 | tr |
| SkyBar | 1 bar (1.5 oz) | 190 | 28 | 25 | 0 |
| ***Nestle*** | | | | | |
| Buncha Crunch | 1 pkg (1.4 oz) | 90 | 26 | 20 | tr |
| Crunch | 1 bar (1.55 oz) | 230 | 29 | 24 | tr |
| Crunch Disk | 1 (1.2 oz) | 180 | 22 | 19 | tr |
| Crunchkins | 5 pieces | 190 | 24 | 21 | tr |
| Jingles Milk Chocolate Butterfinger | 5 pieces | 180 | 26 | 20 | tr |
| Jingles Milk Chocolate Crunch | 7 pieces | 220 | 28 | 23 | tr |

| FOOD | PORTION | CALS | CARB | SUGAR | FIBER |
|---|---|---|---|---|---|
| Jingles White Crunch | 7 pieces | 230 | 24 | 21 | 0 |
| Milk Chocolate | 1 bar (1.45 oz) | 220 | 26 | 24 | tr |
| Nesteggs Milk Chocolate Butterfinger | 5 pieces | 210 | 28 | 23 | tr |
| Nesteggs Milk Chocolate Crunch | 5 pieces | 190 | 24 | 21 | tr |
| Nesteggs White Crunch | 7 pieces | 230 | 24 | 21 | 0 |
| Pearson's Egg Nog | 2 pieces | 60 | 11 | 7 | 0 |
| Treasures Butterfinger | 3 pieces | 180 | 24 | 19 | tr |
| Treasures Crunch | 4 pieces (1.4 oz) | 210 | 26 | 21 | tr |
| Treasures Peanut Butter | 4 pieces | 250 | 23 | 21 | 1 |
| Turtles | 2 pieces (1.2 oz) | 160 | 20 | 15 | tr |
| Turtles Bite Size | 1 piece (0.4 oz) | 50 | 6 | 5 | tr |
| White Crunch | 1 bar (1.4 oz) | 220 | 23 | 20 | 0 |
| ***Newman's Own*** | | | | | |
| Organic Peanut Butter Cups Dark Chocolate | 3 pieces (1.2 oz) | 180 | 18 | 14 | tr |
| Organic Peanut Butter Cups Milk Chocolate | 3 pieces (1.2 oz) | 180 | 18 | 14 | tr |
| Organic Peppermint Cups | 3 pieces (1.2 oz) | 180 | 20 | 18 | tr |
| ***Nibs*** | | | | | |
| Cherry | 1 pkg (0.49 oz) | 45 | 11 | – | – |
| Licorice | 1 pkg (0.49 oz) | 40 | 10 | – | – |
| ***Nips*** | | | | | |
| Butter Rum | 2 pieces | 60 | 11 | 7 | 0 |
| Caramel | 2 pieces | 60 | 11 | 7 | 0 |
| Chocolate | 2 pieces | 60 | 11 | 7 | 0 |
| Chocolate Parfait | 2 pieces | 60 | 10 | 7 | 0 |
| Coffee | 2 pieces | 50 | 10 | 7 | 0 |
| Vanilla Almond Cafe | 2 pieces | 50 | 10 | 7 | 0 |
| ***Oh Henry!*** | | | | | |
| Bar | 1 (1.8 oz) | 120 | 16 | 12 | 0 |

| FOOD | PORTION | CALS | CARB | SUGAR | FIBER |
|---|---|---|---|---|---|
| ***Pearson's*** | | | | | |
| Irish Cream Parfait | 2 pieces | 60 | 10 | 6 | 0 |
| Mint Patties | 1 | 30 | 6 | 5 | tr |
| ***Perlege*** | | | | | |
| Sugar Free Belgium Chocolate All Flavors | 1 bar (3.5 oz) | 532 | 14 | 0 | 3 |
| Sugar Free Cream Filled Belgian Chocolate All Flavors | 1 bar (1.5 oz) | 226 | 22 | 0 | 0 |
| ***Pez*** | | | | | |
| Candy | 1 roll (0.3 oz) | 35 | 9 | 9 | – |
| Candy Sugar Free | 1 roll (0.3 oz) | 30 | 8 | 0 | – |
| ***Planters*** | | | | | |
| Original Peanut Bar | 1 pkg (1.6 oz) | 230 | 22 | 13 | 2 |
| ***Pure De-Lite*** | | | | | |
| Caramel | 1 bar | 120 | 19 | 0 | 1 |
| Caramel Crisp | 1 bar | 120 | 18 | 0 | 1 |
| Caramel Nougat | 1 bar | 110 | 20 | 0 | 1 |
| Caramel Peanut Butter | 1 bar | 120 | 17 | 0 | 1 |
| Caramel Pecan | 1 bar | 130 | 17 | 0 | 1 |
| Sugar Free Dark Chocolate | 1 bar | 173 | 1 | 0 | 4 |
| Sugar Free Milk Choclate w/ Mint | 1 bar | 187 | 3 | 0 | 1 |
| Sugar Free Milk Chocolate | 1 bar | 187 | 3 | 0 | 1 |
| Sugar Free Milk Chocolate w/ Almonds | 1 bar | 190 | 4 | 0 | 2 |
| Sugar Free Milk Chocolate w/ Coconut | 1 bar | 190 | 4 | 0 | 1 |
| Sugar Free Milk Chocolate w/ Orange | 1 bar | 187 | 3 | 0 | 1 |
| Sugar Free Milk Chocolate w/ Peanuts | 1 bar | 190 | 4 | 0 | 1 |
| Sugar Free White Chocolate | 1 bar | 187 | 3 | 0 | 0 |
| Truffle Bar Caramel | 1 bar | 140 | 16 | 0 | 0 |
| Truffle Bar Dark Mint | 1 bar | 160 | 13 | 0 | 1 |
| Truffle Bar Hazelnut | 1 bar | 160 | 12 | 0 | 1 |
| Truffle Bar Peanut Butter | 1 bar | 160 | 13 | 0 | 1 |
| ***Raisinets*** | | | | | |
| Candy | 1 pkg (1.58 oz) | 200 | 31 | 28 | 1 |

| FOOD | PORTION | CALS | CARB | SUGAR | FIBER |
|---|---|---|---|---|---|
| Fun Size | 3 pkg (1.7 oz) | 200 | 43 | 29 | 2 |
| ***Reese's*** | | | | | |
| FastBreak | 1 bar (2 oz) | 270 | 34 | 30 | 2 |
| Nutrageous | 1 bar (0.6 oz) | 95 | 9 | 8 | 1 |
| Peanut Butter Cups | 1 (0.28 oz) | 40 | 4 | – | – |
| Peanut Butter Cups Miniature | 1 (0.3 oz) | 42 | 4 | 4 | tr |
| Pieces | 25 (0.7 oz) | 100 | 12 | – | – |
| ResseSticks Peanut Butter | 2 pieces (1.2 oz) | 190 | 19 | 14 | 1 |
| ***Ritter Sport*** | | | | | |
| Dark Chocolate Whole Hazelnuts | 6 pieces (1.3 oz) | 210 | 16 | 14 | 7 |
| ***Rokeach*** | | | | | |
| Cotton Candy | 2 cups (1 oz) | 110 | 28 | 28 | 0 |
| ***Rolo*** | | | | | |
| Caramels in Milk Chocolate | 3 pieces (0.64 oz) | 90 | 12 | – | – |
| ***Russell Stover*** | | | | | |
| Low Carb Pecan Delights | 1 pkg (1 oz) | 130 | 16 | 0 | tr |
| Peanut Butter & Grape Jelly | 1 piece (0.8 oz) | 100 | 10 | 8 | tr |
| Peanut Butter & Red Raspberry Cups | 2 (1.2 oz) | 140 | 14 | 12 | tr |
| Pecan Delights | 1 pkg (2 oz) | 280 | 27 | 20 | tr |
| Pecan Roll | 1 (1.75 oz) | 260 | 23 | 19 | 2 |
| S'mores | 3 (1.4 oz) | 210 | 22 | 18 | tr |
| Sugar Free Peanut Butter Cups | 4 pieces (1.3 oz) | 200 | 17 | – | 2 |
| Sugar Free Pecans & Caramel | 2 pieces (1.2 oz) | 170 | 17 | – | 0 |
| ***Smucker's*** | | | | | |
| Fruit Fillers Strawberry | 1 pkg (0.9 oz) | 80 | 19 | 13 | – |
| ***Snickers*** | | | | | |
| Cruncher | 3 fun size (1.4 oz) | 230 | 25 | 18 | 1 |
| ***Sno Caps*** | | | | | |
| Candies | 1 pkg (2.3 oz) | 300 | 48 | 38 | 3 |

| FOOD | PORTION | CALS | CARB | SUGAR | FIBER |
|---|---|---|---|---|---|
| ***Speakeasy*** | | | | | |
| Organic Mints All Flavors | 4 pieces (2 g) | 10 | 2 | 2 | – |
| ***Steel's*** | | | | | |
| Salt Water Taffy Assorted | 3 pieces (1 oz) | 90 | 22 | 16 | 0 |
| ***Symphony*** | | | | | |
| Bar | 1 (0.6 oz) | 100 | 10 | – | – |
| w/ Almonds & Chocolate Chips | 1 bar (0.6 oz) | 90 | 9 | – | – |
| ***Tobler*** | | | | | |
| Orange Dark Chocolate | 5 pieces (1.5 oz) | 240 | 28 | 25 | 3 |
| ***Toblerone*** | | | | | |
| Milk Chocolate w/ Honey & Almond Nougat | ⅓ bar (1.76 oz) | 170 | 21 | 18 | tr |
| ***Tom's*** | | | | | |
| Cherry Sours | 1 pkg (2.25 oz) | 210 | 53 | 38 | 0 |
| Jelly Beans | 1 pkg (2.25 oz) | 230 | 58 | 44 | 0 |
| ***Tootsie*** | | | | | |
| Pop | 1 | 60 | 12 | 11 | – |
| ***Torras*** | | | | | |
| Sugar Free Dark Chocolate | 1 oz | 136 | 15 | 0 | 0 |
| Sugar Free Milk Chocolate | 1 oz | 140 | 17 | 0 | 0 |
| Sugar Free Milk Chocolate w/ Almonds | 1 oz | 146 | 15 | 0 | 0 |
| Sugar Free Milk Chocolate w/ Hazelnuts | 1 oz | 148 | 15 | 0 | 0 |
| Sugar Free White Chocolate | 1 oz | 138 | 17 | 0 | 0 |
| ***Tropical Source*** | | | | | |
| Butterscotch Dream | 4 pieces (0.5 oz) | 60 | 14 | 11 | 0 |
| Chocolate Dairy Free California Raisin & Currant | ½ bar (1.5 oz) | 230 | 25 | 25 | 1 |
| Chocolate Dairy Free Hazelnut Espresso Crunch | ½ bar (1.5 oz) | 250 | 21 | 19 | 1 |
| Chocolate Dairy Free Maple Almond Granola | ½ bar (1.5 oz) | 230 | 24 | 23 | 1 |
| Chocolate Dairy Free Mint Candy Crunch | ½ bar (1.5 oz) | 220 | 24 | 24 | 1 |

| FOOD | PORTION | CALS | CARB | SUGAR | FIBER |
|---|---|---|---|---|---|
| Chocolate Dairy Free Red Raspberry Crush | ½ bar (1.5 oz) | 230 | 22 | 22 | 1 |
| Chocolate Dairy Free Sundried Jungle Banana | ½ bar (1.5 oz) | 230 | 26 | 22 | 2 |
| Chocolate Dairy Free Toasted Almond | ½ bar (1.5 oz) | 250 | 21 | 19 | 1 |
| Chocolate Dairy Free Wild Rice Crisp | ½ bar (1.5 oz) | 230 | 26 | 23 | 1 |
| Cool Peppermint | 4 pieces (0.5 oz) | 60 | 14 | 11 | 0 |
| Lollipops All Flavors | 1 | 24 | 6 | 4 | 0 |
| Mango Papaya | 4 pieces (0.5 oz) | 60 | 14 | 11 | 0 |
| ***Twizzlers*** | | | | | |
| Cherry | 1 piece | 35 | 9 | – | – |
| Chocolate | 1 piece | 30 | 7 | – | – |
| Licorice | 1 piece | 35 | 9 | – | – |
| Pull'n'Peel Cherry | 1 piece (1 oz) | 90 | 19 | – | – |
| Strawberry | 1 piece | 35 | 9 | – | – |
| ***Unique Origin*** | | | | | |
| Guaranda Dark Chocolate | 1 piece (0.3 oz) | 54 | 4 | 3 | 1 |
| ***Werther's*** | | | | | |
| Original | 3 pieces (0.5 oz) | 60 | 13 | 11 | 0 |
| ***Whatchamacallit*** | | | | | |
| Bar | 1 (0.58 oz) | 80 | 10 | – | – |
| ***Whoppers*** | | | | | |
| Malted Milk Balls | 1 pkg (0.7 oz) | 100 | 16 | 13 | 0 |
| ***York*** | | | | | |
| Chocolate Covered Peppermint Bites | 15 pieces (1 oz) | 150 | 31 | 29 | tr |
| Peppermint Patty | 1 (0.49 oz) | 50 | 11 | 8 | – |
| **CANTALOUPE** | | | | | |
| dried | 3.5 pieces (1.4 oz) | 140 | 34 | 32 | 1 |
| fresh cubed | 1 cup | 57 | 13 | – | 1 |
| fresh half | ½ | 94 | 22 | – | 2 |

| FOOD | PORTION | CALS | CARB | SUGAR | FIBER |
|---|---|---|---|---|---|
| ***Chiquita*** | | | | | |
| Wedge | ¼ med (4.7 oz) | 50 | 12 | 11 | 1 |
| **CARAWAY** | | | | | |
| seed | 1 tsp | 7 | 1 | – | – |
| **CARDAMOM** | | | | | |
| ground | 1 tsp | 6 | 1 | – | – |
| **CARDOON** | | | | | |
| fresh cooked | 3 ½ oz | 22 | 5 | – | – |
| fresh shredded | ½ cup | 36 | 4 | – | – |
| **CARIBOU** | | | | | |
| roasted | 3 oz | 142 | 0 | 0 | 0 |
| **CARISSA** | | | | | |
| fresh | 1 | 12 | 3 | – | – |
| **CAROB** | | | | | |
| carob mix | 3 tsp | 45 | 11 | – | – |
| carob mix as prep w/ whole milk | 9 oz | 195 | 23 | – | – |
| flour | 1 tbsp | 14 | 7 | – | – |
| flour | 1 cup | 185 | 92 | – | – |
| ***Sunspire*** | | | | | |
| Carob Chips Unsweetened | 13 pieces (0.5 oz) | 70 | 8 | 5 | 0 |
| Carob Chips Vegan | 13 pieces (0.5 oz) | 70 | 11 | 5 | 0 |
| **CARP** | | | | | |
| fresh | 3 oz | 108 | 0 | 0 | 0 |
| fresh cooked | 1 fillet (6 oz) | 276 | 0 | 0 | 0 |
| fresh cooked | 3 oz | 138 | 0 | 0 | 0 |
| roe raw | 1 oz | 37 | tr | – | – |
| roe salted in olive oil | 2 tbsp (1 oz) | 40 | 6 | – | 0 |
| **CARROT JUICE** | | | | | |
| canned | 6 oz | 73 | 17 | – | – |
| **CARROTS** | | | | | |
| **CANNED** | | | | | |
| slices | ½ cup | 17 | 4 | – | 1 |

| FOOD | PORTION | CALS | CARB | SUGAR | FIBER |
|---|---|---|---|---|---|
| slices low sodium | ½ cup | 17 | 4 | – | 1 |
| ***Del Monte*** | | | | | |
| Sliced | ½ cup (4.3 oz) | 35 | 8 | 5 | 3 |
| ***S&W*** | | | | | |
| Julienne | ½ cup (4.3 oz) | 30 | 5 | 4 | 2 |
| Sliced | ½ cup (4.3 oz) | 30 | 5 | 4 | 2 |
| Whole Small | ½ cup (4.3 oz) | 30 | 5 | 4 | 2 |
| **FRESH** | | | | | |
| baby raw | 1 (½ oz) | 6 | 1 | – | – |
| raw | 1 (2.5 oz) | 31 | 7 | – | 2 |
| raw shredded | ½ cup | 24 | 6 | – | 2 |
| slices cooked | ½ cup | 35 | 8 | – | – |
| ***Dole*** | | | | | |
| Shredded | 1 cups (3 oz) | 40 | 9 | 5 | 2 |
| ***Earthbound Farms*** | | | | | |
| Organic Mini Peeled | ½ cup | 30 | 7 | 4 | 3 |
| **FROZEN** | | | | | |
| slices cooked | ½ cup | 26 | 6 | – | – |
| ***Fresh Like*** | | | | | |
| Carrots Slice | 3.5 oz | 42 | 10 | – | – |
| **CASABA** | | | | | |
| cubed | 1 cup | 45 | 11 | – | – |
| fresh | 1/10 | 43 | 10 | – | – |
| **CASHEWS** | | | | | |
| cashew butter w/o salt | 1 tbsp | 94 | 4 | – | – |
| dry roasted salted | 1 oz | 163 | 9 | – | – |
| dry roasted w/ salt | 18 nuts (1 oz) | 160 | 9 | – | 1 |
| oil roasted | 1 oz | 163 | 8 | – | – |
| oil roasted salted | 1 oz | 163 | 8 | – | – |
| ***Frito Lay*** | | | | | |
| Salted | 1 oz | 180 | 7 | 2 | 1 |
| ***Lance*** | | | | | |
| Cashews | 1 pkg (1⅛ oz) | 200 | 8 | 3 | 3 |
| ***Maranatha*** | | | | | |
| Cashew Butter | 2 tbsp | 190 | 11 | 2 | 2 |
| Tamari Cashews | ¼ cup | 160 | 9 | 2 | 1 |
| ***Sweet Delights*** | | | | | |
| Cashew Roasters | ⅓ pkg (1 oz) | 170 | 10 | 1 | 2 |

| FOOD | PORTION | CALS | CARB | SUGAR | FIBER |
|---|---|---|---|---|---|
| **CASSAVA** | | | | | |
| fresh | 3½ oz | 120 | 27 | – | – |
| **CATFISH** | | | | | |
| channel breaded & fried | 3 oz | 194 | 7 | – | – |
| channel raw | 3 oz | 99 | 0 | 0 | 0 |
| **CAULIFLOWER** | | | | | |
| **FRESH** | | | | | |
| cooked | ½ cup (2.2 oz) | 14 | 3 | – | 1 |
| flowerets cooked | 3 (2 oz) | 12 | 2 | – | 1 |
| flowerets raw | 3 (2 oz) | 14 | 3 | – | 1 |
| green cooked | 1½ cup (3.2 oz) | 29 | 6 | – | 3 |
| green raw | 1 head 7 in diam (18 oz) | 158 | 31 | – | 16 |
| green raw | 1 cup (2.2 oz) | 20 | 4 | – | 2 |
| green raw floweret | 1 (0.9 oz) | 8 | 2 | – | 1 |
| raw | ½ cup (1.8 oz) | 13 | 3 | – | 1 |
| **FROZEN** | | | | | |
| cooked | ½ cup | 17 | 3 | – | – |
| ***Fresh Like*** | | | | | |
| Florets | 3.5 oz | 26 | 5 | – | 1 |
| **CAVIAR** | | | | | |
| black | 1 tbsp | 40 | 1 | – | – |
| red | 1 tbsp | 40 | 1 | – | – |
| **CELERIAC** | | | | | |
| fresh cooked | 3½ oz | 25 | 6 | – | – |
| raw | ½ cup | 31 | 7 | – | – |
| **CELERY** | | | | | |
| diced cooked | ½ cup | 13 | 3 | – | – |
| fresh | 1 stalk (1.3 oz) | 6 | 1 | – | 1 |
| raw diced | ½ cup | 10 | 2 | – | 1 |
| seed | 1 tsp | 8 | 1 | – | – |
| ***McCormick*** | | | | | |
| Celery Salt | ¼ tsp | 0 | 0 | 0 | 0 |
| **CELTUCE** | | | | | |
| raw | 3½ oz | 22 | 4 | – | – |

| FOOD | PORTION | CALS | CARB | SUGAR | FIBER |
|---|---|---|---|---|---|
| **CEREAL** | | | | | |
| bran flakes | ¾ cup (1 oz) | 90 | 22 | – | – |
| corn flakes | 1¼ cup (1 oz) | 110 | 24 | – | – |
| corn flakes low sodium | 1 cup (0.9 oz) | 100 | 22 | – | tr |
| corn grits white regular & quick as prep w/ water & salt | ¾ cup (6.4 oz) | 109 | 24 | – | tr |
| corn grits white regular or quick as prep | ¾ cup (6.4 oz) | 109 | 24 | – | tr |
| corn grits yellow regular & quick as prep w/ water & salt | ¾ cup (6.4 oz) | 109 | 24 | – | tr |
| corn grits yellow regular & quick not prep | 1 cup (5.5 oz) | 579 | 124 | – | 3 |
| crispy rice | 1 cup (1 oz) | 111 | 25 | – | tr |
| crispy rice low sodium | 1 cup (0.9 oz) | 105 | 23 | – | tr |
| farina as prep w/ water | ¾ cup (6.1 oz) | 88 | 19 | – | 2 |
| farina not prep | 1 tbsp (0.4 oz) | 40 | 9 | – | tr |
| granola | ½ cup (2.1 oz) | 285 | 32 | – | 6 |
| oatmeal instant w/ cinnamon & spice as prep w/ water | 1 pkg (5.6 oz) | 177 | 35 | – | 3 |
| oatmeal instant w/ raisins & spice as prep w/ water | 1 cup (5.5 oz) | 161 | 32 | – | 2 |
| oatmeal instant w/ bran & raisins as prep w/ water | 1 pkg (6.8 oz) | 158 | 30 | – | 6 |
| oatmeal istant as prep w/ water | 1 cup (8.2 oz) | 138 | 24 | – | 4 |
| oatmeal regular & quick as prep w/ water | ¾ cup (6.1 oz) | 149 | 19 | – | 3 |
| oatmeal regular & quick not prep | ⅓ cup (0.9 oz) | 104 | 18 | – | 3 |
| oatmeal instant cooked w/o salt | 1 cup | 145 | 25 | – | – |
| oatmeal quick cooked w/o salt | 1 cup | 145 | 25 | – | – |
| oatmeal regular cooked w/o salt | 1 cup | 145 | 25 | – | – |
| puffed rice | 1 cup (0.5 oz) | 56 | 13 | – | tr |
| puffed wheat | 1 cup (0.4 oz) | 44 | 10 | – | 1 |
| shredded mini wheats | 1 cup (1.1 oz) | 107 | 24 | – | 3 |
| shredded wheat rectangular | 1 biscuit (0.8 oz) | 85 | 19 | – | 2 |

| FOOD | PORTION | CALS | CARB | SUGAR | FIBER |
|---|---|---|---|---|---|
| shredded wheat round | 2 biscuits (1.3 oz) | 136 | 31 | – | 4 |
| sugar-coated corn flakes | ¾ cup (1 oz) | 110 | 26 | – | – |
| whole wheat hot natural as prep w/ water | ¾ cup (6.4 oz) | 113 | 25 | – | 3 |
| ***Albers*** | | | | | |
| Hominy Quick Grits uncooked | ¼ cup | 140 | 31 | 0 | 1 |
| ***Alpen*** | | | | | |
| Corn Flakes | 1 serv (1 oz) | 110 | 25 | 0 | tr |
| No Salt No Sugar | 1 serv (2 oz) | 200 | 34 | 10 | 6 |
| Regular | 1 serv (2 oz) | 200 | 37 | 17 | 4 |
| ***Atkins*** | | | | | |
| Banana Nut Harvest | ⅔ cup | 100 | 11 | 1 | 6 |
| Blueberry Bounty w/ Almonds | ⅔ cup | 100 | 10 | 1 | 6 |
| Crunchy Almond Crisp | ⅔ cup | 100 | 8 | 1 | 5 |
| ***Aunt Paula's*** | | | | | |
| Hot Flax Cereal | 1 serv (1½ oz) | 100 | 8 | 0 | 5 |
| ***Back To Nature*** | | | | | |
| Hi-Protein | ⅔ cup | 140 | 25 | 10 | 3 |
| Muesli | ½ cup | 160 | 32 | 11 | 4 |
| Puff Wheat | ½ cup | 160 | 32 | 11 | 4 |
| Ultra Flax | ¾ cup | 150 | 28 | 11 | 3 |
| ***Barbara's Bakery*** | | | | | |
| Apple Cinnamon O's | ¾ cup | 110 | 24 | 11 | 2 |
| Bite Size Shredded Oats | 1¼ cups (2 oz) | 220 | 46 | 12 | 6 |
| Cinnamon Puffins | 1¼ cup (2 oz) | 100 | 26 | 6 | 6 |
| Cocoa Crunch Stars | 1 cup (1 oz) | 110 | 26 | 8 | 1 |
| Frosted Corn Flakes | 1 cup (1 oz) | 110 | 27 | 8 | 4 |
| Fruit Juice Sweetened Breakfast O's | 1 cup (1 oz) | 120 | 22 | 2 | 3 |
| Fruit Juice Sweetened Brown Rice Crisps | 1 cup (1 oz) | 120 | 25 | 2 | 1 |
| Fruit Juice Sweetened Corn Flakes | 1 cup (1 oz) | 110 | 26 | 3 | 2 |
| GrainShop | ⅔ cup (1 oz) | 90 | 24 | 5 | 8 |
| Honey Crunch Stars | 1 cup (1 oz) | 110 | 26 | 8 | 2 |
| Honey Nut Toasted O's | ¾ cup | 120 | 23 | 11 | 2 |
| Organic Fruity Punch | 1 cup (1 oz) | 110 | 26 | 8 | 0 |

| FOOD | PORTION | CALS | CARB | SUGAR | FIBER |
|---|---|---|---|---|---|
| Organic Soy Essence | ¾ cup (1 oz) | 100 | 25 | 5 | 5 |
| Puffins | ¾ cup (0.9 oz) | 90 | 23 | 5 | 5 |
| Shredded Spoonfuls | ¾ cup (1.1 oz) | 110 | 23 | 5 | 4 |
| Shredded Wheat | 2 biscuits (1.4 oz) | 140 | 31 | 0 | 5 |
| ***Carbsense*** | | | | | |
| Hot Cereal Country Spice not prep | ½ cup | 130 | 15 | 0 | 12 |
| Hot Cereal Roasted Hazelnut not prep | ½ cup | 140 | 15 | 0 | 12 |
| ***Erewhon*** | | | | | |
| Apple Stroodles | ¾ cup | 110 | 25 | 4 | 1 |
| Aztec | 1 cup | 110 | 26 | 1 | 1 |
| Banana O's | ¾ cup | 110 | 26 | 7 | 2 |
| Brown Rice Cream | ¼ cup | 170 | 36 | 0 | 1 |
| Corn Flakes | 1¼ cups | 210 | 45 | tr | 3 |
| Crispy Brown Rice | 1 cup | 110 | 25 | 1 | 1 |
| Crispy Brown Rice No Salt Added | 1 cup | 110 | 25 | 1 | 1 |
| Fruit'n Wheat | ¾ cup | 170 | 39 | 12 | 5 |
| Kamut Flakes | ⅔ cup | 110 | 25 | 1 | 4 |
| Raisin Bran | 1 cup | 170 | 40 | 10 | 6 |
| Rice Twice | ¾ cup | 120 | 28 | 8 | 0 |
| Whole Wheat Flakes | 1 cup | 180 | 42 | tr | 6 |
| ***Expert Foods*** | | | | | |
| Low Carb Hot Cereal Sub | ½ cup | 24 | 2 | – | – |
| ***General Mills*** | | | | | |
| Basic 4 | 1 cup (1.9 oz) | 200 | 42 | 14 | 3 |
| Boo Berry | 1 cup (1 oz) | 120 | 27 | 14 | – |
| Cheerios | 1 cup (1 oz) | 110 | 22 | 1 | 3 |
| Cheerios Apple Cinnamon | ¾ cup (1 oz) | 120 | 25 | 13 | 1 |
| Cheerios Frosted | 1 cup (1 oz) | 120 | 25 | 13 | 1 |
| Cheerios Honey Nut | 1 cup (1 oz) | 120 | 24 | 11 | 2 |
| Cheerios Multi-Grain | 1 cup (1 oz) | 110 | 24 | 8 | 3 |
| Cheerios Team | 1 cup (1 oz) | 120 | 25 | 11 | 1 |
| Chex Corn | 1 cup (1 oz) | 110 | 26 | 3 | 0 |
| Chex Honey Nut | ¾ cup | 120 | 26 | 9 | – |

| FOOD | PORTION | CALS | CARB | SUGAR | FIBER |
|---|---|---|---|---|---|
| Chex Morning Mix Cinnamon | 1 pkg (1.1 oz) | 130 | 24 | 8 | 1 |
| Chex Morning Mix Fruit & Nut | 1 pkg (1.1 oz) | 180 | 24 | 8 | 1 |
| Chex Morning Mix Honey Nut | 1 pkg (1.1 oz) | 130 | 24 | 8 | 1 |
| Chex Multi-Bran | 1 cup (2 oz) | 200 | 49 | 12 | 8 |
| Chex Rice | 1¼ cup (1.1 oz) | 120 | 27 | 2 | 0 |
| Cinnamon Grahams | ¾ cup (1 oz) | 120 | 26 | 11 | 1 |
| Cinnamon Toast Crunch | ¾ cup (1 oz) | 130 | 24 | 10 | 1 |
| Cocoa Puffs | 1 cup (1 oz) | 120 | 26 | 14 | – |
| Cookie Crisp | 1 cup (1 oz) | 120 | 26 | 13 | 0 |
| Count Chocula | 1 cup (1 oz) | 120 | 26 | 14 | 0 |
| Country Corn Flakes | 1 cup (1 oz) | 120 | 26 | 2 | – |
| Fiber One | ½ cup (1 oz) | 60 | 24 | 0 | 14 |
| Franken Berry | 1 cup (1 oz) | 120 | 27 | 14 | – |
| French Toast Crunch | ¾ cup (1 oz) | 120 | 26 | 12 | 0 |
| Gold Medal Raisin Bran | 1⅓ cups (1.9 oz) | 170 | 41 | 12 | 6 |
| Golden Grahams | ¾ cup (1 oz) | 120 | 25 | 10 | 1 |
| Harmony | 1¼ cups (1.9 oz) | 200 | 44 | 13 | 2 |
| Honey Nut Clusters | 1 cup (1.9 oz) | 210 | 46 | 17 | 3 |
| Kaboom | 1¼ cup (1 oz) | 120 | 24 | 8 | 1 |
| Kix | 1⅓ cup (1 oz) | 120 | 26 | 3 | 1 |
| Kix Berry Berry | ¾ cup (1 oz) | 120 | 26 | 9 | 0 |
| Lucky Charms | 1 cup (1 oz) | 120 | 25 | 13 | 1 |
| Nature Valley Low Fat Fruit Granola | ⅔ cup (1.9 oz) | 210 | 44 | 19 | 3 |
| Newquick | ¾ cup (1 oz) | 120 | 25 | 12 | – |
| Oatmeal Crisp Almond | 1 cup (1.9 oz) | 220 | 42 | 16 | 4 |
| Oatmeal Crisp Apple Cinnamon | 1 cup (1.9 oz) | 210 | 45 | 19 | 4 |
| Oatmeal Crisp Raisin | 1 cup (1.9 oz) | 210 | 44 | 18 | 4 |
| Para Su Familia Cinnamon Stars | 1 cup (1 oz) | 120 | 28 | 6 | – |
| Para Su Familia Fruitis | 1 cup (1 oz) | 120 | 25 | 6 | – |
| Para Su Familia Raisin Bran | 1¼ cups (2 oz) | 170 | 41 | 12 | 6 |
| Raisin Nut Bran | ¾ cup (1.9 oz) | 200 | 41 | 18 | 4 |
| Reese's Puffs | ¾ cup | 130 | 23 | 13 | 0 |
| Snack'N Dash Cinnamon Toast Crunch | 1 pkg (1.2 oz) | 140 | 27 | 12 | 1 |
| Snack'N Dash Honey Nut Cheerios | 1 pkg (1 oz) | 110 | 23 | 10 | 2 |

| FOOD | PORTION | CALS | CARB | SUGAR | FIBER |
|---|---|---|---|---|---|
| Snack'N Dash Lucky Charms | 1 pkg (1 oz) | 110 | 24 | 12 | 1 |
| Sunrise Organic | ¾ cup (1 oz) | 110 | 26 | 10 | 1 |
| Total Brown Sugar & Oat | ¾ cup (1 oz) | 110 | 23 | 9 | 1 |
| Total Corn Flakes | 1⅓ cup (1 oz) | 110 | 24 | 4 | – |
| Total Raisin Bran | 1 cup (1.9 oz) | 170 | 41 | 20 | 5 |
| Total Whole Grain | ¾ cup (1 oz) | 110 | 23 | 5 | 3 |
| Trix | 1 cup (1 oz) | 120 | 27 | 13 | 1 |
| Wheat Hearts | ¼ cup (1.3 oz) | 130 | 26 | 1 | 2 |
| Wheaties | 1 cup (1 oz) | 110 | 24 | 4 | 3 |
| Wheaties Energy Crunch | 1 cup (1.9 oz) | 210 | 42 | 13 | 4 |
| Wheaties Frosted | ¾ cup (1 oz) | 110 | 27 | 12 | – |
| Wheaties Raisin Bran | 1 cup (1.9 oz) | 180 | 45 | 18 | 5 |
| ***Grainfield's*** | | | | | |
| Brown Rice | 1 serv (1 oz) | 110 | 24 | 1 | tr |
| Crisp Rice | 1 serv (1 oz) | 112 | 25 | 0 | tr |
| Raisin Bran | 1 serv (1 oz) | 90 | 20 | tr | 2 |
| Wheat Flakes | 1 serv (1 oz) | 100 | 20 | tr | 2 |
| ***Gram's Gourmet*** | | | | | |
| Cream Of Flax not prep | ½ cup | 142 | 11 | 1 | 8 |
| Crunch Granolas All Flavors | ½ cup | 349 | 10 | 1 | 6 |
| ***Hansen's*** | | | | | |
| Orange & Chocolate | ½ cup | 230 | 35 | 6 | 4 |
| Strawberry & Yogurt | ½ cup | 230 | 30 | 11 | 6 |
| Toasted Nut Crunch | ½ cup | 230 | 39 | 6 | 7 |
| Tropical Cluster | ½ cup | 210 | 36 | 15 | 6 |
| ***Health Valley*** | | | | | |
| 10 Bran O's Apple Cinnamon | ¾ cup | 100 | 23 | 4 | 3 |
| Bran w/ Apples & Cinnamon | ¾ cup | 160 | 41 | 10 | 7 |
| Golden Flax | ½ cup | 190 | 38 | 8 | 6 |
| Granola 98% Fat Free Date Almond | ⅔ cup | 180 | 43 | 10 | 6 |
| Healthy Crunches & Flakes Almond | ¾ cup | 130 | 31 | 4 | 4 |
| Healthy Crunches & Flakes Apple Cinnamon | ¾ cup | 130 | 31 | 4 | 4 |
| Healthy Crunches & Flakes Honey Crunch | ¾ cup | 130 | 31 | 4 | 4 |
| Hot Cereal Cups Amazing Apple! | 1 pkg | 220 | 43 | 9 | 4 |

| FOOD | PORTION | CALS | CARB | SUGAR | FIBER |
|---|---|---|---|---|---|
| Hot Cereal Cups Banana Gone Nuts! | 1 pkg | 240 | 45 | 9 | 4 |
| Hot Cereal Cups Maple Madness! | 1 pkg | 240 | 47 | 19 | 4 |
| Hot Cereal Cups Terrific 10 Grain! | 1 pkg | 220 | 41 | 8 | 5 |
| Oat Bran O'S | ¾ cup | 100 | 23 | 5 | 3 |
| Organic Amaranth Flakes | ¾ cup | 100 | 24 | 4 | 4 |
| Organic Blue Corn Bran Flakes | ¾ cup | 100 | 24 | 4 | 4 |
| Organic Bran w/ Raisin | ¾ cup | 160 | 40 | 10 | 6 |
| Organic Fiber 7 Flakes | ¾ cup | 100 | 24 | 4 | 4 |
| Organic Healthy Fiber Flakes | ¾ cup | 100 | 23 | 3 | 4 |
| Organic Oat Bran Flakes | ¾ cup | 100 | 24 | 4 | 4 |
| Organic Oat Bran Flakes w/ Raisins | ¾ cup | 110 | 26 | 6 | 4 |
| Puffed Honey Sweetened Corn | 1 cup | 110 | 28 | 7 | 2 |
| Puffed Honey Sweetened Crisp Brown Rice | 1 cup | 110 | 28 | 5 | 2 |
| Raisin Bran Flakes | 1¼ cup | 190 | 47 | 13 | 5 |
| Real Oat Bran | ½ cup | 200 | 34 | 9 | 5 |
| ***Hi-Lo*** | | | | | |
| Low Carb Cereal | ½ cup | 90 | 11 | 1 | 6 |
| ***Hodgson Mill*** | | | | | |
| Bulgur Wheat w/ Soy Grits | ¼ cup | 116 | 22 | 0 | 3 |
| Cracked Wheat | ¼ cup | 110 | 26 | 0 | 8 |
| Multi Grain w/ Flaxseed & Soy | ⅓ cup | 160 | 25 | 1 | 6 |
| ***Kashi*** | | | | | |
| Breakfast Pilaf as prep | ½ cup (4.9 oz) | 170 | 30 | 0 | 6 |
| Go Apple Spice | ½ cup (4.9 oz) | 270 | 56 | 10 | 6 |
| Go Banana Almond | ½ cup (4.9 oz) | 280 | 57 | 11 | 6 |
| Go Berry Tart | ½ cup (4.9 oz) | 260 | 55 | 8 | 6 |
| Go Blueberry Bliss | ½ cup (4.9 oz) | 260 | 55 | 8 | 6 |
| Go Cherry Vanilla | ½ cup (4.9 oz) | 260 | 54 | 15 | 6 |
| Go Just Peachy | ½ cup (4.9 oz) | 260 | 54 | 17 | 6 |
| GoLean | ¾ cup (1.4 oz) | 120 | 28 | 7 | 10 |
| Good Friends | ¾ cup (1 oz) | 90 | 24 | 6 | 8 |
| Honey Puffed | 1 cup (1 oz) | 120 | 25 | 7 | 2 |
| Medley | ½ cup (1 oz) | 100 | 20 | 5 | 2 |
| Pillows Apple | ¾ cup (1.9 oz) | 200 | 45 | 19 | 2 |
| Pillows Chocolate | ¾ cup (1.9 oz) | 200 | 45 | 19 | 2 |

| FOOD | PORTION | CALS | CARB | SUGAR | FIBER |
|---|---|---|---|---|---|
| Pillows Strawberry Crisp | ¾ cup (1.9 oz) | 200 | 46 | 19 | 2 |
| Puffed | 1 cup (0.9 oz) | 70 | 13 | 0 | 2 |
| ***Kellogg's*** | | | | | |
| Corn Pops K-Sentials | 1 oz | 100 | 25 | 13 | 0 |
| Froot Loops K-Sentials | 1 oz | 100 | 24 | 11 | 0 |
| ***Keto*** | | | | | |
| Cocoa Crisp | ½ cup | 110 | 4 | 0 | 1 |
| Frosted Flakes All Flavors | ¾ cup | 110 | 9 | tr | 2 |
| Hot Cereal Apple Cinnamon | 2 scoops | 150 | 12 | tr | 9 |
| Hot Cereal Strawberry & Creme | 2 scoops | 150 | 12 | tr | 9 |
| Low Carb Crispy Soy | ¾ cup | 110 | 2 | 0 | 0 |
| Oatmeal Old Fashioned | 2 scoops | 150 | 12 | tr | 9 |
| ***Lundberg*** | | | | | |
| Purely Organic Hot'n Creamy Rice | ⅓ cup | 190 | 43 | 0 | 3 |
| ***McCann's*** | | | | | |
| Irish Oatmeal Instant Apples & Cinnamon | 1 pkg (1 oz) | 130 | 26 | 13 | 2 |
| Irish Oatmeal Instant Maple & Brown Sugar | 1 pkg (1 oz) | 160 | 32 | 14 | 3 |
| Irish Oatmeal Instant Regular | 1 pkg (1 oz) | 100 | 18 | 1 | 3 |
| ***MiniCarb*** | | | | | |
| Milk Chocolate Hot Cereal not prep | ½ cup | 140 | 17 | 2 | 13 |
| ***Post*** | | | | | |
| Alpha-Bits Marshmallow | 1 cup (1 oz) | 120 | 25 | 14 | 0 |
| Grape-Nuts Flakes | ¾ cup (1 oz) | 100 | 24 | 5 | 3 |
| Selects Blueberry Morning | ¾ cup (1.3 oz) | 140 | 30 | 9 | 2 |
| ***Quaker*** | | | | | |
| Oatmeal Instant Apples & Cinnamon | 1 pkg (1.2 oz) | 130 | 27 | 12 | 3 |
| Oatmeal Instant Cinnamon & Spice | 1 pkg (1.6 oz) | 170 | 35 | 16 | 3 |
| Oatmeal Instant Maple & Brown Sugar | 1 pkg (1.5 oz) | 160 | 32 | 13 | 3 |
| Oatmeal Nutrition for Women Golden Brown Sugar | 1 pkg (1.6 oz) | 170 | 33 | 13 | 3 |
| ***Sunbelt*** | | | | | |
| Berry Basic | ½ cup (1.9 oz) | 220 | 40 | 12 | 5 |
| Granola Banana Nut | ½ cup (1.9 oz) | 250 | 37 | 13 | 4 |

| FOOD | PORTION | CALS | CARB | SUGAR | FIBER |
|---|---|---|---|---|---|
| Granola Cinnamon Raisins | ½ cup (1.9 oz) | 200 | 42 | 20 | 4 |
| Granola Fruit & Nut | ½ cup (1.9 oz) | 240 | 40 | 21 | 3 |
| Muesli 5 Whole Grains | ½ cup (1.9 oz) | 210 | 44 | 17 | 3 |
| ***Uncle Sam*** | | | | | |
| Cereal | 1 cup (1.9 oz) | 190 | 38 | tr | 10 |
| ***Weetabix*** | | | | | |
| Cereal | 2 biscuits (1.2 oz) | 100 | 21 | 2 | 3 |
| ***Wheatena*** | | | | | |
| Cereal | ⅓ cup (1.4 oz) | 150 | 33 | 0 | 5 |
| **CEREAL BARS** *(see also* ENERGY BARS*)* | | | | | |
| granola | 1 (1 oz) | 134 | 18 | 7 | 2 |
| ***Barbara's Bakery*** | | | | | |
| Nature's Choice Apple Cinnamon | 1 bar (1.3 oz) | 120 | 27 | 11 | 2 |
| Nature's Choice Blueberry | 1 bar (⅓ oz) | 120 | 27 | 11 | 2 |
| Nature's Choice Cherry | 1 bar (1.3 oz) | 120 | 27 | 11 | 2 |
| Nature's Choice Granola Carob Chip | 1 bar (0.7 oz) | 80 | 16 | 8 | 2 |
| Nature's Choice Granola Cinnamon & Raisin | 1 bar (0.7 oz) | 80 | 16 | 7 | 3 |
| Nature's Choice Granola Oats 'N Honey | 1 bar (0.7 oz) | 80 | 15 | 7 | 2 |
| Nature's Choice Granola Peanut Butter | 1 bar (0.7 oz) | 80 | 14 | 7 | 2 |
| Nature's Choice Raspberry | 1 bar (1.3 oz) | 120 | 27 | 11 | 2 |
| Nature's Choice Strawberry | 1 bar (1.3 oz) | 120 | 27 | 11 | 2 |
| Nature's Choice Triple Berry | 1 bar (1.3 oz) | 120 | 27 | 11 | 2 |
| ***Dolly Madison*** | | | | | |
| Apple | 1 (1.3 oz) | 120 | 25 | 14 | 1 |
| Blueberry | 1 (1.3 oz) | 120 | 25 | 14 | 1 |
| Raspberry | 1 (1.3 oz) | 120 | 24 | 14 | 1 |
| Strawberry | 1 (1.3 oz) | 120 | 24 | 14 | 1 |
| ***Entenmann's*** | | | | | |
| Apple Cinnamon | 1 (1.3 oz) | 140 | 25 | 15 | tr |
| Blueberry | 1 (1.3 oz) | 140 | 25 | 15 | tr |
| Multi-Grain Chocolate Chip | 1 | 140 | 28 | 16 | 2 |
| Multi-Grain Rainbow Chip | 1 | 180 | 26 | 15 | tr |
| Multi-Grain Real Raspberry | 1 | 140 | 26 | 16 | 1 |

| FOOD | PORTION | CALS | CARB | SUGAR | FIBER |
|---|---|---|---|---|---|
| Oatmeal Apple Cinnamon | 1 (1.3 oz) | 140 | 27 | 15 | 1 |
| Oatmeal Apple Raisin | 1 (1.3 oz) | 140 | 27 | 15 | 1 |
| Raspberry | 1 (1.3 oz) | 140 | 27 | 15 | 1 |
| Strawberry | 1 (1.3 oz) | 140 | 25 | 15 | tr |
| ***Estee*** | | | | | |
| Rice Crunchie Chocolate | 1 (0.7 oz) | 50 | 15 | 0 | tr |
| Rice Crunchie Chocolate Chip | 1 (0.7 oz) | 50 | 15 | 0 | 0 |
| Rice Crunchie Peanut Butter | 1 (0.7 oz) | 60 | 15 | 0 | 0 |
| Rice Crunchie Vanilla | 1 (0.7 oz) | 60 | 14 | 0 | 0 |
| ***General Mills*** | | | | | |
| Milk 'N Cereal Bars Chex | 1 bar (1.6 oz) | 160 | 26 | 13 | – |
| Milk 'N Cereal Bars Cinnamon Toast Crunch | 1 bar (1.6 oz) | 180 | 30 | 19 | 1 |
| Oatmeal Crisp Apple | 1 bar (1.4 oz) | 150 | 31 | 15 | 1 |
| Oatmeal Crisp Strawberry | 1 bar (1.4 oz) | 140 | 30 | 14 | 1 |
| ***Glenny's*** | | | | | |
| Chocolate Crunch Creamy Low Fat | 1 bar (1.75 oz) | 190 | 36 | 17 | 4 |
| Chocolate Crunch Roasted Peanut | 1 bar (1.75 oz) | 200 | 36 | 14 | 6 |
| Chocolate Crunch Toasted Almond | 1 bar (1.75 oz) | 200 | 36 | 14 | 6 |
| ***Health Valley*** | | | | | |
| 98% Fat Free Raisin Cinnamon | ⅔ cup | 180 | 43 | 10 | 6 |
| 98% Fat Free Tropical | ⅔ cup | 180 | 43 | 10 | 6 |
| Blueberry | 1 | 140 | 35 | 14 | 3 |
| Breakfast Bakes Apple Cinnamon | 1 bar | 110 | 26 | 13 | 3 |
| Breakfast Bakes California Strawberry | 1 bar | 110 | 26 | 13 | 3 |
| Breakfast Bakes Mountain Blueberry | 1 bar | 110 | 26 | 13 | 3 |
| Breakfast Bakes Red Raspberry | 1 bar | 110 | 26 | 13 | 3 |
| Chocolate Chip | 1 | 140 | 35 | 14 | 3 |
| Crisp Rice Bars Apple Cinnamon | 1 | 110 | 26 | 15 | 1 |
| Crisp Rice Bars Orange Date | 1 | 110 | 26 | 15 | 1 |
| Crisp Rice Bars Tropical Fruit | 1 | 110 | 26 | 15 | 1 |
| Date Almond | 1 | 140 | 35 | 14 | 3 |

| FOOD | PORTION | CALS | CARB | SUGAR | FIBER |
|---|---|---|---|---|---|
| Fiber 7 Flakes w/ Strawberry | 1 bar | 110 | 26 | 13 | 3 |
| O's Almond | ¾ cup | 120 | 26 | 3 | 3 |
| O's Apple Cinnamon | ¾ cup | 120 | 26 | 3 | 3 |
| O's Honey Crunch | ¾ cup | 120 | 26 | 3 | 3 |
| Oat Bran Flakes w/ Blueberry | 1 bar | 110 | 26 | 13 | 3 |
| Raisin | 1 | 140 | 35 | 14 | 3 |
| Raisin Bran Flakes w/ Apple Raisin | 1 bar | 110 | 26 | 13 | 3 |
| Raspberry | 1 | 140 | 35 | 14 | 3 |
| Strawberry | 1 | 140 | 35 | 14 | 3 |
| ***Hershey's*** | | | | | |
| Crispy Rice Snacks Peanut Butter | 1 bar (0.5 oz) | 60 | 9 | 5 | tr |
| ***Hostess*** | | | | | |
| Apple | 1 (1.3 oz) | 120 | 25 | 14 | 1 |
| Banana Nut | 1 (1.3 oz) | 120 | 25 | 14 | 2 |
| Blueberry | 1 (1.3 oz) | 120 | 25 | 14 | 1 |
| Raspberry | 1 (1.3 oz) | 120 | 24 | 14 | 1 |
| Strawberry | 1 (1.3 oz) | 120 | 24 | 14 | 1 |
| ***Kudos*** | | | | | |
| Chocolate Coated Chocolate Chip | 1 | 120 | 20 | 13 | 1 |
| Chocolate Coated Peanut Butter | 1 | 90 | 17 | 9 | 1 |
| Snickers | 1 | 100 | 16 | 10 | 0 |
| With M&M's | 1 | 90 | 17 | 9 | 1 |
| ***Little Debbie*** | | | | | |
| Raspberry | 1 (1.3 oz) | 130 | 28 | 18 | tr |
| S'mores Granola Treats | 1 (1 oz) | 130 | 21 | 12 | 1 |
| Strawberry | 1 (1.3 oz) | 130 | 28 | 18 | tr |
| ***Nabisco*** | | | | | |
| Nutter Butter Granola Bar | 1 (1 oz) | 120 | 21 | 9 | tr |
| Oreo Granola Bar | 1 (1 oz) | 120 | 21 | 9 | 1 |
| ***Nature Valley*** | | | | | |
| Low Fat Chewy Orchard Blend | 1 bar (1 oz) | 110 | 22 | 8 | 1 |
| ***Nutri-Grain*** | | | | | |
| Fruit-full Squares Apple | 1 (1.7 oz) | 180 | 35 | 17 | 1 |
| Fruit-full Squares Banana | 1 (1.7 oz) | 190 | 35 | 17 | 1 |
| Fruit-full Squares Cinnamon Raisin | 1 (1.7 oz) | 180 | 35 | 17 | 1 |
| Minis Strawberry | 1 pkg (1.5 oz) | 160 | 32 | 18 | 1 |

| FOOD | PORTION | CALS | CARB | SUGAR | FIBER |
|---|---|---|---|---|---|
| Twists Low Fat Apple Cinnamon | 1 (1.3 oz) | 140 | 27 | 12 | 1 |
| Twists Low Fat Banana Strawberry | 1 (1.3 oz) | 140 | 26 | 14 | 1 |
| Twists Low Fat Strawberry Blueberry | 1 (1.3 oz) | 140 | 27 | 12 | 1 |
| ***Quaker*** | | | | | |
| Chewy Chocolate Chip | 1 (1 oz) | 120 | 21 | 9 | 1 |
| Chewy Cookies 'n Cream | 1 (1 oz) | 110 | 22 | 10 | 1 |
| Chewy Peanut Butter Chocolate Chunk | 1 (1 oz) | 120 | 20 | 9 | 1 |
| Chewy Graham Slam Chocolate Chip | 1 (1 oz) | 110 | 22 | 10 | 1 |
| Chewy Graham Slam Peanut Butter | 1 (1 oz) | 110 | 22 | 9 | 1 |
| Chewy Low Fat Chocolate Chunk | 1 (1 oz) | 110 | 22 | 10 | 1 |
| Chewy Low Fat Oatmeal Raisin | 1 (1 oz) | 110 | 22 | 10 | 1 |
| Chewy Low Fat S'mores | 1 (1 oz) | 110 | 22 | 10 | 1 |
| Fruit & Oatmeal Apple Cinnamon | 1 (1.3 oz) | 130 | 26 | 15 | 1 |
| Fruit & Oatmeal Bites Apple Crisp | 1 pkg | 140 | 27 | 15 | 1 |
| Fruit & Oatmeal Bites Strawberry | 1 pkg | 140 | 27 | 14 | 1 |
| Fruit & Oatmeal Bites Very Berry | 1 pkg | 140 | 27 | 14 | 1 |
| Fruit & Oatmeal Low Fat Cherry Cobbler | 1 (1.3 oz) | 140 | 26 | 15 | 1 |
| Fruit & Oatmeal Low Fat Strawberry | 1 (1.3 oz) | 140 | 26 | 15 | 1 |
| Fruit & Oatmeal Low Fat Strawberry Banana | 1 (1.3 oz) | 130 | 26 | 15 | tr |
| Fruit & Oatmeal Low Fat Strawberry Cheesecake | 1 (1.3 oz) | 130 | 26 | 14 | tr |
| ***Rice Krispies*** | | | | | |
| Treats | 1 (0.8 oz) | 90 | 18 | 8 | 0 |
| Treats Peanut Butter Chocolate | 1 (0.8 oz) | 110 | 16 | 9 | 0 |
| Treats Cocoa | 1 (0.8 oz) | 100 | 16 | 7 | 0 |
| ***SnackWell's*** | | | | | |
| Country Fruit Medley | 1 (1.3 oz) | 130 | 27 | 13 | tr |

| FOOD | PORTION | CALS | CARB | SUGAR | FIBER |
|---|---|---|---|---|---|
| Fat Free Apple Cinnamon | 1 (1.3 oz) | 120 | 28 | 15 | 1 |
| Fat Free Blueberry | 1 (1.3 oz) | 120 | 28 | 15 | 1 |
| Fat Free Strawberry | 1 (1.3 oz) | 120 | 28 | 16 | 1 |
| Hearty Fruit'n Grain Crisp Autumn Apple | 1 (1.3 oz) | 130 | 25 | 14 | 1 |
| Hearty Fruit'n Grain Mixed Berry | 1 (1.3 oz) | 120 | 25 | 14 | 1 |
| Hearty Fruit'n Grain Orchard Cherry | 1 (1.3 oz) | 130 | 26 | 14 | 1 |
| ***Sunbelt*** | | | | | |
| Apple | 1 (1.3 oz) | 130 | 28 | 18 | tr |
| Blueberry | 1 (1.3 oz) | 130 | 28 | 18 | tr |
| Chewy Granola Almond | 1 (1 oz) | 130 | 17 | 8 | 1 |
| Chewy Granola Apple Cinnamon | 1 (1.2 oz) | 140 | 28 | 14 | 2 |
| Chewy Granola Chocolate Chip | 1 (1.2 oz) | 160 | 23 | 12 | 2 |
| Chewy Granola Oatmeal Raisin | 1 (1.2 oz) | 130 | 27 | 15 | 1 |
| Chewy Granola Oats & Honey | 1 (1 oz) | 120 | 19 | 9 | 1 |
| Granola Fudge Dipped Chocolate Chip | 1 (1.5 oz) | 200 | 27 | 16 | 2 |
| Granola Fudge Dipped Macaroon | 1 (1.4 oz) | 190 | 24 | 14 | 1 |
| ***Weight Watchers*** | | | | | |
| Apple Cinnamon | 1 (1 oz) | 100 | 21 | 12 | 2 |
| Blueberry | 1 (1 oz) | 100 | 21 | 10 | 1 |
| Raspberry | 1 (1 oz) | 100 | 21 | 12 | 2 |
| **CHAMPAGNE** | | | | | |
| mimosa | 1 serv | 117 | 12 | – | tr |
| punch | 1 serv | 113 | 5 | – | 0 |
| sekt german champagne | 3.5 fl oz | 84 | 5 | – | – |
| ***Andre*** | | | | | |
| Blush | 4 fl oz | 88 | 4 | – | – |
| Brut | 4 fl oz | 84 | 4 | – | – |
| Cold Duck | 4 fl oz | 100 | 8 | – | – |
| Extra Dry | 4 fl oz | 92 | 4 | – | – |
| ***Ballatore*** | | | | | |
| Spumante | 4 fl oz | 92 | 8 | – | – |

| FOOD | PORTION | CALS | CARB | SUGAR | FIBER |
|---|---|---|---|---|---|
| ***Eden Roc*** | | | | | |
| Brut | 4 fl oz | 92 | 4 | – | – |
| Brut Rosé | 4 fl oz | 99 | 8 | – | – |
| Extra Dry | 4 fl oz | 84 | 4 | – | – |
| ***Tott's*** | | | | | |
| Blanc de Noir | 4 fl oz | 88 | 8 | – | – |
| Brut | 4 fl oz | 80 | tr | – | – |
| Extra Dry | 4 fl oz | 84 | 4 | – | – |
| **CHAYOTE** | | | | | |
| fresh cooked | 1 cup | 38 | 8 | – | – |
| raw | 1 (7 oz) | 49 | 11 | – | – |
| **CHEESE** *(see also* CHEESE DISHES, CHEESE SUBSTITUTES, COTTAGE CHEESE, CREAM CHEESE, NEUFCHATEL*)* | | | | | |
| american | 1 oz | 93 | 2 | – | – |
| american cheese food | 1 pkg (8 oz) | 745 | 17 | – | – |
| american cheese spread | 1 jar (5 oz) | 412 | 12 | – | – |
| american cold pack | 1 pkg (8 oz) | 752 | 19 | – | – |
| american cheese spread | 1 oz | 82 | 2 | – | – |
| beaufort | 1 oz | 115 | tr | tr | 0 |
| bel paese | 1 oz | 112 | 0 | 0 | 0 |
| blue | 1 oz | 100 | 1 | – | – |
| blue crumbled | 1 cup (4.7 oz) | 477 | 3 | – | – |
| brick | 1 oz | 105 | 1 | – | – |
| brie | 1 oz | 95 | tr | – | – |
| cacio di roma sheep's milk cheese | 1 oz | 130 | 0 | 0 | 0 |
| caerphilly | 1.4 oz | 150 | 0 | 0 | 0 |
| camembert | 1 oz | 85 | tr | – | – |
| camembert | 1 wedge (1⅓ oz) | 114 | tr | – | – |
| cantal | 1 oz | 105 | tr | tr | 0 |
| caraway | 1 oz | 107 | 1 | – | – |
| chabichou | 1 oz | 95 | tr | tr | 0 |
| chaource | 1 oz | 83 | tr | tr | 0 |
| cheddar | 1 oz | 114 | tr | – | – |
| cheddar low fat | 1 oz | 49 | 1 | – | – |
| cheddar low sodium | 1 oz | 113 | 1 | – | – |
| cheddar reduced fat | 1.4 oz | 104 | 0 | 0 | 0 |
| cheddar shredded | 1 cup | 455 | 1 | – | – |

| FOOD | PORTION | CALS | CARB | SUGAR | FIBER |
|---|---|---|---|---|---|
| cheshire | 1 oz | 110 | 1 | – | – |
| cheshire reduced fat | 1.4 oz | 108 | tr | – | 0 |
| colby | 1 oz | 112 | 1 | – | – |
| colby low fat | 1 oz | 49 | 1 | – | – |
| colby low sodium | 1 oz | 113 | 1 | – | – |
| comte | 1 oz | 114 | tr | tr | 0 |
| coulommiers | 1 oz | 88 | tr | tr | 0 |
| crottin | 1 oz | 105 | tr | tr | 0 |
| derby | 1.4 oz | 161 | 0 | 0 | 0 |
| edam | 1 oz | 101 | tr | – | – |
| edam reduced fat | 1.4 oz | 92 | tr | – | 0 |
| emmentaler | 1 oz | 115 | tr | – | – |
| feta | 1 oz | 75 | 1 | – | – |
| fontina | 1 oz | 110 | tr | – | – |
| frais | 1.6 oz | 51 | 3 | – | 0 |
| gjetost | 1 oz | 132 | 12 | – | – |
| gloucester double | 1.4 oz | 162 | 0 | 0 | 0 |
| goat fresh | 1 oz | 23 | tr | tr | 0 |
| goat hard | 1 oz | 128 | 1 | – | – |
| goat semisoft | 1 oz | 103 | 1 | – | – |
| goat soft | 1 oz | 76 | tr | – | – |
| gorgonzola | 1 oz | 107 | tr | – | – |
| gouda | 1 oz | 101 | 1 | – | – |
| gruyere | 1 oz | 117 | tr | – | – |
| lancashire | 1.4 oz | 149 | 0 | 0 | 0 |
| leicester | 1.4 oz | 160 | 0 | 0 | 0 |
| limburger | 1 oz | 93 | tr | – | – |
| lymeswold | 1.4 oz | 170 | tr | – | 0 |
| maroilles | 1 oz | 97 | tr | tr | 0 |
| monterey | 1 oz | 106 | tr | – | – |
| morbier | 1 oz | 99 | tr | tr | 0 |
| mozzarella | 1 oz | 80 | 1 | – | – |
| mozzarella | 1 lb | 1276 | 10 | – | – |
| mozzarella fresh | 1 oz | 80 | tr | 0 | 0 |
| mozzarella low moisture | 1 oz | 90 | 1 | – | – |
| mozzarella part skim | 1 oz | 72 | 1 | – | – |
| muenster | 1 oz | 104 | tr | – | – |
| parmesan grated | 1 oz | 129 | 1 | – | – |
| parmesan grated | 1 tbsp (5 g) | 23 | tr | – | – |
| parmesan hard | 1 oz | 111 | 1 | – | – |

| FOOD | PORTION | CALS | CARB | SUGAR | FIBER |
|---|---|---|---|---|---|
| picodon | 1 oz | 99 | tr | tr | 0 |
| pimento | 1 oz | 106 | tr | – | – |
| pont l'eveque | 1 oz | 86 | tr | tr | 0 |
| port du salut | 1 oz | 100 | tr | – | – |
| provolone | 1 oz | 100 | 1 | – | – |
| pyrenees | 1 oz | 101 | tr | tr | 0 |
| quark 20% fat | 1 oz | 33 | 1 | – | – |
| quark 40% fat | 1 oz | 48 | 1 | – | – |
| quark made w/ skim milk | 1 oz | 22 | 1 | – | – |
| queso anego | 1 oz | 106 | 1 | – | – |
| queso asadero | 1 oz | 101 | 1 | – | – |
| queso chihuahua | 1 oz | 106 | 2 | – | – |
| queso fresco | 1 oz | 41 | 1 | – | 0 |
| queso manchego | 1 oz | 107 | tr | – | 0 |
| queso panela | 1 oz | 74 | 1 | – | 0 |
| raclette | 1 oz | 102 | tr | tr | 0 |
| reblochon | 1 oz | 88 | tr | tr | 0 |
| ricotta part skim | ½ cup (4.4 oz) | 171 | 6 | – | – |
| ricotta part skim | 1 cup (8.6 oz) | 340 | 13 | – | – |
| ricotta whole milk | 1 cup (8.6 oz) | 428 | 7 | – | – |
| ricotta whole milk | ½ cup (4.4 oz) | 216 | 4 | – | – |
| romadur 40% fat | 1 oz | 83 | tr | – | – |
| romano | 1 oz | 110 | 1 | – | – |
| roquefort | 1 oz | 105 | 1 | – | – |
| rouy | 1 oz | 95 | tr | tr | 0 |
| saint marcellin | 1 oz | 94 | tr | tr | 0 |
| saint nectaire | 1 oz | 97 | tr | tr | 0 |
| saint paulin | 1 oz | 85 | tr | tr | 0 |
| sainte maure | 1 oz | 99 | tr | tr | 0 |
| selles sur cher | 1 oz | 93 | tr | tr | 0 |
| stilton blue | 1.4 oz | 164 | 0 | 0 | 0 |
| stilton white | 1.4 oz | 145 | 0 | 0 | 0 |
| swiss | 1 oz | 107 | 1 | – | – |
| swiss cheese food | 1 pkg (8 oz) | 734 | 10 | – | – |
| swiss processed | 1 oz | 95 | 1 | – | – |
| tilsit | 1 oz | 96 | 1 | – | – |
| tome | 1 oz | 92 | tr | tr | 0 |
| triple creme | 1 oz | 113 | tr | tr | 0 |
| vacherin | 1 oz | 92 | tr | tr | 0 |
| wensleydale | 1.4 oz | 151 | 0 | 0 | 0 |

| FOOD | PORTION | CALS | CARB | SUGAR | FIBER |
|---|---|---|---|---|---|
| whey cheese | 1 oz | 126 | 9 | 0 | 0 |
| yogurt cheese | 1 oz | 80 | 0 | 0 | 0 |
| ***Alouette*** | | | | | |
| Garlic & Herbs | 2 tbsp (0.8 oz) | 70 | 1 | tr | 0 |
| ***Alpine Lace*** | | | | | |
| American Jalapeno Peppers | 1 slice (1 oz) | 80 | 2 | 0 | 0 |
| American Less Fat Less Sodium White | 1 slice (1 oz) | 50 | 2 | 0 | 0 |
| American Less Fat Less Sodium Yellow | 1 slice (1 oz) | 80 | 2 | 0 | 0 |
| Cheddar Reduced Fat | 1 slice (1 oz) | 70 | 1 | 0 | 0 |
| Colby Reduced Fat | 1 slice (1 oz) | 80 | 1 | 0 | 0 |
| Fat Free Parmesan | 2 tsp (5 g) | 10 | 0 | 0 | 0 |
| Feta Reduced Fat | 1 oz | 50 | 1 | 0 | 0 |
| Feta Reduced Fat Sun Dried Tomato & Basil | 1 oz | 50 | 1 | 0 | 0 |
| Goat Reduced Fat | 1 oz | 40 | tr | 0 | 0 |
| Mozzarella Reduced Fat | 1 oz | 70 | 1 | 0 | 0 |
| Muenster Reduced Sodium | 1 slice (1 oz) | 100 | 1 | 0 | 0 |
| Provolone Smoked Reduced Fat | 1 slice (1 oz) | 70 | 1 | 0 | 0 |
| Swiss Reduced Fat | 1 slice (1 oz) | 90 | 1 | 0 | 0 |
| ***Athenos*** | | | | | |
| Feta | 1 oz | 80 | tr | 0 | 0 |
| ***Boar's Head*** | | | | | |
| American | 1 oz | 100 | 1 | 0 | 0 |
| Baby Swiss | 1 oz | 110 | tr | 0 | 0 |
| Canadian Cheddar | 1 oz | 110 | 0 | 0 | 0 |
| Double Gloucester Yellow | 1 oz | 110 | 0 | 0 | 0 |
| Feta | 1 oz | 60 | 1 | 0 | 0 |
| Havarti | 1 oz | 110 | 0 | 0 | 0 |
| Havarti w/ Dill | 1 oz | 110 | 0 | 0 | 0 |
| Havarti w/ Jalapeno | 1 oz | 110 | 0 | 0 | 0 |
| Lacey Swiss | 1 oz | 90 | 0 | 0 | 0 |
| Longhorn Colby | 1 oz | 110 | tr | 0 | 0 |
| Monterey Jack | 1 oz | 100 | 0 | 0 | 0 |
| Monterey Jack w/ Jalapeno | 1 oz | 100 | 0 | 0 | 0 |
| Mozzarella | 1 oz | 90 | tr | 0 | 0 |
| Muenster | 1 oz | 100 | 0 | 0 | 0 |

| FOOD | PORTION | CALS | CARB | SUGAR | FIBER |
|---|---|---|---|---|---|
| Muenster Low Sodium | 1 oz | 100 | 0 | 0 | 0 |
| Provolone Picante Sharp | 1 oz | 100 | 1 | 0 | 0 |
| Swiss | 1 oz | 110 | tr | 0 | 0 |
| Swiss No Salt Added | 1 oz | 110 | tr | 0 | 0 |
| ***Bonbel*** | | | | | |
| Mini Babybel | 1 piece (0.7 oz) | 70 | 0 | 0 | 0 |
| ***Boursin*** | | | | | |
| Garlic & Fine Herbs | 2 tbsp | 120 | tr | – | – |
| ***Cabot*** | | | | | |
| American | 1 slice (0.7 oz) | 80 | 1 | 0 | 0 |
| Cheddar | 1 oz | 110 | tr | 0 | 0 |
| Cheddar Smoked | 1 oz | 110 | tr | 0 | 0 |
| Cheddar Light 50% Reduced Fat | 1 oz | 70 | 1 | 0 | 0 |
| Cheddar Light 50% Reduced Fat Jalapeno | 1 oz | 70 | 1 | 0 | 0 |
| Cheddar Light 75% Reduced Fat | 1 oz | 60 | tr | 0 | 0 |
| Colby Jack | 1 oz | 110 | 7 | 0 | 0 |
| Fancy Blend Shredded | ¼ cup | 100 | 1 | 0 | 0 |
| Monterey Jack | 1 oz | 110 | tr | 0 | 0 |
| Mozzarella Shredded | ¼ cup | 80 | 1 | 0 | 0 |
| Pepper Jack | 1 oz | 110 | tr | 0 | 0 |
| Swiss Slices | 1 slice (1 oz) | 110 | 1 | 0 | 0 |
| ***Cedar Grove*** | | | | | |
| Marble Colby | 1 oz | 110 | 0 | 0 | 0 |
| Organic Tomato Basil Cheddar | 1 oz | 110 | 0 | 0 | 0 |
| ***Chavrie*** | | | | | |
| Goat's Milk | 2 tbsp | 50 | 1 | 1 | 0 |
| ***Connoisseur*** | | | | | |
| Asiago Spread | 1 tbsp | 90 | 2 | 2 | 0 |
| ***Fleurs De France*** | | | | | |
| Brie | 3.5 oz | 311 | tr | 0 | tr |
| ***Friendship*** | | | | | |
| Farmer | 2 tbsp (1 oz) | 50 | 0 | 0 | 0 |
| ***Hollow Road Farms*** | | | | | |
| Sheep's Milk | 1 oz | 45 | 1 | – | – |

| FOOD | PORTION | CALS | CARB | SUGAR | FIBER |
|---|---|---|---|---|---|
| ***Land O Lakes*** | | | | | |
| American | 1 slice (0.7 oz) | 80 | 1 | 0 | 0 |
| American Jalapeno | 1 slice (0.6 oz) | 70 | 1 | tr | 0 |
| American Light | 1 oz | 70 | 2 | 0 | 0 |
| American Reduced Salt | 1 oz | 110 | tr | 0 | 0 |
| American Sharp | 2 slices (1 oz) | 100 | 1 | tr | 0 |
| American & Swiss | 1 slice (0.6 oz) | 70 | 1 | 0 | 0 |
| Baby Swiss | 1 oz | 110 | 0 | 0 | 0 |
| Chedarella | 1 oz | 100 | 0 | 0 | 0 |
| Cheddar | 1 oz | 100 | tr | 0 | 0 |
| Cheddar Extra Sharp | 1 oz | 110 | tr | 0 | 0 |
| Cheddar Sharp | 1 oz | 110 | tr | 0 | 0 |
| Cheese Spread Golden Velvet | 1 oz | 80 | 2 | 2 | 0 |
| Colby | 1 oz | 110 | tr | 0 | 0 |
| Jalapeno Light | 1 oz | 70 | 1 | 0 | 0 |
| Monterey Jack | 1 oz | 110 | tr | 0 | 0 |
| Monterey Jack Hot Pepper | 1 oz | 110 | tr | 0 | 0 |
| Mozzarella | 1 oz | 80 | tr | 0 | 0 |
| Muenster | 1 oz | 100 | 0 | 0 | 0 |
| Parmesan Grated | 1 tbsp | 35 | 0 | 0 | 0 |
| Provolone | 1 oz | 100 | tr | 0 | 0 |
| Swiss | 1 oz | 110 | tr | 0 | 0 |
| Swiss Light | 1 oz | 80 | tr | 0 | 0 |
| ***Organic Valley*** | | | | | |
| Aged Swiss Unpasteurized | 1 oz | 100 | tr | 0 | 0 |
| Cheddar Reduced Fat Low Sodium | 1 oz | 90 | 1 | 0 | 0 |
| Cheddar Sharp & Mild | 1 oz | 110 | 1 | 0 | 0 |
| Cheddar Sharp & Mild Unpasteurized | 1 oz | 110 | 1 | 0 | 0 |
| Colby | 1 oz | 110 | 1 | 0 | 0 |
| Colby Unpasteurized | 1 oz | 110 | 1 | 0 | 0 |
| Farmer Reduced Fat | 1 oz | 90 | 1 | 0 | 0 |
| Feta | 1 oz | 90 | 0 | 0 | 0 |
| Monterey Jack | 1 oz | 100 | 1 | 0 | 0 |
| Monterey Jack Reduced Fat | 1 oz | 80 | 1 | 0 | 0 |
| Mozzarella Part Skim | 1 oz | 80 | 1 | 0 | 0 |

| FOOD | PORTION | CALS | CARB | SUGAR | FIBER |
|---|---|---|---|---|---|
| Muenster | 1 oz | 100 | 1 | 0 | 0 |
| Pepper Jack | 1 oz | 110 | 1 | 0 | 0 |
| Provolone | 1 oz | 100 | 1 | 0 | 0 |
| String Part Skim | 1 oz | 80 | 1 | 0 | 0 |
| Wisconsin Raw Milk Cheese | 1 oz | 100 | 1 | 0 | 0 |
| ***Rouge Et Noir*** | | | | | |
| Breakfast | 1 oz | 86 | 1 | – | – |
| Brie | 1 oz | 86 | 1 | – | – |
| Camembert | 1 oz | 86 | 1 | – | – |
| Schloss | 1 oz | 86 | 1 | – | – |
| ***Sargento*** | | | | | |
| Blue Crumbled | ¼ cup (1 oz) | 100 | 1 | 0 | 0 |
| Cheddar Extra Sharp | 1 oz | 110 | 1 | 0 | 0 |
| Cheddar Shredded | ¼ cup (1 oz) | 110 | 1 | tr | 0 |
| Cheese For Nachos & Tacos Shredded | ¼ cup (1 oz) | 110 | 1 | 0 | 0 |
| Cheese For Pizza Shredded | ¼ cup (1 oz) | 90 | 0 | 0 | 0 |
| Cheese For Tacos Shredded | ¼ cup (1 oz) | 110 | 1 | 0 | 0 |
| Colby | 1 slice (1 oz) | 110 | 0 | 0 | 0 |
| Colby-Jack Shredded | ¼ cup (1 oz) | 110 | tr | 0 | 0 |
| Jarlsberg | 1 slice (1.2 oz) | 120 | 1 | 0 | 0 |
| Monterey Jack | 1 slice (1 oz) | 100 | 0 | 0 | 0 |
| Monterey Jack Shredded | ¼ cup (1 oz) | 100 | 0 | 0 | 0 |
| MooTown Snackers Cheddar | 1 piece (0.8 oz) | 100 | 1 | 0 | 0 |
| MooTown Snackers Cheddar Mild Light | 1 piece (0.8 oz) | 60 | tr | 0 | 0 |
| MooTown Snackers Cheese & Pretzels | 1 pkg (0.9 oz) | 90 | 12 | 1 | 0 |
| MooTown Snackers Colby-Jack | 1 piece (0.8 oz) | 90 | tr | 0 | 0 |
| MooTown Snackers Pizza Cheese & Sticks | 1 pkg (1 oz) | 100 | 13 | 3 | 0 |
| MooTown Snackers String | 1 piece (0.8 oz) | 70 | tr | 0 | 0 |
| MooTown Snackers String Light | 1 piece (0.8 oz) | 60 | tr | 0 | 0 |
| Mozzarella | 1 slice (1.5 oz) | 130 | 2 | 0 | 0 |

| FOOD | PORTION | CALS | CARB | SUGAR | FIBER |
|---|---|---|---|---|---|
| Mozzarella Shredded | ¼ cup (1 oz) | 80 | 1 | 0 | 0 |
| Muenster | 1 slice (1 oz) | 100 | tr | 0 | 0 |
| Parmesan Grated | 1 tbsp (5 g) | 25 | 0 | 0 | 0 |
| Parmesan Shredded | ¼ cup (1 oz) | 110 | 1 | 0 | 0 |
| Parmesan & Romano Shredded | ¼ cup (1 oz) | 110 | 1 | 0 | 0 |
| Parmesan & Romano Grated | 1 tbsp (5 g) | 25 | 0 | 0 | 0 |
| Pizza Double Cheese Shredded | ¼ cup (1 oz) | 90 | 1 | 0 | 0 |
| Preferred Light Cheddar Mild Shredded | ¼ cup (1 oz) | 70 | tr | 0 | 0 |
| Preferred Light Mozzarella | 1 slice (1.5 oz) | 90 | 0 | 0 | 0 |
| Preferred Light Mozzarella Shredded | ¼ cup (1 oz) | 70 | tr | 0 | 0 |
| Preferred Light Swiss | 1 slice (1 oz) | 80 | tr | 0 | 0 |
| Provolone | 1 slice (1 oz) | 100 | 0 | 0 | 0 |
| Recipe Blend 4 Cheese Mexican Shredded | ¼ cup (1 oz) | 110 | tr | 0 | 0 |
| Recipe Blend 6 Cheese Italian Shredded | ¼ cup (1 oz) | 90 | 0 | 0 | 0 |
| Reduced Fat 4 Cheese Mexican Shredded | ¼ cup (1 oz) | 80 | tr | 0 | 0 |
| Ricotta Light | ¼ cup (2.2 oz) | 60 | 3 | 3 | 0 |
| Ricotta Old Fashioned | ¼ cup (2.2 oz) | 90 | 3 | 3 | 0 |
| Ricotta Part Skim | ¼ cup (2.2 oz) | 80 | 2 | 3 | 0 |
| Swiss | 1 slice (0.7 oz) | 80 | 0 | 0 | 0 |
| Swiss Shredded | ¼ cup (1 oz) | 110 | 0 | 0 | 0 |
| Swiss Wafer Thin | 2 slices (1 oz) | 110 | 0 | 0 | 0 |
| Mozzarella Part Skim Jalapeno | 1 oz | 80 | 1 | 0 | 0 |
| Pizza Cheese Shredded | ¼ cup | 90 | 1 | 0 | 0 |
| ***Suisse Delicat*** | | | | | |
| Healthy Swiss | 1 oz | 90 | 0 | 0 | 0 |
| ***Tree Of Life*** | | | | | |
| Cheddar 33% Reduced Fat Organic Milk | 1 oz | 90 | 1 | – | – |
| Colby | 1 oz | 110 | 1 | – | – |
| Colby Organic Milk | 1 oz | 120 | 1 | – | – |
| Farmer Part Skim Organic Milk | 1 oz | 90 | 1 | – | – |
| Jalapeno Organic Milk | 1 oz | 110 | 1 | – | – |

| FOOD | PORTION | CALS | CARB | SUGAR | FIBER |
|---|---|---|---|---|---|
| Monterey Jack 35% Reduced Fat Organic Milk | 1 oz | 80 | 1 | – | – |
| Monterey Jack Organic Milk | 1 oz | 100 | 1 | – | – |
| Mozzarella Organic Milk | 1 oz | 80 | 1 | – | – |
| Muenster Organic Milk | 1 oz | 100 | 1 | – | – |
| Provolone | 1 oz | 100 | 1 | – | – |
| ***Weight Watchers*** | | | | | |
| Cheddar Mild Yellow | 1 oz | 80 | 1 | 0 | 0 |
| Cheddar Sharp Yellow | 1 oz | 80 | 1 | 0 | 0 |
| Fat Free Grated Italian Topping | 1 tbsp | 20 | 2 | 1 | 0 |
| Fat Free Reduced Sodium Yellow | 2 slices (0.75 oz) | 30 | 3 | 2 | 0 |
| Fat Free Sharp Cheddar | 2 slices (0.75 oz) | 30 | 3 | 2 | 0 |
| Fat Free Swiss | 2 slices (0.75 oz) | 30 | 2 | 2 | 0 |
| Fat Free White | 2 slices (0.75 oz) | 30 | 3 | 2 | 0 |
| Fat Free Yellow | 2 slices (0.75 oz) | 30 | 3 | 2 | 0 |
| ***Wholesome Valley*** | | | | | |
| Organic American Reduced Fat | 1 slice (0.7 oz) | 50 | 2 | 2 | 0 |
| **CHEESE DISHES** | | | | | |
| **FROZEN** | | | | | |
| ***Banquet*** | | | | | |
| Mozzeralla Nuggets | 6 | 260 | 19 | 3 | 1 |
| ***Fillo Factory*** | | | | | |
| Tyropita Cheese Fillo Appetizers | 5 (5 oz) | 340 | 44 | 1 | 2 |
| ***Health Is Wealth*** | | | | | |
| Mozzarella Stick | 2 (1.3 oz) | 120 | 14 | 0 | 0 |
| **TAKE-OUT** | | | | | |
| cheese omelette as prep w/ 2 eggs | 1 (6.8 oz) | 519 | tr | – | 0 |
| fondue | ½ cup (3.8 oz) | 247 | 4 | – | – |
| souffle | 1 serv (7 oz) | 504 | 18 | 5 | 1 |
| welsh rarebit | 1 slice | 228 | 14 | – | 1 |

| FOOD | PORTION | CALS | CARB | SUGAR | FIBER |
|---|---|---|---|---|---|
| **CHEESE SUBSTITUTES** | | | | | |
| mozzarella | 1 oz | 70 | 7 | – | – |
| ***Sargento*** | | | | | |
| Cheddar Shredded | ¼ cup (1 oz) | 90 | 2 | 0 | 0 |
| Mozzarella Shredded | ¼ cup (1 oz) | 80 | tr | 0 | 0 |
| ***Yves*** | | | | | |
| Good Slice American | 1 slice (0.7 oz) | 35 | 0 | 0 | 0 |
| Good Slice Cheddar | 1 slice (0.7 oz) | 35 | 1 | 0 | 1 |
| Good Slice Jalapeno Jack | 1 slice (0.7 oz) | 35 | 0 | 0 | 0 |
| Good Slice Mozzarella | 1 slice (0.7 oz) | 30 | 0 | 0 | 0 |
| Good Slice Swiss | 1 slice (0.7 oz) | 35 | 1 | 0 | 0 |
| **CHERIMOYA** | | | | | |
| fresh | 1 | 515 | 131 | – | – |
| **CHERRIES** | | | | | |
| **CANNED** | | | | | |
| sour in heavy syrup | ½ cup | 232 | 60 | – | – |
| sour in light syrup | ½ cup | 189 | 49 | – | – |
| sour water packed | 1 cup | 87 | 22 | – | – |
| sweet in heavy syrup | ½ cup | 107 | 27 | – | – |
| sweet in light syrup | ½ cup | 85 | 22 | – | – |
| sweet juice pack | ½ cup | 68 | 17 | – | – |
| sweet water pack | ½ cup | 57 | 15 | – | – |
| ***Del Monte*** | | | | | |
| Dark Pitted in Heavy Syrup | ½ cup (4.2 oz) | 100 | 24 | 24 | 1 |
| **DRIED** | | | | | |
| bing unsulfured | ¼ cup | 130 | 31 | 21 | 2 |
| montmorency tart pitted | ⅓ cup | 160 | 36 | 24 | 2 |
| yogurt covered | ¼ cup | 170 | 29 | 22 | 5 |
| **FRESH** | | | | | |
| sour | 1 cup | 51 | 13 | – | – |
| sweet | 10 | 49 | 11 | – | – |
| ***Chiquita*** | | | | | |
| Cherries | 21 | 90 | 22 | 19 | 9 |

| FOOD | PORTION | CALS | CARB | SUGAR | FIBER |
|---|---|---|---|---|---|
| **FROZEN** | | | | | |
| sour unsweetened | 1 cup | 72 | 17 | – | – |
| sweet sweetened | 1 cup | 232 | 58 | – | – |
| **CHERRY JUICE** | | | | | |
| ***Eden*** | | | | | |
| Montmorency Juice | 8 oz | 140 | 33 | 25 | 0 |
| ***Juicy Juice*** | | | | | |
| Drink | 1 box (8.5 oz) | 140 | 34 | 32 | 0 |
| Drink | 1 box (4.23 oz) | 70 | 17 | 16 | 0 |
| ***Mott's*** | | | | | |
| Cherry | 1 box (8 oz) | 120 | 31 | – | – |
| ***Ocean Spray*** | | | | | |
| Black Cherry Blast | 8 oz | 140 | 33 | 33 | 0 |
| ***Squeezit*** | | | | | |
| Cherry Cola | 1 bottle (7 oz) | 110 | 27 | 25 | 0 |
| Chucklin' Cherry | 1 bottle (7 oz) | 110 | 28 | 26 | 0 |
| **CHERVIL** | | | | | |
| seed | 1 tsp | 1 | tr | – | – |
| **CHESTNUTS** | | | | | |
| chinese cooked | 1 oz | 44 | 10 | – | – |
| chinese dried | 1 oz | 103 | 23 | – | – |
| chinese raw | 1 oz | 64 | 14 | – | – |
| chinese roasted | 1 oz | 68 | 15 | – | – |
| cooked | 1 oz | 37 | 8 | – | – |
| creme de marrons | 1 oz | 73 | 18 | 10 | 1 |
| dried peeled | 1 oz | 105 | 22 | – | – |
| japanese cooked | 1 oz | 16 | 4 | – | – |
| japanese dried | 1 oz | 102 | 23 | – | – |
| japanese raw | 1 oz | 44 | 10 | – | – |
| japanese roasted | 1 oz | 57 | 13 | – | – |
| roasted | 2 to 3 (1 oz) | 70 | 15 | – | – |
| roasted | 1 cup | 350 | 76 | – | – |
| **CHEWING GUM** | | | | | |
| bubble gum | 1 block (8 g) | 27 | 8 | – | – |
| stick | 1 (3 g) | 10 | 3 | – | – |
| ***Aquafresh*** | | | | | |
| Peppermint | 2 pieces | 5 | 2 | – | – |

| FOOD | PORTION | CALS | CARB | SUGAR | FIBER |
|---|---|---|---|---|---|
| ***Arm & Hammer*** | | | | | |
| Dental Care Spearmint or Peppermint | 2 pieces (2.5 g) | 5 | 2 | – | – |
| ***Big Red*** | | | | | |
| Stick | 1 | 10 | 2 | – | – |
| ***CareFree*** | | | | | |
| Koolerz Lemonaide | 1 piece | 5 | 2 | 0 | 0 |
| ***Dentyne*** | | | | | |
| Ice Peppermint | 2 pieces (3 g) | 5 | 2 | 0 | – |
| ***Doublemint*** | | | | | |
| Chewing Gum | 1 piece | 10 | 2 | – | – |
| ***Eclipse*** | | | | | |
| Spearmint | 2 pieces | 5 | 2 | – | – |
| ***Extra Sugar Free*** | | | | | |
| Cinnamon | 1 piece | 8 | tr | – | – |
| Spearmint & Peppermint | 1 stick | 8 | tr | – | – |
| Winter Fresh | 1 piece | 8 | tr | – | – |
| ***Freedent*** | | | | | |
| Spearmint Peppermint & Cinnamon | 1 stick | 10 | 3 | – | – |
| ***Hubba Bubba*** | | | | | |
| Bubble Gum Cola | 1 piece | 23 | 6 | – | – |
| Bubble Gum Sugarfree Grape | 1 piece | 13 | tr | – | – |
| Bubble Gum Sugarfree Original | 1 piece | 14 | tr | – | – |
| Original | 1 piece | 23 | 6 | – | – |
| Strawberry Grape Raspberry | 1 piece | 23 | 6 | – | – |
| ***Juicy Fruit*** | | | | | |
| Stick | 1 | 10 | 2 | – | – |
| ***Lance*** | | | | | |
| Big Red Cinnamon | 1 piece (3 g) | 10 | 2 | 2 | 0 |
| Double Bubble | 1 piece (7 g) | 25 | 6 | 5 | 0 |
| Double Mint | 1 piece (3 g) | 10 | 2 | 2 | 0 |
| ***Speakeasy*** | | | | | |
| Natural Rainforest All Flavors | 2 pieces | 10 | 2 | 2 | – |
| ***Wrigley's*** | | | | | |
| Orbit | 1 piece | 5 | 1 | – | – |
| Spearmint | 1 stick | 10 | 2 | – | – |
| ***Xylichew*** | | | | | |
| Licorice | 2 pieces | 4 | 2 | 0 | 0 |

| FOOD | PORTION | CALS | CARB | SUGAR | FIBER |
|---|---|---|---|---|---|
| **CHIA SEEDS** | | | | | |
| dried | 1 oz | 134 | 14 | – | – |
| **CHICKEN** (*see also* CHICKEN DISHES, CHICKEN SUBSTITUTES, DINNER, HOT DOGS) | | | | | |
| **CANNED** | | | | | |
| chicken spread | 1 tbsp | 25 | 1 | – | – |
| chicken spread | 1 oz | 55 | 2 | – | – |
| chicken spread barbeque flavored | 1 oz | 55 | 2 | – | – |
| w/ broth | ½ can (2.5 oz) | 117 | 0 | 0 | 0 |
| w/ broth | 1 can (5 oz) | 234 | 0 | 0 | 0 |
| **FRESH** | | | | | |
| broiler/fryer back w/o skin fried | ½ back (2 oz) | 167 | 3 | – | – |
| broiler/fryer breast w/ skin batter dipped & fried | 2.9 oz | 218 | 8 | – | – |
| broiler/fryer breast w/ skin batter dipped & fried | ½ breast (4.9 oz) | 364 | 13 | – | – |
| broiler/fryer breast w/ skin roasted | 2 oz | 115 | 0 | 0 | 0 |
| broiler/fryer breast w/ skin roasted | ½ breast (3.4 oz) | 193 | 0 | 0 | 0 |
| broiler/fryer breast w/ skin stewed | ½ breast (3.9 oz) | 202 | 0 | 0 | 0 |
| broiler/fryer breast w/o skin fried | ½ breast (3 oz) | 161 | tr | 0 | 0 |
| broiler/fryer breast w/o skin roasted | ½ breast (3 oz) | 142 | 0 | 0 | 0 |
| broiler/fryer breast w/o skin stewed | 2 oz | 86 | 0 | 0 | 0 |
| broiler/fryer drumstick w/ skin batter dipped & fried | 1 (2.6 oz) | 193 | 6 | – | – |
| broiler/fryer drumstick w/ skin floured & fried | 1 (1.7 oz) | 120 | 1 | – | – |
| broiler/fryer drumstick w/ skin roasted | 1 (1.8 oz) | 112 | 0 | 0 | 0 |
| broiler/fryer drumstick w/ skin stewed | 1 (2 oz) | 116 | 0 | 0 | 0 |
| broiler/fryer drumstick w/o skin fried | 1 (1.5 oz) | 82 | 0 | 0 | 0 |

| FOOD | PORTION | CALS | CARB | SUGAR | FIBER |
|---|---|---|---|---|---|
| broiler/fryer drumstick w/o skin roasted | 1 (1.5 oz) | 76 | 0 | 0 | 0 |
| broiler/fryer drumstick w/o skin stewed | 1 (1.6 oz) | 78 | 0 | 0 | 0 |
| broiler/fryer leg w/ skin batter dipped & fried | 1 (5.5 oz) | 431 | 14 | – | – |
| broiler/fryer leg w/ skin floured & fried | 1 (3.9 oz) | 285 | 3 | – | – |
| broiler/fryer leg w/ skin roasted | 1 (4 oz) | 265 | 0 | 0 | 0 |
| broiler/fryer leg w/ skin stewed | 1 (4.4 oz) | 275 | 0 | 0 | 0 |
| broiler/fryer leg w/o skin fried | 1 (3.3 oz) | 195 | 1 | – | – |
| broiler/fryer leg w/o skin roasted | 1 (3.3 oz) | 182 | 0 | 0 | 0 |
| broiler/fryer leg w/o skin stewed | 1 (3.5 oz) | 187 | 0 | 0 | 0 |
| broiler/fryer neck w/ skin stewed | 1 (1.3 oz) | 94 | 0 | 0 | 0 |
| broiler/fryer neck w/o skin stewed | 1 (.6 oz) | 32 | 0 | 0 | 0 |
| broiler/fryer skin batter dipped & fried | from ½ chicken (6.7 oz) | 748 | 44 | – | – |
| broiler/fryer skin floured & fried | from ½ chicken (2 oz) | 281 | 5 | – | – |
| broiler/fryer skin roasted | from ½ chicken (2 oz) | 254 | 0 | 0 | 0 |
| broiler/fryer skin stewed | from ½ chicken (2.5 oz) | 261 | 0 | 0 | 0 |
| broiler/fryer thigh w/ skin batter dipped & fried | 1 (3 oz) | 238 | 8 | – | – |
| broiler/fryer thigh w/ skin floured & fried | 1 (2.2 oz) | 162 | 2 | – | – |
| broiler/fryer thigh w/ skin roasted | 1 (2.2 oz) | 153 | 0 | 0 | 0 |
| broiler/fryer thigh w/ skin stewed | 1 (2.4 oz) | 158 | 0 | 0 | 0 |
| broiler/fryer | 1 (1.8 oz) | 113 | 1 | – | – |

| FOOD | PORTION | CALS | CARB | SUGAR | FIBER |
|---|---|---|---|---|---|
| thigh w/o skin fried broiler/fryer | 1 (1.8 oz) | 109 | 0 | 0 | 0 |
| thigh w/o skin roasted broiler/fryer | 1 (1.9 oz) | 107 | 0 | 0 | 0 |
| thigh w/o skin stewed broiler/fryer w/ skin floured & fried | ½ chicken (11 oz) | 844 | 10 | – | – |
| broiler/fryer w/ skin fried | ½ chicken (16.4 oz) | 1347 | 44 | – | – |
| broiler/fryer w/ skin roasted | ½ chicken (10.5 oz) | 715 | 0 | 0 | 0 |
| broiler/fryer w/ skin stewed | ½ chicken (11.7 oz) | 730 | 0 | 0 | 0 |
| broiler/fryer w/ skin neck & giblets batter dipped & fried | 1 chicken (2.3 lbs) | 2987 | 93 | – | – |
| broiler/fryer w/ skin neck & giblets roasted | 1 chicken (1.5 lbs) | 1598 | tr | – | – |
| broiler/fryer w/ skin neck & giblets stewed | 1 chicken (1.6 lbs) | 1625 | tr | – | – |
| broiler/fryer w/o skin fried | 1 cup | 307 | 2 | – | – |
| broiler/fryer w/o skin roasted | 1 cup (5 oz) | 266 | 0 | 0 | 0 |
| broiler/fryer w/o skin stewed | 1 cup (5 oz) | 248 | 0 | 0 | 0 |
| broiler/fryer w/o skin stewed | 1 oz | 54 | 0 | 0 | 0 |
| broiler/fryer wing w/ skin batter dipped & fried | 1 (1.7 oz) | 159 | 5 | – | – |
| broiler/fryer wing w/ skin floured & fried | 1 (1.1 oz) | 103 | 1 | – | – |
| broiler/fryer wing w/ skin roasted | 1 (1.2 oz) | 99 | 0 | 0 | 0 |
| broiler/fryer wing w/ skin stewed | 1 (1.4 oz) | 100 | 0 | 0 | 0 |
| capon w/ skin neck & giblets roasted | 1 chicken (3.1 lbs) | 3211 | 1 | – | – |
| cornish hen w/ skin roasted | 1 hen (8 oz) | 595 | 0 | 0 | 0 |
| cornish hen w/o skin & bone roasted | ½ hen (2 oz) | 72 | 0 | 0 | 0 |
| cornish hen w/o skin & bone roasted | 1 hen (3.8 oz) | 144 | 0 | 0 | 0 |
| cornish hen w/ skin roasted | ½ hen (4 oz) | 296 | 0 | 0 | 0 |

| FOOD | PORTION | CALS | CARB | SUGAR | FIBER |
|---|---|---|---|---|---|
| roaster dark meat w/o skin roasted | 1 cup (5 oz) | 250 | 0 | 0 | 0 |
| roaster light meat w/o skin roasted | 1 cup (5 oz) | 214 | 0 | 0 | 0 |
| roaster w/ skin neck & giblets roasted | 1 chicken (2.4 lbs) | 2363 | 1 | – | – |
| roaster w/ skin roasted | ½ chicken (1.1 lbs) | 1071 | 0 | 0 | 0 |
| roaster w/o skin roasted | 1 cup (5 oz) | 469 | 0 | 0 | 0 |
| stewing dark meat w/o skin stewed | 1 cup (5 oz) | 361 | 0 | 0 | 0 |
| stewing w/ skin neck & giblets stewed | 1 chicken (1.3 lbs) | 1636 | tr | – | – |
| stewing w/ skin stewed | ½ chicken (9.2 oz) | 744 | 0 | 0 | 0 |
| stewing w/ skin stewed | 6.2 oz | 507 | 0 | 0 | 0 |
| ***Amish Select*** | | | | | |
| Boneless Skinless Breast w/ Honey Dijon Mustard | 1 serv (4 oz) | 130 | 4 | 3 | 0 |
| ***Perdue*** | | | | | |
| Boneless Skinless Breasts Cooked | 3 oz | 110 | 0 | – | – |
| Boneless Breast Roasted Garlic Herb | 1 piece (3 oz) | 90 | 3 | – | – |
| Breaded Breast Strips Barbecue | 3 oz | 120 | 16 | 4 | – |
| Breaded Breast Strips Hot & Spicy | 3 oz | 110 | 13 | 1 | – |
| Breaded Breast Strips Original | 3 oz | 120 | 14 | 1 | – |
| Burger Cooked | 1 (3 oz) | 160 | 0 | – | – |
| Chicken Breast Seasoned Italian Cooked | 1 piece (3 oz) | 90 | 3 | 1 | – |
| Chicken Breast Seasoned Teriyaki Cooked | 1 piece (3 oz) | 90 | 3 | 1 | – |
| Ground Cooked | 3 oz | 170 | 0 | – | – |
| Ground Breast Cooked | 3 oz | 80 | 0 | – | – |
| Honey Rotisserie Dark Meat | 3 oz | 200 | 1 | 1 | – |
| Honey Rotisserie White Meat | 3 oz | 140 | 1 | 1 | – |
| Oven Stuffer Dark Meat Roasted | 3 oz | 210 | 0 | – | – |

| FOOD | PORTION | CALS | CARB | SUGAR | FIBER |
|---|---|---|---|---|---|
| Oven Stuffer Drumbstick Roasted | 1 (3.6 oz) | 190 | 0 | – | – |
| Oven Stuffer White Meat Roasted | 3 oz | 170 | 0 | – | – |
| Oven Stuffer Wingette Roasted | 3 (3.4 oz) | 220 | 0 | – | – |
| Ovenables Breast Lemon Pepper Cooked | 1 piece (3 oz) | 90 | 2 | – | – |
| Seasoned Roasting Chicken Toasted Garlic Dark Meat | 3 oz | 190 | 1 | – | – |
| Seasoned Roasting Chicken Toasted Garlic White Meat | 3 oz | 160 | 1 | – | – |
| Seasoned Strips Parmesan Garlic cooked | 3 oz | 100 | 2 | – | – |
| Seasoned Strips Savory Classic cooked | 3 oz | 90 | 1 | 0 | – |
| Seasoned Strips Spicy Fiesta cooked | 3 oz | 140 | 3 | 1 | – |
| Split Breast Cooked | 1 piece (6.8 oz) | 370 | 0 | – | – |
| Thin Sliced Breast Rosemary Garlic Thyme | 1 piece (3 oz) | 90 | 1 | – | – |
| Thin Sliced Breast Tomato Herb | 1 piece (3 oz) | 90 | 1 | – | – |
| Whole Dark Meat Cooked | 3 oz | 150 | 0 | – | – |
| Whole White Meat Cooked | 3 oz | 170 | 0 | – | 0 |
| Wings Roasted | 2 (3.2 oz) | 210 | 0 | – | – |
| ***Tyson*** | | | | | |
| Broth Marinated Breast Filet | 1 (4.7 oz) | 140 | 0 | 0 | 0 |
| Broth Marinated Drums | 2 (4 oz) | 140 | 0 | 0 | 0 |
| Broth Marinated Thighs | 1 (4.9 oz) | 380 | 1 | 1 | 0 |
| Broth Marinated Wings | 4 pieces (4.2 oz) | 240 | 0 | 0 | 0 |
| Chicken Broccoli & Cheese | 1 piece (5.9 oz) | 320 | 23 | 3 | 3 |
| Chicken Stuffed w/ Wild Rice & Mushroom | 1 piece (5.9 oz) | 300 | 25 | 4 | 1 |
| Cordon Bleu | 1 piece (5.9 oz) | 350 | 24 | 3 | 3 |
| Cornish Hen | 1 serv (4 oz) | 180 | 0 | 0 | 0 |

| FOOD | PORTION | CALS | CARB | SUGAR | FIBER |
|---|---|---|---|---|---|
| Kiev | 1 piece (5.9 oz) | 460 | 24 | 3 | 2 |
| ***Wampler*** | | | | | |
| Breast Tenders | 4 oz | 130 | 0 | – | – |
| **FROZEN** | | | | | |
| ***Banquet*** | | | | | |
| Breast Nuggets | 7 | 280 | 11 | 2 | 1 |
| Breast Patties Grilled Honey BBQ | 1 | 110 | 3 | 2 | 0 |
| Breast Patties Grilled Honey Mustard | 1 | 120 | 5 | 3 | 0 |
| Breast Tenders Our Original | 3 | 250 | 15 | 1 | tr |
| Breast Tenders Southern | 3 pieces | 260 | 16 | 1 | 1 |
| Country Fried | 1 serv (3 oz) | 270 | 13 | 1 | 1 |
| Fat Free Baked Breast Patties | 1 | 100 | 15 | 3 | 1 |
| Fried Our Original | 1 serv (3 oz) | 280 | 15 | 1 | 1 |
| Honey BBQ Skinless Fried | 1 serv (3 oz) | 230 | 9 | 1 | 1 |
| Hot 'n Spicy Fried | 1 serv (3 oz) | 260 | 13 | 1 | 1 |
| Nuggets Our Original | 6 | 270 | 12 | 2 | 1 |
| Nuggets Southern Fried | 5 | 270 | 16 | 4 | 2 |
| Patties Our Original | 1 | 190 | 10 | 2 | 1 |
| Patties Southern Fried | 1 | 190 | 10 | tr | tr |
| Skinless Fried | 1 serv (3 oz) | 220 | 7 | 1 | 2 |
| Smokehouse Big Wings | 2 | 200 | 4 | 3 | 0 |
| Southern Fried | 1 serv (3 oz) | 280 | 15 | 1 | 1 |
| Wings Firehouse Big | 2 | 190 | 1 | 0 | 0 |
| Wings Honey BBQ | 4 | 380 | 15 | 4 | 1 |
| Wings Hot & Spicy | 4 pieces | 280 | 9 | 0 | tr |
| ***Bell & Evans*** | | | | | |
| Breaded Breast Nuggets | 1 serv (4 oz) | 190 | 13 | 1 | 1 |
| Breaded Whole Breast Tenders | 1 (4 oz) | 190 | 13 | 1 | 1 |
| Burgers | 1 (3 oz) | 120 | tr | 0 | 0 |
| Chicken Sandwich Steaks | 1 serv (2 oz) | 60 | tr | 0 | 0 |
| ***Country Skillet*** | | | | | |
| Bites | 5 | 270 | 18 | 2 | 1 |
| Breast Tenders | 3 | 240 | 16 | 1 | 1 |
| Chunks | 5 | 270 | 18 | 2 | 1 |
| Fried | 3 oz | 270 | 13 | 1 | 1 |
| Nuggets | 10 | 280 | 16 | 2 | 1 |

| FOOD | PORTION | CALS | CARB | SUGAR | FIBER |
|---|---|---|---|---|---|
| Patties | 1 | 190 | 12 | 3 | 1 |
| Southern Fried Chunks | 5 | 270 | 17 | 4 | 1 |
| Southern Fried Patties | 1 | 190 | 12 | 3 | 1 |
| ***Health Is Wealth*** | | | | | |
| Nuggets | 4 (3 oz) | 150 | 9 | 0 | 0 |
| Patties | 1 (3 oz) | 150 | 9 | 0 | 0 |
| Tenders | 3 (3 oz) | 130 | 11 | 0 | 0 |
| ***Kid Cuisine*** | | | | | |
| Dino Mite Nuggets | 4 pieces | 300 | 10 | 3 | 1 |
| Radical Racin' Nuggets w/ Cheese | 4 pieces | 300 | 12 | 3 | tr |
| ***Weaver*** | | | | | |
| Breast Strips | 3 pieces (3.3 oz) | 210 | 13 | 1 | 2 |
| Breast Tenders | 5 pieces (3 oz) | 220 | 8 | 0 | 1 |
| Croquettes | 1 serv (3.5 oz) | 290 | 22 | 4 | 2 |
| Dutch Frye Nuggets | 5 pieces (3.3 oz) | 280 | 12 | 0 | 2 |
| Honey Battered Tenders | 5 pieces (2.9 oz) | 230 | 12 | 3 | 1 |
| Hot Wings Buffalo Style | 3 pieces (2.7 oz) | 190 | 0 | 0 | 0 |
| Mini Drums Crispy | 5 pieces (3.3 oz) | 250 | 14 | 2 | 1 |
| Nuggets | 4 pieces (2.7 oz) | 210 | 9 | 0 | 1 |
| Patties | 1 (2.6 oz) | 180 | 10 | 1 | 1 |
| Rondelet | 1 (2.6 oz) | 170 | 10 | 1 | 1 |
| Rondelet Dutch Frye | 1 (2.6 oz) | 230 | 10 | 1 | 1 |
| Rondelet Italian | 1 (2.6 oz) | 210 | 12 | 1 | 1 |
| **READY-TO-EAT** | | | | | |
| chicken roll light meat | 2 oz | 90 | 1 | – | – |
| chicken roll light meat | 1 pkg (6 oz) | 271 | 4 | – | – |
| poultry salad sandwich spread | 1 tbsp (13 g) | 109 | 1 | – | – |
| poultry salad sandwich spread | 1 oz | 238 | 2 | – | – |
| ***Banquet*** | | | | | |
| Fat Free Baked Breast Tenders | 3 | 120 | 16 | 0 | 2 |

| FOOD | PORTION | CALS | CARB | SUGAR | FIBER |
|---|---|---|---|---|---|
| ***Boar's Head*** | | | | | |
| Breast Hickory Smoked | 2 oz | 60 | tr | 0 | 0 |
| Breast Oven Roasted | 2 oz | 50 | tr | 0 | 0 |
| Breast Bar B Q Sauce Basted | 2 oz | 60 | 3 | 1 | 0 |
| ***Butterball*** | | | | | |
| Crispy Baked Breasts Italian Style Herb | 1 piece (0.5 oz) | 190 | 16 | 0 | 1 |
| Crispy Baked Breasts Lemon Pepper | 1 piece (0.5 oz) | 200 | 16 | 2 | tr |
| Crispy Baked Breasts Original | 1 piece (0.5 oz) | 180 | 16 | 2 | 1 |
| Crispy Baked Breasts Parmesan | 1 piece (0.5 oz) | 200 | 16 | 5 | tr |
| Crispy Baked Breasts Southwestern | 1 piece (0.5 oz) | 170 | 13 | 0 | 2 |
| Tenders Baked Breast | 3 pieces | 170 | 15 | 2 | 1 |
| Tenders Hickory Smoked Grilled | 4 pieces + sauce | 160 | 12 | 9 | 1 |
| Tenders Oriental Grilled | 4 pieces + sauce | 160 | 12 | 10 | 1 |
| ***Carl Buddig*** | | | | | |
| Chicken Sliced | 1 pkg (2.5 oz) | 110 | 1 | 1 | – |
| Lean Slices Honey Smoked Breast | 1 pkg (2.5 oz) | 70 | 3 | 3 | – |
| Lean Slices Roasted Breast | 1 pkg (2.5 oz) | 60 | 1 | 1 | – |
| ***Perdue*** | | | | | |
| Breast Cutlets Homestyle | 1 (2.9 oz) | 110 | 12 | – | – |
| Breast Cutlets Italian Style | 1 (2.9 oz) | 120 | 11 | – | – |
| Breast Filets in Barbecue Sauce | 1 piece + 3 tbsp sauce (5.9 oz) | 200 | 24 | 23 | – |
| Breast Strips in Garlic & Herb Sauce | 1 serv (5 oz) | 100 | 4 | 1 | 2 |
| Breast Strips in Marinara Sauce | 1 serv (5 oz) | 120 | 5 | 1 | – |
| Breast Strips in Teriyaki Sauce | 1 serv (5 oz) | 190 | 26 | 22 | – |
| Carved Breast Honey Roasted | ½ cup (2.5 oz) | 100 | 2 | 1 | – |
| Carved Breast Original Roasted | ½ cup (2.5 oz) | 90 | 1 | – | – |
| Cutlets Cooked | 1 (3.5 oz) | 220 | 15 | – | – |
| Nuggets | 5 (3.4 oz) | 210 | 15 | – | – |
| Nuggets Chicken & Cheese | 5 (3.4 oz) | 230 | 15 | – | – |

| FOOD | PORTION | CALS | CARB | SUGAR | FIBER |
|---|---|---|---|---|---|
| Short Cuts Entrees in Teriyaki Sauce | 5 oz | 190 | 26 | 22 | – |
| Short Cuts Italian | ½ cup (2.5 oz) | 100 | 0 | – | – |
| Short Cuts Lemon Pepper | ½ cup (2.5 oz) | 100 | 1 | – | – |
| Short Cuts Southwestern | ½ cup (2.5 oz) | 100 | 1 | – | – |
| ***Tyson*** | | | | | |
| Breaded Breast Chunks | 6 pieces (2.9 oz) | 230 | 13 | 0 | 1 |
| Breaded Breast Fillet | 2 pieces (2.8 oz) | 180 | 15 | 0 | 1 |
| Breaded Breast Pattie | 1 (2.6 oz) | 190 | 9 | 2 | 1 |
| Breaded Breast Tenders | 5 pieces (3 oz) | 220 | 8 | 0 | 1 |
| Breaded Chicken Chunks | 6 pieces (3 oz) | 220 | 11 | 1 | 0 |
| Chick'n Quick Chick'n Cheddar | 1 patty (2.6 oz) | 220 | 12 | 1 | 0 |
| Chicken Bits Southern Fried | 6 pieces (2.9 oz) | 260 | 11 | 0 | 1 |
| Chicken Strips Southwestern | 1 serv (3 oz) | 110 | 2 | 1 | 0 |
| Country Fried Chicken Fritter | 5 pieces (2.9 oz) | 260 | 13 | 0 | 1 |
| Drumsticks Hot BBQ Style | 2 (3.5 oz) | 160 | 3 | 2 | 1 |
| Glazed Grilled Breast Pattie | 1 (2.7 oz) | 120 | 1 | 0 | 0 |
| Grilled Breast Strips | 1 serv (3 oz) | 110 | 2 | 2 | 0 |
| Grilled Chicken Pattie | 1 (2.9 oz) | 170 | 1 | 0 | 0 |
| Nuggets Breaded White Meat | 6 pieces (2.9 oz) | 250 | 12 | 0 | 1 |
| Patties Southern Fried | 1 (2.9 oz) | 260 | 11 | 0 | 1 |
| Roasted Drumsticks | 3 (5.6 oz) | 320 | 2 | 2 | 0 |
| Roasted Drumsticks w/o Skin | 2 (3.3 oz) | 140 | 1 | 1 | 0 |
| Roasted Half Chicken | 1 serv (3 oz) | 160 | 1 | 1 | 0 |
| Roasted Whole Chicken | 1 serv (3 oz) | 160 | 1 | 1 | 0 |
| Roasted Breast Boneless w/o Skin | 1 (3.7 oz) | 130 | 1 | 1 | 0 |
| Roasted Breast Half w/o Skin | 1 (4.3 oz) | 150 | 1 | 1 | 0 |
| Roasted Half Breast w/ Skin | 1 (5.1 oz) | 260 | 1 | 1 | 0 |
| Roasted Half Chicken w/o Skin | 1 serv (3 oz) | 120 | 1 | 1 | 0 |

| FOOD | PORTION | CALS | CARB | SUGAR | FIBER |
|---|---|---|---|---|---|
| Roasted Tabasco Wings | 3 (3 oz) | 190 | 1 | 1 | 1 |
| Roasted Thigh w/ Skin | 1 (3.6 oz) | 270 | 1 | 1 | 0 |
| Roasted Thighs w/o Skin | 1 (2.9 oz) | 150 | 1 | 1 | 0 |
| Roll White Meat | 2 oz | 90 | 0 | 0 | 0 |
| Southern Fried Breaded Breast Pattie | 1 (2.6 oz) | 180 | 8 | 0 | 0 |
| Southern Fried Breast Fillets | 2 pieces (3.4 oz) | 210 | 14 | 0 | 1 |
| Southern Fried Chunks | 6 pieces (2.9 oz) | 260 | 11 | 0 | 1 |
| Tenders Breaded Honey Battered | 5 pieces (2.9 oz) | 230 | 12 | 3 | 1 |
| Tenders Breaded Pattie | 3 pieces (3.2 oz) | 100 | 11 | 1 | 1 |
| Thick'n Crispy Pattie | 1 (2.6 oz) | 200 | 10 | 1 | 1 |
| Wings BBQ | 3 pieces (3.2 oz) | 200 | 2 | 2 | 0 |
| Wings Hot N'Spicy | 4 (3.2 oz) | 210 | 1 | 0 | 0 |
| Wings Teriyaki | 4 pieces (3.4 oz) | 190 | 2 | 1 | 2 |
| Wings Of Fire | 4 pieces (3.4 oz) | 220 | 1 | 0 | 0 |
| **TAKE-OUT** | | | | | |
| oven roasted breast of chicken | 2 oz | 60 | 0 | 0 | 0 |

## CHICKEN DISHES

| FOOD | PORTION | CALS | CARB | SUGAR | FIBER |
|---|---|---|---|---|---|
| **CANNED** | | | | | |
| ***Bumble Bee*** | | | | | |
| Chicken Salad | 1 pkg (3.5 oz) | 230 | 25 | 8 | 0 |
| **MIX** | | | | | |
| ***Chicken Skillet Helper*** | | | | | |
| Stir-Fried Chicken as prep | 1 cup | 270 | 30 | 1 | 1 |
| ***Hamburger Helper*** | | | | | |
| Reduced Sodium Cheddar Spirals Chicken Recipe as prep | 1 cup | 240 | 27 | 6 | 0 |
| Reduced Sodium Italian Herb Chicken Recipe as prep | 1 cup | 200 | 29 | 6 | 2 |
| Reduced Sodium Southwestern Beef Chicken Recipe as prep | 1 cup | 220 | 32 | 6 | 2 |

| FOOD | PORTION | CALS | CARB | SUGAR | FIBER |
|---|---|---|---|---|---|
| ***Tyson*** | | | | | |
| Mandarin Wrap Kit | 1½ wraps (14.6 oz) | 630 | 92 | 8 | 5 |
| **REFRIGERATED** | | | | | |
| salad low fat | ⅓ cup | 90 | 9 | – | – |
| ***Lloyd's*** | | | | | |
| Barbecue Shredded Chicken | ¼ cup (2 oz) | 90 | 11 | 9 | – |
| ***Oscar Mayer*** | | | | | |
| Lunchables Chicken Wraps | 1 pkg | 440 | 64 | 25 | 3 |
| ***Tyson*** | | | | | |
| Chicken Breast Medallions in Tomato & Herb Sauce | 1 serv (5 oz) | 120 | 5 | 2 | 0 |
| ***Wampler*** | | | | | |
| Cacciatore | 1 cup | 260 | 10 | – | – |
| Fajitas | 1 cup | 210 | 13 | – | – |
| Salad | ⅓ cup | 200 | 9 | – | – |
| Salad Lite | ⅓ cup | 130 | 9 | – | – |
| Smokey Barbecue Chicken | 1 cup | 430 | 31 | – | – |
| Sweet-n-Sour | 1 cup | 250 | 35 | – | – |
| **SHELF-STABLE** | | | | | |
| ***Lunch Bucket*** | | | | | |
| Chicken Fiesta | 1 pkg (7.5 oz) | 160 | 30 | 6 | 5 |
| Dumplings'n Chicken | 1 pkg (7.5 oz) | 140 | 21 | 2 | 1 |
| ***TastyBite*** | | | | | |
| Chicken Moglai | 1 pkg (9.5 oz) | 300 | 20 | 5 | 3 |
| **TAKE-OUT** | | | | | |
| boneless breaded & fried w/ barbecue sauce | 6 pieces (4.6 oz) | 330 | 25 | – | – |
| boneless breaded & fried w/ honey | 6 pieces (4 oz) | 339 | 27 | – | – |
| boneless breaded & fried w/ mustard sauce | 6 pieces (4.6 oz) | 323 | 21 | – | – |
| boneless breaded & fried w/ sweet & sour sauce | 6 pieces (4.6 oz) | 346 | 29 | – | – |
| boneless breast w/ apple stuffing | 1 serv (5 oz) | 260 | 10 | 2 | 1 |
| breast & wing breaded & fried | 2 pieces (5.7 oz) | 494 | 20 | – | – |
| chicken & dumplings | ¾ cup | 256 | 12 | – | tr |
| chicken & noodles | 1 cup | 365 | 26 | – | – |

| FOOD | PORTION | CALS | CARB | SUGAR | FIBER |
|---|---|---|---|---|---|
| chicken a la king | 1 cup | 470 | 12 | – | – |
| chicken cacciatore | ¾ cup | 394 | 9 | – | 2 |
| chicken pie w/ top crust | 1 slice (5.6 oz) | 472 | 32 | – | 1 |
| chicken cordon blue | 1 serv (5 oz) | 280 | 10 | 0 | 0 |
| drumstick breaded & fried | 2 pieces (5.2 oz) | 430 | 16 | – | – |
| groundnut stew hkatenkwan | 1 serv (15.7 oz) | 576 | 18 | 3 | 4 |
| jamaican jerk wings | 4 wings (9.9 oz) | 709 | 3 | tr | tr |
| sancocho de pollo dominican chicken stew | 1 serv | 702 | 34 | 4 | 1 |
| thigh breaded & fried | 2 pieces (5.2 oz) | 430 | 16 | – | – |
| **CHICKEN SUBSTITUTES** | | | | | |
| ***Health Is Wealth*** | | | | | |
| Buffalo Wings | 3 pieces (2.2 oz) | 100 | 11 | 0 | 3 |
| Chicken-Free Nuggets | 3 pieces (2.25 oz) | 90 | 11 | 0 | 2 |
| Chicken-Free Patties | 1 (3 oz) | 120 | 15 | 0 | 2 |
| ***Loma Linda*** | | | | | |
| Chicken Supreme Mix not prep | ⅓ cup (0.9 oz) | 90 | 6 | 0 | 4 |
| Chik Nuggets | 5 pieces (3 oz) | 240 | 13 | tr | 5 |
| Fried Chik'n w/ Gravy | 2 pieces (2.8 oz) | 160 | 4 | tr | 2 |
| ***Morningstar Farms*** | | | | | |
| Chik Nuggets | 4 pieces (3 oz) | 160 | 17 | 2 | 5 |
| Chik Patties | 1 (2.5 oz) | 150 | 15 | 1 | 2 |
| Meatless Buffalo Wings | 5 pieces (3 oz) | 200 | 16 | 1 | 3 |
| ***Quorn*** | | | | | |
| Cutlets | 1 (3.5 oz) | 200 | 20 | 2 | 4 |
| Naked Cutlets | 1 (2.4 oz) | 80 | 5 | 0 | 2 |
| Nuggets | 3-4 pieces (3 oz) | 180 | 18 | 2 | 3 |

| FOOD | PORTION | CALS | CARB | SUGAR | FIBER |
|---|---|---|---|---|---|
| Patties | 1 patty (2.6 oz) | 160 | 12 | 2 | 3 |
| Tenders | 1 cup (3 oz) | 90 | 8 | 1 | 3 |
| ***Worthington*** | | | | | |
| Chic-Ketts | 2 slices (1.9 oz) | 120 | 2 | 0 | 2 |
| Chicken Sliced or Roll | 2 slices (2 oz) | 80 | 1 | 0 | tr |
| ChikStiks | 1 (1.6 oz) | 110 | 3 | tr | 2 |
| CrispyChik Patties | 1 (2.5 oz) | 150 | 15 | 1 | 2 |
| Cutlets | 1 slice (2.1 oz) | 70 | 3 | 0 | 2 |
| Diced Chik | ¼ cup (1.9 oz) | 40 | 1 | 0 | 1 |
| FriChik | 2 pieces (3.2 oz) | 120 | 1 | 0 | 1 |
| FriChik Low Fat | 2 pieces (3 oz) | 80 | 2 | 0 | 1 |
| Golden Croquettes | 4 pieces (3 oz) | 210 | 14 | 1 | 6 |
| ***Yves*** | | | | | |
| Veggie Chicken Burgers | 1 (3 oz) | 120 | 6 | 1 | 3 |
| **CHICKPEAS** | | | | | |
| **CANNED** | | | | | |
| chickpeas | 1 cup | 285 | 54 | – | – |
| ***Progresso*** | | | | | |
| Chick Peas | ½ cup (4.6 oz) | 120 | 20 | 3 | 5 |
| Garbanzo | ½ cup (4.4 oz) | 110 | 18 | tr | 5 |
| **DRIED** | | | | | |
| cooked | 1 cup | 269 | 45 | – | – |
| **CHICORY** | | | | | |
| greens raw chopped | ½ cup | 21 | 4 | – | – |
| root raw | 1 (2.1 oz) | 44 | 11 | – | – |
| roots raw cut up | ½ cup (1.6 oz) | 33 | 8 | – | – |
| witloof head raw | 1 (1.9 oz) | 9 | 2 | – | – |
| witloof raw | ½ cup (1.6 oz) | 8 | 2 | – | – |
| **CHILI** | | | | | |
| chile pepper paste | 1 tbsp | 6 | 1 | – | 1 |
| chili w/ beans | 1 cup | 286 | 30 | – | – |
| dried ancho | 1 tsp | 3 | 1 | – | tr |

| FOOD | PORTION | CALS | CARB | SUGAR | FIBER |
|---|---|---|---|---|---|
| dried casabel | 1 tsp | 3 | 1 | – | tr |
| dried guajillo | 1 tsp | 3 | 1 | – | tr |
| dried mulato | 1 tsp | 3 | 1 | – | tr |
| dried pasilla | 1 tsp | 3 | 1 | – | tr |
| dried smoked chipotle | 1 tsp | 3 | 1 | – | tr |
| powder | 1 tsp | 8 | 1 | – | – |
| ***Amy's*** | | | | | |
| Chili & Cornbread | 1 pkg (10.5 oz) | 320 | 59 | 14 | 8 |
| Organic Black Bean | 1 cup | 200 | 31 | 3 | 15 |
| Organic Medium | 1 cup | 190 | 26 | 5 | 7 |
| Organic Medium w/ Vegetables | 1 cup | 190 | 29 | 6 | 8 |
| ***Armour*** | | | | | |
| Chili No Beans | 1 cup (8.7 oz) | 390 | 18 | 0 | 0 |
| Chili W/ Beans Western Style | 1 cup (8.8 oz) | 370 | 29 | 4 | 9 |
| Chili w/ Beans | 1 cup (8.9 oz) | 370 | 33 | 2 | 10 |
| Chili w/ Beans Hot | 1 cup (8.9 oz) | 370 | 33 | 2 | 10 |
| Vienna Sausage & Chili | 1 cup (8.7 oz) | 410 | 27 | 4 | 15 |
| ***Carroll Shelby's*** | | | | | |
| Original Texas Chili Kit | 2 tbsp | 60 | 12 | 0 | 0 |
| ***Chef Boyardee*** | | | | | |
| Chili Mac | ½ can (7 oz) | 260 | 30 | 5 | 3 |
| ***Chili Man*** | | | | | |
| Seasoning Mix | 1 tbsp (7 g) | 25 | 4 | – | 2 |
| ***Del Monte*** | | | | | |
| Sauce | 1 tbsp (0.6 oz) | 20 | 5 | 4 | 0 |
| ***Gebhardt*** | | | | | |
| Chili Powder | ¼ tsp (0.3 g) | 1 | tr | tr | tr |
| Chili Quik Seasoning | 1 tbsp (0.3 oz) | 43 | 8 | 1 | 2 |
| Plain | 1 cup (9.4 oz) | 232 | 11 | 0 | 3 |
| With Beans | 1 cup (9.4 oz) | 322 | 32 | tr | 15 |
| ***Gringo Billy's*** | | | | | |
| Chili Mix | 1 tbsp | 24 | 2 | 0 | 2 |
| ***Health Valley*** | | | | | |
| Burrito | 1 cup | 160 | 28 | 7 | 12 |
| Enchilada | 1 cup | 160 | 28 | 7 | 12 |
| Fajita | 1 cup | 80 | 15 | 4 | 7 |
| in A Cup Black Bean Mild | ¾ cup | 120 | 21 | 3 | 6 |

| FOOD | PORTION | CALS | CARB | SUGAR | FIBER |
|---|---|---|---|---|---|
| in A Cup Texas Style Spicy | ¾ cup | 120 | 21 | 3 | 6 |
| Vegetarian Lentil Mild | 1 cup | 160 | 28 | 6 | 12 |
| Vegetarian Lentil No Salt | 1 cup | 80 | 14 | 3 | 6 |
| Vegetarian Mild | 1 cup | 160 | 28 | 7 | 12 |
| Vegetarian Mild No Salt | 1 cup | 160 | 28 | 7 | 12 |
| Vegetarian Spicy | 1 cup | 160 | 28 | 7 | 12 |
| Vegetarian Spicy No Salt | 1 cup | 160 | 28 | 7 | 12 |
| Vegetarian w/ 3 Beans Mild | 1 cup | 160 | 28 | 7 | 12 |
| Vegetarian w/ Black Beans Mild | 1 cup | 160 | 28 | 7 | 12 |
| Vegetarian w/ Black Beans Spicy | 1 cup | 160 | 28 | 7 | 12 |
| ***Healthy Choice*** | | | | | |
| Bowls Chili & Cornbread | 1 meal (9.5 oz) | 350 | 49 | 18 | 8 |
| ***Hunt's*** | | | | | |
| Chili Beans | ½ cup (4.5 oz) | 87 | 17 | 8 | 6 |
| Chili Sauce | 2 tbsp (1.2 oz) | 35 | 8 | 8 | 1 |
| ***Instant India*** | | | | | |
| Chili Ginger Paste | 2 tbsp (1 oz) | 90 | 6 | 5 | 0 |
| ***Just Rite*** | | | | | |
| With Beans | 1 cup (9 oz) | 379 | 31 | 0 | 13 |
| ***Lean Cuisine*** | | | | | |
| Everyday Favorites Three Bean Chili w/ Rice | 1 pkg (10 oz) (10 oz) | 250 | 37 | 7 | 9 |
| ***Lunch Bucket*** | | | | | |
| Chili With Beans | 1 pkg (7.5 oz) | 260 | 25 | 1 | 8 |
| ***Manwich*** | | | | | |
| Homestyle Fixins | ½ cup (4.6 oz) | 84 | 19 | 7 | 6 |
| ***Marie Callender's*** | | | | | |
| Chili & Cornbread | 1 meal (16 oz) | 560 | 67 | 25 | 7 |
| ***McCormick*** | | | | | |
| Mexican Style Chili Powder | ¼ tsp | 0 | 0 | 0 | 0 |
| Original Chili Seasoning | 1⅓ tbsp (9 g) | 30 | 5 | tr | 2 |
| ***Natural Choice*** | | | | | |
| Organic Vegan Three Bean | ½ cup (4.6 oz) | 140 | 24 | 4 | 7 |
| ***Natural Touch*** | | | | | |
| Vegetarian | 1 cup (8.1 oz) | 170 | 21 | 2 | 11 |

| FOOD | PORTION | CALS | CARB | SUGAR | FIBER |
|---|---|---|---|---|---|
| ***Nature's Entree*** | | | | | |
| Texas Chili | 1 pkg (12 oz) | 320 | 43 | 5 | 11 |
| ***Open Range*** | | | | | |
| Plain | 1 cup (8.8 oz) | 353 | 19 | 6 | 6 |
| With Beans | 1 cup (9 oz) | 281 | 25 | 7 | 10 |
| ***Soy7*** | | | | | |
| Chili Mix as prep | 1 cup | 150 | 24 | 3 | 7 |
| ***Ultimate*** | | | | | |
| No Beans Hot | 1 cup (8.7 oz) | 420 | 18 | 4 | 5 |
| Turkey w/ Beans | 1 cup (8.7 oz) | 260 | 28 | 4 | 9 |
| W/ Beans | 1 cup (8.7 oz) | 320 | 25 | 4 | 9 |
| W/ Beans Hot | 1 cup (8.7 oz) | 320 | 25 | 4 | 9 |
| ***Van Camp*** | | | | | |
| Beanee Weenee Chilee | 1 cup (7.7 oz) | 240 | 27 | 1 | 9 |
| Chili With Beans | 1 cup (8.9 oz) | 350 | 28 | 1 | 7 |
| Mexican Style Chili Beans | ½ cup (4.6 oz) | 110 | 21 | 1 | 8 |
| ***Wampler*** | | | | | |
| Turkey | 1 cup | 250 | 22 | – | – |
| ***Wick Fowler's*** | | | | | |
| 2 Alarm Chili Kit | 3 tbsp | 60 | 10 | 0 | 0 |
| False Alarm Chili Kit | 2 tbsp | 50 | 9 | 0 | 0 |
| ***Worthington*** | | | | | |
| Chili | 1 cup (8.1 oz) | 290 | 21 | 2 | 9 |
| Low Fat | 1 cup (8.1 oz) | 170 | 21 | 2 | 11 |
| ***Yves*** | | | | | |
| Veggie Chili | 1 pkg (10.5 oz) | 230 | 37 | 7 | 14 |
| **TAKE-OUT** | | | | | |
| con carne w/ beans | 8.9 oz | 254 | 22 | – | – |

**CHILI PEPPER** *(see* PEPPERS*)*

**CHINESE FOOD** *(see* ASIAN FOOD*)*

| FOOD | PORTION | CALS | CARB | SUGAR | FIBER |
|---|---|---|---|---|---|
| **CHINESE PRESERVING MELON** | | | | | |
| cooked | ½ cup | 11 | 3 | – | – |
| **CHIPS** | | | | | |
| barbecue | 1 bag (7 oz) | 971 | 105 | – | – |
| barbecue | 1 oz | 139 | 15 | – | – |
| corn | 1 bag (7 oz) | 1067 | 113 | – | 9 |
| corn | 1 oz | 153 | 16 | – | 1 |

| FOOD | PORTION | CALS | CARB | SUGAR | FIBER |
|---|---|---|---|---|---|
| corn barbecue | 1 bag (7 oz) | 1036 | 111 | – | 10 |
| corn barbecue | 1 oz | 148 | 16 | – | 1 |
| corn cones | 1 oz | 145 | 18 | – | – |
| corn cones nacho | 1 oz | 152 | 17 | – | – |
| corn onion | 1 oz | 142 | 19 | – | – |
| potato | 1 oz | 152 | 15 | – | – |
| potato | 1 bag (8 oz) | 1217 | 120 | – | – |
| potato cheese | 1 oz | 140 | 16 | – | – |
| potato cheese | 1 bag (6 oz) | 842 | 98 | – | – |
| potato light | 1 bag (6 oz) | 801 | 114 | – | – |
| potato light | 1 oz | 134 | 19 | – | – |
| potato sour cream & onion | 1 bag (7 oz) | 1051 | 102 | – | – |
| potato sour cream & onion | 1 oz | 150 | 15 | – | – |
| potato sticks | ½ cup (0.6 oz) | 94 | 10 | – | 1 |
| potato sticks | 1 oz | 148 | 15 | – | 1 |
| potato sticks | 1 pkg (1 oz) | 148 | 15 | – | – |
| taco | 1 oz | 136 | 18 | – | – |
| taco | 1 bag (8 oz) | 1089 | 143 | – | – |
| taro | 10 (0.8 oz) | 115 | 16 | – | – |
| taro | 1 oz | 141 | 19 | – | – |
| tortilla | 1 bag (7.5 oz) | 1067 | 134 | – | 14 |
| tortilla | 1 oz | 142 | 18 | – | 2 |
| tortilla nacho | 1 bag (8 oz) | 1131 | 142 | – | 12 |
| tortilla nacho | 1 oz | 141 | 18 | – | 2 |
| tortilla nacho light | 1 oz | 126 | 20 | – | – |
| tortilla nacho light | 1 bag (6 oz) | 757 | 122 | – | – |
| tortilla ranch | 1 oz | 139 | 18 | – | – |
| tortilla ranch | 1 bag (7 oz) | 969 | 128 | – | – |
| ***Atkins*** | | | | | |
| Crunchers Barbeque | 1 pkg (1 oz) | 100 | 8 | 0 | 4 |
| Crunchers Nacho Cheese | 1 pkg (1 oz) | 100 | 8 | 1 | 3 |
| Crunchers Original | 1 pkg (1 oz) | 90 | 8 | 0 | 4 |
| Crunchers Sour Cream & Onion | 1 pkg (1 oz) | 100 | 8 | 0 | 3 |
| ***Barbara's Bakery*** | | | | | |
| Potato | 1¼ cup (1 oz) | 150 | 15 | 0 | 1 |
| Potato No Salt Added | 1¼ cups (1 oz) | 150 | 15 | 0 | 1 |
| Potato Ripple | 1¼ cup (1 oz) | 150 | 15 | 0 | 1 |
| Potato Yogurt & Green Onion | 1¼ cup (1 oz) | 150 | 15 | tr | 1 |
| Tortilla Blue Corn | 15 chips (1 oz) | 140 | 16 | tr | 1 |

| FOOD | PORTION | CALS | CARB | SUGAR | FIBER |
|---|---|---|---|---|---|
| Tortilla Blue Corn No Salt | 15 chips (1 oz) | 140 | 16 | tr | 1 |
| Tortilla Pinta Salsa | 15 chips (1 oz) | 130 | 19 | 0 | 2 |
| ***Bruno & Luigi's*** | | | | | |
| Pasta Chips Garlic & Herb | 1 oz | 117 | 23 | 0 | 1 |
| ***Cape Cod*** | | | | | |
| Potato Golden Russet | 1 pkg (0.5 oz) | 70 | 8 | 0 | tr |
| ***Chester's*** | | | | | |
| Flamin'Hot | 1 oz | 140 | 17 | 6 | tr |
| Salsa | 1 oz | 140 | 18 | 0 | tr |
| ***Doritos*** | | | | | |
| 3D's Cooler Ranch | 27 (1 oz) | 140 | 18 | 2 | 1 |
| 3D's Nacho Cheesier | 27 (1 oz) | 140 | 17 | 2 | 1 |
| Cooler Ranch | 12 (1 oz) | 140 | 18 | tr | 1 |
| Flamin' Hot | 11 (1 oz) | 140 | 17 | 3 | 1 |
| Nacho Cheesier | 11 (1 oz) | 140 | 17 | 2 | 1 |
| Salsa Verde | 12 (1 oz) | 150 | 20 | 1 | 1 |
| Smokey Red | 12 (1 oz) | 150 | 21 | 1 | 1 |
| Spicy Nacho | 12 (1 oz) | 140 | 18 | 1 | 1 |
| Toasted Corn | 13 (1 oz) | 140 | 18 | 0 | 1 |
| ***Durangos*** | | | | | |
| Tortilla | 15 (1 oz) | 150 | 20 | 0 | 2 |
| ***Eden*** | | | | | |
| Brown Rice Chips | 1 oz | 150 | 19 | 0 | 0 |
| Sea Vegetable Chips | 1 oz | 140 | 23 | 2 | 0 |
| ***Fritos*** | | | | | |
| Chili Cheese | 31 (1 oz) | 160 | 16 | tr | 1 |
| Corn Chips BBQ | 29 (1 oz) | 150 | 16 | tr | 1 |
| Corn Chips King Size | 12 (1 oz) | 150 | 16 | 0 | 1 |
| Corn Chips Sabrositas Flamin' Hot | 30 (1 oz) | 150 | 16 | 1 | 1 |
| Corn Chips Sabrositas Lime'N Chile | 28 (1 oz) | 150 | 17 | 0 | 1 |
| Corn Chips Wild N'Mild Ranch | 28 (1 oz) | 160 | 15 | tr | 1 |
| Original | 32 (1 oz) | 160 | 15 | tr | 1 |
| Scoops | 11 (1 oz) | 160 | 17 | 0 | 1 |
| Texas Grill Honey BBQ | 15 (1 oz) | 150 | 16 | 1 | 1 |
| ***GeniSoy*** | | | | | |
| Soy Crisps | 1 oz | 110 | 14 | 1 | 2 |

| FOOD | PORTION | CALS | CARB | SUGAR | FIBER |
|---|---|---|---|---|---|
| Soy Crisps Apple Cinnamon Crunch | 1 oz | 120 | 17 | 4 | 2 |
| Soy Crisps Creamy Ranch | 1 oz | 110 | 15 | 1 | 2 |
| Soy Crisps Deep Sea Salt | 1 oz | 110 | 14 | 1 | 2 |
| Soy Crisps Rich Cheddar Cheese | 1 oz | 110 | 14 | 1 | 2 |
| Soy Crisps Roasted Garlic & Onion | 1 oz | 100 | 14 | 1 | 2 |
| Soy Crisps Zesty Barbeque | 1 oz | 110 | 17 | 2 | 2 |
| ***Guiltless Gourmet*** | | | | | |
| Tortilla Baked Chili Lime | 18 (1 oz) | 110 | 22 | 2 | 2 |
| Tortilla Baked Mucho Nacho | 18 (1 oz) | 110 | 22 | 2 | 2 |
| Tortilla Baked Organic Blue Corn | 18 (1 oz) | 110 | 22 | 0 | 2 |
| Tortilla Baked Picante Ranch | 18 (1 oz) | 110 | 22 | 2 | 2 |
| Tortilla Baked Red Corn | 18 (1 oz) | 110 | 22 | 2 | 2 |
| Tortilla Baked Spicy Black Bean | 18 (1 oz) | 110 | 22 | 0 | 2 |
| Tortilla Baked Sweet White Corn | 18 (1 oz) | 110 | 22 | 0 | 2 |
| Tortilla Baked Yellow Corn | 18 (1 oz) | 110 | 22 | 0 | 2 |
| Tortilla Baked Yellow Corn Unsalted | 18 (1 oz) | 110 | 22 | 0 | 2 |
| ***Husman's*** | | | | | |
| Deli Style Tortilla | 11 chips | 150 | 19 | 0 | 1 |
| Potato | 18 (1 oz) | 160 | 14 | 0 | 1 |
| Potato Sour Cream & Onion | 18 (1 oz) | 150 | 14 | 1 | 1 |
| Potato Sweet N'Sassy | 18 (1 oz) | 155 | 15 | 1 | 1 |
| ***Keto*** | | | | | |
| Low Carb Tortilla All Flavors | 1 oz | 150 | 8 | 0 | 4 |
| ***Lance*** | | | | | |
| BBQ | 22 (1 oz) | 160 | 15 | 1 | 1 |
| Cajun | 15 (1 oz) | 150 | 14 | 0 | 1 |
| Corn Chips | 39 (1.25 oz) | 200 | 14 | 0 | 1 |
| Corn Chips Hot BBQ | 35 (1.25 oz) | 210 | 20 | 0 | 1 |
| Hot Fries | 1 pkg (0.9 oz) | 140 | 11 | 0 | 1 |
| Mesquite BBQ | 22 (1 oz) | 150 | 15 | 0 | 1 |
| Potato | 23 (1 oz) | 160 | 15 | 0 | 1 |
| Ripple | 15 (1 oz) | 160 | 14 | 0 | 1 |
| Salt & Vinegar | 22 (1 oz) | 160 | 14 | 0 | 2 |
| Sour Cream & Onion | 22 (1 oz) | 160 | 15 | 1 | 1 |
| Tortilla Fiesta Salsa Triangle | 16 (1 oz) | 140 | 18 | 0 | 2 |

| FOOD | PORTION | CALS | CARB | SUGAR | FIBER |
|---|---|---|---|---|---|
| Tortilla Nacho Mini Round | 46 (1.5 oz) | 180 | 21 | 0 | 2 |
| Tortilla Nacho Triangles | 15 (1 oz) | 140 | 18 | 1 | 1 |
| ***Lay's*** | | | | | |
| Adobadas | 16 (1 oz) | 170 | 18 | 1 | 1 |
| Baked KC Masterpiece BBQ | 11 (1 oz) | 120 | 22 | 2 | 2 |
| Baked Original | 11 (1 oz) | 110 | 23 | 2 | 2 |
| Baked Roasted Herb | 12 (1 oz) | 130 | 25 | 2 | 2 |
| Baked Sour Cream & Onion | 12 (1 oz) | 120 | 21 | 3 | 2 |
| Classic | 20 (1 oz) | 150 | 15 | 0 | 1 |
| Deli Style Hot N'Tangy BBQ | 18 (1 oz) | 150 | 16 | 1 | 1 |
| Deli Style Jalapeno | 17 (1 oz) | 150 | 16 | 0 | 1 |
| Deli Style Original | 17 (1 oz) | 140 | 16 | 0 | 1 |
| Deli Style Salt & Vinegar | 16 (1 oz) | 90 | 16 | 1 | 1 |
| Flamin' Hot | 17 pieces (1 oz) | 150 | 16 | 5 | 1 |
| KC Masterpiece BBQ | 15 (1 oz) | 150 | 15 | 2 | 1 |
| Onion & Garlic | 19 (1 oz) | 150 | 16 | 1 | 1 |
| Original Baked | 1 pkg 1⅛ oz | 130 | 26 | 2 | 2 |
| Salt & Vinegar | 17 pieces (1 oz) | 150 | 15 | 1 | 1 |
| Sour Cream & Onion | 17 pieces (1 oz) | 160 | 12 | 1 | 1 |
| Toasted Onion & Cheese | 17 pieces (1 oz) | 160 | 14 | 0 | 1 |
| Wavy Au Gratin | 13 (1 oz) | 150 | 14 | tr | 1 |
| Wavy Original | 11 pieces (1 oz) | 160 | 15 | 0 | 1 |
| Wavy Ranch | 11 (1 oz) | 160 | 14 | 0 | 1 |
| Wow Mesquite BBQ | 20 (1 oz) | 75 | 17 | 1 | 1 |
| Wow Mesquite BBQ | 20 (1 oz) | 75 | 17 | 1 | 1 |
| Wow Original | 20 (1 oz) | 75 | 18 | 0 | 1 |
| Wow Sour Cream & Chive | 19 (1 oz) | 80 | 17 | tr | 1 |
| Wow Sour Cream & Chive | 19 (1 oz) | 80 | 17 | tr | 1 |
| ***Met-Rx*** | | | | | |
| Pro Chips Bar-B-Que | 1 pkg (2 oz) | 260 | 8 | 4 | 0 |
| Pro Chips Nacho | 1 pkg (2 oz) | 260 | 6 | 2 | 0 |
| ***Old Dutch Foods*** | | | | | |
| Potato | 12-15 chips (1 oz) | 150 | 16 | 1 | 1 |

| FOOD | PORTION | CALS | CARB | SUGAR | FIBER |
|---|---|---|---|---|---|
| Potato BBQ | 12-15 chips (1 oz) | 150 | 15 | 1 | 1 |
| Potato BBQ Ripple | 12-15 chips (1 oz) | 150 | 16 | 1 | tr |
| Potato Cajun Ripple | 12-15 chips (1 oz) | 150 | 15 | tr | 1 |
| Potato Cheddar & Sour Cream Ripple | 12-15 chips (1 oz) | 160 | 16 | tr | 1 |
| Potato Cheddar & Sour Cream Ripples | 12-15 chips (1 oz) | 150 | 15 | 1 | 1 |
| Potato Dill | 12-15 chips (1 oz) | 140 | 16 | 2 | 1 |
| Potato Dutch Crunch | 15-20 chips (1 oz) | 130 | 18 | 0 | 2 |
| Potato French Onion Ripple | 12-15 chips (1 oz) | 150 | 15 | 2 | 1 |
| Potato Jalapeno & Cheddar Dutch Crunch | 15-20 chips (1 oz) | 130 | 17 | 0 | 1 |
| Potato Jalapeno Cheese | 12-15 chips (1 oz) | 150 | 16 | tr | 1 |
| Potato Mesquite BBQ Dutch Crunch | 15-20 chips (1 oz) | 130 | 19 | 1 | 2 |
| Potato Onion & Garlic | 12-15 chips (1 oz) | 140 | 16 | 1 | 1 |
| Potato Outback Spicy BBQ | 12-15 chips (1 oz) | 150 | 15 | 1 | 1 |
| Potato Ripples | 12-15 chips (1 oz) | 150 | 15 | 0 | 1 |
| Potato Salt & Vinegar Dutch Crunch | 15-20 chips (1 oz) | 130 | 18 | 1 | 1 |
| Potato Sour Cream & Onion | 12-15 chips (1 oz) | 150 | 15 | 2 | 1 |
| Tortilla Bite Size White Corn | 20 chips (1 oz) | 150 | 18 | 0 | 1 |
| Tortilla Nacho Cheese | 15 chips (1 oz) | 150 | 19 | 0 | 1 |
| Tortilla Restaurant Style White | 9 chips (1 oz) | 140 | 20 | 0 | 2 |
| Tostados White Corn | 11 chips (1 oz) | 140 | 20 | 0 | 2 |

| FOOD | PORTION | CALS | CARB | SUGAR | FIBER |
|---|---|---|---|---|---|
| Tostados Yellow | 11 chips (1 oz) | 140 | 21 | 0 | 1 |
| ***Pita-Snax*** | | | | | |
| Cheddar Cheese | 34 (1 oz) | 110 | 21 | 1 | tr |
| Chili & Lime | 34 (1 oz) | 120 | 20 | 1 | tr |
| Cinnamon | 34 (1 oz) | 120 | 22 | 2 | tr |
| Dill Ranch | 34 (1 oz) | 120 | 21 | 0 | tr |
| Garlic | 34 (1 oz) | 120 | 22 | 0 | tr |
| Lightly Salted | 34 (1 oz) | 110 | 22 | 0 | tr |
| ***Pringles*** | | | | | |
| BBQ | 14 chips (1 oz) | 150 | 15 | 1 | 1 |
| Cheese & Onion | 14 chips (1 oz) | 160 | 15 | 1 | 1 |
| Cheez-ums | 14 chips (1 oz) | 150 | 14 | 1 | 1 |
| Original | 14 chips (1 oz) | 160 | 15 | – | 1 |
| Pizzalicious | 14 chips (1 oz) | 160 | 14 | 1 | 1 |
| Ranch | 14 chips (1 oz) | 150 | 15 | 1 | 1 |
| Salt & Vinegar | 14 chips (1 oz) | 160 | 15 | 1 | 1 |
| Sour Cream & Onion | 14 chips (1 oz) | 160 | 15 | 1 | 1 |
| ***Racquet*** | | | | | |
| Wheat Chips All Flavors | 6 chips | 30 | 4 | 0 | 0 |
| ***Revival*** | | | | | |
| Baked Soy Pasta Chips Lightly Salted Sunshine | 1 bag (0.9 oz) | 100 | 13 | 0 | 0 |
| Baked Soy Pasta Chips Naturally Nice | 1 bag (0.9 oz) | 80 | 12 | 0 | 0 |
| Baked Soy Pasta Chips Rev It Up Ranch | 1 bag (0.9 oz) | 105 | 12 | 1 | 0 |
| ***Ruffles*** | | | | | |
| Baked | 10 (1 oz) | 110 | 23 | 2 | 2 |
| Baked Cheddar & Sour Cream | 9 (1 oz) | 120 | 21 | 2 | 2 |
| Buffalo Style | 11 chips (1 oz) | 160 | 16 | 0 | 1 |

| FOOD | PORTION | CALS | CARB | SUGAR | FIBER |
|---|---|---|---|---|---|
| Cheddar & Sour Cream | 11 chips (1 oz) | 160 | 14 | 2 | 1 |
| French Onion | 11 (1 oz) | 150 | 15 | tr | 1 |
| MC Masterpiece Mesquite BBQ | 11 (1 oz) | 150 | 15 | tr | 1 |
| Original | 12 chips (1 oz) | 150 | 14 | 0 | 1 |
| Original | 1 pkg (1.5 oz) | 240 | 22 | 0 | 2 |
| Ranch | 13 (1 oz) | 150 | 15 | 1 | 1 |
| Reduced Fat | 16 (1 oz) | 130 | 18 | 0 | 1 |
| The Works | 12 (1 oz) | 160 | 14 | 2 | 1 |
| Wow Cheddar & Sour Cream | 15 (1 oz) | 75 | 16 | tr | 1 |
| Wow Cheddar & Sour Cream | 15 (1 oz) | 75 | 16 | tr | 1 |
| Wow Original | 17 (1 oz) | 75 | 17 | 0 | 1 |
| ***Santitas*** | | | | | |
| 100% White Corn | 6 (1 oz) | 130 | 19 | 0 | 1 |
| Restaurant Style Chips | 7 (1 oz) | 130 | 19 | 0 | 1 |
| Restaurant Style Strips | 10 (1 oz) | 130 | 19 | 0 | 1 |
| ***Skinny*** | | | | | |
| BBQ | 1½ cups | 90 | 17 | 1 | 1 |
| Corn | 1½ cups | 90 | 17 | 0 | 1 |
| Nacho Cheese | 1½ cups | 90 | 15 | 1 | 1 |
| Sour Cream & Onion | 1½ cups | 90 | 17 | 1 | 1 |
| Sticks Garden Veggie | 1 oz | 140 | 17 | 2 | 1 |
| Sticks Island Lime Chili | 1 oz | 140 | 17 | 2 | 1 |
| Sticks Maui Wowie | 1 oz | 140 | 17 | 2 | 1 |
| Sticks Original Spud | 1 oz | 140 | 17 | 2 | 1 |
| ***Snyder's Of Hanover*** | | | | | |
| BBQ Rib | 1 oz | 140 | 17 | tr | tr |
| Barbeque Corn | 1.5 oz | 230 | 22 | 0 | 2 |
| Cheddar Bacon | 1 oz | 150 | 20 | tr | 3 |
| Corn Chips | 1.5 oz | 230 | 22 | 0 | 2 |
| Grilled Steak & Onion | 1 oz | 140 | 20 | 0 | 4 |
| Hot Buffalo | 1 oz | 150 | 20 | 0 | 4 |
| Kosher Dill | 1 oz | 140 | 20 | 1 | 3 |
| No Salt | 1 oz | 140 | 19 | 0 | 3 |
| Potato | 1 oz | 140 | 19 | 0 | 3 |
| Ripple | 1 oz | 140 | 18 | 0 | 4 |
| Salt & Vinegar | 1 oz | 140 | 19 | tr | 4 |
| Sausage Pizza | 1 oz | 150 | 20 | tr | 4 |
| Sour Cream & Onion | 1 oz | 150 | 19 | tr | 4 |

| FOOD | PORTION | CALS | CARB | SUGAR | FIBER |
|---|---|---|---|---|---|
| Tasty Veggie Potato Chips | 1 oz | 150 | 20 | 1 | 4 |
| Tortilla Nacho | 1 oz | 140 | 19 | tr | 1 |
| Tortilla No Salt Yellow Corn | 1 oz | 140 | 19 | tr | 1 |
| Tortilla White Corn | 1 oz | 140 | 20 | tr | 1 |
| Tortilla Yellow Corn | 1 oz | 140 | 19 | tr | 1 |
| Tortilla Yellow Corn Mini | 1 oz | 160 | 20 | tr | 1 |
| Veggie Crisps | 1 pkg (1.5 oz) | 190 | 26 | 0 | 2 |
| ***Soya King*** | | | | | |
| Soy Mongolian BBQ | 23 chips (1 oz) | 140 | 19 | – | 3 |
| Soy Original | 23 chips (1 oz) | 140 | 19 | – | 3 |
| Soy Sour Cream & Onion | 23 chips (1 oz) | 140 | 19 | – | 3 |
| Soy Taco | 23 chips (1 oz) | 140 | 19 | – | 3 |
| ***Stacy's*** | | | | | |
| Pita Chips Cinnamon Sugar | 1 oz | 130 | 18 | – | 3 |
| Pita Chips Parmesan Garlic & Herb | 1 oz | 130 | 18 | – | 3 |
| Pita Chips Simply Naked | 1 oz | 130 | 18 | – | 3 |
| Twisted Pasta Low Fat | 1 oz | 110 | 21 | 1 | 1 |
| ***Sunchips*** | | | | | |
| French Onion | 13 (1 oz) | 140 | 18 | 2 | 2 |
| Harvest Cheddar | 13 (1 oz) | 140 | 19 | 2 | 2 |
| Original | 14 (1 oz) | 140 | 19 | 2 | 2 |
| ***Torengos*** | | | | | |
| Chips | 13 chips (1 oz) | 140 | 15 | 0 | 1 |
| ***Tostitos*** | | | | | |
| Baked Bite Size | 20 (1 oz) | 110 | 24 | 0 | 2 |
| Baked Bite Size Salsa & Cream Cheese | 16 (1 oz) | 120 | 21 | 1 | 1 |
| Baked Original | 13 (1 oz) | 110 | 21 | 0 | 1 |
| Bite Size | 15 (1 oz) | 140 | 17 | 0 | 1 |
| Crispy Rounds | 13 (1 oz) | 150 | 17 | tr | 1 |
| Nacho Style | 6 (1 oz) | 140 | 19 | tr | 1 |
| Restaurant Style | 7 (1 oz) | 140 | 19 | 0 | 1 |
| Restaurant Style Hint of Lime | 6 (1 oz) | 140 | 19 | tr | 1 |
| Santa Fe Gold | 7 (1 oz) | 140 | 19 | 0 | 1 |

| FOOD | PORTION | CALS | CARB | SUGAR | FIBER |
|---|---|---|---|---|---|
| Wow Original | 6 (1 oz) | 90 | 20 | 0 | 1 |
| ***Tyson*** | | | | | |
| Tortilla Salted | 13 (1 oz) | 150 | 20 | 0 | 2 |
| Tortilla Yellow Corn Salted | 13 (1 oz) | 150 | 20 | 0 | 2 |
| ***Utz*** | | | | | |
| Baked Crisps | 12 (1 oz) | 110 | 23 | 2 | 2 |
| Carolina Barbeque | 20 (1 oz) | 150 | 14 | tr | 1 |
| Cheddar & Sour Cream | 20 (1 oz) | 160 | 14 | tr | 1 |
| Corn Chips | 24 (1 oz) | 160 | 16 | 0 | 1 |
| Corn Chips Barbecue | 24 (1 oz) | 160 | 16 | tr | 1 |
| Grandma | 20 (1 oz) | 140 | 14 | 0 | 1 |
| Grandma BBQ | 20 (1 oz) | 140 | 15 | 2 | 1 |
| Home Style Kettle | 20 (1 oz) | 140 | 14 | 0 | 1 |
| Home Style Kettle BBQ | 20 (1 oz) | 140 | 15 | 2 | 1 |
| Kettle Classics Crunchy | 20 (1 oz) | 150 | 15 | 0 | 1 |
| Kettle Classics Crunchy Mesquite BBQ | 20 (1 oz) | 150 | 15 | 2 | 1 |
| No Salt Added | 20 (1 oz) | 150 | 14 | 0 | 1 |
| Onion & Garlic | 20 (1 oz) | 150 | 14 | tr | 1 |
| Potato | 20 (1 oz) | 150 | 14 | 0 | 1 |
| Reduced Fat BBQ | 22 (1 oz) | 140 | 19 | 1 | 1 |
| Reducted Fat Ripple | 24 (1 oz) | 140 | 18 | 0 | 1 |
| Ripple | 20 (1 oz) | 150 | 14 | 0 | 1 |
| Ripple Sour Cream & Onion | 20 (1 oz) | 160 | 14 | tr | 1 |
| Ripple Barbeque | 20 (1 oz) | 150 | 14 | 1 | 1 |
| Salt'N Vinegar | 20 (1 oz) | 150 | 14 | tr | 1 |
| The Crab Chip | 20 (1 oz) | 150 | 14 | tr | 1 |
| Tortilla Black Bean & Salsa | 13 (1 oz) | 150 | 19 | 1 | 1 |
| Tortilla Low Fat Baked | 10 (1 oz) | 120 | 24 | 0 | 2 |
| Tortilla Nacho | 13 (1 oz) | 150 | 19 | tr | 1 |
| Tortilla Restaurant Style | 6 (1 oz) | 140 | 18 | 0 | 1 |
| Tortilla Spicy Nacho | 13 (1 oz) | 150 | 19 | tr | 1 |
| Tortilla White Corn | 12 (1 oz) | 140 | 18 | 0 | 1 |
| Wavy | 20 chips (1 oz) | 150 | 14 | 0 | 1 |
| Yes! Fat Free | 20 (1 oz) | 75 | 17 | 0 | 1 |
| Yes! Fat Free Barbeque | 20 (1 oz) | 75 | 16 | 1 | 1 |
| Yes! Fat Free Ripple | 20 (1 oz) | 75 | 17 | 0 | 1 |

| FOOD | PORTION | CALS | CARB | SUGAR | FIBER |
|---|---|---|---|---|---|
| **CHITTERLINGS** | | | | | |
| pork cooked | 3 oz | 258 | 0 | 0 | 0 |
| **CHIVES** | | | | | |
| freeze-dried | 1 tbsp | 1 | tr | – | – |
| fresh chopped | 1 tbsp | 1 | tr | – | – |
| fresh chopped | 1 tsp | 0 | tr | – | – |
| **CHOCOLATE** *(see also* CANDY, COCOA, ICE CREAM TOPPINGS, MILK DRINKS*)* | | | | | |
| ***Twist*** | | | | | |
| Sugar Free Chocolate Spread | 2 tbsp | 170 | 2 | 0 | 0 |
| **BAKING** | | | | | |
| baking | 1 oz | 145 | 8 | – | – |
| grated unsweetened | 1 cup | 689 | 37 | – | 20 |
| liquid unsweetened | 1 oz | 134 | 10 | – | 5 |
| squares unsweetened | 1 square (1 oz) | 146 | 8 | – | 4 |
| ***Nestle*** | | | | | |
| Choco Bake | ½ oz | 80 | 5 | 0 | 2 |
| Premier White Bar | ½ oz | 80 | 8 | 8 | 0 |
| Premier White Morsels | 1 tbsp | 80 | 9 | 9 | 0 |
| Semi-Sweet Bar | ½ oz | 70 | 9 | 8 | tr |
| Unsweetened Bar | ½ oz | 80 | 4 | 0 | 2 |
| **CHIPS** | | | | | |
| milk chocolate | 1 cup (6 oz) | 862 | 100 | – | – |
| semisweet | 60 pieces (1 oz) | 136 | 18 | – | – |
| semisweet | 1 cup (6 oz) | 804 | 106 | – | – |
| ***Cloud Nine*** | | | | | |
| Double Dark Chocolate | 13 pieces (0.5 oz) | 80 | 9 | 9 | 0 |
| ***Ghirardelli*** | | | | | |
| Semi-Sweet | 33 pieces (0.5 oz) | 70 | 9 | 7 | tr |
| ***Hershey*** | | | | | |
| Almond Joy Bits | 1 tbsp (0.5 oz) | 60 | 7 | – | – |
| Chocolate & Peanut Butter Chips | 1 tbsp (0.5 oz) | 70 | 10 | – | – |
| Holiday Baking Bits | 1 tbsp (0.5 oz) | 70 | 11 | – | – |

| FOOD | PORTION | CALS | CARB | SUGAR | FIBER |
|---|---|---|---|---|---|
| Milk Chocolate | 1 tbsp (0.5 oz) | 80 | 9 | – | – |
| Mini Kisses For Baking | 11 pieces (0.5 oz) | 80 | 9 | – | – |
| Mint Chocolate | 1 tbsp (0.5 oz) | 80 | 10 | – | – |
| Premier White Milk Chips | 1 tbsp (0.5 oz) | 80 | 9 | – | – |
| Raspberry Chips | 1 tbsp (0.5 oz) | 80 | 10 | – | – |
| Semi-Sweet | 1 tbsp (0.5 oz) | 80 | 10 | – | – |
| Semi-Sweet Mini | 1 tbsp (0.5 oz) | 80 | 10 | – | – |
| Skor English Toffee Baking Bits | 1 tbsp (0.5 oz) | 70 | 7 | – | – |
| ***Nestle*** | | | | | |
| Crunch Baking Pieces | 1½ tbsp | 80 | 10 | 8 | 0 |
| Milk Chocolate Morsels | 1 tbsp | 70 | 9 | 8 | 0 |
| Mint Chocolate Morsels | 1 tbsp | 70 | 9 | 8 | tr |
| Morsels Semi-Sweet | 1 tbsp | 70 | 9 | 8 | tr |
| Semi-Sweet Mega Morsels | 1 tbsp | 70 | 9 | 8 | tr |
| Semi-Sweet Mini Morsels | 1 tbsp | 70 | 9 | 8 | tr |
| ***Sunspire*** | | | | | |
| Chocolate Sundrops | 47 pieces (1.4 oz) | 190 | 27 | 26 | 1 |
| Dark Chocolate Grain Sweetened | 13 pieces (0.5 oz) | 70 | 10 | 5 | 1 |
| Organic | 13 pieces (0.5 oz) | 70 | 9 | 7 | 0 |
| ***Tropical Source*** | | | | | |
| Espresso Roast Dairy Free | 13 pieces (1.5 oz) | 70 | 9 | 9 | 1 |
| Semi-Sweet Dairy Free | 13 pieces (1.5 oz) | 80 | 9 | 9 | 0 |
| **MIX** | | | | | |
| powder | 2-3 heaping tsp | 75 | 20 | – | – |
| powder as prep w/ whole milk | 9 oz | 226 | 31 | – | – |

| FOOD | PORTION | CALS | CARB | SUGAR | FIBER |
|---|---|---|---|---|---|
| ***Quik*** | | | | | |
| Chocolate Powder | 2 tbsp (0.8 oz) | 90 | 19 | 18 | 1 |
| Chocolate Powder No Sugar | 2 tbsp (0.4 oz) | 40 | 7 | 1 | 2 |

**CHOCOLATE MILK** *(see* MILK DRINKS*)*

## CHOCOLATE SYRUP

| FOOD | PORTION | CALS | CARB | SUGAR | FIBER |
|---|---|---|---|---|---|
| chocolate fudge | 1 cup (11.9 oz) | 1176 | 200 | – | – |
| chocolate fudge | 1 tbsp (0.7 oz) | 73 | 12 | – | – |
| syrup | 1 cup | 653 | 177 | – | – |
| syrup | 2 tbsp | 82 | 22 | – | – |
| syrup as prep w/ whole milk | 9 oz | 232 | 34 | – | – |
| ***Ah!Laska*** | | | | | |
| Organic | 2 tbsp | 85 | 20 | 18 | – |
| ***Colac*** | | | | | |
| Chocolate Topping | 1 tbsp | 37 | 15 | 0 | 0 |
| ***DaVinci Gourmet*** | | | | | |
| Sugar Free | 2 tbsp | 15 | 5 | 0 | 1 |
| ***Estee*** | | | | | |
| Chocolate | 2 tbsp | 15 | 5 | – | 0 |
| ***Hershey*** | | | | | |
| Chocolate Fudge | 1 tbsp (0.7 oz) | 70 | 10 | – | – |
| Chocolate Malt | 2 tbsp (1.4 oz) | 100 | 25 | – | – |
| Lite | 2 tbsp (1.2 oz) | 50 | 12 | – | – |
| Syrup | 2 tbsp (1.4 oz) | 100 | 24 | – | – |
| ***Quik*** | | | | | |
| Chocolate | 2 tbsp (1.3 oz) | 100 | 23 | 17 | tr |
| ***Smucker's*** | | | | | |
| Plate Scapers Chocolate | 2 tbsp | 100 | 23 | 11 | 1 |
| ***Toll House*** | | | | | |
| Mint Chocolate | 2 tbsp (1.5 oz) | 130 | 25 | 22 | 1 |

| FOOD | PORTION | CALS | CARB | SUGAR | FIBER |
|---|---|---|---|---|---|
| Semi-Sweet | 2 tbsp (1.5 oz) | 130 | 24 | 22 | 1 |
| ***Walden Farms*** | | | | | |
| Sugar Free | 2 tbsp | 0 | 0 | 0 | 0 |
| **CHUTNEY** | | | | | |
| apple | 1.2 oz | 68 | 18 | – | 1 |
| apple cranberry | 1 tbsp | 16 | 4 | – | – |
| coconut | ¼ cup | 74 | 4 | – | 2 |
| mango | 1 tbsp | 54 | 10 | – | tr |
| tomato | 1 tbsp | 32 | 8 | – | tr |
| ***Wild Thyme Farms*** | | | | | |
| Apricot Cranberry Walnut | 1 tbsp | 15 | 3 | 3 | – |
| Pineapple Peach Lime | 1 tbsp | 14 | 6 | 5 | – |
| **CILANTRO** | | | | | |
| fresh | 1 tsp (2 g) | tr | tr | – | tr |
| fresh | 1 cup (1.6 oz) | 11 | 2 | – | 1 |
| **CINNAMON** | | | | | |
| ground | 1 tsp | 6 | 2 | – | – |
| sticks | 0.5 oz | 39 | 8 | 0 | 3 |
| ***Gringo Billy's*** | | | | | |
| Cinnamon Sweetener | ½ tsp | 0 | 0 | 0 | 0 |
| **CISCO** | | | | | |
| smoked | 1 oz | 50 | 0 | 0 | 0 |
| smoked | 3 oz | 151 | 0 | 0 | 0 |
| **CLAMS** | | | | | |
| **CANNED** | | | | | |
| liquid only | 1 cup | 6 | tr | – | – |
| liquid only | 3 oz | 2 | tr | – | – |
| meat only | 1 cup | 236 | 8 | – | – |
| meat only | 3 oz | 126 | 4 | – | – |
| ***Bumble Bee*** | | | | | |
| Baby | 2 oz | 50 | 2 | 0 | 0 |
| ***Progresso*** | | | | | |
| Creamy Clam Sauce | ½ cup (4.2 oz) | 110 | 8 | 0 | 0 |
| Minced | ¼ cup (2.1 oz) | 25 | 2 | 0 | 0 |
| Red Clam Sauce | ½ cup (4.4 oz) | 60 | 8 | 4 | 1 |
| White Clam Sauce | ½ cup (4.4 oz) | 150 | 5 | tr | 0 |

| FOOD | PORTION | CALS | CARB | SUGAR | FIBER |
|---|---|---|---|---|---|
| **FRESH** | | | | | |
| cooked | 3 oz | 126 | 4 | – | – |
| cooked | 20 sm | 133 | 5 | – | – |
| raw | 9 lg (6.3 oz) | 133 | 5 | – | – |
| raw | 20 sm (6.3 oz) | 133 | 5 | – | – |
| raw | 3 oz | 63 | 2 | – | – |
| **TAKE-OUT** | | | | | |
| breaded & fried | 20 sm | 379 | 19 | – | – |
| **CLEMENTINES** | | | | | |
| ***Haddon House*** | | | | | |
| in Light Syrup | ½ cup | 80 | 19 | 18 | 1 |
| **CLOVES** | | | | | |
| ground | 1 tsp | 7 | 1 | – | – |
| **COCOA** *(see also* HOT COCOA) | | | | | |
| powder unsweetened | 1 tbsp (5 g) | 11 | 3 | – | 2 |
| powder unsweetened | 1 cup (3 oz) | 197 | 47 | – | 29 |
| ***Ah!Laska*** | | | | | |
| Organic | 2 tbsp | 100 | 23 | 20 | 5 |
| Organic Bakers Cocoa | 1 tbsp | 20 | 3 | – | 1 |
| ***Hershey*** | | | | | |
| Cocoa | 1 tbsp (5 g) | 20 | 3 | – | – |
| European Cocoa | 1 tbsp (5 g) | 20 | 3 | – | – |
| ***Nestle*** | | | | | |
| Cocoa | 1 tbsp | 15 | 3 | 0 | 1 |
| **COCONUT** | | | | | |
| coconut water | 1 tbsp | 3 | 1 | – | – |
| coconut water | 1 cup | 46 | 9 | – | – |
| cream canned | 1 cup | 568 | 25 | – | – |
| cream canned | 1 tbsp | 36 | 2 | – | – |
| dried sweetened flaked | 1 cup | 351 | 35 | – | – |
| dried sweetened flaked | 7 oz pkg | 944 | 95 | – | – |
| dried sweetened flaked canned | 1 cup | 341 | 32 | – | – |
| dried sweetened shredded | 7 oz pkg | 997 | 95 | – | – |
| dried sweetened shredded | 1 cup | 466 | 44 | – | – |
| dried toasted | 1 oz | 168 | 13 | – | – |
| dried unsweetened | 1 oz | 187 | 7 | – | – |
| fresh | 1 piece (1.5 oz) | 159 | 7 | – | 4 |

| FOOD | PORTION | CALS | CARB | SUGAR | FIBER |
|---|---|---|---|---|---|
| fresh shredded | 1 cup | 283 | 12 | – | 7 |
| milk canned | 1 cup | 445 | 6 | – | – |
| milk canned | 1 tbsp | 30 | tr | – | – |
| milk frozen | 1 cup | 486 | 13 | – | – |
| milk frozen | 1 tbsp | 30 | 1 | – | – |
| ***Thai Kitchen*** | | | | | |
| Milk | 2 oz | 124 | 3 | 1 | 0 |
| **COD** | | | | | |
| atlantic canned | 3 oz | 89 | 0 | 0 | 0 |
| atlantic canned | 1 can (11 oz) | 327 | 0 | 0 | 0 |
| atlantic dried | 3 oz | 246 | 0 | 0 | 0 |
| atlantic fresh cooked | 1 fillet (6.3 oz) | 189 | 0 | 0 | 0 |
| atlantic fresh cooked | 3 oz | 89 | 0 | 0 | 0 |
| atlantic fresh raw | 3 oz | 70 | 0 | 0 | 0 |
| pacific fresh baked | 3 oz | 95 | 0 | 0 | 0 |
| roe canned | 1 oz | 34 | tr | – | – |
| roe baked w/ butter & lemon juice | 1 oz | 36 | tr | – | – |
| roe raw | 1 oz | 37 | tr | – | – |
| roe tarama | 3.5 oz | 547 | 6 | tr | – |
| **COFFEE** (*see also* COFFEE BEVERAGES, COFFEE SUBSTITUTES) | | | | | |
| **INSTANT** | | | | | |
| decaffeinated | 1 rounded tsp | 4 | 1 | – | – |
| decaffeinated as prep | 6 oz | 4 | 1 | – | – |
| regular as prep | 1 cup (6 oz) | 4 | 1 | – | 0 |
| regular w/ chicory | 1 rounded tsp | 6 | 1 | – | – |
| regular w/ chicory as prep | 6 oz | 6 | 1 | – | – |
| ***Nescafe*** | | | | | |
| Decafe | 1 tsp (2 g) | 0 | tr | 0 | 0 |
| Decafe w/ Chicory | 1 tsp (2 g) | 0 | tr | 0 | 0 |
| French Vanilla | 1 tsp (2 g) | 5 | 1 | 0 | 0 |
| French Vanilla Decaf | 1 tsp (2 g) | 5 | 1 | 0 | 0 |
| Hazelnut | 1 tsp (2 g) | 5 | 1 | 0 | 0 |
| Irish Creme | 1 tsp (2 g) | 5 | 1 | 0 | 0 |
| Regular | 1 tsp (2 g) | 0 | tr | 0 | 0 |
| With Chicory | 1 tsp (2 g) | 5 | 1 | 0 | 0 |

| FOOD | PORTION | CALS | CARB | SUGAR | FIBER |
|---|---|---|---|---|---|
| **REGULAR** | | | | | |
| brewed | 8 oz | 2 | tr | – | – |
| roasted beans | 1 oz | 64 | 18 | – | 2 |
| ***Nescafe*** | | | | | |
| Cafe Mocha | 1 can (10 oz) | 140 | 27 | 24 | 1 |
| Caffe Latte | 1 can (10 oz) | 130 | 22 | 20 | 1 |
| Caffe Latte Decaffeinated | 1 can (10 oz) | 130 | 22 | 20 | 0 |
| Espresso | 1 tsp (2 g) | 0 | tr | 0 | 0 |
| Espresso Cafe Latte | 1 pkg (0.6 oz) | 70 | 10 | 6 | 0 |
| Espresso Cafe Mocha | 1 pkg (1 oz) | 110 | 20 | 15 | 1 |
| Espresso Cappuccino | 1 pkg (0.6 oz) | 80 | 11 | 6 | 0 |
| Espresso Roast | 1 can (10 oz) | 90 | 21 | 14 | 0 |
| French Vanilla | 1 can (10 oz) | 150 | 25 | 21 | 2 |
| Hazelnut | 1 can (10 oz) | 130 | 22 | 20 | 0 |
| Roasted Ground Decaffeinated as prep | 1 cup (6 oz) | 0 | tr | 0 | 0 |
| Roasted Ground as prep | 1 cup (6 oz) | 0 | tr | 0 | 0 |
| ***Revival*** | | | | | |
| Soy Caramal Corn | 1 cup (8 oz) | 0 | 0 | 0 | 0 |
| Soy Hazelnut | 1 cup (8 oz) | 0 | 0 | 0 | 0 |
| Soy Original Roast | 1 cup (8 oz) | 0 | 0 | 0 | 0 |
| **TAKE-OUT** | | | | | |
| cafe amaretto w/ alcohol | 1 serv | 192 | 15 | – | 0 |
| cafe au lait | 1 cup (8 fl oz) | 77 | 6 | 7 | – |
| cafe brulot | 1 cup | 48 | 3 | 3 | – |
| cafe brulot w/ alcohol | 1 serv | 130 | 16 | – | 3 |
| cappuccino | 1 cup (8 fl oz) | 77 | 6 | 7 | – |
| coffee con leche | 1 cup (8 fl oz) | 77 | 6 | 7 | – |
| espresso | 1 cup (3 fl oz) | 2 | tr | 0 | – |
| irish coffee | 1 serv | 226 | 6 | – | 0 |
| latte w/ skim milk | 13 oz | 88 | 12 | 11 | 0 |
| latte w/ whole milk | 13 oz | 152 | 12 | 11 | 0 |
| mocha | 1 mug (9.6 fl oz) | 202 | 17 | 12 | – |

## COFFEE BEVERAGES

| | | | | | |
|---|---|---|---|---|---|
| cappuccino mix as prep | 7 oz | 62 | 11 | – | – |
| french mix as prep | 7 oz | 57 | 7 | – | – |
| mocha mix as prep | 7 oz | 51 | 8 | – | – |

| FOOD | PORTION | CALS | CARB | SUGAR | FIBER |
|---|---|---|---|---|---|
| ***AchievONE*** | | | | | |
| All Flavors | 1 bottle (9.5 oz) | 120 | 5 | 4 | – |
| ***Arizona*** | | | | | |
| Iced Latte Supreme | 8 oz | 110 | 21 | 16 | 1 |
| Iced Mocha Latte | 8 oz | 110 | 21 | 19 | 1 |
| ***Chock full o'Nuts*** | | | | | |
| New York Cappuccino French Vanilla | 1 pkg (0.9 oz) | 90 | 19 | 14 | 0 |
| New York Cappuccino Hazelnut | 1 pkg. (0.9 oz) | 90 | 19 | 14 | 0 |
| ***Coffee House USA*** | | | | | |
| All Flavors | 1 bottle (9.5 oz) | 100 | 29 | 28 | tr |
| ***Flavour Creations*** | | | | | |
| Coffee Flavoring Tablets All Flavors | 1 tablet | 0 | tr | tr | 0 |
| ***Gehl's*** | | | | | |
| Iced Cappuccino | 1 can (11 oz) | 190 | 33 | 31 | 0 |
| ***Jakada*** | | | | | |
| Latte Mocha | 1 bottle (10.5 oz) | 180 | 33 | 32 | 0 |
| Latte Vanilla | 1 bottle (10.5 oz) | 180 | 32 | 31 | 0 |
| ***Silk*** | | | | | |
| Coffee Soylatte | 1 bottle (11 oz) | 220 | 38 | 31 | 0 |
| ***Sipper Sweets*** | | | | | |
| Sugar Free Low Carb Cappuccino | 1 serv | 50 | 3 | 0 | 0 |
| ***Starbucks*** | | | | | |
| Frappuccino | 1 bottle (9.5 oz) | 190 | 39 | 30 | 0 |
| Frappuccino Mocha | 1 bottle (9.5 oz) | 190 | 39 | 30 | 0 |
| Frappuccino Vanilla | 1 bottle (9.5 oz) | 190 | 39 | 30 | 0 |

## COFFEE SUBSTITUTES

| | | | | | |
|---|---|---|---|---|---|
| powder | 1 tsp | 9 | 2 | – | – |

| FOOD | PORTION | CALS | CARB | SUGAR | FIBER |
|---|---|---|---|---|---|
| powder as prep | 6 oz | 9 | 2 | – | – |
| powder as prep w/ milk | 6 oz | 121 | 10 | – | – |
| ***Natural Touch*** | | | | | |
| Kaffree Roma | 1 tsp (2 g) | 10 | 2 | 0 | 0 |
| Roma Cappuccino | 3 tbsp (0.4 oz) | 50 | 5 | 4 | 0 |
| **COFFEE WHITENERS** | | | | | |
| liquid nondairy frzn | 1 tbsp (0.5 oz) | 20 | 2 | – | – |
| powder nondairy | 1 tsp | 11 | 1 | – | – |
| ***N-Rich*** | | | | | |
| Coffee Creamer | 1 tsp (2 g) | 10 | 1 | 0 | 0 |
| ***Silk*** | | | | | |
| Creamer | 1 tbsp | 15 | 1 | 0 | 0 |
| Creamer French Vanilla | 1 tbsp | 20 | 3 | 3 | 0 |
| Creamer Hazelnut | 1 tbsp | 15 | 1 | 0 | 0 |
| **COLESLAW** | | | | | |
| **TAKE-OUT** | | | | | |
| coleslaw w/ dressing | ½ cup | 42 | 7 | – | – |
| vinegar & oil coleslaw | 3.5 oz | 150 | 16 | – | – |
| **COLLARDS** | | | | | |
| fresh cooked | ½ cup | 17 | 4 | – | – |
| frzn chopped cooked | ½ cup | 31 | 6 | – | – |
| ***Birds Eye*** | | | | | |
| Chopped Greens frzn | 1 cup | 30 | 2 | 1 | 2 |
| **COOKIES** | | | | | |
| **MIX** | | | | | |
| chocolate chip | 1 (0.56 oz) | 79 | 10 | – | – |
| oatmeal | 1 (0.6 oz) | 74 | 10 | – | tr |
| oatmeal raisin | 1 (0.6 oz) | 74 | 10 | – | tr |
| ***Aunt Paula's*** | | | | | |
| Low Carb Chef Chocolate Chip as prep | 1 | 66 | 4 | 0 | 1 |
| Low Carb Chef Peanut Butter as prep | 1 | 66 | 4 | 0 | 1 |
| ***Betty Crocker*** | | | | | |
| Chocolate Peanut Butter as prep | 1 bar | 180 | 25 | 18 | – |

| FOOD | PORTION | CALS | CARB | SUGAR | FIBER |
|---|---|---|---|---|---|
| Date Bar as prep | 1 bar | 150 | 23 | 14 | 1 |
| Oatmeal as prep | 2 | 150 | 22 | 12 | 1 |
| ***GoldnBrown*** | | | | | |
| Fat Free | 1 (1.1 oz) | 120 | 27 | 15 | 0 |
| ***Keto*** | | | | | |
| Chocolate Chip as prep | 1 | 47 | 2 | 1 | 1 |
| Oatmeal Raisin as prep | 2 | 59 | 2 | 0 | 1 |
| ***MiniCarb*** | | | | | |
| All Flavors as prep | 1 | 110 | 7 | 1 | 5 |
| **READY-TO-EAT** | | | | | |
| animal | 11 crackers (1 oz) | 126 | 21 | – | – |
| animal crackers | 1 box (2.4 oz) | 299 | 51 | – | – |
| animal crackers | 1 (2.5 g) | 11 | 2 | – | – |
| australian anzac biscuit | 1 | 98 | 17 | – | 1 |
| butter | 1 (5 g) | 23 | 3 | – | tr |
| chocolate chip | 1 (0.4 oz) | 48 | 7 | – | tr |
| chocolate chip | 1 box (1.9 oz) | 233 | 36 | – | – |
| chocolate chip low fat | 1 (0.25 oz) | 45 | 7 | – | – |
| chocolate chip low sugar low sodium | 1 (0.24 oz) | 31 | 5 | – | – |
| chocolate chip soft-type | 1 (0.5 oz) | 69 | 9 | – | tr |
| chocolate w/ creme filling | 1 (0.35 oz) | 47 | 7 | – | tr |
| chocolate w/ creme filling chocolate coated | 1 (0.60 oz) | 82 | 11 | – | – |
| chocolate w/ creme filling sugar free low sodium | 1 (0.35 oz) | 46 | 7 | – | – |
| chocolate w/ extra creme filling | 1 (0.46 oz) | 65 | 9 | – | – |
| chocolate wafer | 1 (0.2 oz) | 26 | 4 | – | – |
| cream cheese | 1 (1.1 oz) | 141 | 14 | 6 | tr |
| digestive biscuits plain | 2 | 141 | 21 | – | 1 |
| fig bars | 1 (0.56 oz) | 56 | 11 | – | 1 |
| fortune | 1 (0.28 oz) | 30 | 7 | – | tr |
| fudge | 1 (0.73 oz) | 73 | 17 | – | tr |
| gingersnaps | 1 (0.24 oz) | 29 | 5 | – | – |
| graham | 1 squares (0.24 oz) | 30 | 5 | – | – |
| graham chocolate covered | 1 (0.49 oz) | 68 | 9 | – | – |
| graham honey | 1 (0.24 oz) | 30 | 5 | – | tr |
| hermits | 1 (1 oz) | 117 | 18 | 10 | 1 |

| FOOD | PORTION | CALS | CARB | SUGAR | FIBER |
|---|---|---|---|---|---|
| jumbles coconut | 1 (1 oz) | 121 | 13 | 7 | 1 |
| ladyfingers | 1 (0.38 oz) | 40 | 7 | – | – |
| macaroons | 1 (0.8 oz) | 97 | 17 | – | – |
| madeleines | 1 (0.8 oz) | 86 | 10 | 5 | tr |
| marshmallow chocolate coated | 1 (0.46 oz) | 55 | 9 | – | – |
| marshmallow pie chocolate coated | 1 (1.4 oz) | 165 | 26 | – | – |
| merinque | 1 (0.3 oz) | 20 | 5 | 5 | 0 |
| molasses | 1 (0.5 oz) | 65 | 11 | – | – |
| neapolitan tri-color cookie | 1 (0.6 oz) | 79 | 8 | 5 | tr |
| oatmeal | 1 (0.6 oz) | 81 | 12 | – | 1 |
| oatmeal | 1 (0.52 oz) | 71 | 9 | – | tr |
| oatmeal soft-type | 1 (0.5 oz) | 61 | 10 | – | tr |
| oatmeal raisin | 1 (0.6 oz) | 81 | 12 | – | 1 |
| oatmeal raisin low sugar no sodium | 1 (0.24 oz) | 31 | 5 | – | – |
| oatmeal raisin soft-type | 1 (0.5 oz) | 61 | 10 | – | tr |
| peanut butter sandwich | 1 (0.5 oz) | 67 | 9 | – | – |
| peanut butter sandwich sugar free low sodium | 1 (0.35 oz) | 54 | 5 | – | – |
| peanut butter softy-type | 1 (0.5 oz) | 69 | 9 | – | tr |
| pinenut cookies | 1 (1.1 oz) | 134 | 11 | 8 | 1 |
| raisin soft-type | 1 (0.5 oz) | 60 | 10 | – | – |
| reginette queen'a biscuit | 1 (0.8 oz) | 86 | 13 | 4 | tr |
| shortbread | 1 (0.28 oz) | 40 | 5 | – | – |
| shortbread pecan | 1 (0.49 oz) | 79 | 8 | – | tr |
| spritz | 1 (0.4 oz) | 42 | 6 | 3 | tr |
| sugar | 1 (0.52 oz) | 72 | 10 | – | – |
| sugar low sugar sodium free | 1 (0.24 oz) | 30 | 5 | – | – |
| sugar wafers w/ creme filling | 1 (0.12 oz) | 18 | 3 | – | – |
| sugar wafers w/ creme filling sugar free sodium free | 1 (0.14 oz) | 20 | 3 | – | – |
| toll house original | 1 (0.8 oz) | 105 | 13 | 9 | tr |
| vanilla sandwich | 1 (0.35 oz) | 48 | 7 | – | tr |
| vanilla wafers | 1 (0.21 oz) | 28 | 4 | – | – |
| zeppole | 1 (0.8 oz) | 78 | 6 | 4 | tr |
| ***Alternative Baking*** | | | | | |
| Vegan Chocolate Chip | 1 serv (2.5 oz) | 280 | 46 | 21 | 1 |
| Vegan Expresso Chocolate Chip | 1 serv (2 oz) | 230 | 35 | 18 | 1 |

| FOOD | PORTION | CALS | CARB | SUGAR | FIBER |
|---|---|---|---|---|---|
| Vegan Lemon | 1 serv (2.25 oz) | 250 | 42 | 19 | 1 |
| Vegan Oatmeal | 1 serv (2.25 oz) | 250 | 35 | 15 | 2 |
| Vegan Peanut Butter | 1 serv (2.25 oz) | 270 | 40 | 17 | 1 |
| Vegan Pumpkin | 1 serv (2 oz) | 200 | 35 | 17 | 1 |
| Vegan Wheat Free Choco Cherry Chunk | 1 serv (1.75 oz) | 190 | 32 | 18 | 1 |
| Vegan Wheat Free Hula Nut | 1 serv (1.75 oz) | 190 | 29 | 10 | 2 |
| Vegan Wheat Free P-nut Fudge Fusion | 1 serv (1.75 oz) | 190 | 29 | 15 | 1 |
| Vegan Wheat Free Snickerdoodle | 1 serv (1.75 oz) | 170 | 35 | 17 | 1 |
| ***Amay's*** | | | | | |
| Chinese Style Almond | 1 (0.5 oz) | 80 | 10 | 4 | 0 |
| ***Archway*** | | | | | |
| Alpine Fudge | 1 (1.3 oz) | 160 | 24 | 15 | tr |
| Carrot Cake | 1 (1 oz) | 130 | 19 | 11 | 0 |
| Chocolate Chip | 1 (0.9 oz) | 120 | 16 | 9 | 0 |
| Chocolate Chip Sugar Free | 1 (0.8 oz) | 110 | 16 | 0 | 0 |
| Coconut Macaroon | 2 (1.4 oz) | 180 | 21 | 16 | 1 |
| Devils Food Chocolate Drop Fat Free | 1 (0.7 oz) | 60 | 15 | 9 | 0 |
| Dutch Cocoa | 1 (0.9 oz) | 100 | 18 | 10 | 0 |
| Frosty Lemon | 1 (0.9 oz) | 100 | 16 | 10 | 0 |
| Fruit & Honey Bar | 1 (0.9 oz) | 110 | 19 | 10 | 0 |
| Fruit Bar Fat Free | 1 (0.9 oz) | 90 | 21 | 11 | 0 |
| Fruit Filled Raspberry | 1 (0.8 oz) | 90 | 15 | 7 | 0 |
| Ginger Snaps | 5 (1 oz) | 120 | 20 | 9 | 0 |
| Homestyle Chocolate Chip | 3 (1 oz) | 130 | 17 | 9 | 1 |
| Iced Spice | 1 (1 oz) | 120 | 19 | 10 | 0 |
| Oatmeal | 1 (0.9 oz) | 100 | 16 | 8 | 0 |
| Oatmeal Apple Filled | 1 (0.9 oz) | 90 | 16 | 8 | 0 |
| Oatmeal Pecan | 1 (0.9 oz) | 110 | 16 | 8 | 1 |
| Oatmeal Raisin Bran | 1 (0.9 oz) | 100 | 18 | 11 | 1 |
| Oatmeal Raspberry Fat Free | 1 (1.1 oz) | 100 | 23 | 13 | 1 |
| Oatmeal Sugar Free | 1 (0.8 oz) | 110 | 16 | 0 | 0 |
| Oatmeal Raisin | 1 (0.9 oz) | 100 | 17 | 10 | 1 |

| FOOD | PORTION | CALS | CARB | SUGAR | FIBER |
|---|---|---|---|---|---|
| Oatmeal Raisin Fat Free | 1 (1.1 oz) | 100 | 24 | 14 | 1 |
| Old Dutch Apple | 1 (0.9 oz) | 110 | 18 | 11 | 0 |
| Peanut Butter | 1 (1 oz) | 150 | 16 | 8 | 0 |
| Peanut Butter Fudge | 1 (1.3 oz) | 220 | 23 | 13 | 1 |
| Peanut Butter Sugar Free | 1 (0.8 oz) | 110 | 14 | 0 | 0 |
| Pecan Crunch | 3 (1.2 oz) | 180 | 20 | 9 | 0 |
| Rocky Road | 1 (0.8 oz) | 110 | 16 | 9 | 0 |
| Rocky Road Sugar Free | 1 (0.8 oz) | 100 | 15 | 0 | tr |
| Shortbread Sugar Free | 1 (0.8 oz) | 110 | 16 | 0 | 0 |
| Strawberry Filled | 1 (0.8 oz) | 90 | 15 | 7 | 0 |
| ***Arnott's*** | | | | | |
| Raspberry Tartlets | 2 | 100 | 17 | 6 | tr |
| ***Atkins*** | | | | | |
| Endulge Wafer Bars Chocolate Creme | 2 bars (1 oz) | 120 | 15 | 0 | 3 |
| Endulge Wafer Bars Mint | 2 bars (1 oz) | 120 | 15 | 0 | 3 |
| Endulge Wafer Bars Peanut Butter | 2 bars (1 oz) | 120 | 14 | 0 | 3 |
| ***BP Gourmet*** | | | | | |
| Biscotti Fat Free Cinnamon Crunch | 6 (1 oz) | 110 | 24 | 15 | 0 |
| Biscotti Fat Free Vanilla Crunch | 4 (1 oz) | 80 | 18 | 6 | 0 |
| Chocolate Fudge Chip Sugar Free | 5 (1 oz) | 100 | 13 | 0 | 0 |
| Dreams Chocolate | 7 (1 oz) | 120 | 21 | 20 | 0 |
| Dreams Fat Free Chocolate Fudge | 13 (1 oz) | 100 | 25 | 25 | 0 |
| Dreams Fat Free Vanilla | 19 (1 oz) | 100 | 25 | 25 | 0 |
| Tangos Fat Free Chocolate Fudge Chip | 4 (1 oz) | 100 | 23 | 18 | 0 |
| ***Bahlsen*** | | | | | |
| Afrika | 8 (1.1 oz) | 170 | 17 | 11 | 2 |
| Butter Leaves | 7 (1 oz) | 140 | 19 | 7 | tr |
| Choco Leibniz | 2 (1 oz) | 140 | 18 | 10 | tr |
| Choco Star Dark Chocolate | 3 (1.1 oz) | 170 | 16 | 10 | 1 |
| Choco Star Milk Chocolate | 3 (1.1 oz) | 180 | 16 | 12 | 1 |
| Chocolate Hearts | 4 (1 oz) | 160 | 18 | 8 | 1 |
| Delice | 6 (1 oz) | 140 | 19 | 5 | tr |
| Deloba | 4 (0.9 oz) | 130 | 19 | 8 | tr |
| Hanover Waffelin | 5 (1 oz) | 160 | 16 | 8 | 0 |

| FOOD | PORTION | CALS | CARB | SUGAR | FIBER |
|---|---|---|---|---|---|
| Hit Chocolate Vanilla Filled | 2 (1 oz) | 140 | 18 | 9 | tr |
| Hit Vanilla Chocolate Filled | 2 (1 oz) | 140 | 19 | 9 | tr |
| Kipferl | 4 (1 oz) | 150 | 16 | 6 | 0 |
| Leibniz | 6 (1 oz) | 130 | 23 | 7 | 1 |
| Nuss Dessert | 3 (1.1 oz) | 180 | 19 | 9 | tr |
| Probiers | 6 (1.1 oz) | 150 | 21 | 9 | tr |
| Twingo | 6 (1.1 oz) | 170 | 18 | 11 | 1 |
| Waffeletten | 4 (1 oz) | 160 | 18 | 10 | 1 |
| ***Baker's Breakfast Cookie*** | | | | | |
| Banana Walnut | 1 (3 oz) | 274 | 52 | 20 | 5 |
| Chocolate Chunk Raisin | 1 (3 oz) | 260 | 54 | 24 | 5 |
| Double Chocolate Chunk | 1 (3 oz) | 250 | 50 | 22 | 5 |
| Fruit & Nut | 1 (3 oz) | 270 | 54 | 26 | 5 |
| Mocha Chocolate Chunk | 1 (3 oz) | 250 | 50 | 22 | 5 |
| Oatmeal Raisin | 1 (3 oz) | 250 | 54 | 24 | 5 |
| Peanut Butter | 1 (3 oz) | 290 | 48 | 20 | 6 |
| Peanut Butter & Jelly | 1 (3 oz) | 320 | 64 | 34 | 6 |
| Pumpkin Spice | 1 (3 oz) | 230 | 52 | 22 | 5 |
| Vegan Peanut Butter Chocolate Chunk | 1 (3 oz) | 310 | 58 | 24 | 6 |
| ***Baker's Harvest*** | | | | | |
| Animal | 12 (0.9 oz) | 130 | 22 | 5 | – |
| Chocolate Graham | 2 (0.9 oz) | 130 | 24 | 7 | 1 |
| Cinnamon Grahams | 2 (0.9 oz) | 130 | 19 | 7 | tr |
| Cinnamon Grahams Low Fat | 2 (0.9 oz) | 110 | 22 | 6 | 1 |
| Fig Bars | 2 (1.2 oz) | 120 | 23 | 14 | 1 |
| Graham | 2 (0.9 oz) | 120 | 21 | 6 | tr |
| Graham Low Fat | 2 (0.9 oz) | 110 | 22 | 6 | 1 |
| Iced Oatmeal | 1 (0.6 oz) | 70 | 11 | 6 | 0 |
| Pecan Shortbread | 1 (0.5 oz) | 80 | 10 | 4 | 0 |
| Vanilla Wafers | 7 (1.1 oz) | 150 | 22 | 10 | 1 |
| ***Barbara's Bakery*** | | | | | |
| Apple Cinnamon Bars Fat Free Whole Wheat | 1 (0.7 oz) | 60 | 14 | 10 | 2 |
| Chocolate Chip | 1 (0.6 oz) | 80 | 10 | 5 | 1 |
| Double Dutch Chocolate | 1 (0.6 oz) | 80 | 10 | 5 | 1 |
| Fig Bars Fat Free Wheat Free | 1 (0.7 oz) | 60 | 15 | 11 | 1 |
| Fig Bars Fat Free Whole Wheat | 1 (0.7 oz) | 60 | 16 | 11 | 2 |
| Nature's Choice Coconut Almond | 1 bar (1 oz) | 120 | 20 | 8 | 1 |

| FOOD | PORTION | CALS | CARB | SUGAR | FIBER |
|---|---|---|---|---|---|
| Nature's Choice Expresso Bean | 1 bar (1 oz) | 120 | 22 | 9 | 1 |
| Nature's Choice Lemon Yogurt | 1 bar (1 oz) | 120 | 22 | 9 | 1 |
| Nature's Choice Roasted Peanut | 1 bar (1 oz) | 130 | 20 | 8 | 1 |
| Old Fashioned Oatmeal | 1 (0.6 oz) | 70 | 11 | 5 | 1 |
| Raspberry Bars Fat Free Wheat Free Raspberry | 1 (0.7 oz) | 60 | 15 | 11 | 1 |
| Snackimals Chocolate Chip | 8 (1 oz) | 120 | 18 | 8 | 1 |
| Snackimals Oatmeal Wheat Free | 8 (1 oz) | 120 | 19 | 6 | 2 |
| Snackimals Vanilla | 8 (1 oz) | 120 | 19 | 7 | 1 |
| Traditional Blueberry Low Fat | 1 (0.7 oz) | 60 | 14 | 9 | 1 |
| Traditional Fig Low Fat | 1 (0.7 oz) | 60 | 14 | 9 | 1 |
| Traditional Shortbread | 1 (0.6 oz) | 80 | 10 | 3 | 1 |
| ***Bed & Breakfast*** | | | | | |
| Cranberry Orange Oatmeal | 1 (0.8 oz) | 110 | 17 | 9 | 1 |
| Enrobed Shortbread | 2 (1.4 oz) | 190 | 24 | 10 | 1 |
| Fruit Center Key Lime | 2 (1.1 oz) | 140 | 22 | 12 | 0 |
| Fruit Center Raspberry | 2 (1.1 oz) | 140 | 22 | 11 | 0 |
| ***Beigel's*** | | | | | |
| Black & White | 1 (1 oz) | 100 | 18 | 15 | 0 |
| ***Breaktime*** | | | | | |
| Chocolate Chip | 1 (0.3 oz) | 37 | 5 | 2 | tr |
| Coconut | 1 (0.3 oz) | 35 | 5 | 3 | tr |
| Ginger | 1 (0.3 oz) | 34 | 6 | 3 | – |
| Oatmeal | 1 (0.3 oz) | 35 | 5 | 3 | tr |
| Sprinkles | 1 (0.3 oz) | 36 | 5 | 3 | – |
| ***Brent & Sam's*** | | | | | |
| Chocolate Chip Pecan | 2 (0.5 oz) | 80 | 9 | 6 | 0 |
| Chocolate Chip Raspberry | 2 (0.5 oz) | 70 | 10 | 7 | 0 |
| Chocolate Chips | 2 (0.5 oz) | 70 | 10 | 7 | 0 |
| Key Lime White Chocolate | 2 (0.5 oz) | 70 | 10 | 8 | 0 |
| Oatmeal Raisin Pecan | 2 (0.5 oz) | 70 | 9 | 6 | 1 |
| Toffee Pecan | 2 (0.5 oz) | 80 | 9 | 5 | 0 |
| White Chocolate Macadamia | 2 (0.5 oz) | 80 | 9 | 6 | 0 |
| ***Bud's Best*** | | | | | |
| Caco Creme | 7 (1 oz) | 140 | 21 | 9 | 2 |
| Chocolate Chip | 6 (1 oz) | 140 | 19 | 9 | 1 |
| French Vanilla | 7 (1 oz) | 150 | 20 | 9 | 2 |
| Oatmeal | 6 (1 oz) | 130 | 20 | 9 | tr |

| FOOD | PORTION | CALS | CARB | SUGAR | FIBER |
|---|---|---|---|---|---|
| ***Cafe*** | | | | | |
| Cinnamony Twists | 1 | 40 | 7 | 4 | 0 |
| Chocolate Chip | (0.5 oz) | | | | |
| Sugar Free California Almond | 4 (1 oz) | 110 | 17 | 0 | 0 |
| Twists Cinnamony | 1 (0.3 oz) | 40 | 7 | 4 | 0 |
| ***Carbolite*** | | | | | |
| Chocolate Chip | 1 (1 oz) | 120 | 12 | 0 | 4 |
| Peanut Butter | 1 (1 oz) | 120 | 12 | 0 | 4 |
| Shortbread | 1 (1 oz) | 180 | 14 | 0 | 5 |
| ***Carr's*** | | | | | |
| Ginger Lemon Cremes | 2 (1 oz) | 140 | 19 | 11 | tr |
| ***Carriage Trade*** | | | | | |
| Finnish Ginger Snaps | 3 | 60 | 21 | 9 | tr |
| ***Cookie Lover's*** | | | | | |
| Chocolate Chip | 1 (0.8 oz) | 90 | 16 | 9 | 0 |
| Creme Supremes | 2 (0.9 oz) | 120 | 18 | 10 | 1 |
| Creme Supremes Mint | 2 (0.9 oz) | 120 | 18 | 10 | 1 |
| Grahams | 2 (1 oz) | 100 | 22 | 5 | 1 |
| Grahams Cinnamon | 2 (1 oz) | 110 | 24 | 6 | 1 |
| Peanut Butter | 1 (0.8 oz) | 100 | 16 | 7 | 0 |
| Shortbread | 1 (0.8 oz) | 120 | 13 | 5 | 0 |
| ***Dare*** | | | | | |
| Blueberry Cheesecake | 1 (0.6 oz) | 90 | 11 | 7 | tr |
| Butter Shortbread | 1 (0.5 oz) | 63 | 7 | 2 | tr |
| Butter Creme | 1 (0.6 oz) | 85 | 11 | 4 | 1 |
| Carrot Cake | 1 (0.6 oz) | 92 | 11 | 7 | tr |
| Chocolate Chip | 1 (0.5 oz) | 77 | 9 | 6 | tr |
| Chocolate Fudge | 1 (0.7 oz) | 97 | 13 | 5 | 1 |
| Cinnamon Danish | 1 (0.4 oz) | 47 | 7 | 2 | tr |
| Coconut Creme | 1 (0.7 oz) | 99 | 12 | 7 | tr |
| French Creme | 1 (0.5 oz) | 80 | 8 | 4 | tr |
| Harvest From The Rain Forest | 1 (0.5 oz) | 70 | 7 | 3 | tr |
| Key Lime Creme | 1 (0.6 oz) | 86 | 12 | 5 | tr |
| Lemon Creme | 1 (0.7 oz) | 95 | 13 | 6 | tr |
| Maple Leaf Creme | 1 (0.6 oz) | 83 | 12 | 5 | tr |
| Maple Walnut Fudge | 1 (0.7 oz) | 99 | 13 | 6 | tr |
| Milk Chocolate Fudge | 1 (0.7 oz) | 99 | 12 | 5 | tr |
| Oatmeal Raisin | 1 (0.4 oz) | 59 | 8 | 3 | tr |
| Social Tea | 1 (0.2 oz) | 26 | 4 | – | tr |
| Sun Maid Raisin Oatmeal | 1 (0.5 oz) | 52 | 8 | 5 | tr |

| FOOD | PORTION | CALS | CARB | SUGAR | FIBER |
|---|---|---|---|---|---|
| ***De Beukelaer*** | | | | | |
| Pirouline | 8 (1 oz) | 130 | 23 | 13 | tr |
| Pirouline Viennese Wafers | 1 (1 oz) | 150 | 20 | 9 | tr |
| ***Delarce*** | | | | | |
| Chocosprits | 1 (0.6 oz) | 90 | 11 | 3 | tr |
| Marquisettes | 3 (0.9 oz) | 140 | 17 | 7 | 1 |
| Roules d'Or | 4 (1 oz) | 180 | 19 | 11 | 0 |
| ***Dunkaroos*** | | | | | |
| Chocolate Graham | 1 pkg | 120 | 20 | 14 | – |
| Cinnamon Graham | 1 pkg | 130 | 21 | 14 | – |
| Honey Graham | 1 pkg | 120 | 20 | 13 | tr |
| ***Dutch Mill*** | | | | | |
| Chocolate Chip | 3 (1.1 oz) | 160 | 18 | 10 | 1 |
| Coconut Macaroons | 3 (1 oz) | 120 | 14 | 12 | 0 |
| Oatmeal Raisin | 3 (1 oz) | 130 | 18 | 10 | 1 |
| ***Eddyleon*** | | | | | |
| Jelly Graham Raspberry | 1 (0.9 oz) | 134 | 15 | 13 | tr |
| Pudding Cookies | 1 (0.9 oz) | 134 | 15 | 13 | tr |
| ***English Bay*** | | | | | |
| Strawberry Fruit Bar | 1 (1.2 oz) | 120 | 22 | 14 | 1 |
| ***Entenmann's*** | | | | | |
| Little Bites Chocolate Chip | 8 (1.8 oz) | 240 | 33 | 19 | 1 |
| Soft Baked Chocolate Chip | 1 (0.7 oz) | 100 | 13 | 8 | tr |
| Soft Baked Double Chocolate Chip | 1 (0.7 oz) | 100 | 14 | 8 | tr |
| Soft Baked Milk Chocolate Chip | 1 (0.7 oz) | 100 | 13 | 8 | tr |
| Soft Baked Original Chocolate Chip | 3 (1 oz) | 150 | 20 | 11 | tr |
| Soft Baked White Chocolate Macadamia Nut | 1 (0.7 oz) | 100 | 12 | 7 | tr |
| Soft Baked Light Chocolately Chip | 2 (1 oz) | 120 | 21 | 13 | tr |
| Soft Baked Light Oatmeal Raisin | 2 (1 oz) | 100 | 23 | 14 | 1 |
| ***Estee*** | | | | | |
| Chocolate Chip | 4 | 150 | 21 | 5 | tr |
| Coconut | 4 | 140 | 19 | 5 | tr |
| Fig Bars | 2 | 100 | 23 | 13 | 3 |
| Fudge | 4 | 150 | 19 | 5 | 1 |
| Lemon Thins | 4 | 140 | 19 | 5 | tr |

| FOOD | PORTION | CALS | CARB | SUGAR | FIBER |
|---|---|---|---|---|---|
| Oatmeal Raisin | 4 | 130 | 19 | 6 | 1 |
| Sandwich Chocolate | 3 | 160 | 24 | 9 | 1 |
| Sandwich Original | 3 | 160 | 24 | 10 | 1 |
| Sandwich Peanut Butter | 3 | 160 | 22 | 7 | 1 |
| Sandwich Vanilla | 3 | 160 | 25 | 7 | tr |
| Shortbread | 4 | 130 | 22 | 5 | tr |
| Sugar Free Chocolate Chip | 3 | 110 | 22 | 0 | 1 |
| Sugar Free Chocolate Walnut | 3 | 110 | 22 | 0 | 1 |
| Sugar Free Coconut | 3 | 110 | 22 | 0 | 1 |
| Sugar Free Grahams Chocolate | 2 | 110 | 27 | 0 | 3 |
| Sugar Free Grahams Cinnamon | 2 | 90 | 18 | 0 | 2 |
| Sugar Free Grahams Old Fashion | 2 | 90 | 17 | 0 | 2 |
| Sugar Free Lemon | 3 | 110 | 22 | 0 | 1 |
| Sugar Free Wafer Banana Split | 5 | 155 | 22 | 0 | 0 |
| Sugar Free Wafer Chocolate | 5 | 150 | 19 | 0 | 0 |
| Sugar Free Wafer Chocolate Peanut Butter Caramel | 5 | 150 | 22 | 0 | 0 |
| Sugar Free Wafer Lemon Creme | 5 | 150 | 22 | 0 | 0 |
| Sugar Free Wafer Peanut Butter Creme | 5 | 150 | 22 | 0 | 0 |
| Sugar Free Wafer Vanilla | 5 | 150 | 21 | 0 | 0 |
| Sugar Free Wafer Vanilla Strawberry | 5 | 150 | 22 | 0 | 0 |
| Vanilla Thins | 4 | 140 | 19 | 5 | tr |
| ***Falcone's*** | | | | | |
| Sorrentini | 1 (1 oz) | 100 | 16 | 6 | 2 |
| ***Famous Amos*** | | | | | |
| Butter Shortie | 1 (0.5 oz) | 80 | 9 | 3 | tr |
| Chocolate Chip | 4 (1 oz) | 140 | 18 | 10 | tr |
| Chocolate Chip & Pecan | 4 (1 oz) | 140 | 18 | 10 | tr |
| Chocolate Chip Toffee | 4 (1 oz) | 130 | 18 | 10 | 0 |
| Chocolate Creme Sandwich | 3 (1.2 oz) | 140 | 22 | 13 | tr |
| Chunky Chocolate Chip | 1 (0.5 oz) | 70 | 9 | 5 | 0 |
| Fat Free Fig Bar | 2 (1 oz) | 90 | 21 | 9 | 1 |
| Fat Free Strawberry Fruit Bar | 2 (1 oz) | 90 | 22 | 11 | 0 |
| Fig Bar | 2 (1.1 oz) | 120 | 22 | 12 | tr |
| Oatmeal Chocolate Chip Walnut | 4 (1 oz) | 140 | 16 | 9 | tr |
| Oatmeal Raisin | 4 (1 oz) | 130 | 20 | 10 | tr |

| FOOD | PORTION | CALS | CARB | SUGAR | FIBER |
|---|---|---|---|---|---|
| Oatmeal Macaroon Creme Sandwich | 3 (1.2 oz) | 160 | 23 | 12 | 1 |
| Peanut Butter Chocolate Chunk | 1 (0.5 oz) | 80 | 9 | 5 | tr |
| Peanut Butter Creme Sandwich | 3 (1.2 oz) | 160 | 19 | 9 | 1 |
| Pecan Shortie | 1 (0.5 oz) | 80 | 9 | 3 | tr |
| Vanilla Creme Sandwich | 3 (1.2 oz) | 160 | 24 | 13 | 0 |
| ***Frookie*** | | | | | |
| Animal Frackers | 14 (1 oz) | 130 | 18 | 10 | 1 |
| Chocolate Chip Wheat & Gluten Free | 3 (1.1 oz) | 140 | 23 | 12 | 1 |
| Double Chocolate Wheat & Gluten Free | 3 (1.1 oz) | 130 | 23 | 13 | 1 |
| Dream Creams Strawberry | 4 (1 oz) | 140 | 18 | 7 | 4 |
| Dream Creams Vanilla | 4 (1 oz) | 140 | 18 | 7 | 4 |
| Funky Monkeys Chocolate | 16 (1 oz) | 120 | 20 | 9 | 1 |
| Funky Monkeys Vanilla | 16 (1 oz) | 120 | 20 | 9 | 1 |
| Graham Cinnamon | 2 (1 oz) | 100 | 17 | 2 | 1 |
| Graham Honey | 2 (1 oz) | 110 | 18 | 2 | 1 |
| Lemon Wafers | 8 (1 oz) | 110 | 26 | 18 | tr |
| Old Fashioned Ginger Snaps | 8 (1 oz) | 120 | 24 | 12 | tr |
| Organic Chocolate Chip | 3 (1.1 oz) | 150 | 20 | 9 | 1 |
| Organic Double Chocolate Chip | 3 (1.1 oz) | 140 | 20 | 11 | 1 |
| Organic Iced Lemon | 3 (1.3 oz) | 165 | 27 | 14 | 0 |
| Organic Oatmeal Raisin | 3 (1.1 oz) | 140 | 22 | 12 | 1 |
| Peanut Butter Chunk Wheat & Gluten Free | 3 (1.1 oz) | 140 | 21 | 12 | 0 |
| Sandwich Chocolate | 2 (0.7 oz) | 100 | 14 | 7 | 1 |
| Sandwich Lemon | 2 (0.7 oz) | 100 | 14 | 7 | 1 |
| Sandwich Peanut Butter | 2 (0.7 oz) | 100 | 14 | 7 | 1 |
| Sandwich Vanilla | 2 (0.7 oz) | 100 | 14 | 7 | 1 |
| Shortbread | 5 (1 oz) | 130 | 20 | 7 | tr |
| Vanilla Wafers | 8 (1 oz) | 110 | 26 | 18 | 0 |
| ***General Henry*** | | | | | |
| Fruit Bars Apple | 1 (0.6 oz) | 60 | 13 | 6 | tr |
| Fruit Bars Blueberry | 1 (0.6 oz) | 60 | 12 | 6 | tr |
| Fruit Bars Figs | 1 (0.6 oz) | 60 | 12 | 6 | tr |
| ***Girl Scout*** | | | | | |
| Apple Cinnamon Reduced Fat | 3 (1 oz) | 120 | 18 | 6 | tr |
| Lemon Drops | 3 (1.2 oz) | 160 | 20 | 6 | 0 |
| Samoas | 2 (1 oz) | 160 | 17 | 12 | 2 |

| FOOD | PORTION | CALS | CARB | SUGAR | FIBER |
|---|---|---|---|---|---|
| Striped Chocolate Chip | 3 (1.2 oz) | 180 | 20 | 11 | tr |
| Tagalongs | 2 (0.9 oz) | 150 | 13 | 8 | 2 |
| Thin Mints | 4 (1 oz) | 140 | 18 | 10 | tr |
| Trefoils | 5 (1.1 oz) | 160 | 20 | 7 | 1 |
| ***Glenny's*** | | | | | |
| Soy Fudgies All Flavors | 3 | 70 | 14 | 0 | 1 |
| ***Godiva*** | | | | | |
| Biscotti Dipped in Milk Chocolate | 1 (0.9 oz) | 120 | 15 | 6 | 0 |
| ***Gol D Lite*** | | | | | |
| Low Carb Pizzelle | 1 (0.3 oz) | 46 | 6 | 0 | 1 |
| ***Golden Grahams Treats*** | | | | | |
| Chocolate Chunk | 1 bar (0.8 oz) | 90 | 17 | 9 | 0 |
| Honey Graham | 1 bar (0.8 oz) | 90 | 17 | 9 | 0 |
| King Size Chocolate Chunk | 1 bar (1.6 oz) | 190 | 35 | 18 | 1 |
| King Size Honey Graham | 1 bar (1.6 oz) | 180 | 36 | 18 | 1 |
| ***Goody Man*** | | | | | |
| Marshmallow Crispy Squares | 1 (1.17 oz) | 130 | 24 | 10 | 0 |
| ***Gourmet*** | | | | | |
| Chocolate Chip | 2 (1.1 oz) | 160 | 19 | 13 | 1 |
| Lemon Creme | 2 (1.4 oz) | 210 | 27 | 17 | 0 |
| Oatmeal Raisin | 2 (0.9 oz) | 120 | 15 | 7 | 1 |
| Peanut Butter Chip | 2 (1 oz) | 150 | 17 | 8 | tr |
| Raspberry Center | 2 (1.1 oz) | 140 | 21 | 12 | tr |
| ***Grandma's*** | | | | | |
| Chocolate Chip | 1 (1.4 oz) | 190 | 25 | 13 | tr |
| Fudge Chocolate Chip | 1 (1.4 oz) | 170 | 26 | 13 | 1 |
| Fudge Sandwich | 3 | 180 | 31 | 15 | tr |
| Fudge Vanilla Sandwich | 3 | 120 | 21 | 10 | tr |
| Mini Fudge | 9 | 150 | 21 | 12 | 1 |
| Mini Peanut Butter | 9 | 150 | 21 | 10 | 1 |
| Mini Vanilla | 9 | 150 | 22 | 10 | tr |
| Oatmeal Raisin | 1 (1.4 oz) | 160 | 26 | 15 | 1 |
| Old Time Molasses | 1 (1.4 oz) | 160 | 29 | 18 | tr |
| Peanut Butter | 1 (1.4 oz) | 190 | 22 | 12 | 1 |
| Peanut Butter Chocolate Chip | 1 (1.4 oz) | 190 | 23 | 15 | 1 |
| Peanut Butter Sandwich | 5 | 210 | 28 | 13 | 1 |
| Rich N'Chewy | 1 pkg | 270 | 39 | 23 | 1 |
| Vanilla Sandwich | 3 | 180 | 32 | 17 | tr |
| Vanilla Sandwich | 5 | 210 | 30 | 15 | tr |

| FOOD | PORTION | CALS | CARB | SUGAR | FIBER |
|---|---|---|---|---|---|
| ***Granny Oats*** | | | | | |
| Low Carb Oatmeal | 4 | 98 | 10 | 0 | 3 |
| ***Health Valley*** | | | | | |
| Apple Spice | 3 | 100 | 24 | 11 | 3 |
| Apricot Delight | 3 | 100 | 24 | 11 | 3 |
| Biscotti Amaretto | 2 | 120 | 23 | 7 | 3 |
| Biscotti Chocolate | 2 | 120 | 23 | 7 | 3 |
| Biscotti Fruit & Nut | 2 | 120 | 23 | 7 | 3 |
| Cheesecake Bars Blueberry | 1 bar | 160 | 34 | 17 | 3 |
| Cheesecake Bars Raspberry | 1 bar | 160 | 34 | 17 | 3 |
| Cheesecake Bars Strawberry | 1 bar | 160 | 34 | 17 | 3 |
| Chips Double Chocolate | 3 | 100 | 24 | 10 | 4 |
| Chips Old Fashioned | 3 | 100 | 24 | 10 | 4 |
| Chips Original | 3 | 100 | 24 | 10 | 4 |
| Chocolate Fudge Center | 2 | 70 | 25 | 10 | 3 |
| Chocolate Sandwich Bar Bavarian Creme | 1 bar | 150 | 35 | 18 | 3 |
| Chocolate Sandwich Bars Caramel Creme | 1 bar | 150 | 35 | 18 | 3 |
| Chocolate Sandwich Bars Vanilla Creme | 1 bar | 150 | 35 | 18 | 3 |
| Date Delight | 3 | 100 | 24 | 11 | 3 |
| Graham Amaranth | 8 | 100 | 23 | 5 | 3 |
| Graham Oat Bran | 8 | 100 | 30 | 5 | 3 |
| Graham Original Amaranth | 6 | 120 | 22 | 4 | 3 |
| Hawaiian Fruit | 3 | 100 | 24 | 11 | 3 |
| Jumbo Apple Raisin | 1 | 80 | 19 | 9 | 3 |
| Jumbo Raisin Raisin | 1 | 80 | 19 | 9 | 3 |
| Jumbo Raspberry | 1 | 80 | 19 | 9 | 3 |
| Marshmallow Bars Chocolate Chip | 1 | 90 | 22 | 11 | 1 |
| Marshmallow Bars Old Fashioned | 1 | 90 | 22 | 11 | 1 |
| Marshmallow Bars Tropical Fruit | 1 | 90 | 22 | 11 | 1 |
| Oat Bran Fruit Bars Raisin Cinnamon | 1 bar | 160 | 34 | 18 | 2 |
| Raisin Oatmeal | 3 | 100 | 24 | 11 | 3 |
| Raspberry Fruit Center | 1 | 70 | 18 | 9 | 2 |
| Tarts Baked Apple Cinnamon | 1 | 150 | 35 | 18 | 3 |

| FOOD | PORTION | CALS | CARB | SUGAR | FIBER |
|---|---|---|---|---|---|
| Tarts California Strawberry | 1 | 150 | 35 | 18 | 3 |
| Tarts Chocolate Fudge | 1 | 150 | 35 | 18 | 3 |
| Tarts Cranberry Apple | 1 | 150 | 35 | 18 | 3 |
| Tarts Mountain Blueberry | 1 | 150 | 35 | 18 | 3 |
| Tarts Red Raspberry | 1 | 150 | 35 | 18 | 3 |
| Tarts Sweet Red Cherry | 1 | 150 | 35 | 18 | 3 |
| ***Heavenly*** | | | | | |
| Meringues All Flavors Sugar Free Fat Free | 1 | 0 | 1 | 0 | 0 |
| ***Hellema*** | | | | | |
| Almond | 1 pkg (0.6 oz) | 90 | 9 | 4 | tr |
| ***Hershey*** | | | | | |
| Cripsy Rice Snacks Peanut Butter | 1 (0.6 oz) | 70 | 10 | 5 | tr |
| ***Jacques Gourmet*** | | | | | |
| Palmier Cinnamon | 3 (1 oz) | 140 | 15 | 5 | 0 |
| Palmier Vanilla | 3 (1 oz) | 140 | 15 | 5 | 0 |
| ***Joseph's*** | | | | | |
| Almond Sugar Free | 2 (0.9 oz) | 100 | 14 | 0 | 0 |
| Chocolate Chip Sugar Free | 2 (0.9 oz) | 100 | 15 | 0 | 0 |
| Chocolate Walnut Sugar Free | 2 (0.9 oz) | 100 | 14 | 0 | 1 |
| Coconut Sugar Free | 2 (0.9 oz) | 105 | 14 | 0 | 0 |
| Lemon Sugar Free | 2 (0.9 oz) | 95 | 15 | 0 | 0 |
| Oatmeal Raisin Sugar Free | 2 (0.9 oz) | 100 | 15 | 0 | 0 |
| Peanut Butter Sugar Free | 2 (0.9 oz) | 95 | 13 | 0 | 1 |
| Pecan Shortbread Sugar Free | 2 (0.9 oz) | 100 | 14 | 0 | 0 |
| ***Keebler*** | | | | | |
| Animal Crackers Chocolate Chip | 7 (1 oz) | 130 | 22 | 6 | 0 |
| Animal Crackers Ernie's | 1 box | 250 | 41 | 14 | 1 |
| Animal Crackers Iced | 6 (1.1 oz) | 150 | 24 | 9 | 0 |
| Animal Crackers Sprinkled | 6 (1.1 oz) | 150 | 24 | 10 | 0 |
| Butter | 5 (1.1 oz) | 150 | 22 | 6 | tr |
| Chips Deluxe | 1 (0.5 oz) | 80 | 9 | 4 | 0 |
| Chips Deluxe Chocolate Lovers | 1 (0.6 oz) | 90 | 11 | 6 | 0 |
| Chips Deluxe Coconut | 1 (0.5 oz) | 80 | 10 | 5 | tr |
| Chips Deluxe Rainbow | 1 (0.6 oz) | 80 | 10 | 5 | tr |
| Chips Deluxe Soft 'n Chewy | 1 (0.6 oz) | 80 | 11 | 5 | 0 |
| Chips Deluxe w/ Peanut Butter Cups | 1 (0.6 oz) | 90 | 9 | 5 | 0 |

| FOOD | PORTION | CALS | CARB | SUGAR | FIBER |
|---|---|---|---|---|---|
| Classic Collection Chocolate Fudge Creme | 1 (0.6 oz) | 80 | 12 | 6 | 0 |
| Classic Collection French Vanilla Creme | 1 (0.6 oz) | 80 | 12 | 6 | 0 |
| Cookie Stix Butter | 5 (1.2 oz) | 160 | 22 | 8 | 1 |
| Cookie Stix Chocolate Chip | 4 (0.9 oz) | 130 | 19 | 9 | tr |
| Cookie Stix Rainbow | 5 (1.2 oz) | 150 | 23 | 9 | tr |
| Danish Wedding | 4 (0.9 oz) | 120 | 20 | 11 | tr |
| Droxies | 3 (1.1 oz) | 140 | 21 | 12 | tr |
| Droxies Reduced Fat | 3 (1.1 oz) | 140 | 23 | 13 | 1 |
| E.L. Fudge Butter w/ Fudge Filling | 2 (0.9 oz) | 120 | 17 | 7 | tr |
| E.L. Fudge Fudge w/ Fudge Filling | 2 (0.9 oz) | 120 | 17 | 7 | tr |
| E.L. Fudge w/ Peanut Butter Filling | 2 (0.9 oz) | 120 | 16 | 7 | tr |
| Fudge Shoppe Deluxe Grahams | 3 (1 oz) | 140 | 19 | 10 | tr |
| Fudge Shoppe Double Fudge 'n Caramel | 2 (1 oz) | 140 | 20 | 12 | tr |
| Fudge Shoppe Fudge Sticks | 3 (1 oz) | 150 | 20 | 15 | tr |
| Fudge Shoppe Fudge Sticks Peanut Butter | 3 (1 oz) | 150 | 18 | 14 | tr |
| Fudge Shoppe Fudge Stripes | 3 (1.1 oz) | 160 | 21 | 10 | tr |
| Fudge Shoppe Fudge Stripes Reduced Fat | 3 (1 oz) | 140 | 21 | 12 | 0 |
| Fudge Shoppe Grasshoppers | 4 (1 oz) | 150 | 20 | 12 | tr |
| Fudge Shoppe S'mores | 3 (1.2 oz) | 160 | 22 | 12 | tr |
| Ginger Snaps | 5 (1.1 oz) | 150 | 24 | 10 | 0 |
| Golden Fruit Cranberry | 1 (0.7 oz) | 80 | 14 | 6 | tr |
| Golden Fruit Raisin | 1 (0.7 oz) | 80 | 15 | 9 | tr |
| Graham Cinnamon Crisp | 8 (1 oz) | 140 | 22 | 9 | 1 |
| Graham Cinnamon Crisp Low Fat | 8 (1 oz) | 110 | 24 | 9 | 1 |
| Graham Honey | 8 (1.1 oz) | 150 | 21 | 6 | 1 |
| Graham Honey Low Fat | 8 (1.1 oz) | 120 | 26 | 9 | 1 |
| Graham Original | 8 (1 oz) | 130 | 23 | 7 | tr |
| Lemon Coolers | 5 (1 oz) | 140 | 21 | 10 | tr |
| Oatmeal Country Style | 2 (0.8 oz) | 120 | 17 | 8 | tr |
| Sandies Almond Shortbread | 1 (0.5 oz) | 80 | 9 | 3 | 0 |
| Sandies Pecan Shortbread | 1 (0.5 oz) | 80 | 9 | 3 | tr |

| FOOD | PORTION | CALS | CARB | SUGAR | FIBER |
|---|---|---|---|---|---|
| Sandies Simply Shortbread | 1 (0.5 oz) | 80 | 9 | 3 | 0 |
| Snack Size Chips Deluxe | 1 pkg (2 oz) | 300 | 36 | 18 | tr |
| Snack Size Chips Deluxe Chocolate Lovers | 1 pkg (2 oz) | 280 | 36 | 20 | 1 |
| Snack Size Mini Fudge Stripes | 1 pkg (2 oz) | 280 | 38 | 16 | 2 |
| Snack Size Rainbow Chips Deluxe | 1 pkg (2 oz) | 290 | 36 | 18 | 1 |
| Snack Size Sandies w/ Pecan | 1 pkg (2 oz) | 300 | 33 | 13 | 1 |
| Snackin' Grahams Cinnamon | 21 (1 oz) | 130 | 23 | 9 | 1 |
| Snackin' Grahams Honey | 23 (1 oz) | 130 | 22 | 8 | tr |
| Soft Batch Chocolate Chip | 1 (0.6 oz) | 80 | 10 | 6 | tr |
| Soft Batch Homestyle Chocolate Chunk | 1 (0.9 oz) | 130 | 17 | 10 | 1 |
| Soft Batch Homestyle Double Chocolate | 1 (0.9 oz) | 130 | 17 | 9 | 1 |
| Soft Batch Homestyle Oatmeal Raisin | 1 (0.9 oz) | 130 | 20 | 11 | tr |
| Soft Batch Oatmeal Raisin | 1 (0.5 oz) | 70 | 10 | 6 | tr |
| Sugar Wafers Creme | 3 (0.9 oz) | 130 | 18 | 13 | tr |
| Sugar Wafers Lemon | 3 (0.9 oz) | 130 | 19 | 14 | 0 |
| Sugar Wafers Peanut Butter | 4 (1.1 oz) | 170 | 19 | 10 | 1 |
| Vanilla Wafers | 8 (1.1 oz) | 150 | 20 | 9 | tr |
| Vanilla Wafers Reduced Fat | 8 (1.1 oz) | 130 | 25 | 11 | tr |
| Vienna Fingers | 2 (1 oz) | 140 | 21 | 8 | tr |
| Vienna Fingers Lemon | 2 (1 oz) | 140 | 21 | 9 | 0 |
| ***Keto*** | | | | | |
| Low Carb Biscotti Chocolate | 1 (1.2 oz) | 157 | 6 | 0 | 3 |
| Low Carb Biscotti Lemon Nut | 1 (1.2 oz) | 157 | 6 | 0 | 3 |
| Low Carb Biscotti Vanilla Almond | 1 (1.2 oz) | 157 | 6 | 0 | 3 |
| ***Knott's Berry Farm*** | | | | | |
| Shortbread Apricot | 3 (1 oz) | 120 | 17 | 7 | 0 |
| Shortbread Boysenberry | 3 (1 oz) | 120 | 17 | 7 | 0 |
| Shortbread Raspberry | 3 (1 oz) | 120 | 17 | 8 | 0 |
| ***LU*** | | | | | |
| Chocolatier | 3 (1 oz) | 150 | 17 | 12 | 1 |
| Le Bastogne | 2 (0.8 oz) | 120 | 18 | 10 | 0 |
| Le Dore | 4 (1 oz) | 140 | 21 | 7 | 0 |
| Le Fondant | 4 (1.1 oz) | 170 | 19 | 9 | 1 |
| Le Palmier | 4 (1.2 oz) | 180 | 20 | 7 | tr |

| FOOD | PORTION | CALS | CARB | SUGAR | FIBER |
|---|---|---|---|---|---|
| Le Petit Beurre | 4 (1.2 oz) | 150 | 26 | 7 | tr |
| Le Petit Ecolier Dark Chocolate | 2 (0.9 oz) | 130 | 17 | 10 | 1 |
| Le Petit Ecolier Extra Dark Chocolate | 2 | 120 | 15 | 7 | 2 |
| Le Petit Ecolier Hazelnut Milk Chocolate | 2 (0.9 oz) | 130 | 16 | 8 | 0 |
| Le Petit Ecolier Milk Chocolate | 2 (0.9 oz) | 130 | 17 | 10 | tr |
| Le Raisin Dore | 4 (1.2 oz) | 160 | 23 | 11 | tr |
| Le Truffe Coconut | 4 (1.2 oz) | 190 | 17 | 12 | 1 |
| Le Truffe Praline Chocolate | 4 (1.2 oz) | 170 | 20 | 15 | 2 |
| Les Varietes | 3 (0.9 oz) | 140 | 17 | 10 | 6 |
| Pim's Orange | 2 (0.9 oz) | 90 | 16 | 12 | tr |
| Pim's Raspberry | 2 (0.9 oz) | 90 | 17 | 14 | tr |
| ***La Choy*** | | | | | |
| Fortune | 4 (1 oz) | 112 | 26 | 11 | 1 |
| ***Lance*** | | | | | |
| Apple Bar Fat Free | 1 (1.75 oz) | 160 | 38 | 29 | tr |
| Apple Oatmeal Bar | 1 (1.8 oz) | 190 | 32 | 10 | 1 |
| Big Town Banana | 1 pkg (2 oz) | 250 | 37 | 21 | 1 |
| Big Town Chocolate | 1 pkg (2 oz) | 250 | 40 | 21 | 1 |
| Big Town Vanilla | 1 pkg (2 oz) | 250 | 37 | 26 | 1 |
| Choc-O-Lunch | 1 pkg (1.5 oz) | 200 | 31 | 17 | 1 |
| Choc-O-Mint | 1 pkg (1¼ oz) | 190 | 24 | 17 | 1 |
| Coated Graham | 1 pkg (1.3 oz) | 190 | 25 | 13 | 1 |
| Fig Bar | 1 (1.75 oz) | 180 | 34 | 23 | 2 |
| Fudge Chocolate Chip | 1 (2 oz) | 130 | 19 | 5 | 1 |
| Gourmet Chocolate Chip | 1 (2 oz) | 130 | 18 | 10 | 1 |
| Lem-O-Lunch | 1 pkg (3.4 oz) | 240 | 32 | 11 | 1 |
| Lemon Nekot | 1 pkg (1.5 oz) | 210 | 28 | 13 | 1 |
| Nut-O-Lunch | 1 pkg (3.3 oz) | 240 | 29 | 8 | 3 |
| Oatmeal | 1 (2 oz) | 130 | 18 | 4 | 1 |
| Oatmeal Creme | 1 (2 oz) | 240 | 35 | 9 | 1 |
| Peanut Butter | 1 (2 oz) | 140 | 14 | 10 | 1 |
| Peanut Butter Creme Wafer | 1 pkg (1.5 oz) | 230 | 26 | 16 | 2 |
| Van-O-Lunch | 1 pkg (1.5 oz) | 210 | 31 | 13 | 0 |
| ***Landies Candies*** | | | | | |
| Sugar Free Dark Royal Pecan Shortbread | 2 | 167 | 16 | 0 | 1 |
| Sugar Free Milk Chocolate Chip | 2 | 173 | 17 | 0 | tr |

| FOOD | PORTION | CALS | CARB | SUGAR | FIBER |
|---|---|---|---|---|---|
| Sugar Free Milk Chocolate Peanut Butter | 2 | 171 | 17 | 0 | tr |
| Sugar Free White Chocolate Lemon | 2 | 177 | 20 | 0 | 0 |
| ***Larzaroni*** | | | | | |
| Arancelli | 8 (1 oz) | 160 | 19 | 8 | tr |
| Calypso | 3 (1 oz) | 150 | 18 | 11 | 1 |
| Limonelli | 5 (1 oz) | 140 | 16 | 7 | 2 |
| Malaika | 5 (1 oz) | 158 | 17 | 10 | 1 |
| Nanette | 4 (1.2 oz) | 170 | 20 | 20 | tr |
| Okla | 3 (1 oz) | 186 | 21 | 18 | 1 |
| Oskar | 10 (1 oz) | 150 | 18 | 11 | tr |
| Samba | 5 (1 oz) | 160 | 14 | 6 | 2 |
| Velieri | 3 (0.9 oz) | 120 | 17 | 10 | tr |
| ***Little Debbie*** | | | | | |
| Apple Flips | 1 (1.2 oz) | 150 | 24 | 13 | tr |
| Caramel Bars | 1 (1.2 oz) | 160 | 22 | 16 | 0 |
| Cherry Cordials | 1 (1.3 oz) | 170 | 23 | 15 | tr |
| Coconut Rounds | 1 (1.2 oz) | 150 | 23 | 13 | tr |
| Cookie Wreaths | 1 (0.6 oz) | 100 | 12 | 7 | 0 |
| Easter Puffs | 1 (1.2 oz) | 140 | 24 | 18 | 0 |
| Fig Bars | 1 (1.5 oz) | 150 | 31 | 20 | 1 |
| Fudge Delights | 1 (1.1 oz) | 110 | 24 | 14 | tr |
| Fudge Rounds | 1 (1.2 oz) | 140 | 23 | 14 | tr |
| German Chocolate Ring | 1 (1 oz) | 140 | 18 | 11 | 1 |
| Ginger | 1 (0.7 oz) | 90 | 15 | 8 | 0 |
| Jelly Creme Pies | 1 (1.2 oz) | 160 | 23 | 15 | 0 |
| Marshmallow Crispy Bar | 1 (1.3 oz) | 140 | 26 | 13 | 0 |
| Marshmallow Supremes | 1 (1.1 oz) | 130 | 22 | 15 | tr |
| Marshmallow Pie Banana | 1 pkg (1.5 oz) | 180 | 30 | 18 | 0 |
| Marshmallow Pie Chocolate | 1 (1.4 oz) | 160 | 27 | 16 | 1 |
| Nutty Bar | 1 (2 oz) | 310 | 32 | 20 | 1 |
| Oatmeal Raisin | 1 (1.3 oz) | 160 | 25 | 14 | tr |
| Oatmeal Creme Pie | 1 (1.3 oz) | 170 | 26 | 14 | tr |
| Oatmeal Delights | 1 (1.1 oz) | 110 | 24 | 15 | tr |
| Oatmeal Lights | 1 (1.3 oz) | 130 | 29 | 16 | tr |
| Peanut Butter Bars | 1 (1.9 oz) | 270 | 32 | 19 | 1 |
| Peanut Butter & Jelly Oatmeal Pie | 1 (1.1 oz) | 130 | 22 | 12 | tr |
| Peanut Clusters | 1 (1.4 oz) | 190 | 23 | 16 | tr |

| FOOD | PORTION | CALS | CARB | SUGAR | FIBER |
|---|---|---|---|---|---|
| Pumpkin Delights | 1 (1.2 oz) | 150 | 24 | 13 | 0 |
| Raisin Creme Pie | 1 (1.2 oz) | 140 | 23 | 16 | 0 |
| Star Crunch | 1 (1.1 oz) | 140 | 22 | 12 | 0 |
| Sugar Free Chocolate Chip | 3 (1.1 oz) | 140 | 21 | 0 | tr |
| Sugar Free Oatmeal | 6 (1.1 oz) | 120 | 23 | 0 | 1 |
| Yo-Yo's | 1 (1.2 oz) | 130 | 21 | 12 | tr |
| ***Low Carb Creations*** | | | | | |
| Chocolate Chip | 1 (1 oz) | 140 | 11 | tr | 1 |
| Coconut | 1 (1 oz) | 140 | 9 | tr | 1 |
| Lemon | 1 (1 oz) | 140 | 9 | tr | 1 |
| Snickerdoodle | 1 (1 oz) | 140 | 9 | tr | 1 |
| ***M&M's*** | | | | | |
| Cookies & Milky Way | 1 bar (1.2 oz) | 180 | 21 | 13 | 1 |
| ***Mamma Says'*** | | | | | |
| Biscotti Almond Pistachio | 1 (0.5 oz) | 50 | 7 | 3 | 1 |
| Biscotti Chocolate Macadamia | 1 (0.5 oz) | 45 | 5 | 3 | 1 |
| Biscotti Orange Citrene | 1 (0.5 oz) | 60 | 8 | 4 | 1 |
| ***Meringue*** | | | | | |
| Minis Chocolate Chip | 13 (1 oz) | 120 | 27 | 26 | 1 |
| ***Milk Lunch Brand*** | | | | | |
| New England Biscuits | 4 (1.1 oz) | 140 | 24 | 3 | 1 |
| ***Miss Meringue*** | | | | | |
| Minis Chocolate Raspberry | 13 (1 oz) | 80 | 20 | 19 | 0 |
| Minis Mint Chocolate Chip | 13 (1 oz) | 120 | 26 | 25 | 1 |
| Minis Mochaccino | 13 (1 oz) | 80 | 20 | 19 | 0 |
| Minis Orange | 13 (1 oz) | 80 | 20 | 20 | 0 |
| Minis Rainbow Vanilla | 13 (1 oz) | 110 | 27 | 27 | 0 |
| Minis Toasted Coconut | 13 (1 oz) | 90 | 19 | 19 | 0 |
| Minis Very Chocolate | 13 (1 oz) | 80 | 20 | 19 | 0 |
| Minis Very Minty | 13 (1 oz) | 80 | 20 | 19 | 0 |
| Minis Very Vanilla | 13 (1 oz) | 80 | 20 | 19 | 0 |
| ***MoonPie*** | | | | | |
| Chocolate | 1 (2.75 oz) | 330 | 56 | 24 | 0 |
| Mini Banana | 1 (1.2 oz) | 152 | 26 | 8 | 0 |
| Mini Chocolate | 1 (1.2 oz) | 152 | 26 | 8 | 0 |
| Mini Vanilla | 1 (1.2 oz) | 152 | 26 | 8 | 0 |
| ***Mother's*** | | | | | |
| Almond Shortbread | 3 | 180 | 19 | 6 | 1 |
| Checkerboard Wafers | 8 | 150 | 20 | 10 | 1 |

| FOOD | PORTION | CALS | CARB | SUGAR | FIBER |
|---|---|---|---|---|---|
| Chocolate Chip | 2 | 160 | 20 | 11 | 0 |
| Chocolate Chip Angel | 3 | 180 | 21 | 8 | 1 |
| Chocolate Chip Parade | 4 | 130 | 19 | 8 | 1 |
| Circus Animals | 6 | 140 | 20 | 12 | 0 |
| Classic Assortments | 2 | 140 | 18 | 9 | 1 |
| Cocadas | 5 | 150 | 20 | 6 | 2 |
| Cookie Parade | 4 | 140 | 18 | 9 | 2 |
| Dinosaur Grrrahams | 2 | 130 | 24 | 7 | 2 |
| Double Fudge | 2 | 180 | 24 | 12 | 2 |
| English Tea | 2 | 180 | 26 | 12 | 1 |
| Flaky Flix Fudge | 2 | 140 | 17 | 12 | 2 |
| Flaky Flix Vanilla | 2 | 140 | 17 | 14 | 1 |
| Gaucho Peanut Butter | 2 | 190 | 22 | 7 | 2 |
| Iced Oatmeal | 2 | 130 | 22 | 10 | 1 |
| Iced Raisin | 2 | 180 | 24 | 12 | 1 |
| MLB Double Header Duplex | 3 | 170 | 23 | 12 | 1 |
| Macaroon | 2 | 150 | 18 | 8 | 2 |
| Marias | 3 | 170 | 28 | 9 | 1 |
| Oatmeal | 2 | 110 | 17 | 14 | 1 |
| Oatmeal Chocolate Chip | 2 | 120 | 19 | 9 | 1 |
| Oatmeal Raisin | 5 | 150 | 20 | 9 | 2 |
| Oatmeal Walnut Chocolate Chip | 2 | 130 | 17 | 9 | 1 |
| Rainbow Wafers | 8 | 150 | 20 | 10 | 1 |
| Striped Shortbread | 3 | 170 | 22 | 8 | 1 |
| Sugar | 2 | 140 | 19 | 8 | 1 |
| Taffy | 2 | 180 | 25 | 11 | 2 |
| Triplet Assortment | 2 | 140 | 18 | 11 | 1 |
| Vanilla Wafers | 6 | 150 | 24 | 14 | 1 |
| Wallops Boysenberry | 1 | 80 | 15 | 9 | 1 |
| Wallops Honey Crust Fig | 1 | 80 | 15 | 9 | 0 |
| Wallops Honey Graham Fig | 1 | 80 | 15 | 9 | 1 |
| Wallops Mixed Berry | 1 | 80 | 15 | 9 | 1 |
| Wallops Peach Apricot | 1 | 80 | 15 | 9 | 1 |
| Wallops Raspberry | 1 | 80 | 15 | 9 | 1 |
| Wallops Strawberry | 1 | 80 | 15 | 9 | 1 |
| Walnut Fudge | 2 | 130 | 16 | 7 | 1 |
| Zoo Pals | 14 | 140 | 23 | 6 | 1 |

| FOOD | PORTION | CALS | CARB | SUGAR | FIBER |
|---|---|---|---|---|---|
| ***Mrs. Alison's*** | | | | | |
| Coconut Bar | 2 (1 oz) | 130 | 19 | 6 | 0 |
| Creme Wafers | 5 (1.1 oz) | 170 | 21 | 13 | tr |
| Duplex Sandwich | 3 (1 oz) | 130 | 20 | 8 | 0 |
| Fudge Fingers | 3 (1 oz) | 160 | 19 | 16 | 0 |
| Ginger Snaps | 4 (1 oz) | 130 | 23 | 10 | tr |
| Jelly Tops | 5 (1 oz) | 140 | 18 | 8 | 0 |
| Lemon Creme | 3 (1 oz) | 130 | 21 | 9 | 0 |
| Macaroons | 2 (1 oz) | 140 | 18 | 8 | tr |
| Pecan | 2 (1 oz) | 140 | 19 | 7 | 0 |
| Shortbread | 5 (1 oz) | 120 | 19 | 5 | 0 |
| Vanilla Sandwich | 3 (1 oz) | 130 | 21 | 9 | 0 |
| ***Murray's*** | | | | | |
| Sugar Free Double Fudge | 3 (1.2 oz) | 140 | 23 | 0 | 3 |
| Sugar Free Ginger Snap | 6 (1 oz) | 110 | 21 | 0 | tr |
| Sugar Free Peanut Butter | 6 (1 oz) | 130 | 17 | 0 | 1 |
| Sugar Free Vanilla Sandwich Creme | 3 (1 oz) | 120 | 21 | 0 | 2 |
| Sugar Free Vanilla Wafers | 9 (1.1 oz) | 120 | 23 | 0 | tr |
| ***Nabisco*** | | | | | |
| Barnum's Animal Crackers | 10 (1 oz) | 130 | 23 | 7 | tr |
| Barnum's Animal Crackers Chocolate | 10 (1 oz) | 130 | 23 | 8 | 1 |
| Biscos Sugar Wafers | 8 (1 oz) | 140 | 21 | 13 | 0 |
| Cafe Cremes Cappuccino | 2 (1.1 oz) | 160 | 22 | 9 | 0 |
| Cafe Cremes Vanilla | 2 (1.1 oz) | 160 | 22 | 10 | 0 |
| Cafe Cremes Vanilla Fudge | 2 (1.1 oz) | 200 | 27 | 14 | tr |
| Cameo | 2 (1 oz) | 130 | 21 | 10 | 0 |
| Chips Ahoy! | 3 (1.1 oz) | 160 | 21 | 10 | 1 |
| Chips Ahoy! Chewy | 3 (1.3 oz) | 170 | 24 | 13 | tr |
| Chips Ahoy! Chunky | 1 (0.5 oz) | 80 | 10 | 6 | 0 |
| Chips Ahoy! Munch Size | 6 (1.1 oz) | 160 | 21 | 10 | 1 |
| Chips Ahoy! Reduced Fat | 3 (1.1 oz) | 140 | 22 | 10 | tr |
| Family Favorites Iced Oatmeal | 1 (0.6 oz) | 80 | 12 | 6 | 0 |
| Family Favorites Oatmeal | 1 (0.6 oz) | 80 | 12 | 5 | 0 |
| Famous Chocolate Wafers | 5 (1.1 oz) | 140 | 24 | 11 | 1 |
| Grahams | 4 (1 oz) | 120 | 22 | 6 | 1 |
| Honey Maid Chocolate | 8 (1 oz) | 120 | 22 | 8 | 1 |
| Honey Maid Cinnamon Grahams | 8 (1 oz) | 120 | 23 | 9 | tr |

| FOOD | PORTION | CALS | CARB | SUGAR | FIBER |
|---|---|---|---|---|---|
| Honey Maid Honey Grahams | 8 (1 oz) | 120 | 22 | 7 | 1 |
| Honey Maid Low Fat Cinnamon Grahams | 8 (1 oz) | 110 | 23 | 10 | tr |
| Honey Maid Low Fat Grahams | 8 (1 oz) | 110 | 23 | 8 | tr |
| Honey Maid Oatmeal Crunch | 8 (1 oz) | 120 | 22 | 7 | 1 |
| Lorna Doone | 4 (1 oz) | 140 | 19 | 6 | tr |
| Mallomars | 2 (0.9 oz) | 120 | 17 | 12 | tr |
| Marshmallow Twirls | 1 (1 oz) | 130 | 20 | 14 | 0 |
| Mystic Mint | 1 (0.5 oz) | 90 | 11 | 8 | 0 |
| National Arrowroot | 1 (5 g) | 20 | 4 | 1 | 0 |
| Newton Fat Free Fig | 2 (1 oz) | 90 | 22 | 12 | 1 |
| Newtons Fig | 2 (1.1 oz) | 110 | 22 | 14 | 1 |
| Newtons Fat Free Apple | 2 (1 oz) | 90 | 21 | 12 | tr |
| Newtons Fat Free Cobblers Apple Cinnamon | 1 (0.8 oz) | 70 | 17 | 10 | tr |
| Newtons Fat Free Cobblers Peach Apricot | 1 (0.8 oz) | 70 | 17 | 10 | 0 |
| Newtons Fat Free Cranberry | 2 (1 oz) | 100 | 22 | 14 | tr |
| Newtons Fat Free Raspberry | 2 (1 oz) | 100 | 23 | 13 | tr |
| Newtons Fat Free Strawberry | 2 (1 oz) | 90 | 21 | 11 | 0 |
| Nilla Wafers | 8 (1.1 oz) | 140 | 24 | 12 | 0 |
| Nilla Wafers Chocolate Reduced Fat | 8 (1 oz) | 110 | 23 | 12 | tr |
| Nilla Wafers Reduced Fat | 8 (1 oz) | 120 | 24 | 12 | 0 |
| Nutter Butter Bites | 10 (1 oz) | 150 | 20 | 9 | 1 |
| Nutter Butter Chocolate Peanut Butter Sandwich | 2 (1 oz) | 130 | 19 | 8 | 1 |
| Nutter Butter Peanut Butter Sandwich | 2 (1 oz) | 130 | 19 | 8 | tr |
| Old Fashioned Ginger Snaps | 4 (1 oz) | 120 | 22 | 9 | tr |
| Oreo | 3 (1.2 oz) | 160 | 23 | 13 | 1 |
| Oreo Double Stuff | 2 (1 oz) | 140 | 19 | 13 | tr |
| Oreo Mini | 1 pkg (0.5 oz) | 65 | 10 | 6 | 1 |
| Oreo Reduced Fat | 3 (1.1 oz) | 130 | 25 | 14 | 1 |
| Oreo Halloween | 2 (1 oz) | 140 | 19 | 13 | tr |
| Pecanz | 1 (0.5 oz) | 90 | 9 | 3 | 0 |
| Pinwheels Chocolate Marshmallow | 1 (1 oz) | 130 | 21 | 15 | tr |
| Rugrats Chocolate Frosted | 8 (1.1 oz) | 150 | 24 | 13 | tr |

| FOOD | PORTION | CALS | CARB | SUGAR | FIBER |
|---|---|---|---|---|---|
| Rugrats Vanilla Frosted | 8 (1.1 oz) | 150 | 24 | 13 | tr |
| Social Tea | 6 (1 oz) | 120 | 20 | 7 | tr |
| Sweet Crispers Chocolate | 18 (1.1 oz) | 130 | 25 | 12 | 1 |
| Sweet Crispers Chocolate Chip | 18 (1.1 oz) | 130 | 23 | 11 | tr |
| Teddy Grahams Chocolate | 24 (1 oz) | 130 | 22 | 9 | 1 |
| Teddy Grahams Chocolately Chip | 24 (1 oz) | 130 | 23 | 8 | tr |
| Teddy Grahams Cinnamon | 24 (1 oz) | 130 | 23 | 8 | 1 |
| Teddy Grahams Honey | 24 (1 oz) | 130 | 23 | 8 | tr |
| Flipz Crunchy Graham White Fudge Chocolate | 8 (1 oz) | 140 | 19 | 12 | 0 |
| ***Nonni's*** | | | | | |
| Biscotti Cioccalati | 1 (1 oz) | 130 | 19 | 11 | 1 |
| Biscotti Decadence | 1 (1.1 oz) | 130 | 19 | 11 | 1 |
| Biscotti Original | 1 (1 oz) | 100 | 15 | 8 | 1 |
| Biscotti Paradiso | 1 (1.1 oz) | 130 | 19 | 12 | 0 |
| ***NutraBalance*** | | | | | |
| Fibre Oatmeal Raisin | 1 (0.7 oz) | 80 | 13 | 6 | 3 |
| Protein Fortified | 1 (2 oz) | 260 | 28 | 12 | 2 |
| ReNeph Spice | 1 (2 oz) | 210 | 29 | 14 | 0 |
| ***Old Brussels*** | | | | | |
| Ginger Crisps | 2 (0.9 oz) | 140 | 23 | 4 | 2 |
| ***Old London*** | | | | | |
| Coffee Toppers Chocolate Creme | 3 (0.5 oz) | 70 | 9 | 3 | 0 |
| Coffee Toppers Vanilla Creme | 3 (0.5 oz) | 70 | 9 | 3 | 0 |
| ***Olde World*** | | | | | |
| Pizzelle Almond | 3 (1 oz) | 90 | 12 | 4 | 0 |
| Pizzelle Anise | 3 (1 oz) | 90 | 12 | 4 | 0 |
| Pizzelle Chocolate | 3 (1 oz) | 100 | 11 | 5 | 0 |
| Pizzelle Lemon | 3 (1 oz) | 90 | 12 | 4 | 0 |
| Pizzelle Vanilla | 3 (1 oz) | 90 | 12 | 4 | 0 |
| ***Otis Spunkmeyer*** | | | | | |
| Butter Sugar | 1 med (1.3 oz) | 160 | 23 | 14 | tr |
| Butter Sugar | 1 (2 oz) | 250 | 35 | 21 | 1 |
| Carnival | 1 med (1.3 oz) | 170 | 25 | 16 | 0 |
| Chocolate Chip | 1 bite size (0.75 oz) | 100 | 14 | 9 | 0 |
| Chocolate Chip | 1 med (1.3 oz) | 170 | 24 | 16 | 0 |
| Chocolate Chip | 1 (2 oz) | 250 | 36 | 21 | tr |

| FOOD | PORTION | CALS | CARB | SUGAR | FIBER |
|---|---|---|---|---|---|
| Chocolate Chip Pecan | 1 med (1.3 oz) | 170 | 22 | 14 | tr |
| Chocolate Chip Walnut | 1 bite size (0.75 oz) | 100 | 13 | 8 | 0 |
| Chocolate Chip Walnut | 1 med (1.3 oz) | 180 | 22 | 14 | tr |
| Chocolate Chip Walnut | 1 (2 oz) | 270 | 34 | 21 | tr |
| Double Chocolate Chip | 1 bite size (0.75 oz) | 100 | 13 | 10 | 1 |
| Double Chocolate Chip | 1 med (1.3 oz) | 180 | 23 | 17 | tr |
| Oatmeal Raisin | 1 bite size (0.75 oz) | 90 | 13 | 6 | tr |
| Oatmeal Raisin | 1 med (1.3 oz) | 160 | 23 | 11 | 1 |
| Otis Express Chocolate Chunk | 1 (2 oz) | 280 | 37 | 22 | 1 |
| Otis Express Double Chocolate Chip | 1 (2 oz) | 270 | 35 | 26 | 1 |
| Otis Express Oatmeal Raisin | 1 (2 oz) | 240 | 35 | 17 | 2 |
| Otis Express Peanut Butter | 1 (2 oz) | 270 | 31 | 17 | 2 |
| Peanut Butter | 1 med (1.3 oz) | 180 | 20 | 11 | 1 |
| Pinnacle Checkpoint Chocolate Almond Coconut | 1 (2.4 oz) | 320 | 37 | 24 | 2 |
| Pinnacle Mach One Mocha Chocolate Chunk | 1 (2.4 oz) | 300 | 43 | 26 | 1 |
| Pinnacle Passport Peanut Butter Chocolate Chunk | 1 (2.4 oz) | 300 | 42 | 28 | 1 |
| Pinnacle Ripcord Rocky Road | 1 (2.4 oz) | 310 | 41 | 27 | 2 |
| Pinnacle Takeoff Triple Chocolate | 1 (2.4 oz) | 300 | 42 | 26 | tr |
| Pinnacle Transatlantic Turtle | 1 (2.4 oz) | 310 | 39 | 26 | 2 |
| Travel Lite Low Fat Apple Cinnamon | 1 (1.3 oz) | 130 | 26 | 15 | tr |
| Travel Lite Low Fat Chocolate Chip | 1 (1.3 oz) | 130 | 27 | 16 | tr |
| Travel Lite Low Fat Ginger Spice | 1 (1.3 oz) | 130 | 26 | 15 | tr |
| Travel Lite Low Fat Oatmeal Rum Raisin | 1 (1.3 oz) | 130 | 26 | 15 | 1 |
| White Chocolate Macadamia Nut | 1 med (1.3 oz) | 180 | 21 | 14 | tr |
| White Chocolate Macadamia Nut | 1 (2 oz) | 280 | 33 | 21 | tr |
| ***Pally*** | | | | | |
| Butter | 5 (1 oz) | 140 | 23 | 6 | 1 |

| FOOD | PORTION | CALS | CARB | SUGAR | FIBER |
|---|---|---|---|---|---|
| Carnival | 5 (1 oz) | 130 | 24 | 9 | 1 |
| Cinnamon Biscuit | 5 (1 oz) | 130 | 23 | 11 | 0 |
| Mariel Biscuit | 6 (1 oz) | 150 | 23 | 6 | 1 |
| Tea Biscuits | 5 (1 oz) | 150 | 23 | 6 | 1 |
| ***Pamela's*** | | | | | |
| Pecan Shortbread Rice Flour | 1 (0.8 oz) | 130 | 15 | 4 | tr |
| ***Parmalat*** | | | | | |
| Grisbi Lemon | 1 (0.6 oz) | 90 | 9 | 5 | 1 |
| Grisbi Lemon | 1 (0.6 oz) | 90 | 9 | 5 | 1 |
| ***Peek Freans*** | | | | | |
| Arrowroot | 4 (1.2 oz) | 150 | 26 | 7 | 1 |
| Assorted Creme | 1 (1 oz) | 130 | 19 | 9 | 0 |
| Dream Puffs | 2 (0.9 oz) | 110 | 18 | 12 | 0 |
| Fruit Creme | 2 (0.9 oz) | 130 | 20 | 10 | 0 |
| Ginger Crisp | 4 (1.2 oz) | 150 | 28 | 11 | tr |
| Nice | 4 (1.2 oz) | 160 | 25 | 9 | 1 |
| Petit Beret Creme Caramel | 2 (0.8 oz) | 110 | 15 | 10 | tr |
| Petit Beret Fudge Truffle | 2 (0.8 oz) | 110 | 15 | 10 | tr |
| Petit Beurre | 4 (1 oz) | 130 | 22 | 5 | tr |
| Rich Tea | 4 (1.2 oz) | 160 | 25 | 7 | tr |
| Shortcake | 2 (0.9 oz) | 140 | 18 | 5 | 0 |
| Traditional Oatmeal | 1 (0.7 oz) | 90 | 15 | 7 | tr |
| Tropical Cremes Calypso Lime | 2 (0.9 oz) | 130 | 20 | 10 | 0 |
| ***Pepperidge Farm*** | | | | | |
| Biscotti Almond | 1 (0.7 oz) | 90 | 12 | 5 | 0 |
| Biscotti Chocolate Hazelnut | 1 (0.7 oz) | 90 | 11 | 5 | 2 |
| Biscotti Cranberry Pistachio | 1 (0.7 oz) | 90 | 13 | 7 | 0 |
| Bordeaux | 4 | 130 | 19 | 12 | tr |
| Brussels | 2 | 100 | 13 | 7 | tr |
| Chantilly Raspberry | 2 (1 oz) | 120 | 23 | 11 | tr |
| Chessman | 3 | 120 | 18 | 5 | tr |
| Chocolate Chunk Soft Baked Double Chocolate | 1 (0.9 oz) | 130 | 15 | 9 | 1 |
| Chocolate Chip | 3 | 140 | 18 | 9 | tr |
| Chocolate Chunk Chesapeake | 1 (0.7 oz) | 140 | 15 | 7 | 0 |
| Chocolate Chunk Minis Nantucket | 1 pkg (1.75 oz) | 260 | 34 | 17 | 0 |
| Chocolate Chunk Minis Sausalito | 4 (1 oz) | 160 | 18 | 10 | 0 |
| Chocolate Chunk Montauk | 1 (0.9 oz) | 130 | 17 | 10 | 0 |

| FOOD | PORTION | CALS | CARB | SUGAR | FIBER |
|---|---|---|---|---|---|
| Chocolate Chunk Nantucket | 1 (0.9 oz) | 140 | 16 | 9 | 0 |
| Chocolate Chunk Sausalito | 1 (0.7 oz) | 140 | 16 | 9 | 0 |
| Chocolate Chunk Soft Baked | 1 | 130 | 16 | 9 | 0 |
| Chocolate Chunk Soft Baked Milk Chocolate Macademia | 1 | 130 | 16 | 9 | 0 |
| Chocolate Chunk Soft Baked Reduced Fat | 1 | 110 | 18 | 8 | tr |
| Chocolate Chunk Soft Baked White Chocolate Pecan | 1 | 120 | 16 | 9 | 1 |
| Chocolate Chunk Tahoe | 1 (0.9 oz) | 130 | 15 | 8 | 0 |
| Fruitful Apricot Raspberry Cup | 3 | 140 | 22 | 10 | tr |
| Fruitful Strawberry Cup | 3 | 140 | 22 | 10 | tr |
| Geneva | 3 | 160 | 19 | 8 | 1 |
| Ginger Man | 4 (1 oz) | 130 | 21 | 11 | tr |
| Goldfish Grahams Cinnamon | 1 pkg (1.75 oz) | 240 | 37 | 13 | 2 |
| Lemon Nut Crunch | 3 | 170 | 18 | 7 | 2 |
| Lido | 1 | 90 | 10 | 5 | 0 |
| Milano | 3 | 180 | 21 | 11 | tr |
| Milano Endless Chocolate | 3 | 180 | 21 | 10 | 1 |
| Milano Milk Chocolate | 3 | 170 | 21 | 13 | tr |
| Milano Double Chocolate | 2 (0.7 oz) | 140 | 17 | 10 | tr |
| Milano Mint | 2 | 130 | 16 | 8 | 1 |
| Milano Orange | 2 | 130 | 16 | 8 | tr |
| Pirouettes Chocolate Laced | 5 (1.1 oz) | 180 | 20 | 13 | tr |
| Pirouettes Traditional | 5 (1.2 oz) | 170 | 20 | 13 | 0 |
| Shortbread | 2 | 140 | 16 | 5 | tr |
| Soft Baked Oatmeal Raisin | 1 (0.9 oz) | 130 | 16 | 9 | 0 |
| Soft Baked Reduced Fat Oatmeal Raisin | 1 (0.9 oz) | 100 | 18 | 8 | tr |
| Spritzers Cool Key Lime | 6 (1.1 oz) | 140 | 21 | 9 | 0 |
| Spritzers Ripe Red Raspberry | 5 (1.1 oz) | 140 | 21 | 9 | 0 |
| Spritzers Zesty Lemon | 5 (1.1 oz) | 140 | 21 | 9 | 0 |
| Sugar | 3 | 140 | 20 | 10 | tr |
| Verona Strawberry | 3 (1.1 oz) | 140 | 22 | 10 | tr |
| ***Pure D-Lite*** | | | | | |
| High Protein Peanut Butter Crunch | 1 (2.2 oz) | 210 | 28 | 0 | 5 |
| High Protein Chocolate Fudge | 1 (2.2 oz) | 210 | 29 | 0 | 5 |

| FOOD | PORTION | CALS | CARB | SUGAR | FIBER |
|---|---|---|---|---|---|
| ***Ralston*** | | | | | |
| Animal | 12 (0.9 oz) | 130 | 22 | 5 | – |
| Chocolate Graham | 2 (0.9 oz) | 130 | 24 | 7 | 1 |
| Cinnamon Grahams | 2 (0.9 oz) | 130 | 19 | 7 | tr |
| Cinnamon Grahams Low Fat | 2 (0.9 oz) | 110 | 22 | 6 | 1 |
| Fig Bars | 2 (1.2 oz) | 120 | 23 | 14 | 1 |
| Vanilla Wafers | 7 (1.1 oz) | 150 | 22 | 10 | 1 |
| ***Real Torino*** | | | | | |
| Lady Fingers | 3 (1 oz) | 110 | 23 | 11 | 0 |
| ***Reko*** | | | | | |
| Pizzelle Maple | 5 (1 oz) | 150 | 20 | 8 | 0 |
| Pizzelle Vanilla | 1 (6 g) | 30 | 4 | 2 | 0 |
| ***Royal*** | | | | | |
| Apple Bars | 1 (1.1 oz) | 100 | 21 | 13 | 1 |
| Apple Cake | 1 (1.1 oz) | 110 | 19 | 8 | 1 |
| Brownie Rounds | 1 (1.1 oz) | 130 | 19 | 11 | 0 |
| Chocolate Chip | 1 (1.1 oz) | 140 | 20 | 11 | 1 |
| Devilfood | 1 (1 oz) | 110 | 17 | 10 | 0 |
| Fig Bars | 1 (1.1 oz) | 100 | 20 | 13 | 1 |
| Oatmeal | 1 (1.1 oz) | 130 | 19 | 10 | 1 |
| Raisin | 1 (1 oz) | 110 | 17 | 10 | 0 |
| Strawberry Bars | 1 (1.1 oz) | 100 | 20 | 12 | 1 |
| ***Salerno*** | | | | | |
| Mini Butter | 25 (1 oz) | 180 | 20 | 8 | tr |
| Mini Dinosaur Chocolate Graham | 16 (1.1 oz) | 140 | 22 | 7 | 1 |
| Scooter Pie | 1 (1.2 oz) | 140 | 23 | 14 | 0 |
| ***Santa Fe Farms*** | | | | | |
| Chocolate Chocolate Chip Fat Free | 2 (1 oz) | 60 | 16 | 7 | 3 |
| Chocolate Mint Fat Free | 2 (1 oz) | 60 | 16 | 7 | 3 |
| Ginger Fat Free | 2 (1 oz) | 70 | 17 | 8 | 2 |
| ***Sargento*** | | | | | |
| MooTown Snackers Honey Graham Sticks & Vanilla Creme w/ Sprinkles | 1 pkg (1 oz) | 140 | 17 | 10 | 0 |
| MooTown Snackers Vanilla Sticks & Chocolate Fudge Creme | 1 pkg (1 oz) | 130 | 18 | 11 | tr |

| FOOD | PORTION | CALS | CARB | SUGAR | FIBER |
|---|---|---|---|---|---|
| ***Savion*** | | | | | |
| Chocolate Biscuits | 5 (1 oz) | 120 | 22 | 6 | 0 |
| Tea Biscuits | 5 (1 oz) | 120 | 22 | 6 | 0 |
| Tea Biscuits Vanilla | 5 (1 oz) | 120 | 22 | 6 | 0 |
| ***Scotto's*** | | | | | |
| Biscotti Fat Free French Vanilla | 4 (1 oz) | 80 | 18 | 6 | 0 |
| ***Season*** | | | | | |
| Hamantashen Poppy | 1 (1 oz) | 150 | 20 | 4 | 1 |
| Hamantasken Apricot | 1 (1 oz) | 150 | 20 | 4 | 1 |
| ***Simple Pleasures*** | | | | | |
| Almond | 1 (0.3 oz) | 37 | 5 | 2 | tr |
| Cinnamon Snaps | 1 (0.2 oz) | 31 | 6 | 2 | tr |
| Digestive | 1 (0.3 oz) | 46 | 6 | 2 | tr |
| Encore Tea Cookie | 1 (0.2 oz) | 29 | 6 | 1 | tr |
| Lemon Social Tea | 1 (0.2 oz) | 29 | 6 | 1 | tr |
| Oatmeal | 1 (0.5 oz) | 74 | 5 | 4 | 1 |
| Spice Snaps | 1 (0.3 oz) | 34 | 6 | 2 | tr |
| Sugar | 1 (0.4 oz) | 45 | 7 | 3 | tr |
| ***SnackWell's*** | | | | | |
| Bite Size Chocolate Chip | 13 (1 oz) | 130 | 22 | 10 | tr |
| Bite Size Double Chocolate Chip | 13 (1 oz) | 130 | 22 | 10 | 1 |
| Chocolate Sandwich | 2 (0.8 oz) | 110 | 20 | 11 | tr |
| Creme Sandwich | 1 pkg (1.7 oz) | 210 | 38 | 18 | tr |
| Fat Free Devil's Food | 1 (0.5 oz) | 50 | 12 | 7 | 0 |
| Golden Devil's Food | 1 (0.5 oz) | 50 | 11 | 7 | 0 |
| Mint Creme | 2 (0.9 oz) | 110 | 19 | 14 | tr |
| Oatmeal Raisin | 2 (0.9 oz) | 110 | 20 | 9 | tr |
| Sugar Free Chocolate Chip | 3 (1.2 oz) | 150 | 23 | 0 | tr |
| Sugar Free Oatmeal | 1 (0.8 oz) | 90 | 17 | 0 | tr |
| ***Soybite*** | | | | | |
| All Flavors | 1 | 79 | 7 | 0 | 1 |
| ***Stella D'Oro*** | | | | | |
| Almond Toast Mandel | 2 (1 oz) | 110 | 21 | 10 | 1 |
| Angel Wings | 2 (0.9 oz) | 140 | 13 | 3 | tr |
| Angelica | 1 (0.8 oz) | 100 | 15 | 6 | 0 |
| Anginetti | 4 (1.1 oz) | 140 | 23 | 17 | tr |
| Anisette Sponge | 2 (0.9 oz) | 90 | 19 | 9 | tr |
| Anisette Toast | 3 (1.2 oz) | 130 | 27 | 17 | tr |
| Biscotti Almond | 1 (0.8 oz) | 100 | 15 | 7 | tr |
| Biscotti Chocolate Almond | 1 (0.8 oz) | 90 | 15 | 7 | 1 |

| FOOD | PORTION | CALS | CARB | SUGAR | FIBER |
|---|---|---|---|---|---|
| Biscotti Chocolate Chunk | 1 (0.8 oz) | 90 | 16 | 9 | 0 |
| Biscotti Hazelnut | 1 (0.8 oz) | 100 | 15 | 8 | 0 |
| Biscottini Cashews | 1 (0.7 oz) | 110 | 13 | 5 | 0 |
| Breakfast Treats | 1 (0.8 oz) | 100 | 16 | 7 | tr |
| Breakfast Treats Chocolate | 1 (0.8 oz) | 100 | 15 | 7 | tr |
| Breakfast Treats Viennese Cinnamon | 1 (0.8 oz) | 100 | 17 | 8 | 0 |
| Chinese Dessert Cookies | 1 (1.2 oz) | 170 | 21 | 8 | tr |
| Chocolate Castelets | 2 (1 oz) | 130 | 19 | 8 | 1 |
| Egg Jumbo | 2 (0.8 oz) | 90 | 18 | 9 | tr |
| Fruit Slices Fat Free | 1 (0.6 oz) | 50 | 12 | 6 | tr |
| Kichel Low Sodium | 21 (1 oz) | 150 | 13 | 1 | 0 |
| Lady Stella Assortment | 3 (1 oz) | 130 | 19 | 10 | 0 |
| Margherite Chocolate | 2 (1.1 oz) | 140 | 22 | 9 | 1 |
| Margherite Vanilla | 2 (1.1 oz) | 140 | 22 | 8 | tr |
| Roman Egg Biscuits | 1 (1.2 oz) | 140 | 21 | 9 | 1 |
| Sesame Regina | 3 (1.1 oz) | 150 | 21 | 8 | 1 |
| Swiss Fudge | 2 (0.9 oz) | 130 | 16 | 9 | 0 |
| ***Stieffenhofer*** | | | | | |
| Choco Minis | 4 (1 oz) | 160 | 19 | 8 | 1 |
| Snaky | 3 (1 oz) | 160 | 19 | 10 | 0 |
| ***Streit's*** | | | | | |
| Wafers | 3 (1 oz) | 160 | 19 | 12 | 1 |
| ***Suissette*** | | | | | |
| Swiss Chocolate Hearts | 4 (1 oz) | 170 | 17 | 11 | – |
| Swiss Delight | 4 (1 oz) | 160 | 19 | 9 | – |
| Swiss Praline | 4 (1 oz) | 150 | 17 | 13 | 1 |
| ***Sunshine*** | | | | | |
| All American Butter | 5 (1.1 oz) | 140 | 21 | 7 | tr |
| All American Lemon Coolers | 5 (1 oz) | 140 | 21 | 10 | tr |
| All American Mini Chip-A-Roos | 5 (1.1 oz) | 160 | 21 | 10 | 1 |
| Animal Crackers | 14 (1.1 oz) | 140 | 24 | 7 | tr |
| Ginger Snaps | 7 (1 oz) | 130 | 22 | 9 | tr |
| Golden Fruit Cranberry | 1 (0.7 oz) | 80 | 14 | 7 | tr |
| Golden Fruit Raisin | 1 (0.7 oz) | 80 | 15 | 9 | tr |
| Hydrox | 3 (1.1 oz) | 150 | 21 | 11 | 1 |
| Hydrox Reduced Fat | 3 (1.1 oz) | 140 | 23 | 13 | 1 |
| Oatmeal Country Style | 2 (0.8 oz) | 120 | 17 | 8 | tr |

| FOOD | PORTION | CALS | CARB | SUGAR | FIBER |
|---|---|---|---|---|---|
| Sugar Wafers Peanut Butter Creme | 4 (1.1 oz) | 170 | 19 | 10 | 1 |
| Sugar Wafers Vanilla Creme | 3 (0.9 oz) | 130 | 18 | 13 | tr |
| Vanilla Wafers | 7 (1.1 oz) | 150 | 21 | 9 | tr |
| Vienna Fingers | 2 (1 oz) | 140 | 21 | 8 | tr |
| Vienna Fingers Lemon | 2 (1 oz) | 140 | 21 | 9 | 0 |
| Vienna Fingers Reduced Fat | 2 (1 oz) | 130 | 22 | 9 | tr |
| ***Super Chip*** | | | | | |
| Chocolate Chip | 2 (0.9 oz) | 100 | 10 | 0 | 3 |
| ***Sweet'N Low*** | | | | | |
| Sugar Free Amaretto Biscotti | 4 (1 oz) | 120 | 17 | 0 | tr |
| Sugar Free Chocolate Chip | 4 (1 oz) | 135 | 17 | 0 | tr |
| Sugar Free Cinnamon Graham | 7 (1 oz) | 120 | 19 | 0 | tr |
| Sugar Free Morning Crunch Bars | 2 (1 oz) | 120 | 19 | 0 | tr |
| Sugar Free Vanilla Wafers | 7 (1 oz) | 120 | 19 | 0 | tr |
| ***Sweetzels*** | | | | | |
| Chocolate Chip | 7 (1 oz) | 160 | 18 | 9 | 0 |
| Ginger Snaps | 4 (1.2 oz) | 140 | 25 | 11 | tr |
| Vanilla Wafers | 7 (1.1 oz) | 137 | 22 | 8 | 0 |
| ***Tastykake*** | | | | | |
| Chocolate Chip | 1 (1.4 oz) | 180 | 26 | 7 | 1 |
| Chocolate Chip Bar | 1 (2 oz) | 270 | 39 | 22 | tr |
| Chocolate Fudge Iced | 1 (1.4 oz) | 170 | 25 | 9 | 1 |
| Fudge Bar | 1 (2 oz) | 250 | 37 | 21 | 1 |
| Lemon Bar | 1 (2 oz) | 260 | 41 | 23 | 1 |
| Oatmeal Raisin Bar | 1 (2 oz) | 260 | 40 | 18 | 2 |
| Oatmeal Raisin Boxed | 3 (0.4 oz) | 130 | 14 | 7 | tr |
| Oatmeal Raisin Iced | 1 (1.4 oz) | 170 | 27 | 13 | 1 |
| Strawberry Bar | 1 (2 oz) | 260 | 41 | 23 | 1 |
| Sugar Boxed | 3 (0.4 oz) | 120 | 18 | 6 | 0 |
| ***The Source*** | | | | | |
| Barry's Raspberry Palmiers | 1 (0.7 oz) | 80 | 14 | 8 | 0 |
| ***Tom's*** | | | | | |
| Animal Crackers | ½ pkg (1 oz) | 120 | 23 | 6 | tr |
| Big Cookie Chocolate Chip | 1 pkg (2.75 oz) | 340 | 49 | 24 | 1 |
| Big Cookie Peanut Butter Chocolate Chip | 1 pkg (2 oz) | 280 | 37 | 18 | 1 |
| Chocolate Chip | 1 pkg (2 oz) | 280 | 37 | 18 | 1 |

| FOOD | PORTION | CALS | CARB | SUGAR | FIBER |
|---|---|---|---|---|---|
| Confetti Chip | 1 pkg (2 oz) | 300 | 40 | 23 | tr |
| Fat Free Apple Bar | 1 pkg (1.75 oz) | 160 | 38 | 22 | 1 |
| Fat Free Fig Bar | 1 pkg (1.75 oz) | 160 | 40 | 20 | 2 |
| Vanilla Wafers | ½ pkg (1 oz) | 130 | 20 | 9 | tr |
| ***Tree Of Life*** | | | | | |
| Fat Free Almond Butter | 1 (0.8 oz) | 60 | 14 | 6 | 1 |
| Fat Free Carrot Cake | 1 (0.8 oz) | 60 | 14 | 6 | 1 |
| Fat Free Devil's Food Chocolate | 1 (0.8 oz) | 70 | 15 | 7 | 1 |
| Fat Free Oatmeal Raisin | 1 (0.8 oz) | 70 | 16 | 7 | 1 |
| Fruit Bars Fat Free Fig | 1 (0.8 oz) | 70 | 16 | 11 | 2 |
| Fruit Bars Fat Free Peach Apricot | 1 (0.8 oz) | 70 | 17 | 9 | 1 |
| Fruit Bars Fat Free Wildberry | 1 (0.8 oz) | 70 | 16 | 7 | 2 |
| Monster Carob Chip | 1 (4.7 oz) | 700 | 95 | 40 | 5 |
| Monster Granola | 1 (4.7 oz) | 700 | 95 | 45 | 5 |
| Monster Macaroon | 1 (4.7 oz) | 750 | 85 | 40 | 5 |
| Monster Peanut Butter | 1 (4.7 oz) | 700 | 85 | 45 | 5 |
| Monster Fat Free Carrot Cake | 1 cookie (3.8 oz) | 240 | 60 | 40 | 4 |
| Monster Fat Free Devil's Food Chocolate | 1 cookie (3.8 oz) | 320 | 80 | 48 | 8 |
| Monster Fat Free Gingerbread | 1 cookie (3.8 oz) | 320 | 76 | 36 | 8 |
| Monster Fat Free Maple Pecan | 1 cookie (3.8 oz) | 360 | 80 | 40 | 8 |
| Oatmeal | 1 (0.8 oz) (0.8 oz) | 100 | 16 | 7 | 0 |
| Sandwich Royal Vanilla | 2 (0.9 oz) | 120 | 17 | 10 | 1 |
| Wheat Free Carob | 1 (0.8 oz) | 100 | 14 | 4 | 6 |
| Wheat Free Maple Walnut | 1 (0.8 oz) | 100 | 13 | 4 | 6 |
| Wheat Free Oatmeal | 1 (0.8 oz) | 90 | 11 | 3 | 1 |
| Wheat Free Peanut Butter | 1 (0.8 oz) | 109 | 8 | 3 | 1 |
| ***Twix*** | | | | | |
| Bars Chocolate Caramel | 1 (0.9 oz) | 140 | 18 | 13 | 0 |
| ***Voortman*** | | | | | |
| Almonette | 2 (1 oz) | 150 | 17 | 6 | tr |
| Chocolate Chip | 1 (0.7 oz) | 100 | 13 | 6 | 0 |
| Chocolate Wafers Sugar Free | 3 (1 oz) | 160 | 18 | 0 | 0 |

| FOOD | PORTION | CALS | CARB | SUGAR | FIBER |
|---|---|---|---|---|---|
| Coconut Delight | 1 (0.6 oz) | 90 | 10 | 6 | 0 |
| Peanut Delight | 1 (0.9 oz) | 130 | 15 | 6 | tr |
| Strawberry Wafers Sugar Free | 3 (1 oz) | 160 | 18 | 0 | 0 |
| Sugar | 1 (0.6 oz) | 80 | 11 | 5 | 0 |
| Turnovers Blueberry | 1 (0.9 oz) | 100 | 16 | 8 | 0 |
| Turnovers Cherry | 1 (0.9 oz) | 100 | 16 | 8 | 0 |
| Turnovers Strawberry | 1 (0.9 oz) | 100 | 16 | 8 | 0 |
| Vanilla Wafers Sugar Free | 3 (1 oz) | 160 | 18 | 0 | 0 |
| Windmill | 1 (0.7 oz) | 90 | 13 | 6 | 0 |
| ***Weight Watchers*** | | | | | |
| Apple Raisin Bar | 1 (0.75 oz) | 70 | 14 | 4 | 2 |
| Chocolate Chip | 2 (1.06 oz) | 140 | 22 | 15 | 1 |
| Chocolate Sandwich | 2 (1.06 oz) | 140 | 23 | 16 | 1 |
| Fruit Filled Fig | 1 (0.7 oz) | 70 | 16 | 9 | 0 |
| Fruit Filled Raspberry | 1 (0.7 oz) | 70 | 16 | 7 | 0 |
| Oatmeal Raisin | 2 (1.06 oz) | 120 | 22 | 13 | 1 |
| ***White Eagle Bakery*** | | | | | |
| Chruscik | 2 (1 oz) | 140 | 16 | 5 | 0 |
| ***Wortz*** | | | | | |
| Animal | 9 (1.1 oz) | 140 | 22 | 17 | 1 |
| Chocolate Graham | 2 (0.9 oz) | 130 | 24 | 7 | 1 |
| Cinnamon Grahams | 2 (0.9 oz) | 130 | 19 | 7 | tr |
| Vanilla Wafers | 7 (1.1 oz) | 150 | 22 | 10 | 1 |
| **REFRIGERATED** | | | | | |
| chocolate chip | 1 (0.42 oz) | 59 | 8 | – | – |
| chocolate chip unbaked | 1 oz | 126 | 17 | – | – |
| oatmeal | 1 (0.4 oz) | 56 | 8 | – | – |
| oatmeal raisin | 1 (0.4 oz) | 56 | 8 | – | – |
| peanut butter | 1 (0.4 oz) | 60 | 7 | – | – |
| peanut butter dough | 1 oz | 130 | 15 | – | – |
| sugar | 1 (0.42 oz) | 58 | 8 | – | – |
| sugar dough | 1 oz | 124 | 17 | – | – |
| ***Pillsbury*** | | | | | |
| Bunny | 2 | 130 | 17 | 7 | 0 |
| Chocolate Chip | 1 (1 oz) | 130 | 17 | 12 | tr |
| Chocolate Chip Reduced Fat | 1 (1 oz) | 110 | 19 | 12 | tr |
| Chocolate Chip w/ Walnuts | 1 (1 oz) | 140 | 17 | 10 | tr |
| Chocolate Chunk | 1 (1 oz) | 130 | 17 | 11 | tr |
| Christmas Tree | 2 | 130 | 17 | 7 | 0 |
| Double Chocolate | 1 (1 oz) | 130 | 17 | 11 | tr |

| FOOD | PORTION | CALS | CARB | SUGAR | FIBER |
|---|---|---|---|---|---|
| Flag | 2 | 130 | 17 | 7 | 0 |
| Frosty | 2 | 130 | 17 | 7 | 0 |
| M&M's | 1 (1 oz) | 130 | 18 | 11 | tr |
| Oatmeal Chocolate Chip | 1 (1 oz) | 120 | 16 | 10 | tr |
| One Step Pan Chocolate Chip | ⅛ pan (1 oz) | 130 | 19 | 13 | tr |
| One Step Pan M&M's | ⅛ pan (1 oz) | 130 | 19 | 12 | tr |
| Peanut Butter | 1 (1 oz) | 120 | 15 | 10 | tr |
| Pumpkin | 2 | 130 | 17 | 7 | 0 |
| Reeses | 1 (1 oz) | 130 | 15 | 10 | tr |
| Shamrock | 2 | 130 | 17 | 7 | 0 |
| Sugar | 2 | 130 | 19 | 10 | 0 |
| Sugar Holiday Red & Green | 2 | 130 | 19 | 10 | 0 |
| Valentine | 2 | 130 | 17 | 7 | 0 |
| White Chocolate Chunk | 1 (1 oz) | 130 | 17 | 11 | 0 |
| **TAKE-OUT** | | | | | |
| biscotti with nuts chocolate dipped | 1 (1.3 oz) | 117 | 16 | 11 | 1 |
| black & white | 1 lg (3 oz) | 302 | 52 | 31 | 1 |
| finikia | 1 (1.2 oz) | 171 | 16 | 5 | 1 |
| koulourakia butter cookie twist | 1 (0.9 oz) | 113 | 14 | 5 | tr |
| linzer tart | 1 (2.4 oz) | 280 | 34 | 12 | 0 |

## CORIANDER

| FOOD | PORTION | CALS | CARB | SUGAR | FIBER |
|---|---|---|---|---|---|
| leaf dried | 1 tsp | 2 | tr | – | – |
| leaf fresh | ¼ cup | 1 | tr | – | – |
| seed | 1 tsp | 5 | 1 | – | – |
| ***Instant India*** | | | | | |
| Tomato Coriander Paste | 2 tbsp (1 oz) | 90 | 8 | 6 | 0 |

## CORN

| FOOD | PORTION | CALS | CARB | SUGAR | FIBER |
|---|---|---|---|---|---|
| **CANNED** | | | | | |
| cream style | ½ cup | 93 | 23 | – | – |
| w/ red & green peppers | ½ cup | 86 | 21 | – | – |
| white | ½ cup | 66 | 15 | – | – |
| yellow | ½ cup | 66 | 15 | – | 1 |
| ***Del Monte*** | | | | | |
| Cream Style Golden | ½ cup (4.4 oz) | 90 | 20 | 5 | 2 |
| Cream Style Golden No Salt Added | ½ cup (4.4 oz) | 60 | 14 | 7 | 2 |
| Cream Style White | ½ cup (4.4 oz) | 100 | 21 | 6 | 2 |
| Fiesta | ½ cup (4.4 oz) | 50 | 12 | 5 | 2 |

| FOOD | PORTION | CALS | CARB | SUGAR | FIBER |
|---|---|---|---|---|---|
| Gold & White Supersweet | ½ cup (4.4 oz) | 80 | 18 | 6 | 2 |
| Whole Kernel Golden | ½ cup (4.4 oz) | 90 | 18 | 6 | 3 |
| Whole Kernel Golden Supersweet No Salt Added | ½ cup (4.4 oz) | 70 | 13 | 4 | 3 |
| Whole Kernel Golden Supersweet No Salt Added | ½ cup (4.4 oz) | 60 | 11 | 7 | 3 |
| Whole Kernel Golden Supersweet No Sugar | ½ cup (4.4 oz) | 60 | 11 | 7 | 3 |
| Whole Kernel Golden Supersweet Vacuum Packed | ½ cup (3.7 oz) | 70 | 13 | 4 | 3 |
| Whole Kernel White Sweet | ½ cup (4.4 oz) | 60 | 11 | 7 | 3 |
| ***S&W*** | | | | | |
| Cream Style | ½ cup (4.4 oz) | 60 | 14 | 7 | 2 |
| Whole Kernel | ⅓ cup (3 oz) | 70 | 12 | 6 | 2 |
| ***Veg-All*** | | | | | |
| Whole Kernel | ½ cup | 80 | 16 | 6 | 2 |
| **FRESH** | | | | | |
| on-the-cob w/ butter cooked | 1 ear | 155 | 32 | – | – |
| white cooked | ½ cup | 89 | 21 | – | – |
| white raw | ½ cup | 66 | 15 | – | – |
| yellow cooked | 1 ear (2.7 oz) | 83 | 19 | – | – |
| yellow cooked | ½ cup | 89 | 21 | – | – |
| yellow raw | ½ cup | 66 | 15 | – | – |
| yellow raw | 1 ear (3 oz) | 77 | 17 | – | – |
| **FROZEN** | | | | | |
| cooked | ½ cup | 67 | 17 | – | – |
| on-the-cob cooked | 1 ear (2.2 oz) | 59 | 14 | – | – |
| ***Birds Eye*** | | | | | |
| Gold & White Blend | ½ cup (3.5 oz) | 60 | 11 | 4 | 2 |
| ***Fresh Like*** | | | | | |
| Cut | 3.5 oz | 85 | 21 | – | 1 |
| On The Cob | 1 ear (3 in) | 96 | 24 | – | 1 |
| ***Tree Of Life*** | | | | | |
| Corn | ⅔ cup (3.2 oz) | 80 | 19 | 5 | 1 |
| **TAKE-OUT** | | | | | |
| fritters | 1 (1 oz) | 62 | 9 | – | 1 |
| scalloped | ½ cup | 258 | 43 | – | – |

**CORN CHIPS** *(see* CHIPS)

**CORNISH HENS** *(see* CHICKEN)

| FOOD | PORTION | CALS | CARB | SUGAR | FIBER |
|---|---|---|---|---|---|
| **CORNMEAL** | | | | | |
| corn grits cooked | 1 cup | 146 | 31 | – | – |
| corn grits uncooked | 1 cup | 579 | 124 | – | – |
| white | 1 cup (4.8 oz) | 505 | 107 | – | 10 |
| whole grain | 1 cup (4.3 oz) | 442 | 94 | – | 9 |
| yellow | 1 cup (4.8 oz) | 505 | 107 | – | 10 |
| yellow self-rising | 1 cup (4.3 oz) | 407 | 86 | – | 8 |
| ***Albers*** | | | | | |
| White | 3 tbsp | 110 | 24 | 0 | tr |
| Yellow | 3 tbsp | 110 | 24 | 0 | tr |
| ***Expert Foods*** | | | | | |
| Low Carb Grits Mix | 1½ tsp | 15 | 2 | – | 2 |
| ***Hodgson Mill*** | | | | | |
| Cornbread Mix Jalapeno Mexican | ¼ cup (1 oz) | 100 | 21 | 1 | 1 |
| Yellow Organic | ¼ cup (1 oz) | 100 | 22 | 0 | 3 |
| Yellow Self Rising | ¼ cup (1 oz) | 90 | 21 | 0 | 3 |
| ***Kentucky Kernel*** | | | | | |
| Sweet Cornbread Mix | ¼ cup (1 oz) | 120 | 24 | 6 | 0 |
| ***McKenzie's*** | | | | | |
| Hush Puppies | 1 serv (1.9 oz) | 190 | 23 | 2 | 2 |
| ***Quaker*** | | | | | |
| Yellow | 3 tbsp (1 oz) | 90 | 21 | – | 2 |
| **TAKE-OUT** | | | | | |
| hush puppies | 1 (0.75 oz) | 74 | 10 | – | 1 |
| **CORNSTARCH** | | | | | |
| cornstarch | 1 cup (4.5 oz) | 488 | 117 | – | 1 |
| ***Argo*** | | | | | |
| Cornstarch | 1 cup (128 g) | 460 | 115 | – | – |
| Cornstarch | 1 tbsp (8g) | 30 | 7 | – | – |
| ***Armour*** | | | | | |
| Cream Cornstarch | 1 tbsp (0.4 oz) | 40 | 9 | 0 | 0 |
| **COTTAGE CHEESE** | | | | | |
| creamed | 1 cup (7.4 oz) | 217 | 6 | – | – |
| creamed | 4 oz | 117 | 3 | – | – |
| creamed w/ fruit | 4 oz | 140 | 15 | – | – |
| dry curd | 1 cup (5.1 oz) | 123 | 3 | – | – |
| dry curd | 4 oz | 96 | 2 | – | – |
| lowfat 1% | 4 oz | 82 | 3 | – | – |

| FOOD | PORTION | CALS | CARB | SUGAR | FIBER |
|---|---|---|---|---|---|
| lowfat 1% | 1 cup (7.9 oz) | 164 | 6 | – | – |
| lowfat 2% | 4 oz | 101 | 4 | – | – |
| lowfat 2% | 1 cup (7.9 oz) | 203 | 8 | – | – |
| ***Breakstone's*** | | | | | |
| Cottage Doubles Peach | 1 pkg (5.5 oz) | 140 | 16 | 13 | tr |
| ***Cabot*** | | | | | |
| Cottage Cheese | ½ cup | 100 | 4 | 4 | 0 |
| No Fat | ½ cup | 70 | 5 | 5 | 0 |
| ***Horizon Organic*** | | | | | |
| Cottage Cheese | ½ cup (3.9 oz) | 110 | 4 | 3 | 0 |
| **COTTONSEED** | | | | | |
| kernels roasted | 1 tbsp | 51 | 2 | – | – |
| **COUSCOUS** | | | | | |
| cooked | 1 cup (5.5 oz) | 176 | 36 | – | 2 |
| dry | 1 cup (6.1 oz) | 650 | 134 | – | 9 |
| ***Near East*** | | | | | |
| Parmesan as prep | 1 cup | 220 | 41 | 3 | 2 |
| **COWPEAS** | | | | | |
| catjang dried cooked | 1 cup (2.9 oz) | 200 | 35 | – | – |
| common canned | 1 cup | 184 | 33 | – | – |
| frozen cooked | ½ cup | 112 | 20 | – | – |
| leafy tips chopped cooked | 1 cup | 12 | 1 | – | – |
| leafy tips raw chopped | 1 cup | 10 | 2 | – | – |
| **CRAB** | | | | | |
| **CANNED** | | | | | |
| blue | 1 cup | 133 | 0 | 0 | 0 |
| blue | 3 oz | 84 | 0 | 0 | 0 |
| ***Bumble Bee*** | | | | | |
| Fancy Lump Meat | ½ can (1.9 oz) | 40 | 0 | 0 | 0 |
| Fancy White Meat | ½ can (1.9 oz) | 28 | 1 | 0 | 0 |
| **FRESH** | | | | | |
| alaska king cooked | 1 leg (4.7 oz) | 129 | 0 | 0 | 0 |
| alaska king cooked | 3 oz | 82 | 0 | 0 | 0 |
| alaska king raw | 3 oz | 71 | 0 | 0 | 0 |
| alaska king raw | 1 leg (6 oz) | 144 | 0 | 0 | 0 |
| blue cooked | 1 cup | 138 | 0 | 0 | 0 |
| blue cooked | 3 oz | 87 | 0 | 0 | 0 |
| blue raw | 3 oz | 74 | tr | – | – |

| FOOD | PORTION | CALS | CARB | SUGAR | FIBER |
|---|---|---|---|---|---|
| blue raw | 1 crab (7 oz) | 18 | tr | – | – |
| dungeness raw | 1 crab (5.7 oz) | 140 | 1 | – | – |
| dungeness raw | 3 oz | 73 | 1 | – | – |
| queen steamed | 3 oz | 98 | 0 | 0 | 0 |
| **TAKE-OUT** | | | | | |
| baked | 1 (3.8 oz) | 160 | 4 | – | – |
| cake | 1 (2 oz) | 160 | 5 | – | – |
| kenagi korean crab cooked | 1 serv (3 oz) | 71 | 0 | 0 | 0 |
| soft-shell fried | 1 (4.4 oz) | 334 | 31 | – | – |

## CRACKER CRUMBS

| FOOD | PORTION | CALS | CARB | SUGAR | FIBER |
|---|---|---|---|---|---|
| chocolate wafer cookie crumbs | ½ cup (5.9 oz) | 728 | 120 | – | – |
| cracker meal | 1 cup (4 oz) | 440 | 93 | – | – |
| graham cracker crumbs | ½ cup (4.4 oz) | 540 | 97 | – | 3 |
| ***Baker's Harvest*** | | | | | |
| Graham | ⅓ cup (1 oz) | 130 | 23 | 7 | 1 |

## CRACKERS

| FOOD | PORTION | CALS | CARB | SUGAR | FIBER |
|---|---|---|---|---|---|
| cheese | 14 (½ oz) | 71 | 8 | – | – |
| cheese | 1 (1 in sq) (1 g) | 5 | 1 | – | – |
| cheese low sodium | 14 (½ oz) | 71 | 8 | – | – |
| cheese low sodium | 1 (1 in sq) (1 g) | 5 | 1 | – | – |
| cheese w/ peanut butter filling | 1 (0.24 oz) | 34 | 4 | – | tr |
| crispbread | 3 | 61 | 9 | – | 1 |
| crispbread rye | 1 (0.35 oz) | 37 | 8 | – | 2 |
| crispbread rye | 3 | 77 | 17 | – | 3 |
| melba toast plain | 1 (5 g) | 19 | 4 | – | tr |
| melba toast pumpernickel | 1 (5 g) | 19 | 4 | – | tr |
| melba toast rye | 1 (5 g) | 19 | 4 | – | tr |
| melba toast wheat | 1 (5 g) | 19 | 4 | – | tr |
| milk | 1 (0.42 oz) | 55 | 8 | – | – |
| oyster cracker | 1 (1 g) | 4 | 1 | – | tr |
| peanut butter sandwich | 1 (7 g) | 34 | 4 | – | – |
| rusk toast | 1 (0.35 oz) | 41 | 7 | – | – |
| rye w/ cheese filling | 1 (0.24 oz) | 34 | 4 | – | – |
| rye wafers plain | 1 (0.9 oz) | 84 | 20 | – | – |
| rye wafers seasoned | 1 (0.8 oz) | 84 | 16 | – | – |
| saltines | 1 (3 g) | 13 | 2 | – | tr |

| FOOD | PORTION | CALS | CARB | SUGAR | FIBER |
|---|---|---|---|---|---|
| saltines fat free low sodium | 3 (0.5 oz) | 59 | 12 | – | – |
| saltines fat free low sodium | 6 (1 oz) | 118 | 25 | – | – |
| saltines low salt | 1 (3 g) | 13 | 2 | – | tr |
| snack cracker | 1 (3 g) | 15 | 2 | – | tr |
| snack cracker low salt | 1 (3 g) | 15 | 2 | – | tr |
| snack cracker w/ cheese filling | 1 (7 g) | 33 | 4 | – | – |
| soup cracker | 1 (1 g) | 4 | 1 | – | tr |
| water biscuits | 3 | 92 | 16 | – | 1 |
| wheat w/ cheese filling | 1 (0.24 oz) | 35 | 4 | – | – |
| wheat w/ peanut butter filling | 1 (0.24 oz) | 35 | 4 | – | – |
| wheat thins | 1 (2 g) | 9 | 1 | – | – |
| wheat thins | 7 (0.5 oz) | 67 | 9 | – | 1 |
| wheat thins low salt | 7 (0.5 oz) | 67 | 9 | – | 1 |
| whole wheat | 1 (4 g) | 18 | 3 | – | – |
| whole wheat low salt | 1 (4 g) | 18 | 3 | – | – |
| zwieback | 1 oz | 107 | 21 | – | 1 |
| ***American Vintage*** | | | | | |
| Wine Biscuits All Flavors | 5 | 140 | 17 | 5 | tr |
| ***Andre's*** | | | | | |
| CarboSave Crackerbread All Flavors | 1 oz | 140 | 8 | 2 | 4 |
| ***Austin*** | | | | | |
| Cracker Sandwich Cheese On Cheese | 6 (1.3 oz) | 170 | 25 | 4 | tr |
| Cracker Sandwich Cheese Peanut Butter | 6 (1.3 oz) | 170 | 24 | 3 | 1 |
| Cracker Sandwich Toasty Peanut Butter | 6 (1.3 oz) | 170 | 24 | 4 | 1 |
| Cracker Sandwich Whole Wheat Cheese | 6 (1.3 oz) | 170 | 25 | 4 | tr |
| ***Baker's Harvest*** | | | | | |
| Cheese | 23 (1 oz) | 150 | 18 | 0 | tr |
| Cheese Reduced Fat | 29 (1 oz) | 130 | 21 | 0 | tr |
| Oyster | 35 (0.5 oz) | 70 | 11 | 0 | 1 |
| Saltines Unsalted | 5 (0.5 oz) | 70 | 11 | – | – |
| Saltines Deluxe | 5 (0.5 oz) | 60 | 10 | – | – |
| Snackers | 9 (1.1 oz) | 160 | 19 | 2 | tr |
| Snackers Reduced Fat | 10 (1.1 oz) | 140 | 23 | 2 | tr |
| Snackers Unsalted | 9 (1.1 oz) | 160 | 19 | 2 | tr |
| Wheat Snacks | 16 (1 oz) | 140 | 20 | 2 | 2 |

| FOOD | PORTION | CALS | CARB | SUGAR | FIBER |
|---|---|---|---|---|---|
| Wheat Snacks Reduced Fat | 16 (1.1 oz) | 140 | 23 | 4 | 1 |
| Woven Wheats | 7 (1.1 oz) | 140 | 21 | 0 | 4 |
| Woven Wheats Reduced Fat | 8 (1.1 oz) | 130 | 24 | 0 | 4 |
| ***Barbara's Bakery*** | | | | | |
| Cheese Bites | 26 (1 oz) | 120 | 24 | 0 | 1 |
| Right Lite Rounds Original | 5 (0.5 oz) | 55 | 12 | 1 | 0 |
| Rite Lite Rounds Savory Poppy | 5 (0.5 oz) | 70 | 11 | tr | 0 |
| Rite Lite Rounds Tamari Sesame | 5 (0.5 oz) | 70 | 12 | tr | 0 |
| Wheatines All Flavors | 1 lg sq (0.5 oz) | 50 | 10 | tr | 1 |
| ***Blue Diamond*** | | | | | |
| Nut Thins Almond | 16 (1 oz) | 130 | 19 | 0 | tr |
| Nut Thins Hazelnut | 16 (1 oz) | 120 | 20 | 0 | 1 |
| Nut Thins Pecan | 16 (1 oz) | 130 | 20 | 0 | tr |
| ***Bran-A-Crisp*** | | | | | |
| Low Carb Wheat Bran | 1 | 20 | 6 | tr | 2 |
| ***Breton*** | | | | | |
| Cabaret | 3 (5 g) | 70 | 9 | 1 | 0 |
| Light | 1 (5 g) | 20 | 3 | tr | tr |
| Minis | 20 (0.6 oz) | 89 | 11 | 1 | tr |
| Minis Cheddar Cheese | 20 (0.6 oz) | 87 | 11 | – | – |
| Minis Garden Vegetable | 20 (0.6 oz) | 87 | 12 | – | 1 |
| Multi-Grain | 3 | 70 | 8 | 2 | 1 |
| Original | 3 | 60 | 8 | 1 | 0 |
| Reduced Fat & Sodium | 3 | 60 | 9 | 1 | tr |
| Sesame | 3 | 60 | 7 | 1 | tr |
| ***Cheeters*** | | | | | |
| Low Carb All Flavors | 1 pkg (1 oz) | 104 | 4 | 1 | 2 |
| ***Cheetos*** | | | | | |
| Bacon Cheddar | 1 pkg | 190 | 25 | 3 | 1 |
| Cheddar Cheese | 1 pkg | 210 | 23 | 5 | 1 |
| Golden Toast | 1 pkg | 240 | 25 | 5 | 1 |
| ***Cheez It*** | | | | | |
| Big | 13 (1 oz) | 150 | 16 | tr | tr |
| Big Reduced Fat | 15 (1 oz) | 140 | 20 | tr | tr |
| Heads & Tails | 37 (1 oz) | 140 | 18 | 1 | 1 |
| Hot & Spicy | 26 (1 oz) | 150 | 17 | 1 | tr |
| Low Sodium | 27 (1 oz) | 160 | 16 | tr | tr |
| Nacho | 28 (1 oz) | 150 | 18 | 0 | tr |
| Original | 27 (1 oz) | 160 | 16 | tr | tr |

| FOOD | PORTION | CALS | CARB | SUGAR | FIBER |
|---|---|---|---|---|---|
| Party Mix | ½ cup (1 oz) | 140 | 19 | 1 | 1 |
| Party Mix Nacho | ½ cup (1 oz) | 130 | 20 | 0 | 1 |
| Party Mix Reduced Fat | ½ cup (1 oz) | 130 | 21 | 1 | 1 |
| Peanut Butter | 1 pkg (1.3 oz) | 190 | 22 | 3 | 1 |
| Reduced Fat | 29 (1 oz) | 140 | 20 | tr | tr |
| Snack Mix | ½ cup (1 oz) | 130 | 21 | 2 | 2 |
| Snack Mix Big Crunch | ¾ cup (1 oz) | 110 | 20 | 1 | tr |
| Snack Mix Double Cheese | ¾ cup (1 oz) | 110 | 19 | 1 | tr |
| White Cheddar | 26 (1 oz) | 150 | 18 | tr | tr |
| ***Courtney's*** | | | | | |
| Sun-Dried Tomato Organic | 4 (0.5 oz) | 60 | 10 | 0 | 0 |
| ***Dare*** | | | | | |
| Vinta | 1 (6 g) | 30 | 4 | 1 | 1 |
| ***Doritos*** | | | | | |
| Jalapeno Cheese | 1 pkg | 230 | 26 | 5 | 1 |
| Nacho Cheddar | 1 pkg | 240 | 25 | 6 | 1 |
| ***Eden*** | | | | | |
| Nori Nori Rice | 15 (1 oz) | 110 | 24 | 0 | 2 |
| ***Estee*** | | | | | |
| Sugar Free Cracked Pepper | 18 | 120 | 24 | 0 | 1 |
| Sugar Free Golden | 10 | 130 | 28 | 0 | 1 |
| Sugar Free Wheat | 17 | 100 | 18 | 0 | 2 |
| ***Frito Lay*** | | | | | |
| Cheddar Snacks | 1 pkg | 200 | 27 | tr | 1 |
| ***Frookie*** | | | | | |
| Cheddar | 17 (1 oz) | 140 | 23 | 1 | 1 |
| Cracked Pepper | 8 (0.7 oz) | 70 | 15 | 1 | 1 |
| Garden Vegetable | 13 (1 oz) | 130 | 19 | 1 | 2 |
| Garlic & Herb | 8 (0.7 oz) | 70 | 16 | 1 | 1 |
| Pizza | 17 (1 oz) | 130 | 24 | 1 | 1 |
| Snack & Party | 10 (1 oz) | 140 | 20 | 3 | 1 |
| Water Crackers | 8 (0.7 oz) | 70 | 16 | 1 | 1 |
| Wheat & Onion | 12 (1 oz) | 120 | 18 | 0 | 2 |
| Wheat & Rye | 13 (1 oz) | 120 | 18 | 1 | 3 |
| ***Gold'n Krackle*** | | | | | |
| Cheese | ½ oz | 65 | 9 | 0 | 0 |
| Cheese & Oregano | ½ oz | 65 | 9 | 0 | 0 |
| Hot & Spicy | ½ oz | 58 | 11 | 0 | 0 |
| Onion & Garlic | ½ oz | 58 | 11 | 0 | 0 |
| Plain | ½ oz | 58 | 11 | 0 | 0 |

| FOOD | PORTION | CALS | CARB | SUGAR | FIBER |
|---|---|---|---|---|---|
| ***Health Valley*** | | | | | |
| Healthy Pizza Garlic & Herb | 6 | 50 | 11 | 1 | 2 |
| Healthy Pizza Italiano | 6 | 50 | 11 | 1 | 2 |
| Healthy Pizza Zesty Cheese | 6 | 50 | 11 | 1 | 2 |
| Low Fat Mild Jalapeno | 6 | 60 | 10 | 1 | 2 |
| Low Fat Mild Ranch | 6 | 60 | 10 | 1 | 2 |
| Low Fat Roasted Garlic | 6 | 60 | 10 | 1 | 2 |
| Original Oat Bran | 6 | 120 | 22 | 3 | 3 |
| Original Rice Bran | 6 | 110 | 19 | 4 | 3 |
| Whole Wheat | 5 | 50 | 11 | 1 | 2 |
| Whole Wheat Cheese | 5 | 50 | 11 | 1 | 2 |
| Whole Wheat Herb | 5 | 50 | 11 | 1 | 2 |
| Whole Wheat No Salt Vegetable | 5 | 50 | 11 | 1 | 2 |
| Whole Wheat Onion | 5 | 50 | 11 | 1 | 2 |
| Whole Wheat Vegetable | 5 | 50 | 11 | 1 | 2 |
| ***Heavenly*** | | | | | |
| All Flavors Cholesterol Free Sugar Free | 1 | 16 | 3 | 0 | 0 |
| ***Kashi*** | | | | | |
| TLC Country Cheddar | 15 (1 oz) | 130 | 21 | 1 | 0 |
| TLC Honey Sesame | 15 (1 oz) | 130 | 22 | 5 | 2 |
| TLC Natural Ranch | 15 (1 oz) | 130 | 22 | 3 | 2 |
| TLC Original 7 Grain | 15 (1 oz) | 130 | 22 | 3 | 2 |
| ***Keebler*** | | | | | |
| Club 33% Reduced Fat | 5 (0.6 oz) | 70 | 12 | 2 | 0 |
| Club 50% Reduced Sodium | 4 (0.5 oz) | 70 | 9 | 1 | tr |
| Club Original | 4 (0.5 oz) | 70 | 9 | 1 | tr |
| Elfin | 23 (1 oz) | 130 | 24 | 8 | tr |
| Export Soda | 3 (0.5 oz) | 60 | 10 | 0 | tr |
| Harvest Bakery Multigrain | 2 (0.6 oz) | 70 | 10 | 2 | tr |
| Munch'ems Cheddar | 39 (1 oz) | 140 | 20 | 1 | 1 |
| Munch'ems Cheddar | 30 (1 oz) | 130 | 21 | 2 | tr |
| Munch'ems Chili Cheese | 28 (1.1 oz) | 130 | 23 | 4 | 1 |
| Munch'ems Mexquite BBQ | 40 (1 oz) | 140 | 22 | 1 | 1 |
| Munch'ems Ranch | 40 (1 oz) | 140 | 20 | 1 | 1 |
| Munch'ems Ranch | 33 (1 oz) | 130 | 21 | 2 | tr |
| Munch'ems Salsa | 28 (1.1 oz) | 130 | 23 | 3 | 1 |
| Munch'ems Seasoned Original | 30 (1 oz) | 130 | 20 | 1 | tr |

| FOOD | PORTION | CALS | CARB | SUGAR | FIBER |
|---|---|---|---|---|---|
| Munch'ems Sour Cream & Onion | 39 (1 oz) | 140 | 20 | 1 | 1 |
| Munch'ems Sour Cream & Onion 55% Reduced Fat | 33 (1 oz) | 130 | 22 | 2 | 0 |
| Paks Cheese & Peanut Butter | 1 pkg | 190 | 22 | 4 | tr |
| Paks Club & Cheddar | 1 pkg | 190 | 20 | 4 | tr |
| Paks Toast & Peanut Butter | 1 pkg | 190 | 23 | 5 | 1 |
| Paks Wheat & Cheddar | 1 pkg (1.3 oz) | 180 | 17 | 5 | 0 |
| Toasteds Buttercrisp | 5 (0.6 oz) | 80 | 10 | 1 | 0 |
| Toasteds Buttercrisp | 9 (1 oz) | 140 | 19 | 2 | tr |
| Toasteds Onion | 9 (1 oz) | 140 | 19 | 3 | tr |
| Toasteds Sesame | 5 (0.6 oz) | 80 | 10 | 1 | tr |
| Toasteds Sesame | 9 (1 oz) | 140 | 19 | 1 | tr |
| Toasteds Sesame Reduced Fat | 10 (1 oz) | 120 | 21 | 2 | 2 |
| Toasteds Wheat | 5 (0.6 oz) | 80 | 10 | 2 | tr |
| Toasteds Wheat | 9 (1 oz) | 140 | 19 | 3 | tr |
| Toasteds Wheat Reduced Fat | 5 (0.5 oz) | 60 | 10 | 2 | tr |
| Toasteds Wheat Reduced Fat | 10 (1 oz) | 120 | 22 | 2 | 1 |
| Town House | 5 (0.6 oz) | 80 | 9 | 1 | tr |
| Town House 50% Reduced Sodium | 5 (0.6 oz) | 80 | 10 | 1 | tr |
| Town House Reduced Fat | 6 (0.6 oz) | 70 | 11 | 2 | tr |
| Town House Wheat | 5 (0.6 oz) | 80 | 10 | 1 | tr |
| Wheatables Honey Wheat | 12 (1 oz) | 140 | 20 | 5 | 1 |
| Wheatables Original | 12 (1 oz) | 140 | 10 | 4 | 1 |
| Wheatables Seven Grain | 12 (1 oz) | 140 | 20 | 3 | 1 |
| Zesta Saltine 50% Reduced Sodium | 5 (0.5 oz) | 60 | 11 | 0 | tr |
| Zesta Saltine Fat Free | 5 (0.5 oz) | 50 | 11 | 0 | 0 |
| Zesta Saltine Original | 5 (0.5 oz) | 60 | 10 | 0 | tr |
| Zesta Saltine Unsalted Top | 5 (0.5 oz) | 70 | 10 | 0 | tr |
| Zesta Soup & Oyster | 42 (0.5 oz) | 80 | 10 | 0 | tr |
| ***Lance*** | | | | | |
| Bonnie | 6 (1⅛ oz) | 160 | 23 | 7 | 0 |
| Captain Wafers w/ Cream Cheese & Chives | 1 pkg (1.3 oz) | 190 | 22 | 6 | 0 |
| Cheese-On-Wheat | 1 pkg (1.3 oz) | 190 | 21 | 4 | 2 |
| Cranberry Bar Fat Free | 1 (1.75 oz) | 160 | 38 | 30 | 1 |
| Lanchee | 1 pkg (1¼ oz) | 190 | 18 | 3 | 1 |
| Malt | 1 pkg (1¼ oz) | 190 | 18 | 2 | 1 |

| FOOD | PORTION | CALS | CARB | SUGAR | FIBER |
|---|---|---|---|---|---|
| Nekot | 1 pkg (1.5 oz) | 210 | 25 | 12 | 1 |
| Nip-Chee | 1 pkg (1.3 oz) | 190 | 21 | 3 | 1 |
| Peanut Butter Wheat | 1 pkg (1.3 oz) | 190 | 20 | 4 | 1 |
| Rye-Chee | 1 pkg (1.4 oz) | 210 | 22 | 5 | 1 |
| Sour Dough w/ Cheddar & Sour Cream | 1 pkg (1.6 oz) | 240 | 23 | 4 | 1 |
| Toastchee | 1 pkg (1.4 oz) | 200 | 19 | 0 | 1 |
| Toasty | 1 pkg (1¼ oz) | 190 | 17 | 3 | 1 |
| Wheat Italian | ¾ cup (1.4 oz) | 200 | 23 | 3 | 1 |
| Wheat Pizza | ¾ cup (1.4 oz) | 200 | 23 | 3 | 1 |
| ***Little Debbie*** | | | | | |
| Cheese Crackers With Peanut Butter | 1 (0.9 oz) | 140 | 16 | 2 | tr |
| Cheese On Cheese Crackers | 1 (0.9 oz) | 140 | 15 | 2 | 0 |
| Cream Cheese & Chive | 1 (0.9 oz) | 140 | 17 | 4 | 0 |
| Toasty Crackers With Peanut Butter | 1 (0.9 oz) | 140 | 16 | 3 | tr |
| Wheat Crackers With Cheddar Cheese | 1 (0.9 oz) | 140 | 15 | 2 | 0 |
| ***Nabisco*** | | | | | |
| Royal Lunch | 1 (0.4 oz) | 60 | 8 | 1 | 0 |
| Zwieback | 1 (8 g) | 35 | 6 | 1 | 0 |
| ***No-Carb Kitchen*** | | | | | |
| Cheese | 1 | 25 | 0 | 0 | 0 |
| ***No-No*** | | | | | |
| Flatbreads Tortilla Corn Low Fat Sugar Free Everything | 3 (1 oz) | 95 | 18 | 0 | 1 |
| ***Pepperidge Farm*** | | | | | |
| Butter Thins | 4 (0.5 oz) | 70 | 10 | 1 | 0 |
| English Water Biscuits | 4 (0.5 oz) | 70 | 13 | 1 | 0 |
| Giant Goldfish Peanut Butter Sandwich | 1 pkg (1.4 oz) | 190 | 22 | 3 | 1 |
| Giant Goldfish Wheat | 14 | 140 | 21 | 3 | 1 |
| Goldfish Cheddar | 55 | 140 | 19 | 0 | tr |
| Goldfish Cheddar 30% Less Sodium | 60 (1.1 oz) | 150 | 18 | 0 | tr |
| Goldfish Cheese Trio | 58 | 140 | 19 | 0 | 1 |
| Goldfish Original | 55 | 140 | 19 | 0 | tr |
| Goldfish Parmesan Cheese | 60 | 140 | 13 | 0 | 1 |

| FOOD | PORTION | CALS | CARB | SUGAR | FIBER |
|---|---|---|---|---|---|
| Goldfish Pizza Flavored | 55 (1 oz) | 140 | 19 | 0 | 1 |
| Goldfish Pretzel | 43 (1 oz) | 120 | 22 | tr | tr |
| Hearty Wheat | 3 (0.6 oz) | 80 | 10 | 2 | 1 |
| Sesame | 3 (0.5 oz) | 70 | 9 | 0 | 2 |
| Snack Mix Fat Free Goldfish | ⅔ cup (0.9 oz) | 90 | 20 | 0 | 0 |
| ***Peter Pan*** | | | | | |
| Cheese Peanut Butter | 1 pkg | 210 | 23 | 3 | 1 |
| Toast Peanut Butter | 1 pkg | 210 | 23 | 3 | tr |
| ***Premium*** | | | | | |
| Saltine Multigrain | 5 (0.5 oz) | 60 | 10 | 0 | tr |
| ***Ralston*** | | | | | |
| Cheese | 23 (1 oz) | 150 | 18 | 0 | tr |
| Cheese Reduced Fat | 29 (1 oz) | 130 | 21 | 0 | tr |
| Oyster | 35 (0.5 oz) | 70 | 11 | 0 | 1 |
| Rich & Crisp | 1 (0.5 oz) | 70 | 9 | 1 | 0 |
| Saltines Fat Free | 5 (0.5 oz) | 60 | 13 | – | – |
| Saltines Deluxe | 5 (0.5 oz) | 60 | 10 | – | – |
| Snackers | 9 (1.1 oz) | 160 | 19 | 2 | tr |
| Snackers Reduced Fat | 10 (1.1 oz) | 140 | 23 | 3 | tr |
| Snackers Unsalted | 9 (1.1 oz) | 160 | 19 | 2 | tr |
| Wheat Snacks | 16 (1 oz) | 140 | 20 | 2 | 2 |
| Wheat Snacks Reduced Fat | 16 (1.1 oz) | 140 | 23 | 4 | 1 |
| Woven Wheats | 7 (1.1 oz) | 140 | 21 | 0 | 4 |
| Woven Wheats Reduced Fat | 8 (1.1 oz) | 130 | 24 | 0 | 4 |
| ***RedOval Farms*** | | | | | |
| Stoned Wheat Thins Cracked Pepper | 4 (0.6 oz) | 70 | 10 | 0 | tr |
| ***Rykrisp*** | | | | | |
| Seasoned | 2 | 60 | 10 | 0 | 3 |
| ***Smucker's*** | | | | | |
| Snackers Grape | 1 pkg (3.3 oz) | 410 | 47 | 23 | 3 |
| Snackers Strawberry | 1 pkg (3.3 oz) | 410 | 47 | 23 | 3 |
| ***Sunshine*** | | | | | |
| Hi Ho | 4 (0.5 oz) | 70 | 8 | 1 | tr |
| Hi Ho Reduced Fat | 5 (0.5 oz) | 70 | 10 | 1 | tr |
| Krispy | 5 (0.5 oz) | 60 | 10 | tr | tr |
| Krispy Fat Free | 5 (0.5 oz) | 50 | 11 | 0 | 0 |
| Krispy Mild Cheddar | 5 (0.5 oz) | 60 | 10 | 0 | tr |
| Krispy Soup & Oyster | 17 (0.5 oz) | 60 | 11 | tr | tr |
| Krispy Unsalted Tops | 5 (0.5 oz) | 60 | 10 | tr | tr |

| FOOD | PORTION | CALS | CARB | SUGAR | FIBER |
|---|---|---|---|---|---|
| Krispy Whole Wheat | 5 (0.5 oz) | 60 | 10 | tr | tr |
| ***Tree Of Life*** | | | | | |
| Bite Size Fat Free Cracked Pepper | 12 (0.5) | 55 | 12 | 1 | 0 |
| Bite Size Fat Free Garden Vegetable | 12 (0.5 oz) | 55 | 12 | 1 | 0 |
| Bite Size Fat Free Garlic & Herb | 12 (0.5 oz) | 55 | 12 | 1 | 0 |
| Bite Size Fat Free Toasted Onion | 12 (0.5 oz) | 55 | 12 | 1 | 0 |
| Oyster | 40 (0.5 oz) | 60 | 13 | 0 | 0 |
| Saltine Cracked Pepper Fat Free | 4 (0.5 oz) | 60 | 13 | 0 | 1 |
| Saltine Fat Free | 4 (0.5 oz) | 50 | 11 | 0 | 0 |
| ***Venus*** | | | | | |
| Fat Free Cracked Pepper | 11 (0.5 oz) | 60 | 12 | 1 | 0 |
| Fat Free Garden Vegetable | 5 (0.5 oz) | 60 | 12 | 1 | 0 |
| Fat Free Garlic & Herb | 11 (0.5 oz) | 60 | 12 | 1 | 0 |
| Fat Free Multi-Grain | 5 (0.5 oz) | 60 | 12 | 1 | tr |
| Fat Free Spicy Chili | 10 (0.5 oz) | 60 | 12 | 1 | tr |
| Fat Free Toasted Onion | 5 (0.5 oz) | 60 | 12 | 1 | 0 |
| Fat Free Toasted Wheat | 5 (0.5 oz) | 60 | 12 | 1 | tr |
| Fat Free Tomato & Basil | 10 (0.5 oz) | 60 | 12 | 1 | tr |
| Fat Free Zesty Italian | 10 (0.5 oz) | 60 | 12 | 1 | tr |
| Garden Vegetable | 6 (1 oz) | 150 | 20 | 3 | 1 |
| Honey Wheat | 1 oz | 140 | 21 | 3 | 1 |
| Low Fat Cracker Bread | 5 (0.5 oz) | 60 | 10 | tr | tr |
| Low Fat Water Crackers | 4 (0.5 oz) | 60 | 12 | 0 | 0 |
| Sesame & Flaxseed | 1 oz | 130 | 23 | 1 | 1 |
| Soup Original | 0.5 oz | 60 | 11 | 1 | 0 |
| Toasted Wheat | 6 (1 oz) | 150 | 18 | 2 | tr |
| Wine Cheese Caviar Original | 0.5 oz | 60 | 11 | 1 | 0 |
| Wine Cheese Caviar Pepper & Poppy | 0.5 oz | 60 | 11 | 1 | 0 |
| ***Wasa*** | | | | | |
| Crispbread Fiber Rye | 1 (0.4 oz) | 30 | 7 | 0 | 2 |
| ***Wheatsworth*** | | | | | |
| Crackers | 5 | 80 | 10 | 1 | tr |
| ***Wisecrackers*** | | | | | |
| Low Fat Poblano Chili & Sweet Onion | 4 (0.5 oz) | 45 | 8 | 1 | tr |
| ***Wortz*** | | | | | |
| Cheese | 23 (1 oz) | 150 | 18 | 0 | tr |

| FOOD | PORTION | CALS | CARB | SUGAR | FIBER |
|---|---|---|---|---|---|
| Oyster | 35 (0.5 oz) | 70 | 11 | 0 | 1 |
| Rich & Crisp | 1 (0.5 oz) | 70 | 9 | 1 | 0 |
| Saltines Fat Free | 5 (0.5 oz) | 60 | 13 | – | – |
| Saltines Deluxe | 5 (0.5 oz) | 60 | 10 | – | – |
| Wheat Snacks | 16 (1 oz) | 140 | 20 | 2 | 2 |
| Wheat Snacks Reduced Fat | 16 (1.1 oz) | 140 | 23 | 4 | 1 |
| Woven Wheats | 7 (1.1 oz) | 140 | 21 | 0 | 4 |
| **CRANBERRIES** | | | | | |
| cranberry sauce sweetened | ½ cup | 209 | 54 | – | – |
| fresh chopped | 1 cup | 54 | 14 | – | – |
| ***Jok'n'Al*** | | | | | |
| Cranberry Sauce | 1 tbsp | 8 | 2 | 1 | – |
| ***Ocean Spray*** | | | | | |
| Craisins | ⅓ cup (1.4 oz) | 130 | 33 | 31 | 2 |
| Cran*Fruit Cranberry Orange | ¼ cup | 120 | 29 | 28 | 1 |
| Cranberry Sauce Jellied | ¼ cup | 110 | 27 | 26 | 1 |
| Fresh | 2 oz | 25 | 6 | 0 | 0 |
| Whole Berry Sauce | ¼ cup | 110 | 28 | 27 | 1 |
| ***Steel's*** | | | | | |
| Spiced Cranberry Sauce | ⅓ cup | 20 | 5 | 4 | 1 |
| ***Wild Thyme Farms*** | | | | | |
| Cranberry Sauce | 1 tbsp | 19 | 5 | 4 | – |
| **CRANBERRY BEANS** | | | | | |
| canned | 1 cup | 216 | 39 | – | 16 |
| dried cooked | 1 cup | 241 | 43 | – | 18 |
| **CRANBERRY JUICE** | | | | | |
| cocktail | 1 cup | 147 | 38 | – | – |
| cranberry juice cocktail | 6 oz | 108 | 27 | – | – |
| cranberry juice cocktail low calorie | 6 oz | 33 | 9 | – | – |
| cranberry juice cocktail frzn | 12 oz can | 821 | 210 | – | – |
| cranberry juice cocktail frzn as prep | 6 oz | 102 | 26 | – | – |
| ***Keto*** | | | | | |
| Kooler | ½ tsp | 0 | 0 | 0 | 0 |
| ***Langers*** | | | | | |
| Cocktail | 8 oz | 140 | 35 | 32 | – |
| Diet | 8 oz | 30 | 9 | 9 | – |

| FOOD | PORTION | CALS | CARB | SUGAR | FIBER |
|---|---|---|---|---|---|
| White | 8 oz | 120 | 28 | 28 | – |
| ***Mott's*** | | | | | |
| Cocktail | 8 fl oz | 150 | 37 | – | – |
| ***Nantucket Nectars*** | | | | | |
| Big Cran | 8 oz | 140 | 34 | 32 | 0 |
| ***Ocean Spray*** | | | | | |
| Cocktail | 8 oz | 140 | 34 | 34 | 0 |
| Cocktail Reduced Calorie | 8 oz | 50 | 13 | 13 | 0 |
| Lightstyle Cranberry Juice Cocktail | 8 oz | 40 | 10 | 10 | 0 |
| White Cranberry | 1 cup (8 oz) | 120 | 29 | 29 | – |
| White Cranberry Peach | 1 cup (8 oz) | 120 | 30 | 30 | – |
| White Cranberry Strawberry | 1 cup (8 oz) | 120 | 31 | 31 | – |
| ***Tropicana*** | | | | | |
| Twister Ruby Red | 1 bottle (10 oz) | 160 | 42 | – | – |
| ***Wellfleet Farms*** | | | | | |
| Cranberry | 8 oz | 130 | 33 | 33 | 0 |
| **CRAYFISH** | | | | | |
| cooked | 3 oz | 97 | 0 | 0 | 0 |
| **CREAM** *(see also* WHIPPED TOPPINGS*)* | | | | | |
| clotted cream | 2 tbsp (1 oz) | 164 | 1 | – | 0 |
| creme fraiche | 2 tbsp (1 oz) | 100 | 1 | – | 0 |
| half & half | 1 cup (8.5 oz) | 315 | 10 | – | – |
| half & half | 1 tbsp (0.5 oz) | 20 | 1 | – | – |
| heavy whipping | 1 tbsp (0.5 oz) | 52 | tr | – | – |
| heavy whipping whipped | 1 cup (4.1 oz) | 411 | 7 | – | – |
| light coffee | 1 cup (8.4 oz) | 496 | 9 | – | – |
| light coffee | 1 tbsp (0.5 oz) | 29 | 1 | – | – |
| light whipping | 1 tbsp (0.5 oz) | 44 | tr | – | – |
| light whipping cream whipped | 1 cup (4.2 oz) | 345 | 7 | – | – |
| ***Cabot*** | | | | | |
| Whipped | 2 tbsp | 30 | 2 | 1 | 0 |
| ***Land O Lakes*** | | | | | |
| Fat Free Half & Half | 2 tbsp (1 oz) | 20 | 3 | 2 | 0 |
| Half & Half | 2 tbsp (1 oz) | 40 | 1 | 1 | 0 |
| Heavy Whipping | 1 tbsp (0.5 oz) | 50 | 0 | 0 | 0 |
| ***Organic Valley*** | | | | | |
| Half & Half | 2 tbsp (1 oz) | 40 | 1 | 1 | 0 |

| FOOD | PORTION | CALS | CARB | SUGAR | FIBER |
|---|---|---|---|---|---|
| **CREAM CHEESE** | | | | | |
| cream cheese | 1 oz | 99 | 1 | – | – |
| cream cheese | 1 pkg (3 oz) | 297 | 2 | – | – |
| ***Alpine Lace*** | | | | | |
| Reduced Fat Roasted Garlic & Herbs | 1 tsp (1 oz) | 60 | 2 | 1 | 0 |
| Reduced Fat Sundried Tomato & Basil | 2 tsp (1 oz) | 70 | 2 | 1 | 0 |
| ***Boar's Head*** | | | | | |
| Cream Cheese | 2 tbsp (1 oz) | 100 | 2 | 2 | 0 |
| ***Galaxy*** | | | | | |
| Slices | 1 slice (1 oz) | 50 | 2 | 1 | 0 |
| ***Horizon Organic*** | | | | | |
| Spreadable | 2 tbsp | 100 | 1 | 0 | 0 |
| ***Organic Valley*** | | | | | |
| Cream Cheese | 1 oz | 100 | 1 | tr | 0 |
| **CREAM OF TARTAR** | | | | | |
| cream of tartar | 1 tsp | 8 | 2 | – | – |
| **CREAM SUBSTITUTES** | | | | | |
| ***ExpertExtras*** | | | | | |
| RealCream | 1 tsp | 14 | tr | – | – |
| **CREPES** | | | | | |
| ***Frieda's*** | | | | | |
| Ready-To-Use | 2 (0.8 oz) | 50 | 9 | 4 | 0 |
| **CROAKER** | | | | | |
| atlantic breaded & fried | 3 oz | 188 | 6 | – | – |
| atlantic raw | 3 oz | 89 | 0 | 0 | 0 |
| **CROCODILE** | | | | | |
| cooked | 3 oz | 78 | 0 | 0 | 0 |
| **CROISSANT** | | | | | |
| apple | 1 (2 oz) | 145 | 21 | – | 1 |
| cheese | 1 (2 oz) | 236 | 27 | – | 2 |
| plain | 1 (2 oz) | 232 | 26 | – | 2 |
| plain | 1 mini (1 oz) | 115 | 13 | – | 1 |
| ***Sara Lee*** | | | | | |
| Broccoli & Cheese | 1 (3.7 oz) | 280 | 30 | 0 | 2 |
| French Style | 1 (1.5 oz) | 170 | 20 | 0 | 1 |

| FOOD | PORTION | CALS | CARB | SUGAR | FIBER |
|---|---|---|---|---|---|
| Ham & Swiss | 1 (3.7 oz) | 300 | 27 | 1 | 2 |
| Petite | 2 (2 oz) | 230 | 26 | 0 | 1 |
| **TAKE-OUT** | | | | | |
| w/ egg & cheese | 1 (4.5 oz) | 368 | 24 | – | – |
| w/ egg cheese & bacon | 1 (4.5 oz) | 413 | 24 | – | – |
| w/ egg cheese & ham | 1 (5.3 oz) | 474 | 24 | – | – |
| w/ egg cheese & sausage | 1 (5.6 oz) | 523 | 25 | – | – |
| **CROUTONS** | | | | | |
| plain | 1 cup (1 oz) | 122 | 22 | – | 2 |
| seasoned | 1 cup (1.4 oz) | 186 | 25 | – | 2 |
| ***Pepperidge Farm*** | | | | | |
| Garlic | 6 (0.2 oz) | 30 | 5 | 0 | 0 |
| Homestyle | 6 (0.2 oz) | 30 | 5 | 0 | 0 |
| Sourdough | 6 (0.2 oz) | 35 | 4 | 0 | 0 |
| ***Up Country Naturals*** | | | | | |
| Organic Whole Wheat Garlic & Herb | ¼ cup (0.3 oz) | 35 | 5 | 0 | tr |
| **CUCUMBER** | | | | | |
| fresh raw | 1 (11 oz) | 38 | 8 | – | 3 |
| fresh raw sliced | ½ cup (1.8 oz) | 7 | 1 | – | 1 |
| ***Chiquita*** | | | | | |
| Cucumber | ⅓ med (3.5 oz) | 15 | 3 | 2 | 1 |
| **TAKE-OUT** | | | | | |
| cucumber salad | 3.5 oz | 50 | 11 | – | – |
| kimchee | ½ cup (1.8 oz) | 36 | 4 | 3 | tr |
| tzatziki | ½ cup (3.4 oz) | 72 | 4 | 3 | 1 |
| **CUMIN** | | | | | |
| seed | 1 tsp | 8 | 1 | – | – |
| **CURRANT JUICE** | | | | | |
| black currant nectar | 7 oz | 110 | 26 | – | – |
| red currant nectar | 7 oz | 108 | 26 | – | – |
| **CURRANTS** | | | | | |
| black fresh | ½ cup | 36 | 9 | – | – |
| zante dried | ½ cup | 204 | 53 | – | – |
| **CUSK** | | | | | |
| fillet baked | 3 oz | 106 | 0 | 0 | 0 |

| FOOD | PORTION | CALS | CARB | SUGAR | FIBER |
|---|---|---|---|---|---|
| **CUSTARD** | | | | | |
| **MIX** | | | | | |
| as prep w/ 2% milk | ½ cup (4.7 oz) | 148 | 24 | – | – |
| as prep w/ 2% milk | 1 recipe 4 serv (18.7 oz) | 595 | 95 | – | – |
| as prep w/ whole milk | 1 recipe 4 serv (18.7 oz) | 652 | 94 | – | – |
| as prep w/ whole milk | ½ cup (4.7 oz) | 163 | 23 | – | – |
| flan as prep w/ 2% milk | 1 recipe 4 serv (18.7 oz) | 542 | 102 | – | – |
| flan as prep w/ 2% milk | ½ cup (4.7 oz) | 135 | 26 | – | – |
| flan as prep w/ whole milk | 1 recipe 4 serv (18.7 oz) | 600 | 102 | – | – |
| flan as prep w/ whole milk | ½ cup (4.7 oz) | 150 | 25 | – | – |
| ***Betty Crocker*** | | | | | |
| Flan w/ Caramel Sauce as prep | 1 serv | 330 | 60 | 23 | – |
| **READY-TO-EAT** | | | | | |
| ***Swiss Miss*** | | | | | |
| Egg Custard | 1 pkg (4 oz) | 153 | 22 | 21 | 0 |
| **TAKE-OUT** | | | | | |
| baked | ½ cup (5 oz) | 148 | 15 | – | – |
| flan | ½ cup (5.4 oz) | 220 | 35 | – | – |
| zabaione | ½ cup (57.2 g) | 135 | 13 | – | 0 |
| **CUTTLEFISH** | | | | | |
| steamed | 3 oz | 134 | 1 | – | – |
| **DANDELION GREENS** | | | | | |
| fresh cooked | ½ cup | 17 | 3 | – | – |
| **DANISH PASTRY** | | | | | |
| **FROZEN** | | | | | |
| ***Morton*** | | | | | |
| Honey Buns | 1 (2.28 oz) | 270 | 35 | 16 | 1 |
| Honey Buns Mini | 1 (1.3 oz) | 160 | 19 | 6 | 1 |
| **READY-TO-EAT** | | | | | |
| plain ring | 1 (12 oz) | 1305 | 152 | – | – |

| FOOD | PORTION | CALS | CARB | SUGAR | FIBER |
|---|---|---|---|---|---|
| ***Dolly Madison*** | | | | | |
| Danish Rollers | 3 (2.8 oz) | 290 | 46 | 21 | 1 |
| ***Tastykake*** | | | | | |
| Cheese | 1 (3 oz) | 290 | 44 | 22 | tr |
| Lemon | 1 (3 oz) | 290 | 44 | 22 | 1 |
| Raspberry | 1 (3 oz) | 290 | 44 | 22 | 1 |
| **TAKE-OUT** | | | | | |
| almond | 1 (4¼ in) (2.3 oz) | 280 | 30 | – | 2 |
| apple | 1 (4¼ in) (2.5 oz) | 264 | 34 | – | 1 |
| cheese | 1 (3.2 oz) | 353 | 29 | – | – |
| cheese | 1 (4¼ in) (2.5 oz) | 266 | 26 | – | – |
| cinnamon | 1 (3.1 oz) | 349 | 47 | – | – |
| cinnamon | 1 (4¼ in) (2.3 oz) | 262 | 29 | – | 1 |
| cinnamon nut | 1 (4¼ in) (2.3 oz) | 280 | 30 | – | 2 |
| fruit | 1 (3.3 oz) | 335 | 45 | – | – |
| lemon | 1 (4¼ in) (2.5 oz) | 264 | 34 | – | 1 |
| raisin | 1 (4¼ in) (2.5 oz) | 264 | 34 | – | 1 |
| raisin nut | 1 (4¼ in) (2.3 oz) | 280 | 30 | – | 2 |
| raspberry | 1 (4¼ in) (2.5 oz) | 264 | 34 | – | 1 |
| strawberry | 1 (4¼ in) (2.5 oz) | 264 | 34 | – | 1 |

## DATES

| FOOD | PORTION | CALS | CARB | SUGAR | FIBER |
|---|---|---|---|---|---|
| dried chopped | 1 cup | 489 | 131 | – | – |
| dried whole | 10 | 228 | 61 | – | – |
| jujube dried | 1 oz | 75 | 19 | – | 2 |
| jujube fresh | 1 oz | 30 | 7 | – | – |
| jujube preserved in sugar | 1 oz | 91 | 22 | – | – |
| medjool | 2-3 (1.4 oz) | 120 | 31 | 25 | 3 |
| ***Calavo*** | | | | | |
| Dried Pitted | 5-6 (1.4 oz) | 120 | 31 | 20 | 3 |

| FOOD | PORTION | CALS | CARB | SUGAR | FIBER |
|---|---|---|---|---|---|
| ***California Redi-Date*** | | | | | |
| Deglet Noor Dried | 5-6 (1.4 oz) | 120 | 31 | 29 | 3 |
| ***Dromedary*** | | | | | |
| Chopped Dried | ¼ cup | 130 | 31 | – | – |

**DEER** *(see* VENISON*)*

**DELI MEATS/COLD CUTS** *(see also* BEEF, CHICKEN, HAM, MEAT SUBSTITUTES, TURKEY*)*

| FOOD | PORTION | CALS | CARB | SUGAR | FIBER |
|---|---|---|---|---|---|
| barbecue loaf pork & beef | 1 slice | 40 | 1 | – | 0 |
| beerwurst beef | 1 slice (2¾ in x 1/16 in) | 20 | tr | – | – |
| beerwurst beef | 1 slice (4 in x ⅛ in) | 75 | tr | – | – |
| beerwurst pork | 1 slice (2¾ in x 1/16 in) | 14 | tr | – | – |
| beerwurst pork | 1 slice (4 in x ⅛ in) | 55 | tr | – | – |
| berliner pork & beef | 1 oz | 65 | 1 | – | – |
| blood sausage | 1 oz | 95 | tr | – | – |
| bologna beef | 1 oz | 88 | tr | – | – |
| bologna beef & pork | 1 oz | 89 | 1 | – | – |
| bologna pork | 1 oz | 70 | tr | – | – |
| braunschweiger pork | 1 slice (2½ in x ¼ in) | 65 | 1 | – | – |
| braunschweiger pork | 1 oz | 102 | 1 | – | – |
| corned beef loaf | 1 oz | 43 | 0 | 0 | 0 |
| dried beef | 1 oz | 47 | tr | – | – |
| dutch brand loaf pork & beef | 1 oz | 68 | 2 | – | – |
| headcheese pork | 1 oz | 60 | tr | – | – |
| honey loaf pork & beef | 1 oz | 36 | 2 | – | – |
| honey roll sausage beef | 1 oz | 42 | 1 | – | – |
| lebanon bologna beef | 1 oz | 60 | 1 | – | – |
| liver cheese pork | 1 oz | 86 | 1 | – | – |
| liverwurst pork | 1 oz | 92 | 1 | – | – |
| luncheon meat beef | 1 oz | 87 | 1 | – | – |
| luncheon meat pork & beef | 1 oz | 100 | 1 | – | – |
| luncheon meat pork canned | 1 oz | 95 | 1 | – | – |
| luncheon sausage pork & beef | 1 oz | 74 | tr | – | – |
| luxury loaf pork | 1 oz | 40 | 1 | – | – |

| FOOD | PORTION | CALS | CARB | SUGAR | FIBER |
|---|---|---|---|---|---|
| mortadella beef & pork | 1 oz | 88 | 1 | – | – |
| mother's loaf pork | 1 oz | 80 | 2 | – | – |
| new england sausage pork & beef | 1 oz | 46 | 1 | – | – |
| olive loaf pork | 1 oz | 67 | 3 | – | – |
| peppered loaf pork & beef | 1 oz | 42 | 1 | – | – |
| pepperoni pork & beef | 1 slice (0.2 oz) | 27 | tr | – | – |
| pepperoni pork & beef | 1 (9 oz) | 1248 | 7 | – | – |
| pickle & pimiento loaf pork | 1 oz | 74 | 2 | – | – |
| picnic loaf pork & beef | 1 oz | 66 | 1 | – | – |
| salami cooked beef & pork | 1 oz | 71 | 1 | – | – |
| salami hard pork | 1 pkg (4 oz) | 460 | 2 | – | – |
| salami hard pork | 1 slice (⅓ oz) | 41 | 3 | – | – |
| salami hard pork & beef | 1 slice (0.3 oz) | 42 | tr | – | – |
| salami hard pork & beef | 1 pkg (4 oz) | 472 | 3 | – | – |
| sandwich spread pork & beef | 1 tbsp | 35 | 2 | – | – |
| sandwich spread pork & beef | 1 oz | 67 | 3 | – | – |
| summer sausage thuringer cervelat | 1 oz | 98 | 1 | – | – |
| ***Boar's Head*** | | | | | |
| Bologna Beef | 2 oz | 150 | 0 | 0 | 0 |
| Bologna Garlic | 2 oz | 150 | 1 | 1 | 0 |
| Bologna Lowered Sodium | 2 oz | 150 | 0 | 0 | 0 |
| Bologna Pork & Beef | 2 oz | 150 | tr | tr | 0 |
| Braunschweiger Lite | 2 oz | 120 | 1 | 0 | 0 |
| Head Cheese | 2 oz | 90 | tr | 0 | 0 |
| Liverwurst Strassburger | 2 oz | 170 | 1 | 1 | 0 |
| Olive Loaf | 2 oz | 130 | tr | tr | 0 |
| Pastrami | 2 oz | 90 | 2 | 0 | 0 |
| Prosciutto | 1 oz | 60 | 0 | 0 | 0 |
| Red Pastrami | 2 oz | 90 | 2 | 0 | 0 |
| Salami Beef | 2 oz | 120 | 0 | 0 | 0 |
| Salami Cooked | 2 oz | 130 | 0 | 0 | 0 |
| Salami Genoa | 2 oz | 180 | 1 | 0 | 0 |
| Salami Hard | 1 oz | 110 | tr | 0 | 0 |
| Spiced Ham | 2 oz | 120 | 1 | 0 | 0 |
| ***Carl Buddig*** | | | | | |
| Beef | 1 pkg (2.5 oz) | 100 | 1 | 1 | – |
| Corned Beef | 1 pkg (2.5 oz) | 100 | tr | tr | – |
| Pastrami | 1 pkg (2.5 oz) | 100 | 1 | 1 | – |

| FOOD | PORTION | CALS | CARB | SUGAR | FIBER |
|---|---|---|---|---|---|
| **TAKE-OUT** | | | | | |
| corned beef | 2 oz | 70 | 0 | 0 | 0 |
| corned beef brisket | 2 oz | 90 | 0 | 0 | 0 |
| **DILL** | | | | | |
| seed | 1 tsp | 6 | 1 | – | – |
| sprigs fresh | 1 cup | 4 | 1 | – | – |
| sprigs fresh | 5 | 0 | tr | – | – |
| weed dry | 1 tsp | 3 | 1 | – | – |
| **DINNER** *(see also* ASIAN FOOD, PASTA DISHES, POT PIES, SPANISH FOOD*)* | | | | | |
| ***Amy's*** | | | | | |
| Country Dinner Vegetable Salisbury Steak | 1 pkg (11 oz) | 380 | 60 | 14 | 9 |
| ***Banquet*** | | | | | |
| Beef Patty w/ Country Style Vegetables | 1 meal (9.5 oz) | 310 | 22 | 6 | 2 |
| Boneless Pork Rib | 1 meal (10 oz) | 400 | 40 | 22 | 4 |
| Boneless White Fried Chicken | 1 meal (8.25 oz) | 540 | 41 | 10 | 3 |
| Chicken Parmigiana | 1 meal (9.5 oz) | 320 | 29 | 7 | 3 |
| Chicken Fingers Meal | 1 meal (7.1 oz) | 740 | 67 | 24 | 6 |
| Chicken Fried Beef Steak | 1 pkg (10 oz) | 420 | 39 | 9 | 4 |
| Chicken Nuggets Meal | 1 meal (6.75 oz) | 430 | 42 | 11 | 4 |
| Extra Helping Boneless Pork Riblet | 1 meal (15.25 oz) | 720 | 62 | 18 | 7 |
| Extra Helping Fried Beef Steak | 1 meal (16 oz) | 820 | 63 | 13 | 6 |
| Extra Helping Fried Chicken | 1 meal (14.7 oz) | 910 | 70 | 8 | 5 |
| Extra Helping Meatloaf | 1 meal (16 oz) | 610 | 34 | 12 | 6 |
| Extra Helping Salisbury Steak | 1 meal (16.5 oz) | 740 | 37 | 7 | 7 |
| Extra Helping Turkey & Gravy w/ Dressing | 1 meal (17 oz) | 620 | 54 | 11 | 10 |

| FOOD | PORTION | CALS | CARB | SUGAR | FIBER |
|---|---|---|---|---|---|
| Extra Helping White Fried Chicken | 1 meal (13 oz) | 690 | 40 | 3 | 8 |
| Extra Helping Yankee Pot Roast | 1 meal (14.5 oz) | 410 | 33 | 25 | 3 |
| Family Size Brown Gravy & Salisbury Steak | 1 serv | 240 | 7 | 2 | 1 |
| Family Size Brown Gravy & Sliced Beef | 1 serv | 140 | 5 | 2 | tr |
| Family Size Chicken & Broccoli Alfredo | 1 serv | 270 | 28 | 3 | 3 |
| Family Size Country Style Chicken & Dumplings | 1 serv | 290 | 30 | 6 | 7 |
| Family Size Creamy Broccoli Chicken Cheese & Rice | 1 serv | 280 | 25 | 6 | 2 |
| Family Size Hearty Beef Stew | 1 cup | 170 | 18 | 4 | 4 |
| Family Size Homestyle Gravy & Sliced Turkey | 2 slices | 140 | 5 | 1 | 1 |
| Family Size Mushroom Gravy & Charbroiled Beef Patties | 1 patty | 250 | 6 | 2 | 2 |
| Family Size Potato Ham & Broccoli Au Gratin | ⅔ cup | 210 | 16 | 6 | 2 |
| Family Size Savory Gravy & Meatloaf | 1 slice | 120 | 7 | 2 | 1 |
| Fish Sticks | 1 meal (6.6 oz) | 290 | 33 | 14 | 4 |
| Grilled Chicken | 1 meal (9.9 oz) | 330 | 37 | 18 | 2 |
| Honey Roast Turkey Breast | 1 meal (9 oz) | 270 | 29 | 8 | 4 |
| Meatloaf | 1 meal (9.5 oz) | 280 | 23 | 9 | 3 |
| Our Original Fried Chicken | 1 meal (9 oz) | 470 | 35 | 4 | 2 |
| Pork Cutlet Meal | 1 meal (10.25 oz) | 420 | 36 | 21 | 4 |
| Salisbury Steak | 1 meal (9.5 oz) | 380 | 28 | 4 | 4 |
| Sliced Beef | 1 meal (9 oz) | 270 | 19 | 12 | 4 |

| FOOD | PORTION | CALS | CARB | SUGAR | FIBER |
|---|---|---|---|---|---|
| Turkey | 1 meal (9.25 oz) | 270 | 30 | 7 | 3 |
| Veal Parmagiana | 1 meal (8.75 oz) | 330 | 37 | 7 | 2 |
| Western Style Beef Patty | 1 meal (9.5 oz) | 360 | 28 | 4 | 3 |
| White Meat Fried Chicken | 1 meal (8.75 oz) | 460 | 40 | 4 | 2 |
| Yankee Pot Roast | 1 meal (9.4 oz) | 230 | 20 | 8 | 4 |
| ***Birds Eye*** | | | | | |
| Easy Recipe Creations Sweet & Sour w/ Pineapple Tidbits | 1⅔ cups | 200 | 45 | 41 | 3 |
| Voila! Zesty Garlic Chicken | 2 cups (6.2 oz) | 260 | 28 | 6 | 1 |
| Voila! Beef Sirloin Steak And Garlic Potatoes | 1 cup | 240 | 26 | 5 | 3 |
| Voila! Chicken Alfredo | 1 cup | 230 | 26 | 5 | 2 |
| Voila! Garden Herb Chicken | 1 cup | 310 | 28 | 8 | 2 |
| Voila! Grilled Salsa Chicken w/ Rice | 1 cup | 240 | 35 | 5 | 3 |
| Voila! Homestyle Turkey w/ Roasted Potatoes | 1 cup | 200 | 24 | 4 | 3 |
| Voila! Teriyaki | 2 cups (6.4 oz) | 240 | 26 | 7 | 2 |
| ***Fillo Factory*** | | | | | |
| Fillo Pie Broccoli & Cheese | ¼ pie (4 oz) | 350 | 50 | 1 | 3 |
| Fillo Pie Spinach & Cheese | ⅕ pie (4.8 oz) | 210 | 27 | 1 | 2 |
| ***Healthy Choice*** | | | | | |
| Beef Pepper Steak Oriental | 1 meal (9.5 oz) | 260 | 34 | 5 | 2 |
| Beef Pot Roast | 1 meal (11 oz) | 300 | 41 | 24 | 6 |
| Beef Stroganoff | 1 meal (11 oz) | 320 | 40 | 14 | 7 |
| Beef Tips Francais | 1 meal (9.5 oz) | 300 | 40 | 6 | 4 |
| Beef Tips Portabello | 1 meal (11.25 oz) | 270 | 34 | 14 | 7 |

| FOOD | PORTION | CALS | CARB | SUGAR | FIBER |
|---|---|---|---|---|---|
| Bowls Chicken Teriyaki w/ Rice | 1 meal (9.5 oz) | 270 | 41 | 7 | 4 |
| Bowls Country Chicken Bake | 1 meal (9.5 oz) | 230 | 22 | 9 | 4 |
| Bowls Fiesta Chicken | 1 meal (9.5 oz) | 220 | 34 | 6 | 3 |
| Bowls Garlic Lemon Chicken w/ Rice | 1 meal (9.5 oz) | 300 | 48 | 6 | 4 |
| Bowls Roasted Potatoes w/ Ham | 1 meal (8.5 oz) | 210 | 26 | 10 | 6 |
| Bowls Southwestern Chicken & Pasta | 1 meal (9.5 oz) | 320 | 39 | 2 | 6 |
| Bowls Turkey Divan | 1 meal (9.5 oz) | 250 | 31 | 7 | 4 |
| Charbroiled Beef Patty | 1 meal (11 oz) | 310 | 40 | 8 | 4 |
| Chicken Cantonese | 1 meal (10.75) | 280 | 34 | 15 | 2 |
| Chicken Parmigiana | 1 meal (11.5 oz) | 330 | 46 | 23 | 3 |
| Chicken & Vegetables Marsala | 1 meal (11.5 oz) | 240 | 32 | 4 | 3 |
| Chicken Broccoli Alfredo | 1 meal (11.5 oz) | 300 | 34 | 5 | 2 |
| Chicken Dijon | 1 meal (11 oz) | 270 | 33 | 6 | 6 |
| Chicken Teriyaki | 1 meal (11 oz) | 270 | 37 | 11 | 3 |
| Country Breaded Chicken | 1 meal (10.25 oz) | 350 | 51 | 20 | 5 |
| Country Glazed Chicken Breast | 1 meal (8.5 oz) | 250 | 31 | 6 | 3 |
| Country Herb Chicken | 1 meal (12.15 oz) | 320 | 44 | 23 | 3 |
| Country Inn Roast Turkey | 1 meal (10 oz) | 250 | 28 | 16 | 4 |
| Garlic Chicken Milano | 1 meal (9.5 oz) | 260 | 34 | 4 | 3 |
| Grilled Chicken Sonoma | 1 meal (9 oz) | 230 | 30 | 9 | 3 |

| FOOD | PORTION | CALS | CARB | SUGAR | FIBER |
|---|---|---|---|---|---|
| Grilled Chicken w/ Mashed Potatoes | 1 meal (8 oz) | 180 | 18 | 3 | 3 |
| Herb Baked Fish | 1 meal (10.9 oz) | 340 | 54 | 11 | 5 |
| Herb Breaded Pork Patty | 1 meal (8 oz) | 280 | 38 | 4 | 4 |
| Homestyle Chicken & Pasta | 1 meal (9 oz) | 270 | 32 | 6 | 5 |
| Honey Glazed Chicken | 1 meal (10 oz) | 270 | 32 | 11 | 4 |
| Honey Mustard Chicken | 1 meal (9.5 oz) | 290 | 38 | 7 | 1 |
| Lemon Pepper Fish | 1 meal (10.7 oz) | 320 | 50 | 20 | 5 |
| Mandarin Chicken | 1 meal (10 oz) | 280 | 44 | 9 | 4 |
| Mesquite Beef w/ Barbecue Sauce | 1 meal (11 oz) | 320 | 36 | 16 | 5 |
| Mesquite Chicken Barbecue | 1 meal (10.5 oz) | 310 | 48 | 15 | 6 |
| Oriental Style Chicken & Vegetable Stir Fry | 1 meal (11.9) | 360 | 57 | 16 | 5 |
| Oven Roasted Beef | 1 meal (10.15 oz) | 280 | 35 | 10 | 4 |
| Roast Turkey Breast | 1 meal (8.5 oz) | 220 | 28 | 0 | 5 |
| Roasted Chicken | 1 meal (11 oz) | 230 | 23 | 9 | 4 |
| Sesame Chicken | 1 meal (10.8 oz) | 360 | 54 | 17 | 4 |
| Shrimp & Vegetables | 1 meal (11.8 oz) | 270 | 39 | 6 | 6 |
| Sweet & Sour Chicken | 1 meal (11 oz) | 360 | 53 | 25 | 5 |
| Traditional Meatloaf | 1 meal (12 oz) | 330 | 52 | 17 | 6 |
| Traditional Breast Of Turkey | 1 meal (10.5 oz) | 290 | 40 | 20 | 5 |
| Traditional Salisbury Steak | 1 meal (11.5 oz) | 330 | 48 | 24 | 6 |

| FOOD | PORTION | CALS | CARB | SUGAR | FIBER |
|---|---|---|---|---|---|
| Tuna Casserole | 1 meal (8 oz) | 240 | 33 | 7 | 4 |
| ***Kid Cuisine*** | | | | | |
| Circus Show Corn Dog | 1 meal (8.8 oz) | 490 | 70 | 46 | 5 |
| Cosmic Chicken Nuggets | 1 meal (9.1 oz) | 500 | 50 | 19 | 5 |
| Futuristic Fish Sticks | 1 meal (8.25 oz) | 410 | 57 | 30 | 4 |
| Game Time Taco Roll Up | 1 meal (7.35 oz) | 420 | 55 | 25 | 4 |
| High Flying Fried Chicken | 1 meal (10.1 oz) | 440 | 48 | 20 | 3 |
| Parachuting Pork Ribettes | 1 meal (7.55 oz) | 390 | 39 | 16 | 3 |
| ***Lean Cuisine*** | | | | | |
| Cafe Classics Baked Chicken | 1 pkg (8.6 oz) | 240 | 33 | 4 | 3 |
| Cafe Classics Baked Fish | 1 pkg (9 oz) | 290 | 40 | 6 | 2 |
| Cafe Classics Beef Peppercorn | 1 pkg (8.75 oz) | 260 | 32 | 5 | 4 |
| Cafe Classics Beef Portobello | 1 pkg (9 oz) | 220 | 24 | 6 | 2 |
| Cafe Classics Beef Pot Roast | 1 pkg (9 oz) | 210 | 25 | 4 | 6 |
| Cafe Classics Chicken Carbonara | 1 pkg (9 oz) | 280 | 36 | 5 | 4 |
| Cafe Classics Chicken Medallions w/ Creamy Cheese Sauce | 1 pkg (9.37 oz) | 300 | 40 | 5 | 2 |
| Cafe Classics Chicken Mediterranean | 1 pkg (10.5 oz) | 260 | 38 | 6 | 4 |
| Cafe Classics Chicken & Vegetables | 1 pkg (10.5 oz) | 240 | 30 | 5 | 4 |
| Cafe Classics Chicken in Peanut Sauce | 1 pkg (9 oz) | 260 | 32 | 7 | 4 |
| Cafe Classics Chicken in Wine Sauce | 1 pkg (8.1 oz) | 220 | 23 | 7 | 2 |
| Cafe Classics Chicken L'Orange | 1 pkg (9 oz) | 230 | 33 | 9 | 2 |
| Cafe Classics Chicken Parmesan | 1 pkg (10.9 oz) | 300 | 41 | 8 | 5 |
| Cafe Classics Chicken Piccata | 1 pkg (9 oz) | 300 | 41 | 9 | 2 |

| FOOD | PORTION | CALS | CARB | SUGAR | FIBER |
|---|---|---|---|---|---|
| Cafe Classics Chicken w/ Basil Cream Sauce | 1 pkg (8.5 oz) | 260 | 33 | 4 | 2 |
| Cafe Classics Country Vegetables & Beef | 1 pkg (9 oz) | 210 | 33 | 9 | 3 |
| Cafe Classics Fiesta Chicken | 1 pkg (9.25 oz) | 270 | 40 | 3 | 3 |
| Cafe Classics Glazed Chicken | 1 pkg (8.5 oz) | 240 | 25 | 7 | 0 |
| Cafe Classics Glazed Turkey Tenderloins | 1 pkg (9 oz) | 260 | 41 | 20 | 4 |
| Cafe Classics Grilled Chicken | 1 pkg (9.4 oz) | 250 | 29 | 6 | 3 |
| Cafe Classics Herb Roasted Chicken | 1 pkg (8 oz) | 190 | 22 | 6 | 4 |
| Cafe Classics Honey Mustard Chicken | 1 pkg (8 oz) | 270 | 40 | 8 | 1 |
| Cafe Classics Honey Roasted Chicken | 1 pkg (8.5 oz) | 270 | 41 | 13 | 5 |
| Cafe Classics Honey Roasted Pork | 1 serv (9.5 oz) | 250 | 32 | 11 | 3 |
| Cafe Classics Meatloaf w/ Whipped Potatoes | 1 pkg (9.4 oz) | 260 | 28 | 5 | 4 |
| Cafe Classics Oriental Beef | 1 pkg (9.25 oz) | 210 | 30 | 8 | 2 |
| Cafe Classics Oven Roasted Beef | 1 pkg (9.25 oz) | 260 | 28 | 7 | 4 |
| Cafe Classics Roasted Turkey Breast | 1 pkg (9.75 oz) | 270 | 49 | 27 | 3 |
| Cafe Classics Salisbury Steak | 1 pkg (9.5 oz) | 280 | 29 | 2 | 4 |
| Cafe Classics Southern Beef Tips | 1 pkg (8.75 oz) | 270 | 37 | 10 | 4 |
| Everyday Favorites Vegetable Lasagna | 1 pkg (10.5 oz) | 260 | 36 | 9 | 5 |
| Everyday Favorite Chicken Florentine | 1 pkg (8 oz) | 220 | 32 | 3 | 3 |
| Everyday Favorites Chicken Chow Mein | 1 pkg (9 oz) | 240 | 37 | 3 | 3 |
| Everyday Favorites Homestyle Turkey | 1 pkg (9.4 oz) | 240 | 27 | 6 | 3 |
| Everyday Favorites Human Beef & Broccoli | 1 pkg (8.5 oz) | 240 | 40 | 9 | 2 |

| FOOD | PORTION | CALS | CARB | SUGAR | FIBER |
|---|---|---|---|---|---|
| Everyday Favorites Mandarin Chicken | 1 pkg (9 oz) | 260 | 38 | 9 | 2 |
| Everyday Favorites Roasted Chicken | 1 pkg (8.1 oz) | 260 | 34 | 3 | 4 |
| Everyday Favorites Stuffed Cabbage | 1 pkg (9.5 oz) | 210 | 25 | 4 | 5 |
| Everyday Favorites Swedish Meatballs | 1 pkg (9.1 oz) | 290 | 35 | 4 | 4 |
| Hearty Portions Cheese & Spinach Manicotti | 1 serv | 370 | 50 | 14 | 8 |
| Hearty Portions Chicken & Barbecue Sauce | 1 serv | 370 | 60 | 31 | 6 |
| Hearty Portions Homestyle Beef Stroganoff | 1 serv | 350 | 44 | 12 | 9 |
| Hearty Portions Jumbo Rigatoni w/ Meatballs | 1 serv | 440 | 64 | 12 | 7 |
| Hearty Portions Oriental Glazed Chicken | 1 serv | 370 | 66 | 12 | 4 |
| Hearty Portions Roasted Chicken w/ Mushrooms | 1 serv | 330 | 49 | 5 | 4 |
| Skillet Sensations Beef Teriyaki & Rice | 1 serv | 280 | 48 | 11 | 5 |
| Skillet Sensations Chicken Primavera | 1 serv | 320 | 50 | 7 | 4 |
| Skillet Sensations Chicken Oriental | 1 serv | 280 | 46 | 10 | 6 |
| Skillet Sensations Fiesta Beef & Rice | 1 serv | 300 | 48 | 6 | 6 |
| Skillet Sensations Garlic Chicken | 1 serv | 340 | 56 | 6 | 4 |
| Skillet Sensations Herb Chicken & Roasted Potatoes | 1 serv | 270 | 39 | 10 | 5 |
| Skillet Sensations Roasted Turkey | 1 serv | 220 | 37 | 10 | 6 |
| Skillet Sensations Savory Beef & Vegetables | 1 serv | 290 | 38 | 9 | 9 |
| Skillet Sensations Three Cheese Chicken | 1 serv | 370 | 45 | 9 | 3 |
| ***Luzianne*** | | | | | |
| Cajun Creole Dirty Rice | 1 serv | 160 | 35 | 0 | 0 |

| FOOD | PORTION | CALS | CARB | SUGAR | FIBER |
|---|---|---|---|---|---|
| Cajun Creole Etouffee | 1 serv | 200 | 42 | 2 | 1 |
| Cajun Creole Gumbo | 1 serv | 160 | 33 | 3 | 1 |
| Cajun Creole Jambalaya | 1 serv | 200 | 43 | 0 | 1 |
| ***Marie Callender's*** | | | | | |
| Beef Stroganoff w/ Noodles | 1 meal (13 oz) | 600 | 59 | 9 | 4 |
| Beef Tips in Mushroom Sauce | 1 meal (13 oz) | 430 | 39 | 11 | 6 |
| Breaded Chicken Parmigiana | 1 meal (16 oz) | 860 | 63 | 18 | 5 |
| Breaded Fish w/ Mac & Cheese | 1 meal (12 oz) | 550 | 53 | 12 | 3 |
| Cheesy Rice w/ Chicken & Broccoli | 1 meal (12 oz) | 390 | 44 | 8 | 6 |
| Chicken & Dumplings | 1 meal (14 oz) | 390 | 34 | 14 | 4 |
| Chicken & Noodles | 1 meal (13 oz) | 520 | 42 | 7 | 5 |
| Chicken Cordon Bleu | 1 meal (13 oz) | 610 | 58 | 9 | 6 |
| Chicken Fried Beef Steak & Gravy | 1 meal (15 oz) | 650 | 50 | 9 | 7 |
| Chicken Teriyaki | 1 meal (13 oz) | 510 | 71 | 22 | 2 |
| Country Fried Chicken & Gravy | 1 meal (16 oz) | 620 | 63 | 16 | 6 |
| Country Fried Pork Chop | 1 meal (15 oz) | 540 | 50 | 23 | 8 |
| Escalloped Noodles & Chicken | 1 meal (13 oz) | 740 | 60 | 10 | 5 |
| Glazed Chicken | 1 meal (13 oz) | 490 | 40 | 2 | 1 |
| Grilled Southwestern Style Chicken | 1 meal (14 oz) | 410 | 43 | 9 | 6 |
| Grilled Chicken & Mashed Potatoes | 1 meal (10 oz) | 340 | 20 | 2 | 1 |
| Grilled Chicken Breast & Rice Pilaf | 1 meal (11.75 oz) | 360 | 36 | 14 | 4 |
| Grilled Chicken in Mushroom Sauce | 1 meal (14 oz) | 480 | 54 | 0 | 7 |

| FOOD | PORTION | CALS | CARB | SUGAR | FIBER |
|---|---|---|---|---|---|
| Grilled Turkey Breast & Rice Pilaf | 1 meal (11.75 oz) | 310 | 34 | 8 | 4 |
| Herb Roasted Chicken & Mashed Potatoes | 1 meal (14 oz) | 580 | 26 | 16 | 7 |
| Homestyle Turkey & Noodles | 1 meal (12 oz) | 600 | 52 | 12 | 5 |
| Honey Roasted Chicken | 1 meal (14 oz) | 440 | 27 | 7 | 7 |
| Honey Smoked Ham Steak w/ Macaroni & Cheese | 1 meal (14 oz) | 490 | 63 | 32 | 5 |
| Meatloaf & Gravy w/ Mashed Potatoes | 1 meal (14 oz) | 540 | 42 | 30 | 5 |
| Old Fashioned Beef Pot Roast & Gravy | 1 meal (15 oz) | 500 | 55 | 13 | 3 |
| Roast Beef | 1 meal (14.5 oz) | 390 | 30 | 7 | 11 |
| Sirloin Salisbury Steak & Gravy | 1 meal (14 oz) | 550 | 51 | 14 | 6 |
| Skillet Meal Au Gratin Potatoes | ⅔ cup (5 oz) | 190 | 19 | 4 | 2 |
| Skillet Meal Beef Pot Roast | ½ pkg | 290 | 33 | 5 | 5 |
| Skillet Meal Beef Stroganoff | ½ pkg | 310 | 31 | 7 | 5 |
| Skillet Meal Chicken & Rice w/ Broccoli & Cheese | ½ pkg | 440 | 47 | 5 | 8 |
| Skillet Meal Chicken Teriyaki | ½ pkg | 340 | 61 | 14 | 5 |
| Skillet Meal Herb Chicken | ½ pkg | 290 | 42 | 1 | 5 |
| Skillet Meal Roasted Chicken & Vegetables | ½ pkg | 260 | 30 | 1 | 7 |
| Skillet Meal White & Wild Rice in Cheese Sauce | 1 cup | 300 | 35 | 7 | 2 |
| Swedish Meatballs | 1 meal (12.5 oz) | 520 | 44 | 3 | 3 |
| Sweet & Sour Chicken | 1 meal (14 oz) | 570 | 66 | 55 | 7 |
| Turkey w/ Gravy & Dressing | 1 meal (14 oz) | 500 | 52 | 11 | 4 |
| ***Morton*** | | | | | |
| Breaded Chicken Pattie | 1 meal (6.75 oz) | 290 | 24 | 12 | 4 |
| Chicken Nuggets | 1 meal (7 oz) | 340 | 31 | 12 | 2 |

| FOOD | PORTION | CALS | CARB | SUGAR | FIBER |
|---|---|---|---|---|---|
| Chili Gravy w/ Beef Enchilada & Tamale | 1 meal (10 oz) | 270 | 40 | 3 | 7 |
| Fried Chicken | 1 meal (9 oz) | 470 | 30 | 4 | 3 |
| Gravy & Charbroiled Beef Patty | 1 meal (9 oz) | 310 | 26 | 3 | 5 |
| Gravy & Salisbury Steak | 1 meal (9 oz) | 310 | 24 | 7 | 3 |
| Gravy & Turkey w/ Stuffing | 1 meal (9 oz) | 240 | 27 | 5 | 4 |
| Tomato Sauce w/ Meat Loaf | 1 meal (9 oz) | 250 | 24 | 17 | 3 |
| Veal Parmigiana w/ Tomato Sauce | 1 meal (8.75 oz) | 290 | 30 | 8 | 4 |
| ***Nature's Choice*** | | | | | |
| Broccoli Parmesan Alfredo | 1 pkg (12 oz) | 270 | 29 | 4 | 5 |
| ***Nature's Entree*** | | | | | |
| Hearty Stew | 1 pkg (12 oz) | 290 | 34 | 6 | 3 |
| Tuscany White Bean | 1 pkg (12 oz) | 330 | 42 | 4 | 4 |
| ***Patio*** | | | | | |
| Ranchera | 1 pkg (13 oz) | 470 | 55 | 4 | 9 |
| ***Swanson*** | | | | | |
| Beef Pot Roast | 1 pkg (14 oz) | 320 | 44 | 15 | 4 |
| Chicken Parmigiana w/ Spaghetti | 1 pkg (11 oz) | 380 | 41 | 18 | 5 |
| Turkey Breast | 1 pkg (11.7 oz) | 330 | 50 | 18 | 4 |
| ***Tamarind Tree*** | | | | | |
| Alu Chole | 1 pkg (9.2 oz) | 350 | 63 | 3 | 9 |
| Channa Dal Masala | 1 pkg (9.2 oz) | 340 | 62 | 4 | 10 |
| Dal Makhini | 1 pkg (9.2 oz) | 330 | 55 | 3 | 14 |
| Dhingri Mutter | 1 pkg (9.2 oz) | 290 | 53 | 6 | 7 |
| Navratan Korma | 1 pkg (9.2 oz) | 430 | 60 | 7 | 7 |
| Palak Paneer | 1 pkg (9.2 oz) | 380 | 46 | 6 | 6 |
| Saag Chole | 1 pkg (9.2 oz) | 370 | 55 | 2 | 13 |
| Vegetable Jalfrazi | 1 pkg (9.2 oz) | 310 | 57 | 7 | 7 |
| ***Tyson*** | | | | | |
| BBQ Chicken Potato & Vegetable Medley | 1 pkg (14.7 oz) | 560 | 73 | 23 | 9 |
| Beef Stir Fry | 1 pkg (14 oz) | 430 | 70 | 25 | 4 |
| Blackened Chicken Spanish Rice & Corn | 1 pkg (8.8 oz) | 260 | 36 | 5 | 4 |
| Chicken Primavera | 1 pkg (11.3 oz) | 350 | 48 | 4 | 5 |

| FOOD | PORTION | CALS | CARB | SUGAR | FIBER |
|---|---|---|---|---|---|
| Chicken Divan Candied Carrots & Pasta | 1 pkg (9.8 oz) | 370 | 38 | 8 | 2 |
| Chicken Francais Sliced Potatoes & Green Beans | 1 pkg (8.8 oz) | 260 | 23 | 5 | 6 |
| Chicken Kiev Rice Pilaf & Broccoli Carrots | 1 pkg (9.1 oz) | 440 | 36 | 4 | 2 |
| Chicken Marsala Carrots & Red Potatoes | 1 pkg (8.8 oz) | 180 | 19 | 6 | 4 |
| Chicken Mesquite Corn & Pea Medley & Au Gratin Potatoes | 1 pkg (8.8 oz) | 320 | 44 | 11 | 4 |
| Chicken Picatta | 1 pkg (8.8 oz) | 190 | 18 | 1 | 5 |
| Chicken Stir Fry Kit | 2¾ cups (14 oz) | 430 | 73 | 24 | 5 |
| Chicken w/ Broccoli & Cheese Carrots & Pasta | 1 pkg (8.8 oz) | 270 | 19 | 5 | 3 |
| Chicken w/ Mushroom Sauce Rice Pilaf & Candied Carrots | 1 pkg (8.8 oz) | 220 | 27 | 8 | 2 |
| Chicken w/ Tabasco BBQ Sauce | 1 pkg (8.8 oz) | 260 | 37 | 11 | 5 |
| Fried Chicken & Gravy w/ Mashed Potatoes & Corn | 1 pkg (10.8 oz) | 360 | 39 | 4 | 4 |
| Grilled Chicken Corn O'Brien & Ranch Beans | 1 pkg (8.8 oz) | 230 | 30 | 4 | 7 |
| Grilled Italian Chicken Pasta & Vegetable Medley | 1 pkg (8.8 oz) | 190 | 19 | 3 | 3 |
| Honey Dijon Chicken Pasta & Pea Medley | 1 pkg (11.3 oz) | 340 | 49 | 5 | 6 |
| Roasted Chicken w/ Garlic Sauce Pasta & Vegetable Medley | 1 pkg (8.8 oz) | 210 | 20 | 2 | 3 |
| ***Weight Watchers*** | | | | | |
| Smart One Grilled Salisbury Steak | 1 pkg (8.5 oz) | 250 | 24 | 3 | 3 |
| Smart Ones Chicken Mirabella | 1 pkg (9.2 oz) | 180 | 30 | 4 | 4 |
| Smart Ones Fiesta Chicken | 1 pkg (8.5 oz) | 210 | 35 | 5 | 5 |
| Smart Ones Honey Mustard Chicken | 1 pkg (8.5 oz) | 200 | 35 | 10 | 3 |
| Smart Ones Lemon Herb Chicken Piccata | 1 pkg (8.5 oz) | 190 | 33 | 5 | 3 |
| Smart Ones Pepper Steak | 1 pkg (10 oz) | 240 | 32 | 4 | 4 |

| FOOD | PORTION | CALS | CARB | SUGAR | FIBER |
|---|---|---|---|---|---|
| Smart Ones Risotto w/ Cheese & Mushrooms | 1 pkg (10 oz) | 290 | 47 | 7 | 4 |
| Smart Ones Roast Turkey Medallions & Mushrooms | 1 pkg (8.5 oz) | 180 | 30 | 3 | 2 |
| Smart Ones Shrimp Marinara | 1 pkg (9 oz) | 180 | 31 | 4 | 4 |
| Smart Ones Stuffed Turkey Breast | 1 pkg (10 oz) | 260 | 37 | 14 | 5 |
| Smart Ones Swedish Meatballs | 1 pkg (9 oz) | 280 | 34 | 2 | 3 |
| ***Yves*** | | | | | |
| Veggie Country Stew | 1 pkg (10.5 oz) | 170 | 24 | 2 | 7 |
| **DIP** | | | | | |
| ***Cabot*** | | | | | |
| Bac'n Horseradish | 2 tbsp | 50 | 1 | tr | 0 |
| Clam | 2 tbsp | 50 | 1 | 0 | 0 |
| French Onion | 2 tbsp | 50 | 1 | 1 | 0 |
| Ranch | 1 tbsp | 50 | 1 | 1 | 0 |
| Salsa Grande | 2 tbsp | 50 | 1 | 1 | 0 |
| ***Fritos*** | | | | | |
| Bean | 2 tbsp (1.2 oz) | 40 | 6 | 0 | 0 |
| Chili Cheese | 1.2 oz | 45 | 3 | 1 | 0 |
| French Onion | 2 tbsp (1.1 oz) | 60 | 4 | 1 | 0 |
| Hot Bean | 2 tbsp (1.2 oz) | 40 | 5 | 0 | 1 |
| Jalapeno & Cheddar Cheese | 2 tbsp (1.2 oz) | 50 | 4 | 2 | 0 |
| ***Gringo Billy's*** | | | | | |
| Guacamole Mix | 1 tsp | 10 | 2 | 0 | 1 |
| ***Guiltless Gourmet*** | | | | | |
| Black Bean Mild | 2 tbsp (1 oz) | 30 | 5 | 1 | 1 |
| Black Bean Spicy | 2 tbsp (1 oz) | 30 | 5 | 1 | 1 |
| ***Racquet*** | | | | | |
| Hot Cheddar Jalapeno | 2 tbsp | 30 | 1 | 0 | 0 |
| ***Ruffles*** | | | | | |
| French Onion | 2 tbsp | 70 | 4 | tr | 1 |
| Ranch | 2 tbsp (1.2 oz) | 70 | 4 | 0 | 0 |
| ***Snyder's Of Hanover*** | | | | | |
| Microwavable Hot Nacho Cheese | 2 tbsp | 48 | 5 | 2 | 0 |
| Microwavable Mild Cheese | 2 tbsp | 45 | 2 | 1 | 0 |
| Mustard Pretzel | 2 tbsp | 60 | 12 | 11 | 0 |
| Sour Cream & Onion | 2 tbsp | 60 | 2 | 1 | 0 |

| FOOD | PORTION | CALS | CARB | SUGAR | FIBER |
|---|---|---|---|---|---|
| ***Tyson*** | | | | | |
| Bleu Cheese For Dipping Wings | 2 tbsp (1.4 oz) | 140 | 3 | 1 | 1 |
| ***Utz*** | | | | | |
| Fat Free Sour Cream & Onion | 2 tbsp (1.1 oz) | 30 | 7 | 3 | 0 |
| Jalapeno & Cheddar | 2 tbsp (1 oz) | 30 | 2 | 0 | 0 |
| Low Fat Desert Garden | 2 tbsp (1.1 oz) | 40 | 5 | 2 | 0 |
| Low Fat Salsa Con Queso | 2 tbsp (1 oz) | 40 | 5 | 2 | 0 |
| Mild Cheddar | 2 tbsp (1 oz) | 45 | 2 | 1 | 0 |
| Sour Cream & Onion | 2 tbsp (1 oz) | 60 | 2 | 1 | 0 |
| ***Walden Farms*** | | | | | |
| Low Carb Bruschetta | 2 tbsp | 35 | 0 | 1 | 0 |
| Low Carb Pesto Bruschetta | 1 tsp | 10 | 9 | 9 | 0 |
| **DOCK** | | | | | |
| fresh cooked | 3½ oz | 20 | 3 | – | – |
| **DOLPHINFISH** | | | | | |
| fresh baked | 3 oz | 93 | 0 | 0 | 0 |
| fresh fillet baked | 5.6 oz | 174 | 0 | 0 | 0 |
| **DOUGHNUTS** | | | | | |
| cake type unsugared | 1 (1.6 oz) | 198 | 23 | – | 1 |
| chocolate glazed | 1 (1.5 oz) | 175 | 24 | – | 1 |
| chocolate sugar | 1 (1.5 oz) | 175 | 24 | – | 1 |
| chocolate coated | 1 (1.5 oz) | 204 | 21 | – | 1 |
| creme filled | 1 (3 oz) | 307 | 26 | – | – |
| french cruller glazed | 1 (1.4 oz) | 169 | 24 | – | – |
| frosted | 1 (1.5 oz) | 204 | 21 | – | 1 |
| honey bun | 1 (2.1 oz) | 242 | 27 | – | 1 |
| jelly | 1 (3 oz) | 289 | 33 | – | – |
| old fashioned | 1 (1.6 oz) | 198 | 23 | – | 1 |
| sugared | 1 (1.6 oz) | 192 | 23 | – | 1 |
| wheat glazed | 1 (1.6 oz) | 162 | 19 | – | – |
| wheat sugared | 1 (1.6 oz) | 162 | 19 | – | – |
| yeast glazed | 1 (2.1 oz) | 242 | 27 | – | 1 |
| ***Dolly Madison*** | | | | | |
| Chocolate Frosted | 1 (1.1 oz) | 140 | 15 | 9 | 1 |
| Donut Gems Chocolate | 4 (2 oz) | 260 | 28 | 17 | 1 |
| Donut Gems Crunch | 3 (2 oz) | 220 | 31 | 21 | 0 |
| Donut Gems Powdered | 4 (2 oz) | 230 | 30 | 14 | 0 |
| English Cruller | 1 (2 oz) | 250 | 31 | 11 | 1 |

| FOOD | PORTION | CALS | CARB | SUGAR | FIBER |
|---|---|---|---|---|---|
| Glazed Whirl | 1 (1.6 oz) | 210 | 25 | 9 | 0 |
| Glazed Yeast | 1 (1.5 oz) | 190 | 23 | 6 | 0 |
| Old Fashioned | 1 (1.5 oz) | 280 | 28 | 23 | 0 |
| Plain | 1 (1.2 oz) | 140 | 15 | 3 | 0 |
| Powdered | 1 (1 oz) | 120 | 14 | 7 | 0 |
| ***Dutch Mill*** | | | | | |
| Cider | 1 (2.1 oz) | 240 | 35 | 23 | 1 |
| Cinnamon | 1 (1.8 oz) | 210 | 26 | 12 | 1 |
| Donut Holes | 3 | 220 | 19 | 5 | 0 |
| Double-Dipped Chocolate | (1.4 oz) | | | | |
| Chocolate | | | | | |
| Donut Holes Shootin' Stars | 3 (1.4 oz) | 190 | 23 | 12 | 0 |
| Double-Dipped Chocolate | 1 (2.1 oz) | 280 | 31 | 9 | 1 |
| Glazed | 1 (2.1 oz) | 250 | 34 | 23 | 1 |
| Glazed Chocolate | 1 (2.4 oz) | 270 | 40 | 10 | 1 |
| Plain | 1 (1.8 oz) | 210 | 25 | 9 | 1 |
| Sugared | 1 (1.8 oz) | 220 | 27 | 12 | 1 |
| ***Hostess*** | | | | | |
| Blueberry | 1 (1.7 oz) | 210 | 21 | 11 | 0 |
| Donettes Crumb | 3 (1.5 oz) | 170 | 23 | 16 | 0 |
| Donettes Frosted | 3 (1.5 oz) | 200 | 21 | 13 | 0 |
| Donettes Powdered | 3 (1.5 oz) | 180 | 23 | 10 | 0 |
| Frosted | 1 (1.4 oz) | 180 | 19 | 12 | 0 |
| O's Raspberry Filled | 1 (2.2 oz) | 230 | 34 | 17 | 1 |
| Old Fashioned Glazed | 1 (2.1 oz) | 260 | 33 | 14 | 1 |
| Plain | 1 (1.1 oz) | 140 | 15 | 3 | 0 |
| Powdered | 1 (1.3 oz) | 150 | 19 | 9 | 0 |
| ***Little Debbie*** | | | | | |
| Donut Sticks | 1 (1.6 oz) | 210 | 24 | 15 | 0 |
| Mini Powdered | 1 pkg (2.5 oz) | 290 | 38 | 19 | 2 |
| ***Snack & Smile*** | | | | | |
| Mini Donuts Chocolate | 6 | 370 | 45 | 23 | 2 |
| Mini Donuts Glazed | 6 | 340 | 46 | 28 | tr |
| Mini Donuts Powdered Sugar | 6 | 320 | 46 | 22 | 1 |
| ***Tastykake*** | | | | | |
| Mini Plain Glaze | 1 pkg (2.5 oz) | 260 | 40 | 23 | 1 |
| Mini Powdered Sugar | 1 pkg (2.5 oz) | 260 | 38 | 21 | tr |
| Mini Rich Frosted | 1 pkg (3 oz) | 370 | 43 | 23 | 3 |

| FOOD | PORTION | CALS | CARB | SUGAR | FIBER |
|---|---|---|---|---|---|
| ***Tom's*** | | | | | |
| Chocolate Gem | 1 pkg (2.5 oz) | 320 | 37 | 19 | 1 |
| Dunkin' Sticks | 1 pkg (2.5 oz) | 370 | 43 | 20 | tr |
| Powdered Gems | 1 pkg (2.5 oz) | 320 | 41 | 23 | 1 |
| **DRINK MIXERS** | | | | | |
| whiskey sour mix not prep | 1 pkg (0.6 oz) | 64 | 16 | – | – |
| whiskey sour mix | 2 oz | 55 | 14 | – | 0 |
| ***Baja Bob's*** | | | | | |
| Sugar Free Margarita Mix | 4 oz | 10 | tr | 0 | – |
| Sugar Free Margarita Mix Desert Lime | 4 oz | 10 | tr | 0 | 0 |
| Sugar Free Margarita Mix Wild Strawberry | 4 oz | 10 | tr | 0 | – |
| Sweet-n-Sour Mix | 4 oz | 10 | tr | 0 | – |
| ***Daily's*** | | | | | |
| Bloody Mary Original | 1 serv (6 oz) | 50 | 14 | 14 | – |
| Margarita Daiquiri Strawberry | 1 serv (4 oz) | 180 | 47 | 45 | 2 |
| Margarita Green Demon | 1 serv (3 oz) | 80 | 19 | 19 | – |
| Pina Colada | 1 serv (3 oz) | 160 | 37 | 36 | 1 |
| **DRUM** | | | | | |
| freshwater fillet baked | 5.4 oz | 236 | 0 | 0 | 0 |
| freshwater baked | 3 oz | 130 | 0 | 0 | 0 |
| **DUCK** | | | | | |
| w/ skin roasted | 1 cup (4.9 oz) | 472 | 0 | 0 | 0 |
| w/ skin w/ bone leg roasted | 3 oz | 184 | 0 | 0 | 0 |
| w/ skin w/o bone breast roasted | 3 oz | 172 | 0 | 0 | 0 |
| w/o skin roasted | 1 cup (4.9 oz) | 281 | 0 | 0 | 0 |
| w/o skin w/ bone leg braised | 1 cup (6.1 oz) | 310 | 0 | 0 | 0 |
| w/o skin w/o bone breast broiled | 1 cup (6.1 oz) | 244 | 0 | 0 | 0 |
| wild w/ skin raw | ½ duck (9.5 oz) | 571 | 0 | 0 | 0 |
| wild w/o skin breast raw | ½ breast (2.9 oz) | 102 | 0 | 0 | 0 |
| ***Grimaud Farms*** | | | | | |
| Muscovy Duck Confit | 1 serv (3 oz) | 170 | tr | – | – |

| FOOD | PORTION | CALS | CARB | SUGAR | FIBER |
|---|---|---|---|---|---|
| **DUMPLING** | | | | | |
| ***Health Is Wealth*** | | | | | |
| Potstickers Chicken Free | 2 (1.6 oz) | 80 | 11 | 1 | 1 |
| Potstickers Pork Free | 2 (1.6 oz) | 80 | 11 | 1 | 1 |
| Potstickers Vegetable | 2 (1.6 oz) | 90 | 11 | 0 | 5 |
| Steamed Dumpling | 2 (1.6 oz) | 50 | 12 | 0 | 1 |
| ***Pepperidge Farm*** | | | | | |
| Apple | 1 (3 oz) | 230 | 30 | 11 | 1 |
| Peach | 1 (3 oz) | 320 | 50 | 15 | 4 |
| **DURIAN** | | | | | |
| fresh | 3.5 oz | 141 | 29 | – | – |
| **EEL** | | | | | |
| fresh cooked | 3 oz | 200 | 0 | 0 | 0 |
| fresh cooked | 1 fillet (5.6 oz) | 375 | 0 | 0 | 0 |
| smoked | 3.5 oz | 330 | 0 | 0 | 0 |
| **EGG** *(see also* EGG DISHES, EGG SUBSTITUTES*)* | | | | | |
| **CHICKEN** | | | | | |
| fresh | 1 | 75 | 1 | – | – |
| frozen | 1 cup | 363 | 3 | – | – |
| frozen | 1 | 75 | 1 | – | – |
| hard cooked | 1 | 77 | 1 | – | – |
| hard cooked chopped | 1 cup | 210 | 2 | – | – |
| poached | 1 | 74 | 1 | – | – |
| white only | 1 | 17 | tr | – | – |
| white only | 1 cup | 121 | 2 | – | – |
| ***Eggology*** | | | | | |
| 100% Organic Egg Whites | ¼ cup | 30 | 1 | – | – |
| ***Horizon Organic*** | | | | | |
| Medium | 1 (1.5 oz) | 70 | 1 | – | – |
| ***Land O Lakes*** | | | | | |
| Brown Extra Large | 1 (2 oz) | 80 | 1 | – | – |
| ***Organic Valley*** | | | | | |
| Brown Extra Large | 1 (2.2 oz) | 90 | tr | – | – |
| Brown Large | 1 (2 oz) | 80 | tr | – | – |
| Brown Medium | 1 (1.8 oz) | 70 | tr | – | – |
| **OTHER POULTRY** | | | | | |
| duck | 1 (2.5 oz) | 130 | 1 | – | 0 |

| FOOD | PORTION | CALS | CARB | SUGAR | FIBER |
|---|---|---|---|---|---|
| duck 100 year old | 1 (1 oz) | 49 | 1 | – | – |
| duck preserved hard core | 1 (1.8 oz) | 80 | 1 | 0 | 0 |
| duck preserved soft core | 1 (1.8 oz) | 80 | 1 | 0 | 0 |
| duck salted | 1 (1 oz) | 54 | 2 | – | – |
| goose | 1 (5 oz) | 267 | 2 | – | – |
| quail | 1 (9 g) | 14 | tr | – | – |
| turkey | 1 (2.7 oz) | 135 | 1 | – | – |
| **EGG DISHES** | | | | | |
| **FROZEN** | | | | | |
| ***Weight Watchers*** | | | | | |
| Handy Ham & Cheese Omelet | 1 (4 oz) | 220 | 30 | 7 | 2 |
| **TAKE-OUT** | | | | | |
| deviled | 2 halves | 145 | 1 | – | – |
| omelette plain | 1 serv (3.5 oz) | 172 | tr | tr | 0 |
| salad | ½ cup | 307 | 2 | – | – |
| scotch egg | 1 (4.2 oz) | 301 | 16 | – | 2 |
| scrambled plain | 2 (3.3 oz) | 199 | 2 | – | 0 |
| scrambled w/ whole milk & margarine | 1 serv | 365 | 5 | – | – |
| sunny side up | 1 | 91 | 1 | – | – |
| **EGG ROLLS** | | | | | |
| egg roll wrapper fresh | 1 | 83 | 16 | – | – |
| ***Chun King*** | | | | | |
| Chicken Mini | 6 | 210 | 25 | 3 | 2 |
| Chicken Restaurant Style | 1 (3 oz) | 190 | 22 | 4 | 2 |
| Pork & Shrimp Mini | 6 | 210 | 27 | 4 | 2 |
| Shrimp Mini | 6 | 190 | 28 | 3 | 2 |
| Shrimp Restaurant Style | 1 (3 oz) | 180 | 25 | 6 | 2 |
| ***Health Is Wealth*** | | | | | |
| Broccoli | 1 (3 oz) | 150 | 23 | 0 | 2 |
| Oriental Vegetable | 1 (3 oz) | 160 | 23 | 0 | 2 |
| Oriental Chicken Free | 1 (3 oz) | 120 | 21 | 0 | 2 |
| Pizza | 1 (3 oz) | 200 | 23 | 0 | 3 |
| Spinach | 1 (3 oz) | 180 | 20 | 0 | 3 |
| Spring Rolls | 1 (1.6 oz) | 70 | 10 | 0 | 5 |
| Veggie | 1 (3 oz) | 130 | 21 | 0 | 3 |
| ***La Choy*** | | | | | |
| Chicken Mini | 6 | 210 | 25 | 3 | 2 |

| FOOD | PORTION | CALS | CARB | SUGAR | FIBER |
|---|---|---|---|---|---|
| Chicken Restaurant Style | 1 (3 oz) | 210 | 25 | 4 | 2 |
| Pork Restaurant Style | 1 (3 oz) | 220 | 24 | 6 | 2 |
| Pork & Shrimp Bite Size | 12 | 210 | 25 | 3 | 2 |
| Pork & Shrimp Mini | 6 | 210 | 27 | 4 | 2 |
| Shrimp Mini | 6 | 190 | 28 | 3 | 2 |
| Shrimp Restaurant Style | 1 (3 oz) | 180 | 25 | 6 | 2 |
| Sweet & Sour Chicken Restaurant Style | 1 (3 oz) | 220 | 29 | 10 | 2 |
| Vegetable w/ Lobster Mini | 6 | 190 | 27 | 3 | 2 |
| **TAKE-OUT** | | | | | |
| lobster | 1 (4.8 oz) | 270 | 43 | 4 | 6 |
| lumpia vegetable & shrimp | 2 (3 oz) | 120 | 26 | 1 | 2 |
| meat & shrimp | 1 (4.8 oz) | 320 | 41 | 3 | 4 |
| pork & shrimp | 1 (5 oz) | 300 | 41 | 6 | 7 |
| shrimp | 1 (3 oz) | 170 | 24 | 5 | 5 |
| spicy pork | 1 (3 oz) | 200 | 23 | 3 | 3 |
| vegetable | 1 (3 oz) | 170 | 28 | 4 | 4 |
| **EGG SUBSTITUTES** | | | | | |
| frozen | ¼ cup | 96 | 2 | – | – |
| frozen | 1 cup | 384 | 8 | – | – |
| liquid | 1 cup (8.8 oz) | 211 | 2 | – | – |
| liquid | 1½ oz | 40 | tr | – | – |
| powder | 0.35 oz | 44 | 2 | – | – |
| powder | 0.7 oz | 88 | 4 | – | – |
| ***Better'n Eggs*** | | | | | |
| Fat Free Cholesterol Free | ¼ cup (2 oz) | 30 | 1 | 1 | 0 |
| ***Deb-El*** | | | | | |
| Just Whites | 2 tsp | 12 | 0 | – | 0 |
| ***Egg Beaters*** | | | | | |
| Egg Substitute | ¼ cup | 30 | 1 | tr | 0 |
| ***Morningstar Farms*** | | | | | |
| Breakfast Sandwich Bagel Scramblers Pattie Cheese | 1 (5.9 oz) (5.9 oz) | 320 | 40 | 6 | 4 |
| Scramblers | ¼ cup (2 oz) | 35 | 2 | 2 | 0 |
| ***Quick Eggs*** | | | | | |
| Fat Free Cholesterol Free | ¼ cup | 30 | 1 | 1 | 0 |
| **EGGNOG** | | | | | |
| eggnog | 1 cup | 342 | 34 | – | – |
| eggnog | 1 qt | 1368 | 138 | – | – |

| FOOD | PORTION | CALS | CARB | SUGAR | FIBER |
|---|---|---|---|---|---|
| eggnog flavor mix as prep w/ milk | 9 oz | 260 | 39 | – | – |
| ***Oberweis*** | | | | | |
| Egg Nog | ½ cup | 240 | 25 | 21 | 0 |
| **TAKE-OUT** | | | | | |
| eggnog | 1 cup | 306 | 16 | – | 0 |
| **EGGNOG SUBSTITUTES** | | | | | |
| ***Silk*** | | | | | |
| Nog | ½ cup | 90 | 15 | 12 | 0 |
| **EGGPLANT** | | | | | |
| cubed cooked | 1 cup | 28 | 7 | 1 | 3 |
| whole peeled raw | 1 (1 lb) | 117 | 28 | – | – |
| ***Progresso*** | | | | | |
| Caponata | 2 tbsp (1 oz) | 25 | 2 | 2 | 2 |
| ***TastyBite*** | | | | | |
| Punjab Eggplant | ½ pkg (5 oz) | 130 | 9 | 3 | 4 |
| **TAKE-OUT** | | | | | |
| baba ghannouj | ¼ cup | 55 | 5 | – | – |
| caponata | 2 tbsp (1 oz) | 30 | 3 | 2 | – |
| iman bayildi eggplant w/ onion & tomato | 1 serv (15.6 oz) | 345 | 25 | 6 | 2 |
| indian eggplant runi | 1 serv | 180 | 13 | 1 | 1 |
| papoutsakis little shoes | 1 serv (15.5 oz) | 245 | 15 | 1 | 1 |
| **ELDERBERRIES** | | | | | |
| fresh | 1 cup | 105 | 27 | – | – |
| **ELDERBERRY JUICE** | | | | | |
| elderberry | 7 oz | 76 | 16 | – | – |
| **ELK** | | | | | |
| roasted | 3 oz | 124 | 0 | 0 | 0 |
| **ENDIVE** | | | | | |
| fresh | 3.5 oz | 9 | tr | – | 2 |
| raw chopped | ½ cup | 4 | 1 | – | – |
| **ENERGY BARS** *(see also* CEREAL BARS, NUTRITION SUPPLEMENTS*)* | | | | | |
| ***AllGoode Organics*** | | | | | |

| FOOD | PORTION | CALS | CARB | SUGAR | FIBER |
|---|---|---|---|---|---|
| Amazin' Peanut Raisin | 1 bar | 210 | 25 | 15 | 3 |
| Banana Nut Nirvana | 1 bar | 190 | 30 | 21 | 3 |
| Cashew Almond Passion | 1 bar | 210 | 25 | 16 | 3 |
| Chocolate Peanut Pleasure | 1 bar | 200 | 29 | 22 | 3 |
| Honey Nut Harvest | 1 bar | 210 | 29 | 17 | 3 |
| Nutty Chocolate Apricot | 1 bar | 200 | 26 | 19 | 5 |
| ***Atkins*** | | | | | |
| Advantage Almond Brownie | 1 bar (1.6 oz) | 220 | 21 | 0 | 7 |
| Advantage Chocolate Coconut | 1 bar (1.6 oz) | 230 | 21 | 0 | 9 |
| Advantage Chocolate Decadence | 1 bar (1.6 oz) | 220 | 25 | 0 | 11 |
| Advantage Chocolate Mocha Crunch | 1 bar (1.6 oz) | 220 | 22 | 0 | 10 |
| Advantage Chocolate Peanut Butter | 1 bar (1.6 oz) | 240 | 21 | 1 | 10 |
| Advantage Cookies 'N Creme | 1 bar (1.6 oz) | 220 | 22 | 0 | 11 |
| Advantage S'mores | 1 bar (1.6 oz) | 220 | 26 | 0 | 11 |
| Morning Start Apple Crisp | 1 bar | 170 | 13 | 1 | 6 |
| Morning Start Blueberry Muffin | 1 bar | 160 | 16 | 1 | 7 |
| Morning Start Chocolate Chip Crisp | 1 bar | 160 | 14 | tr | 5 |
| ***Back To Nature*** | | | | | |
| 10th Tee Chocolate Fudge | 1 bar | 200 | 31 | 18 | 1 |
| 10th Tee Peanut Honey | 1 bar | 260 | 32 | 16 | 2 |
| 1st Tee Chocolate Peanut | 1 bar | 290 | 44 | 16 | 1 |
| 1st Tee Oatmeal Raisin | 1 bar | 280 | 44 | 16 | 1 |
| ***Balance*** | | | | | |
| Oasis Strawberry Cheesecake | 1 bar (1.69 oz) | 180 | 28 | 16 | tr |
| ***Be Natural*** | | | | | |
| Almond & Apricot | 1 bar | 218 | 21 | 15 | 4 |
| Almond & Coconut | 1 bar | 248 | 19 | 15 | 1 |
| Banana & Wheat Bran | 1 bar | 201 | 29 | 19 | 4 |
| Fruit & Nut Delight | 1 bar | 225 | 21 | 14 | 3 |
| Macadamia & Apricot | 1 bar | 224 | 21 | 16 | 3 |
| Nut Delight | 1 bar | 266 | 20 | 10 | 3 |
| Sesame Nut Split | 1 bar | 256 | 20 | 15 | 2 |
| Walnut & Date | 1 bar | 147 | 29 | 10 | 1 |
| Yogurt Coated Almond & Apricot | 1 bar | 233 | 23 | 20 | 2 |

| FOOD | PORTION | CALS | CARB | SUGAR | FIBER |
|---|---|---|---|---|---|
| Yogurt Coated Fruit & Nut | 1 bar | 190 | 19 | 15 | 1 |
| ***Benecol*** | | | | | |
| Chocolate Crisp | 1 bar (1.2 oz) | 130 | 23 | 14 | 2 |
| Chocolate Crisp | 1 bar (1.2 oz) | 130 | 23 | 14 | 2 |
| Peanut Crisp | 1 bar (1.2 oz) | 140 | 23 | 14 | 1 |
| ***Better Bar*** | | | | | |
| Chocolate Coated Caramel Pecan | 1 bar (1.8 oz) | 180 | 15 | 10 | 0 |
| Chocolate Coated Peanut | 1 bar (1.8 oz) | 180 | 15 | 10 | 0 |
| Yogurt Coated Raspberry | 1 bar (1.8 oz) | 180 | 15 | 11 | 0 |
| ***Boost*** | | | | | |
| Chocolate Crunch | 1 bar (1.5 oz) | 190 | 29 | 19 | tr |
| ***Breakthru*** | | | | | |
| Organic Chocolate Fudge | 1 bar (2.1 oz) | 230 | 39 | 17 | 3 |
| Organic Cinnamon Crunch | 1 bar (2.1 oz) | 220 | 37 | 16 | 3 |
| Organic Honey Graham | 1 bar (2.1 oz) | 220 | 37 | 16 | 3 |
| Organic Mocha Fudge | 1 bar (2.1 oz) | 230 | 39 | 17 | 3 |
| ***Carb Options*** | | | | | |
| Chocolate Chip | 1 bar | 200 | 17 | 0 | tr |
| Chocolate Peanut | 1 bar | 200 | 17 | tr | tr |
| Cinnamon Delight | 1 bar | 200 | 17 | 0 | 0 |
| ***CarbWise*** | | | | | |
| Chocolate S'Mores Crunch | 1 bar | 240 | 24 | 0 | 1 |
| ***Carbolite*** | | | | | |
| Chocolate Peanut Butter Butter Sugar Free | 1 bar (1 oz) | 144 | 2 | 0 | 0 |
| ***Centrum*** | | | | | |
| Energy Chocolate Nougat | 1 (1.98 oz) | 220 | 34 | 25 | tr |
| Energy Chocolate Peanut Butter | 1 (1.98 oz) | 220 | 34 | 25 | tr |
| ***Choice*** | | | | | |
| Berry Almond Crispy | 1 bar | 50 | 10 | 3 | 0 |
| Fudge Brownie | 1 bar | 140 | 19 | 3 | 3 |
| Peanut Butter Crispy | 1 bar | 60 | 10 | 2 | tr |
| Peanutty Chocolate | 1 bar | 140 | 19 | 9 | 3 |
| ***Clif Bar*** | | | | | |
| Apricot | 1 bar (2.4 oz) | 220 | 43 | 21 | 5 |
| Carrot Cake | 1 bar (2.4 oz) | 240 | 43 | 21 | 5 |
| Chocolate Brownie | 1 bar (2.4 oz) | 240 | 41 | 20 | 6 |
| Chocolate Almond Fudge | 1 bar (2.4 oz) | 230 | 36 | 20 | 5 |

| FOOD | PORTION | CALS | CARB | SUGAR | FIBER |
|---|---|---|---|---|---|
| Chocolate Chip | 1 bar (2.4 oz) | 240 | 41 | 21 | 5 |
| Chocolate Chip Peanut Crunch | 1 bar (2.4 oz) | 240 | 39 | 20 | 5 |
| Cookies'N Cream | 1 bar (2.4 oz) | 230 | 39 | 21 | 5 |
| Cranberry Apple Cherry | 1 bar (2.4 oz) | 220 | 44 | 22 | 5 |
| Crunchy Peanut Butter | 1 bar (2.4 oz) | 240 | 39 | 18 | 5 |
| GingerSnap | 1 bar (2.4 oz) | 230 | 42 | 20 | 6 |
| ***DrSoy*** | | | | | |
| Double Chocolate | 1 bar (1.76 oz) | 180 | 27 | 9 | 1 |
| ***Ensure*** | | | | | |
| All Flavors | 1 bar (2.1 oz) | 230 | 35 | 23 | 1 |
| ***Extend*** | | | | | |
| Chocolate Chip Crunch | 1 bar (1.4 oz) | 160 | 31 | 8 | tr |
| Peanut Butter Crunch | 1 bar (1.4 oz) | 160 | 30 | 10 | 0 |
| ***Fast Fuel Up*** | | | | | |
| Natural Chocolate Espresso | 1 bar (2.3 oz) | 300 | 32 | 13 | 3 |
| Natural Chocolate Crunch | 1 bar (2.3 oz) | 300 | 32 | 13 | 3 |
| Organic Chocolate Espresso | 1 bar (1.8 oz) | 230 | 24 | 10 | 2 |
| Organic Chocolate Crunch | 1 bar (1.8 oz) | 230 | 24 | 10 | 2 |
| ***Gatorade*** | | | | | |
| All Flavors | 1 bar (2.3 oz) | 260 | 46 | 20 | 2 |
| ***GeniSoy*** | | | | | |
| Soy Protein Arctic Frost Crispy Chocolate Mint | 1 bar (2.2 oz) | 230 | 33 | 27 | 2 |
| Soy Protein Dutch Crunch Sour Apple Crisp | 1 bar (2.2 oz) | 230 | 33 | 26 | 1 |
| Soy Protein Fair Trade Arabica Cafe Mocha Fudge | 1 bar (2.2 oz) | 220 | 33 | 27 | 1 |
| Soy Protein New York Style Blueberry Cheesecake | 1 bar (2.2 oz) | 220 | 34 | 28 | 1 |
| Soy Protein Obsession Fudge Cookies & Cream | 1 bar (2.2 oz) | 230 | 33 | 27 | 2 |
| Soy Protein Pure Golden Honey Creamy Peanut Yogurt | 1 bar (2.2 oz) | 230 | 33 | 28 | 1 |
| Soy Protein Southern Style Chunky Peanut Butter Fudge | 1 bar (2.2 oz) | 240 | 32 | 24 | 1 |
| Soy Protein Ultimate Chocolate Fudge Brownie | 1 bar (2.2 oz) | 230 | 33 | 27 | 2 |
| Xtreme Carrot Cake Quake | 1 bar (1.6 oz) | 190 | 24 | 18 | 1 |
| Xtreme Peanut Butter Fix | 1 bar (1.6 oz) | 200 | 23 | 16 | 2 |

| FOOD | PORTION | CALS | CARB | SUGAR | FIBER |
|---|---|---|---|---|---|
| Xtreme Raspberry Rush | 1 bar (1.6 oz) | 190 | 24 | 18 | 2 |
| Xtreme Rocky Roadtrip | 1 bar (1.6 oz) | 190 | 23 | 16 | 2 |
| ***Glucerna*** | | | | | |
| All Flavors | 1 bar (1.3 oz) | 140 | 24 | 7 | 4 |
| ***Hansen's*** | | | | | |
| Chocolate Banana Crunch | 1 bar | 180 | 37 | 19 | 2 |
| Chocolate Orchard Crunch | 1 bar | 170 | 37 | 19 | 2 |
| Natural Bar Tropical Fruit Crunch | 1 bar | 170 | 35 | 20 | 1 |
| Natural Bar Yogurt Strawberry Crunch | 1 bar | 190 | 38 | 21 | 1 |
| ***HeartBar*** | | | | | |
| Cranberry | 1 bar (1.8 oz) | 190 | 27 | 21 | 3 |
| Original | 1 bar (1.76 oz) | 180 | 26 | 15 | 3 |
| ***Ideal*** | | | | | |
| Mixed Berry Tart | 1 bar (1.7 oz) | 200 | 20 | 13 | 0 |
| ***Jenny Craig*** | | | | | |
| Meal Bar Chocolate Peanut | 1 bar (2 oz) | 220 | 33 | 20 | 1 |
| Meal Bar Lemon Meringue | 1 bar (2 oz) | 210 | 31 | 23 | 0 |
| Meal Bar Milk Chocolate | 1 bar (2 oz) | 210 | 33 | 20 | 1 |
| Meal Bar Oatmeal Raisin | 1 bar (1.97 oz) | 210 | 35 | 22 | 3 |
| Meal Bar Yogurt Peanut | 1 bar (2 oz) | 220 | 33 | 20 | 0 |
| ***Kashi*** | | | | | |
| GoLean Chocolate Almond Toffee | 1 (2.7 oz) | 290 | 45 | 31 | – |
| GoLean Cookies 'N Cream | 1 (2.7 oz) | 290 | 50 | 35 | 6 |
| GoLean Frosted Spice Cake | 1 (2.7 oz) | 290 | 49 | 33 | 6 |
| GoLean Honey Vanilla Yogurt | 1 (2.7 oz) | 290 | 49 | 32 | 6 |
| GoLean Malted Chocolate Chip | 1 (2.7 oz) | 290 | 49 | 35 | 6 |
| GoLean Oatmeal Raisin Cookie | 1 (2.7 oz) | 280 | 49 | 33 | 6 |
| GoLean Peanut Butter & Chocolate | 1 (2.7 oz) | 290 | 48 | 31 | 5 |
| GoLean Strawberries 'N Cream | 1 (2.7 oz) | 290 | 50 | 33 | 6 |
| GoLean Strawberry Vanilla Yogurt | 1 (2.7 oz) | 280 | 53 | 28 | 6 |

| FOOD | PORTION | CALS | CARB | SUGAR | FIBER |
|---|---|---|---|---|---|
| GoLean Crunchy Chocolate Caramel Karma | 1 (1.6 oz) | 140 | 26 | 15 | 5 |
| GoLean Crunchy Chocolate Peanut Bliss | 1 (1.8 oz) | 270 | 30 | 13 | 5 |
| GoLean Crunchy Sublime Lemon Lime | 1 (1.8 oz) | 670 | 32 | 13 | 5 |
| ***Lean Body For Her*** | | | | | |
| Chocolate Honey Peanut | 1 bar (1.76 oz) | 190 | 10 | 6 | tr |
| ***Luna*** | | | | | |
| Chai Tea | 1 bar (1.7 oz) | 180 | 27 | 12 | 2 |
| Chocolate Pecan Pie | 1 bar (1.7 oz) | 180 | 24 | 12 | 2 |
| LemonZest | 1 bar (1.7 oz) | 180 | 24 | 12 | 2 |
| Nutz Over Chocolate | 1 bar (1.7 oz) | 180 | 24 | 12 | 2 |
| S'Mores | 1 bar (1.7 oz) | 180 | 26 | 12 | 2 |
| Sesame Raisin Crunch | 1 bar (1.7 oz) | 170 | 26 | 13 | 2 |
| Toasted Nuts 'n Cranberry | 1 bar (1.7 oz) | 170 | 26 | 12 | 2 |
| Tropical Crisp | 1 bar (1.7 oz) | 180 | 24 | 11 | 2 |
| ***Met-Rx*** | | | | | |
| Big 100 Gram Bar Peanut Butter | 1 bar (3.5 oz) | 340 | 52 | 38 | 2 |
| Source/One Chocolate Cheesecake | 1 bar (2.1 oz) | 160 | 21 | 4 | tr |
| ***Moto Bar*** | | | | | |
| Bodacious Banana Split | 1 bar | 300 | 54 | 16 | 6 |
| Charming Cherry Almond | 1 bar (2.9 oz) | 300 | 54 | 18 | 3 |
| Cozy Pumpkin Pie | 1 bar | 300 | 54 | 16 | 6 |
| Jazzy Peanut Butter & Jelly | 1 bar | 300 | 52 | 20 | 4 |
| Kooky Cappuccino | 1 bar | 300 | 54 | 16 | 8 |
| Luscious Lemon Blueberry | 1 bar | 300 | 54 | 16 | 4 |
| Saucy Apple Cinnamon | 1 bar | 280 | 54 | 18 | 6 |
| Zany Cranberry Orange | 1 bar | 300 | 54 | 18 | 4 |
| ***New You*** | | | | | |
| Chocolate Crisp | 1 bar (1.65 oz) | 180 | 25 | 11 | 3 |
| ***NuGo*** | | | | | |
| Banana Chocolate Protein | 1 bar | 190 | 26 | 13 | 3 |
| Blue Berry Boom | 1 bar | 180 | 26 | 13 | 3 |
| Chocolate Blast | 1 bar | 180 | 26 | 13 | 3 |
| Coffee Break | 1 bar | 180 | 26 | 13 | 3 |

| FOOD | PORTION | CALS | CARB | SUGAR | FIBER |
|---|---|---|---|---|---|
| Orange Smoothie Protein | 1 bar | 190 | 25 | 13 | 1 |
| Peanut Butter Pleaser | 1 bar | 180 | 26 | 13 | 3 |
| ***Nutiva*** | | | | | |
| Flaxseed & Raisin Organic | 1 bar (1.4 oz) | 280 | 12 | 5 | 6 |
| Hempseed Bar Organic | 1 bar (1.4 oz) | 210 | 11 | 5 | 5 |
| ***Nutribar*** | | | | | |
| Chocolate Covered Belgian Chocolate | 1 bar (2.3 oz) | 252 | 33 | – | 2 |
| Chocolate Covered Caramel | 1 bar (2.3 oz) | 261 | 34 | – | tr |
| Chocolate Covered Chocolate Fudge | 1 bar (2.3 oz) | 267 | 35 | – | 2 |
| Chocolate Covered Hazelnut | 1 bar (2.3 oz) | 261 | 34 | – | 1 |
| Chocolate Covered Mocha Almond | 1 bar (2.3 oz) | 261 | 34 | – | tr |
| Chocolate Covered Peanut | 1 bar (2.3 oz) | 262 | 34 | – | 1 |
| Yogurt Covered Peach Apricot | 1 bar (2.3 oz) | 261 | 34 | – | tr |
| Yogurt Covered Raspberry | 1 bar (2.3 oz) | 261 | 34 | – | tr |
| Yogurt Covered Wildberry | 1 bar (2.3 oz) | 261 | 34 | – | tr |
| ***Odwalla Bar!*** | | | | | |
| Peanut Crunch | 1 bar (2.2 oz) | 260 | 40 | 17 | 3 |
| ***Peacekeeper*** | | | | | |
| Nuts About Peace All Flavors | 1 bar (1.4 oz) | 180 | 21 | 11 | 2 |
| ***PermaLean*** | | | | | |
| Protein Crunch Chocoholic Chocolate | 1 bar (1.8 oz) | 170 | 10 | 1 | tr |
| Protein Crunch Chocolate Raspberry | 1 bar (1.8 oz) | 180 | 9 | 1 | 0 |
| Protein Crunch Stark Raving Peanutz | 1 bar (1.8 oz) | 180 | 9 | 2 | 0 |
| ***PowerBar*** | | | | | |
| Apple Cinnamon | 1 bar (2.3 oz) | 230 | 45 | 20 | 3 |
| Banana | 1 bar (2.3 oz) | 230 | 45 | 20 | 3 |
| Chocolate | 1 bar (2.3 oz) | 230 | 45 | 14 | 3 |
| Essentials Chocolate | 1 bar (1.9 oz) | 180 | 28 | 20 | 3 |
| Harvest Blueberry | 1 bar (2.3 oz) | 240 | 45 | 18 | 4 |
| Harvest Strawberry | 1 bar (2.3 oz) | 240 | 45 | 18 | 4 |
| Malt-Nut | 1 bar (2.3 oz) | 230 | 45 | 18 | 3 |
| Mocha | 1 bar (2.3 oz) | 230 | 45 | 17 | 3 |
| Oatmeal Raisin | 1 bar (2.3 oz) | 230 | 45 | 20 | 3 |

| FOOD | PORTION | CALS | CARB | SUGAR | FIBER |
|---|---|---|---|---|---|
| Peanut Butter | 1 bar (2.3 oz) | 230 | 45 | 20 | 3 |
| Power Gel Strawberry Banana | 1 pkg | 110 | 28 | 5 | – |
| Pria Chocolate Honey Graham | 1 bar (1 oz) | 110 | 16 | 10 | – |
| Pria Chocolate Peanut Crunch | 1 bar (1 oz) | 110 | 16 | 10 | – |
| Pria Double Chocolate Cookie | 1 bar (1 oz) | 110 | 16 | 10 | – |
| Pria French Vanilla Crisp | 1 bar (1 oz) | 110 | 16 | 10 | – |
| Vanilla Crisp | 1 bar (2.3 oz) | 230 | 45 | 20 | 3 |
| Wild Berry | 1 bar (2.3 oz) | 230 | 45 | 14 | 3 |
| ***Pure Protein*** | | | | | |
| Blueberry Cheesecake | 1 bar | 190 | 23 | 3 | 0 |
| ***Revival*** | | | | | |
| Soy Apple Cinnamon Celebration | 1 bar | 200 | 28 | 2 | 1 |
| Soy Autumn Frost Low Carb | 1 bar | 200 | 28 | 2 | 1 |
| Soy Chocolate Raspberry Zing Low Carb | 1 bar | 200 | 28 | tr | 2 |
| Soy Chocolate Temptation | 1 bar | 220 | 30 | 16 | tr |
| Soy Marshmallow Krunch | 1 bar | 220 | 33 | 21 | tr |
| Soy Peanut Butter Chocolate Pal | 1 bar | 240 | 32 | 18 | 1 |
| Soy Peanut Butter Pal | 1 bar | 240 | 31 | 19 | tr |
| ***Slim-Fast*** | | | | | |
| Crispy Peanut Caramel | 1 bar | 120 | 21 | 13 | tr |
| Dutch Chocolate | 1 bar | 140 | 20 | 13 | 2 |
| Meal On-The-Go Apple Cobbler | 1 bar | 220 | 33 | 23 | 2 |
| Meal On-The-Go Chocolate Cookie Dough | 1 bar | 220 | 35 | 22 | 2 |
| Meal On-The-Go Honey Peanut | 1 bar | 220 | 34 | 23 | 2 |
| Meal On-The-Go Milk Chocolate Peanut | 1 bar | 220 | 36 | 24 | 2 |
| Meal On-The-Go Oatmeal Raisin | 1 bar | 220 | 36 | 19 | 2 |
| Meal On-The-Go Rich Chocolate Brownie | 1 bar | 220 | 34 | 23 | 2 |
| Meal On-The-Go Toasted Oat & Spice | 1 bar | 220 | 35 | 20 | 2 |
| Peanut Butter | 1 bar | 150 | 19 | 10 | 2 |
| Peanut Butter Crunch | 1 bar | 130 | 21 | 20 | tr |
| Rich Chewy Caramel | 1 bar | 120 | 22 | 11 | 2 |

| FOOD | PORTION | CALS | CARB | SUGAR | FIBER |
|---|---|---|---|---|---|
| ***SoBe*** | | | | | |
| Milk Chocolate | 1 bar (1.75 oz) | 240 | 28 | 24 | tr |
| ***Strive*** | | | | | |
| Crunchy Chocolate Smores | 1 bar (2.1 oz) | 200 | 25 | 0 | 0 |
| ***Sweet Success*** | | | | | |
| Chewy Chocolate Brownie | 1 bar (1.2 oz) | 120 | 23 | 12 | 3 |
| ***Think!*** | | | | | |
| Apple Spice | 1 bar (2 oz) | 205 | 40 | 15 | 7 |
| Chocolate Almond Coconut Raisin | 1 bar (2 oz) | 243 | 39 | 13 | 2 |
| Chocolate Fruit Harvest | 1 bar (2 oz) | 217 | 43 | 18 | 7 |
| ***ZonePerfect*** | | | | | |
| Honey Peanut | 1 bar (1.8 oz) | 200 | 22 | 20 | 1 |

## ENERGY DRINKS

| FOOD | PORTION | CALS | CARB | SUGAR | FIBER |
|---|---|---|---|---|---|
| ***AMP*** | | | | | |
| Energy Drink | 1 can (8.4 oz) | 120 | 32 | 30 | 0 |
| ***Arizona*** | | | | | |
| Extreme Energy Shot | 1 bottle (8.3 oz) | 130 | 34 | 33 | – |
| ***Atkins*** | | | | | |
| Cafe Au Lait | 1 can (11 oz) | 170 | 5 | 1 | 3 |
| Chocolate | 1 can (11 oz) | 170 | 5 | 2 | 3 |
| Chocolate Royale | 1 can (11 oz) | 170 | 6 | 4 | 1 |
| Strawberry | 1 can (11 oz) | 170 | 4 | 2 | 2 |
| Vanilla | 1 can (11 oz) | 170 | 4 | 2 | 2 |
| ***Boost*** | | | | | |
| High Protein Vanilla | 1 can (8 oz) | 240 | 33 | 16 | 0 |
| Vanilla | 8 oz | 240 | 41 | 23 | 0 |
| ***Choice*** | | | | | |
| Chocolate | 1 can (8 oz) | 220 | 24 | 10 | 3 |
| Chocolate Fudge Sugar Free | 1 pkg (11 oz) | 125 | 11 | 0 | 9 |
| French Vanilla Sugar Free | 1 pkg (11 oz) | 100 | 7 | 0 | 6 |
| Strawberries'n Cream Sugar Free | 1 pkg (11 oz) | 100 | 7 | 0 | 6 |
| Vanilla | 1 can (8 oz) | 220 | 24 | 9 | 3 |
| ***Crunk*** | | | | | |
| Energy Drink | 1 can | 120 | 29 | 29 | – |

| FOOD | PORTION | CALS | CARB | SUGAR | FIBER |
|---|---|---|---|---|---|
| ***Fuze*** | | | | | |
| Energize Blackberry Grape | 8 oz | 100 | 26 | 24 | – |
| Energize Exotic Punch | 8 oz | 100 | 26 | 24 | – |
| Energize Mojo Mango | 8 oz | 100 | 28 | 24 | – |
| Essential Cranberry Grapefruit | 8 oz | 90 | 25 | 24 | – |
| Focus Orange Carrot | 8 oz | 90 | 24 | 23 | – |
| Refresh Banana Colada | 8 oz | 90 | 24 | 22 | – |
| Refresh Mixed Berry | 8 oz | 90 | 25 | 23 | – |
| Refresh Peach Mango | 8 oz | 90 | 24 | 22 | – |
| Replenish Agave Cactus | 8 oz | 90 | 24 | 23 | – |
| Slenderize Tropical Punch | 8 oz | 10 | 2 | 2 | – |
| Stamina Grape & Aronia Punch | 8 oz | 80 | 23 | 23 | – |
| Vitaboost Citrus Starfruit Punch | 8 oz | 90 | 24 | 21 | – |
| ***Gatorade*** | | | | | |
| All Flavors | 1 cup (8 oz) | 50 | 14 | 14 | – |
| Energy Drink All Flavors | 1 bottle (12 oz) | 310 | 78 | 24 | – |
| Nutrition Shake All Flavors | 1 can (11 oz) | 370 | 62 | 43 | 1 |
| ***GeniSoy*** | | | | | |
| Soy Protein Shake Chocolate | 1 scoop (1.2 oz) | 120 | 17 | 15 | 2 |
| Soy Protein Shake Vanilla | 1 scoop (1.2 oz) | 130 | 18 | 13 | 0 |
| Soy Protein Shake Strawberry Banana | 1 scoop | 130 | 17 | 14 | 1 |
| ***Hansen's*** | | | | | |
| Energy Kiwi Strawberry | 8 oz | 120 | 30 | 30 | – |
| Energy Peach | 8 oz | 130 | 33 | 30 | – |
| Energy Punch | 8 oz | 120 | 30 | 30 | – |
| Healthy Start Carrot Orange Antioxidant Blend | 8 oz | 130 | 30 | 29 | – |
| Healthy Start Citrus Punch Focus Blend | 8 oz | 130 | 34 | 30 | – |
| Healthy Start Cranberry Grape Defense Blend | 8 oz | 110 | 28 | 26 | – |
| Healthy Start Tropical Orange Vitamix Blend | 8 oz | 110 | 30 | 26 | – |
| ***Healthy Pleasures*** | | | | | |
| Chocolate Irish Cream | 1 bottle (10.5 oz) | 260 | 45 | 45 | 0 |

| FOOD | PORTION | CALS | CARB | SUGAR | FIBER |
|---|---|---|---|---|---|
| ***Hype*** | | | | | |
| Classic Energy | 1 can (8.3 oz) | 110 | 26 | 26 | – |
| ***Impulse*** | | | | | |
| Energy Drink | 1 can (8.3 oz) | 110 | 28 | 27 | – |
| Sugar Free | 1 can (8.3 oz) | 5 | 1 | 0 | – |
| ***Invigor8*** | | | | | |
| Energy Boost | 1 can | 110 | 27 | 20 | 1 |
| Nutrition Boost | 1 can | 110 | 27 | 20 | 1 |
| ***Jugular*** | | | | | |
| Energy Drink | 1 can (8.3 oz) | 49 | 9 | 9 | – |
| ***Kashi*** | | | | | |
| GoLean Shake Mix Vanilla | 2 scoops | 220 | 32 | 22 | 7 |
| GoLean Shake Mix Woman Chocolate | 2 scoops | 220 | 31 | 22 | 7 |
| Shake Chocolate | 1 can | 230 | 38 | 30 | 7 |
| Shake Vanilla | 1 can | 220 | 36 | 29 | 7 |
| ***Kindercal*** | | | | | |
| Vanilla | 1 can (8 oz) | 250 | 32 | – | 0 |
| ***Nantucket Nectars*** | | | | | |
| Super Nectars Ginkgo Mango | 8 oz | 150 | 38 | 37 | – |
| Super Nectars Green Angel | 8 oz | 140 | 35 | 29 | – |
| Super Nectars Protein Smoothie | 8 oz | 170 | 38 | 34 | – |
| Super Nectars Red Guarana Tea | 8 oz | 110 | 26 | 25 | – |
| Super Nectars Vital C | 8 oz | 130 | 32 | 27 | – |
| ***New York Minute*** | | | | | |
| Energy Drink | 1 can (8.4 oz) | 130 | 33 | 33 | – |
| ***Nitro2Go*** | | | | | |
| High Energy | 1 can | 110 | 28 | 27 | – |
| High Energy Lite | 1 can | 20 | 5 | 4 | 0 |
| ***NutraShake*** | | | | | |
| Citrus | 1 pkg (4 oz) | 200 | 44 | – | – |
| Citrus Free | 1 serv (4 oz) | 200 | 44 | 4 | 0 |
| Vanilla | 1 serv (8 oz) | 400 | 62 | – | – |
| Vanilla No Added Sugar | 1 serv (4 oz) | 200 | 25 | – | – |
| ***Odwalla*** | | | | | |
| Blueberry B Monster | 8 fl oz | 140 | 33 | 26 | 2 |
| C Monster | 8 fl oz | 150 | 33 | 30 | 2 |
| Femme Vitale | 8 fl oz | 130 | 29 | 28 | 1 |
| Glorious Morning | 8 fl oz | 130 | 31 | 22 | 3 |
| Mango Tango | 8 fl oz | 150 | 31 | 28 | 0 |

| FOOD | PORTION | CALS | CARB | SUGAR | FIBER |
|---|---|---|---|---|---|
| Mo Beta | 8 fl oz | 140 | 34 | 26 | 1 |
| Serious Energy | 8 fl oz | 150 | 36 | 21 | 1 |
| Strawberry C Monster | 8 fl oz | 150 | 34 | 27 | tr |
| Super Protein | 8 fl oz | 170 | 33 | 28 | 2 |
| Superfood | 8 fl oz | 140 | 32 | 26 | 2 |
| Wellness | 8 fl oz | 150 | 33 | – | 1 |
| ***Pimp Juice*** | | | | | |
| Energy Drink | 1 can | 140 | 35 | 34 | – |
| ***Pink*** | | | | | |
| Diet | 1 can | 10 | 2 | 0 | – |
| ***Piranha*** | | | | | |
| Phunky Fruit Punch | 1 can (8.4 oz) | 140 | 35 | 35 | 0 |
| ***Pounds Off*** | | | | | |
| Dark Chocolate Ecstasy | 1 can (11 oz) | 200 | 39 | 32 | 6 |
| French Vanilla | 1 can (11 oz) | 220 | 41 | 35 | 5 |
| ***Powerade*** | | | | | |
| Fruit Punch | 8 fl oz | 70 | 19 | 15 | – |
| Lemon Lime | 8 fl oz | 70 | 19 | 15 | – |
| Mountain Blast | 8 fl oz | 70 | 19 | 15 | – |
| ***Pure Power*** | | | | | |
| Energy Drink | 1 can (8.4 oz) | 110 | 28 | – | – |
| Shotz | 1 can (5.75 oz) | 80 | 19 | 19 | 0 |
| ***Red Bull*** | | | | | |
| Energy Drink | 1 can (8.3 oz) | 110 | 28 | 27 | – |
| Sugar Free | 1 can | 10 | 3 | 0 | – |
| ***Slim-Fast*** | | | | | |
| Chocolate as prep w/ fat free milk | 1 serv | 190 | 32 | 29 | 2 |
| Chocolate Malt as prep w/ fat free milk | 1 serv | 190 | 32 | 29 | 2 |
| JumpStart Chocolate as prep w/ fat free milk | 1 serv | 240 | 39 | 33 | 5 |
| Strawberry as prep w/ fat free milk | 1 serv | 190 | 32 | 30 | 2 |
| Vanilla as prep w/ fat free milk | 1 serv | 190 | 32 | 30 | 2 |
| ***Snapple*** | | | | | |
| Meal Replacement All Flavors | 1 bottle (11.5 oz) | 210 | 43 | 36 | 5 |

| FOOD | PORTION | CALS | CARB | SUGAR | FIBER |
|---|---|---|---|---|---|
| ***SoBe*** | | | | | |
| Adrenaline Rush | 1 can (8.3 oz) | 140 | 36 | 34 | – |
| Black & Blue Berry Brew | 8 oz | 120 | 31 | 31 | – |
| Courage Cherry Citrus | 8 oz | 110 | 33 | 30 | – |
| Drive | 8 oz | 120 | 32 | 31 | – |
| Elixir Cranberry Grapefruit | 8 oz | 110 | 29 | 28 | – |
| Elixir Orange Carrot 3C | 8 oz | 90 | 24 | 23 | – |
| Elixir Pomegranate Cranberry | 8 oz | 100 | 26 | 25 | – |
| Energy | 8 oz | 120 | 32 | 30 | – |
| Fuerte | 8 oz | 130 | 35 | 33 | – |
| Karma | 8 oz | 120 | 33 | 31 | – |
| Long John Lizard's Grape Grog | 8 oz | 120 | 31 | 30 | – |
| Power | 8 oz | 120 | 32 | 31 | – |
| Tsunami | 8 oz | 110 | 29 | 27 | – |
| Wisdom | 8.5 oz | 110 | 30 | 29 | – |
| Zen Blend | 8.5 oz | 90 | 24 | 23 | – |
| ***Stevita*** | | | | | |
| All Flavors | 2 tsp | 0 | 0 | 0 | 0 |
| ***Sweet Success*** | | | | | |
| Creamy Milk Chocolate | 1 can | 200 | 36 | 30 | 3 |
| Creamy Milk Chocolate as prep w/ skim milk | 1 serv | 180 | 36 | 8 | 6 |
| ***TwinLab*** | | | | | |
| Hydra Fuel | 16 fl oz | 132 | 33 | – | – |
| Nitro Fuel | 16 oz | 460 | 100 | – | – |
| Ultra Fuel | 1 bottle (16 oz) | 400 | 100 | 30 | – |
| ***XO*** | | | | | |
| Balance | 8 oz | 50 | 13 | 12 | – |
| Berry | 1 bottle | 90 | 22 | 19 | – |
| Citrus | 1 bottle | 90 | 22 | 19 | – |
| Defense | 8 oz | 40 | 9 | 8 | – |
| Diet | 1 bottle | 15 | 2 | 0 | – |
| Endurance | 8 oz | 50 | 14 | 12 | – |
| Energy | 8 oz | 40 | 9 | 8 | – |
| Essential | 8 oz | 40 | 9 | 8 | – |
| Focus | 8 oz | 40 | 9 | 8 | – |
| Grape | 1 Bottle | 90 | 21 | 18 | – |
| Multi-V | 8 oz | 40 | 9 | 8 | – |

| FOOD | PORTION | CALS | CARB | SUGAR | FIBER |
|---|---|---|---|---|---|
| Original | 1 bottle | 110 | 28 | 28 | – |
| Peach | 1 bottle | 90 | 21 | 19 | – |
| Power-C | 8 oz | 40 | 9 | 8 | – |
| Rescue | 8 oz | 40 | 9 | 8 | – |
| Revive | 8 oz | 50 | 13 | 12 | – |
| Stress-B | 8 oz | 40 | 9 | 8 | – |
| Vanilla | 1 bottle | 90 | 21 | 20 | – |
| ***YET*** | | | | | |
| Your Energy Drink | 1 can | 8 | 0 | 0 | – |
| **ENGLISH MUFFIN** | | | | | |
| **FROZEN** | | | | | |
| ***Weight Watchers*** | | | | | |
| Sandwich | 1 (4 oz) | 210 | 28 | 1 | 2 |
| **READY-TO-EAT** | | | | | |
| apple cinnamon | 1 | 138 | 28 | – | – |
| crumpets | 1 (1.5 oz) | 80 | 16 | 1 | tr |
| granola | 1 | 155 | 31 | – | – |
| mixed grain | 1 | 155 | 31 | – | – |
| plain | 1 | 134 | 26 | – | – |
| plain toasted | 1 | 133 | 26 | – | – |
| raisin cinnamon | 1 | 138 | 28 | – | – |
| sourdough | 1 | 134 | 26 | – | – |
| wheat | 1 | 127 | 26 | – | – |
| whole wheat | 1 | 134 | 27 | – | 4 |
| ***Milton's*** | | | | | |
| Multi-Grain | 1 (2 oz) | 150 | 33 | 7 | 3 |
| ***Pepperidge Farm*** | | | | | |
| Original | 1 | 130 | 26 | tr | 2 |
| ***Thomas'*** | | | | | |
| Blueberry | 1 | 140 | 29 | 5 | 1 |
| Original | 1 | 120 | 25 | 1 | 1 |
| Raisin Bran | 1 | 150 | 30 | 7 | 2 |
| Raisin Cinnamon | 1 | 140 | 30 | 8 | 1 |
| Sourdough | 1 | 120 | 25 | 2 | 1 |
| Super Size | 1 (3.2 oz) | 200 | 41 | 2 | 2 |
| ***Wonder*** | | | | | |
| Cinnamon Raisin | 1 (2.1 oz) | 140 | 26 | 11 | 2 |
| Original | 1 (2 oz) | 130 | 25 | 4 | 1 |
| Sourdough | 1 (2 oz) | 130 | 25 | 1 | 1 |

| FOOD | PORTION | CALS | CARB | SUGAR | FIBER |
|---|---|---|---|---|---|
| **TAKE-OUT** | | | | | |
| w/ butter | 1 (2.2 oz) | 189 | 30 | – | – |
| w/ cheese & sausage | 1 (4 oz) | 393 | 29 | – | – |
| w/ egg cheese & canadian bacon | 1 (4.8 oz) | 289 | 28 | – | 2 |
| w/ egg cheese & sausage | 1 (5.8 oz) | 487 | 31 | – | – |
| **EPAZOTE** | | | | | |
| fresh | 1 tbsp (1 g) | tr | tr | – | tr |
| fresh sprig | 1 (2 g) | 1 | tr | – | tr |
| **EPPAW** | | | | | |
| raw | ½ cup | 75 | 16 | – | – |
| **FALAFEL** | | | | | |
| **TAKE-OUT** | | | | | |
| falafel | 1 (1.2 oz) | 57 | 5 | – | – |
| **FAT** *(see also* BUTTER, BUTTER SUBSTITUTES, MARGARINE, OIL*)* | | | | | |
| beef cooked | 1 oz | 193 | 0 | 0 | 0 |
| beef suet | 1 oz | 242 | 0 | 0 | 0 |
| beef tallow | 1 tbsp (13 g) | 115 | 0 | 0 | 0 |
| chicken | 1 cup | 1846 | 0 | 0 | 0 |
| chicken | 1 tbsp | 115 | 0 | 0 | 0 |
| cocoa butter | 1 tbsp | 120 | 0 | 0 | 0 |
| duck | 1 tbsp (13 g) | 115 | 0 | 0 | 0 |
| goose | 1 tbsp | 115 | 0 | 0 | 0 |
| goose | 1 oz | 257 | 0 | 0 | 0 |
| lamb new zealand | 1 oz | 182 | 0 | 0 | 0 |
| lard | 1 tbsp (13 g) | 115 | 0 | 0 | 0 |
| lard | 1 cup (205 g) | 1849 | 0 | 0 | 0 |
| nutmeg butter | 1 tbsp | 120 | 0 | 0 | 0 |
| pork backfat | 1 oz | 230 | 0 | 0 | 0 |
| pork cooked | 1 oz | 178 | 0 | 0 | 0 |
| salt pork | 1 oz | 212 | 0 | 0 | 0 |
| shortening | 1 cup | 1812 | 0 | 0 | 0 |
| shortening | 1 tbsp | 113 | 0 | 0 | 0 |
| turkey | 1 tbsp | 115 | 0 | 0 | 0 |
| ucuhuba butter | 1 tbsp | 120 | 0 | 0 | 0 |

| FOOD | PORTION | CALS | CARB | SUGAR | FIBER |
|---|---|---|---|---|---|
| **FAT SUBSTITUTES** | | | | | |
| ***Smucker's*** | | | | | |
| Baking Healthy 100% Fat Free | 1 tbsp | 30 | 7 | 4 | 0 |
| **FAVA BEANS** | | | | | |
| ***Progresso*** | | | | | |
| Fava Beans | ½ cup (4.6 oz) | 110 | 20 | 0 | 5 |
| **FEIJOA** | | | | | |
| fresh | 1 (1.75 oz) | 25 | 5 | – | – |
| puree | 1 cup | 119 | 26 | – | – |
| **FENNEL** | | | | | |
| fresh bulb | 1 (8.2 oz) | 72 | 17 | – | – |
| fresh sliced | 1 cup | 27 | 6 | – | – |
| leaves | 1 oz | 7 | 1 | – | 1 |
| seed | 1 tsp | 7 | 1 | – | – |
| **FENUGREEK** | | | | | |
| seed | 1 tsp | 12 | 2 | – | – |
| **FIBER** | | | | | |
| ***Apple Fiber*** | | | | | |
| Pure | 2 tbsp (7 g) | 16 | 7 | – | 4 |
| ***Benefiber*** | | | | | |
| Supplement | 1 pkg (4 g) | 20 | 4 | – | 3 |
| ***Choice*** | | | | | |
| Fiber Burst Lemon Lime | 3 pieces | 45 | 12 | 0 | 3 |
| Fiber Burst Tropical Fruit | 3 pieces | 45 | 11 | 0 | 3 |
| ***Metamucil*** | | | | | |
| Fiber Wafers Apple Crisp | 2 | 120 | 17 | – | 6 |
| ***ND Labs*** | | | | | |
| Pure Apple Fiber | 1 tbsp (7 g) | 16 | 7 | – | 4 |
| **FIDDLEHEAD FERNS** | | | | | |
| fresh | 3.5 oz | 34 | 6 | – | – |
| **FIGS** | | | | | |
| calimyrna | 3 (5.4 oz) | 120 | 28 | 11 | 4 |
| canned in heavy syrup | 3 | 75 | 19 | – | – |
| canned in light syrup | 3 | 58 | 15 | – | – |
| canned water pack | 3 | 42 | 11 | – | – |
| dried cooked | ½ cup | 140 | 16 | – | – |

| FOOD | PORTION | CALS | CARB | SUGAR | FIBER |
|---|---|---|---|---|---|
| dried whole | 10 | 477 | 122 | – | 17 |
| fresh | 1 med | 50 | 10 | – | – |
| **FIREWEED** | | | | | |
| leaves chopped | 1 cup (0.8 oz) | 24 | 4 | – | 2 |
| **FISH** *(see also* FISH SUBSTITUTES, *individual names,* SUSHI*)* | | | | | |
| **FROZEN** | | | | | |
| breaded fillet | 1 (2 oz) | 155 | 14 | – | – |
| sticks | 1 stick (1 oz) | 76 | 7 | – | – |
| ***Gorton's*** | | | | | |
| Baked Au Gratin | 1 piece (4.6 oz) | 130 | 7 | 1 | – |
| Baked Broccoli Cheddar | 1 piece (4.6 oz) | 130 | 7 | 1 | – |
| Baked Primavera | 1 piece (4.6 oz) | 120 | 4 | 2 | – |
| Batter Dipped Portions | 1 piece (2.5 oz) | 170 | 12 | 2 | – |
| Crunchy Golden Fillets Breaded | 2 (3.8 oz) | 250 | 21 | 3 | – |
| Crunchy Golden Sticks | 6 (3.8 oz) | 250 | 21 | 3 | – |
| Garlic & Herb | 2 pieces (3.6 oz) | 220 | 21 | 6 | – |
| Garlic Butter Crumb | 1 piece (4.6 oz) | 170 | 5 | 1 | – |
| Grilled Cajun Blackened | 1 piece (3.8 oz) | 120 | 1 | 1 | – |
| Grilled Garlic Butter | 1 piece (3.8 oz) | 120 | 1 | 1 | – |
| Grilled Italian Herb | 1 piece (3.8 oz) | 130 | 2 | 2 | – |
| Grilled Lemon Butter | 1 piece (3.8 oz) | 120 | 1 | 1 | – |
| Grilled Lemon Pepper | 1 piece (3.8 oz) | 120 | 1 | 1 | – |
| Parmesan | 2 pieces (3.6 oz) | 260 | 20 | 4 | – |
| Ranch | 1 piece (3.6 oz) | 240 | 22 | 3 | – |
| Southern Fried Country Style | 2 pieces (3.6 oz) | 230 | 16 | 3 | – |

| FOOD | PORTION | CALS | CARB | SUGAR | FIBER |
|---|---|---|---|---|---|
| Tenders | 3.5 pieces (4 oz) | 250 | 20 | 2 | – |
| Tenders Extra Crunchy | 3.5 pieces (4 oz) | 270 | 29 | 4 | – |
| **TAKE-OUT** | | | | | |
| fish cake | 1 (4.7 oz) | 166 | 6 | – | – |
| jamaican brown fish stew | 1 serv | 426 | 9 | – | 2 |
| kedgeree | 5.6 oz | 242 | 15 | – | 1 |
| mousse | 1 serv (3.5 oz) | 185 | 3 | tr | tr |
| stew | 1 cup (7.9 oz) | 157 | 10 | – | – |
| taramasalata | 2 tbsp | 124 | 1 | – | – |
| **FISH OIL** | | | | | |
| cod liver | 1 tbsp | 123 | 0 | 0 | 0 |
| herring | 1 tbsp | 123 | 0 | 0 | 0 |
| menhaden | 1 tbsp | 123 | 0 | 0 | 0 |
| salmon | 1 tbsp | 123 | 0 | 0 | 0 |
| sardine | 1 tbsp | 123 | 0 | 0 | 0 |
| shark | 1 oz | 270 | 0 | 0 | 0 |
| whale | 1 oz | 270 | 0 | 0 | 0 |
| **FISH PASTE** | | | | | |
| fish paste | 2 tsp | 15 | tr | – | 0 |
| **FISH SUBSTITUTES** | | | | | |
| ***Loma Linda*** | | | | | |
| Ocean Platter not prep | ⅓ cup (0.9 oz) | 90 | 8 | 0 | 4 |
| ***Worthington*** | | | | | |
| Fillets | 2 (3 oz) | 180 | 8 | tr | 4 |
| **FLAXSEED** | | | | | |
| ***Arrowhead*** | | | | | |
| Organic Flax Seeds | ¼ cup | 140 | 10 | 0 | 6 |
| ***Bite Me*** | | | | | |
| Flax Bar | 1 bar (1.8 oz) | 242 | 30 | 5 | 12 |
| ***Bob's Red Mill*** | | | | | |
| Flax Seed Meal | 2 tbsp | 60 | 4 | 0 | 4 |
| ***Cracker Flax*** | | | | | |
| Organic Apple Raisin | 1 oz | 130 | 16 | 4 | 9 |
| ***Hodgson Mill*** | | | | | |
| Milled | 2 tbsp | 60 | 4 | 0 | 4 |

| FOOD | PORTION | CALS | CARB | SUGAR | FIBER |
|---|---|---|---|---|---|
| **FLOUNDER** | | | | | |
| **FRESH** | | | | | |
| cooked | 1 fillet (4.5 oz) | 148 | 0 | 0 | 0 |
| cooked | 3 oz | 99 | 0 | 0 | 0 |
| **TAKE-OUT** | | | | | |
| battered & fried | 3.2 oz | 211 | 15 | – | – |
| breaded & fried | 3.2 oz | 211 | 15 | – | – |
| **FLOUR** | | | | | |
| buckwheat whole groat | 1 cup (4.2 oz) | 402 | 85 | – | 12 |
| corn masa | 1 cup (4 oz) | 416 | 87 | – | 11 |
| cottonseed low fat | 1 oz | 94 | 10 | – | – |
| peanut defatted | 1 cup | 196 | 21 | – | – |
| peanut defatted | 1 oz | 92 | 10 | – | – |
| peanut lowfat | 1 cup | 257 | 19 | – | – |
| potato | 1 cup (6.3 oz) | 628 | 143 | – | – |
| rice brown | 1 cup (5.5 oz) | 574 | 121 | – | 7 |
| rice white | 1 cup (5.5 oz) | 578 | 127 | – | 4 |
| rye dark | 1 cup (4.5 oz) | 415 | 88 | – | 29 |
| rye light | 1 cup (3.6 oz) | 374 | 82 | – | 15 |
| rye medium | 1 cup (3.6 oz) | 361 | 79 | – | 15 |
| sesame lowfat | 1 oz | 95 | 10 | – | – |
| triticale whole grain | 1 cup (4.6 oz) | 439 | 95 | – | 19 |
| white all purpose | 1 cup (4.4 oz) | 455 | 95 | – | 2 |
| white bread | 1 cup (4.8 oz) | 495 | 99 | – | 3 |
| white cake unsifted | 1 cup (4.8 oz) | 496 | 107 | – | 2 |
| white self-rising | 1 cup (4.4 oz) | 443 | 93 | – | 3 |
| white unbleached | 1 cup (4.4 oz) | 455 | 95 | – | 3 |
| whole wheat | 1 cup (4.2 oz) | 407 | 87 | – | 15 |
| ***All Trump*** | | | | | |
| Flour | ¼ cup (1 oz) | 100 | 22 | tr | tr |
| ***Arrowhead*** | | | | | |
| Whole Grain Oat | ⅓ cup | 120 | 18 | 0 | 3 |
| ***Betty Crocker*** | | | | | |
| Softasilk Velvet Cake Flour | ¼ cup (1 oz) | 100 | 23 | tr | tr |
| ***Gold Medal*** | | | | | |
| All Purpose | ¼ cup (1 oz) | 100 | 22 | tr | tr |
| Better For Bread | ¼ cup (1 oz) | 100 | 22 | 0 | tr |
| Organic All Purpose | ¼ cup (1 oz) | 100 | 22 | – | tr |
| Self Rising | ¼ cup (1 oz) | 100 | 22 | – | tr |

| FOOD | PORTION | CALS | CARB | SUGAR | FIBER |
|---|---|---|---|---|---|
| Unbleached | ¼ cup (1 oz) | 100 | 22 | tr | tr |
| Wondra | ¼ cup | 100 | 23 | – | tr |
| ***Heckers*** | | | | | |
| All Purpose Unbleached | ¼ cup | 100 | 22 | tr | tr |
| Whole Wheat | ¼ cup | 100 | 21 | 0 | 3 |
| ***Hodgson Mill*** | | | | | |
| White Unbleached Organic | ¼ cup (1 oz) | 100 | 23 | 0 | 3 |
| Whole Wheat Graham Organic | ¼ cup (1 oz) | 100 | 22 | 0 | 3 |
| ***La Pina*** | | | | | |
| Flour | ¼ cup (1 oz) | 100 | 23 | tr | 1 |
| ***Red Band*** | | | | | |
| All Purpose | ¼ cup (1 oz) | 100 | 23 | – | tr |
| Self-Rising | ¼ cup (1 oz) | 100 | 22 | – | tr |
| ***Robin Hood*** | | | | | |
| All Purpose | ¼ cup (1 oz) | 100 | 22 | tr | tr |
| Self-Rising | ¼ cup (1 oz) | 100 | 22 | tr | tr |
| Unbleached | ¼ cup (1 oz) | 100 | 22 | tr | tr |
| Whole Wheat | ¼ cup (1 oz) | 90 | 21 | – | 3 |
| **FRENCH BEANS** | | | | | |
| dried cooked | 1 cup | 228 | 43 | – | 17 |
| **FRENCH FRIES** *(see* POTATOES*)* | | | | | |
| **FRENCH TOAST** | | | | | |
| **FROZEN** | | | | | |
| french toast | 1 slice (2 oz) | 126 | 19 | – | 2 |
| **TAKE-OUT** | | | | | |
| plain | 1 slice | 151 | 16 | – | – |
| sticks | 5 (4.9 oz) | 513 | 58 | – | 3 |
| w/ butter | 2 slices (4.7 oz) | 356 | 36 | – | – |
| **FROG'S LEGS** | | | | | |
| **TAKE-OUT** | | | | | |
| as prep w/ seasoned flour & fried | 1 (0.8) | 70 | 15 | – | – |
| **FRUCTOSE** | | | | | |
| ***Estee*** | | | | | |
| Fructose | 1 tsp | 15 | 4 | 4 | 0 |

| FOOD | PORTION | CALS | CARB | SUGAR | FIBER |
|---|---|---|---|---|---|
| Packet | 1 pkg | 10 | 3 | 3 | 0 |
| **FRUIT DRINKS** *(see also individual names)* | | | | | |
| **FROZEN** | | | | | |
| ***Tree Of Life*** | | | | | |
| Organic Smoothie Banana Raspberry Strawberry | ⅔ cup (5 oz) | 90 | 23 | 15 | 3 |
| Organic Smoothie Mango Strawberry Raspberry | ⅔ cup (5 oz) | 70 | 18 | 15 | 4 |
| Organic Smoothie Strawberry Banana | ⅔ cup (5 oz) | 90 | 23 | 15 | 3 |
| Organic Smoothie Strawberry Blueberry Banana | ⅔ cup (5 oz) | 90 | 22 | 12 | 3 |
| **READY-TO-DRINK** | | | | | |
| fruit punch | 6 fl oz | 87 | 22 | – | – |
| pineapple & orange drink | 8 fl oz | 125 | 29 | – | – |
| ***Apple & Eve*** | | | | | |
| Apple Cranberry | 8 oz | 120 | 30 | 26 | – |
| ***Citrus Squeeze*** | | | | | |
| California Punch | 8 oz | 130 | 33 | 33 | – |
| Florida Punch | 8 oz | 120 | 30 | 30 | – |
| ***Del Monte*** | | | | | |
| Peach Raspberry | 5.5 fl oz | 160 | 40 | 33 | 3 |
| Pineapple Banana Orange | 5.5 fl oz | 170 | 44 | 34 | 1 |
| Strawberry Peach Banana | 5.5 fl oz | 150 | 39 | 30 | 1 |
| ***Dole*** | | | | | |
| Apple Berry Burst | 8 fl oz | 120 | 31 | – | – |
| Cranberry Apple | 8 fl oz | 120 | 30 | – | – |
| Fruit Fiesta | 8 fl oz | 140 | 34 | – | – |
| Fruit Punch | 1 carton (10 oz) | 160 | 39 | – | – |
| Mountain Cherry | 8 fl oz | 150 | 30 | 28 | – |
| Orange Peach Mango | 8 oz | 120 | 28 | – | – |
| Orange Strawberry Banana | 8 oz | 120 | 28 | – | – |
| Orchard Peach | 8 oz | 140 | 34 | 28 | – |
| Pineapple Orange | 8 oz | 120 | 27 | – | – |
| Pineapple Orange Strawberry | 8 oz | 130 | 32 | – | – |
| Tropical Fruit | 8 oz | 160 | 38 | – | 0 |
| ***Eden*** | | | | | |
| Organic Apple Cherry Juice | 8 oz | 120 | 30 | 29 | 1 |

| FOOD | PORTION | CALS | CARB | SUGAR | FIBER |
|---|---|---|---|---|---|
| ***Fresh Samantha*** | | | | | |
| Banana Strawberry | 1 cup (8 oz) | 130 | 11 | – | 6 |
| Carrot Orange | 1 cup (8 oz) | 100 | 8 | – | 4 |
| Desperately Seeking C | 1 cup (8 oz) | 110 | 9 | – | 7 |
| Protein Blast | 1 cup (8 oz) | 160 | 10 | – | 8 |
| Super Juice | 1 cup (8 oz) | 140 | 11 | – | 8 |
| The Big Bang | 1 cup (8 oz) | 100 | 8 | – | 8 |
| ***Guzzler*** | | | | | |
| Citrus Punch | 8 fl oz | 140 | 25 | 25 | – |
| Island Punch | 8 fl oz | 140 | 29 | 22 | 0 |
| ***Hansen's*** | | | | | |
| Fruit Punch 100% Juice | 1 box (4.23 oz) | 60 | 15 | 14 | – |
| Juice Slam Wild Berry | 1 box | 120 | 29 | 25 | – |
| Smoothie Apricot Nectar | 1 can | 170 | 43 | 43 | – |
| Smoothie Cranberry Twist | 1 can | 180 | 45 | 44 | – |
| Smoothie Energy Island Blast | 1 can | 170 | 40 | 40 | – |
| Smoothie Guava Strawberry | 1 can | 170 | 43 | 43 | – |
| Smoothie Mango Pineapple | 1 can | 170 | 43 | 43 | – |
| Smoothie Peach Berry | 1 can | 170 | 43 | 43 | – |
| Smoothie Pineapple Coconut | 1 can | 180 | 43 | 43 | – |
| Smoothie Strawberry Banana | 1 can | 180 | 44 | 43 | – |
| Smoothie Tropical Passion | 1 can | 170 | 44 | 43 | – |
| Smoothie Whipped Orange | 1 can | 180 | 44 | 44 | – |
| Smoothie Lite Cranberry Raspberry | 1 can | 50 | 13 | 13 | – |
| ***Juicy Juice*** | | | | | |
| Apple Grape | 1 box (8.45 oz) | 140 | 34 | 32 | 0 |
| Berry | 1 box (8.45 oz) | 130 | 37 | 31 | 0 |
| Punch | 1 box (8.45 oz) | 140 | 34 | 32 | 0 |
| Punch | 1 box (4.23 oz) | 70 | 17 | 15 | 0 |
| Tropical | 1 box (8.45 oz) | 140 | 34 | 31 | 0 |
| ***Langers*** | | | | | |
| 100% Juice Pineapple Coconut | 8 oz | 140 | 28 | 27 | 1 |
| Blueberry Cranberry | 8 oz | 135 | 34 | 34 | – |

| FOOD | PORTION | CALS | CARB | SUGAR | FIBER |
|---|---|---|---|---|---|
| Cranberry Berry | 8 oz | 135 | 34 | 31 | – |
| Cranberry Fuji | 8 oz | 160 | 39 | 35 | – |
| Cranberry Grape | 8 oz | 165 | 41 | 37 | – |
| Cranberry Grape Cocktail | 8 oz | 165 | 41 | 37 | – |
| Cranberry Orange | 8 oz | 130 | 33 | 30 | – |
| Diet Cranberry Berry | 8 oz | 30 | 8 | 8 | – |
| Diet Cranberry Grape | 8 oz | 30 | 8 | 8 | – |
| Fruit Punch Cocktail | 8 oz | 120 | 30 | 30 | – |
| Kiwi Raspberry Cocktail | 8 oz | 120 | 29 | 26 | – |
| Kiwi Strawberry Cocktail | 8 oz | 120 | 29 | 26 | – |
| Mango Orange | 8 oz | 130 | 33 | 30 | – |
| Mixed Berry 100% Juice | 8 oz | 120 | 30 | 27 | – |
| Pineapple Orange Guava | 8 oz | 130 | 30 | 30 | – |
| Ruby Orange | 8 oz | 130 | 33 | 30 | – |
| Tropical Ruby | 8 oz | 135 | 34 | 34 | – |
| White Cranberry Raspberry | 8 oz | 120 | 28 | 28 | – |
| ***Mauna La'i*** | | | | | |
| Island Guava | 8 oz | 130 | 32 | 32 | 0 |
| Paradise Passion | 8 oz | 130 | 32 | 32 | 0 |
| ***Mott's*** | | | | | |
| Berry | 1 box (8 oz) | 100 | 26 | – | – |
| Fruit Punch | 8 fl oz | 130 | 32 | – | – |
| Fruit Punch | 1 box (8 oz) | 110 | 27 | – | – |
| ***Nantucket Nectars*** | | | | | |
| Apple Raspberry | 8 oz | 140 | 34 | 31 | – |
| California Melonberry | 8 oz | 110 | 28 | 28 | – |
| Cranberry Apple | 8 oz | 140 | 36 | 34 | – |
| Fruit Punch | 8 oz | 130 | 32 | 30 | – |
| Kiwi Berry | 8 oz | 120 | 30 | 26 | – |
| Orange Passionfruit | 8 oz | 120 | 29 | 27 | – |
| Orange Mango | 8 oz | 130 | 32 | 29 | 0 |
| Peach Orange | 8 oz | 130 | 31 | 26 | 1 |
| Pineapple Orange Banana | 8 oz | 140 | 35 | 29 | – |
| Pineapple Orange Guava | 8 oz | 120 | 31 | 28 | – |
| Watermelon Strawberry | 8 oz | 120 | 30 | 27 | – |
| ***Oberweis*** | | | | | |
| Fruit Punch | 8 oz | 120 | 30 | 29 | 0 |
| ***Ocean Spray*** | | | | | |
| Cran*Blueberry | 8 oz | 160 | 41 | 41 | 0 |
| Cran*Cherry | 8 oz | 160 | 39 | 39 | 0 |

| FOOD | PORTION | CALS | CARB | SUGAR | FIBER |
|---|---|---|---|---|---|
| Cran*Currant | 8 oz | 140 | 33 | 33 | 0 |
| Cran*Grape | 8 oz | 170 | 41 | 41 | 0 |
| Cran*Mango | 8 oz | 130 | 33 | 33 | 0 |
| Cran*Raspberry | 8 oz | 140 | 36 | 36 | 0 |
| Cran*Raspberry Reduced Calorie | 8 oz | 50 | 13 | 13 | 0 |
| Cran*Strawberry | 8 oz | 140 | 36 | 35 | 1 |
| Cran*Tangerine | 8 oz | 130 | 33 | 33 | 0 |
| Cranapple | 8 oz | 160 | 41 | 40 | 1 |
| Cranapple Reduced Calorie | 8 oz | 50 | 13 | 13 | 0 |
| Cranicot | 8 oz | 160 | 40 | 40 | 0 |
| Crazy Kiwi Passion | 8 oz | 130 | 32 | 32 | 0 |
| Fruit Punch | 8 oz | 130 | 32 | 32 | 0 |
| Kiwi Strawberry | 8 oz | 120 | 31 | 31 | 0 |
| Lightstyle Cran*Grape | 8 oz | 40 | 9 | 9 | 0 |
| Lightstyle Cran*Mango | 8 oz | 40 | 10 | 10 | 0 |
| Lightstyle Cran*Raspberry | 8 oz | 40 | 10 | 10 | 0 |
| Mandarin Magic | 8 oz | 120 | 31 | 31 | 0 |
| Ruby Red & Tangerine Grapefruit | 8 oz | 130 | 32 | 32 | 0 |
| Ruby Red & Mango | 8 oz | 130 | 33 | 33 | 0 |
| ***Odwalla*** | | | | | |
| Blackberry Fruit Shake | 8 fl oz | 140 | 35 | 30 | 1 |
| Rooty Fruity | 8 fl oz | 110 | 24 | 21 | 0 |
| Strawberry Banana | 8 fl oz | 120 | 31 | 26 | 3 |
| ***Snapple*** | | | | | |
| Cranberry Raspberry | 8 fl oz | 120 | 29 | 27 | – |
| Diet Cranberry Raspberry | 8 fl oz | 10 | 2 | 2 | – |
| Fruit Punch | 8 fl oz | 110 | 29 | 27 | – |
| Kiwi Strawberry | 8 fl oz | 110 | 28 | 26 | – |
| Snapricot Orange | 8 fl oz | 120 | 30 | 28 | – |
| ***Squeezit*** | | | | | |
| Berry B. Wild | 1 bottle (7 oz) | 110 | 28 | 27 | 0 |
| Lemon Lime | 1 bottle (7 oz) | 110 | 28 | 25 | 0 |
| Rockin' Red Puncher | 1 bottle (7 oz) | 110 | 24 | 23 | 0 |
| Tropical Punch | 1 bottle (7 oz) | 110 | 28 | 26 | 0 |
| ***Tropicana*** | | | | | |
| Berry Punch | 8 fl oz | 130 | 32 | – | – |
| Citrus Punch | 8 fl oz | 140 | 36 | 33 | – |
| Fruit Punch | 8 oz | 130 | 32 | – | – |

| FOOD | PORTION | CALS | CARB | SUGAR | FIBER |
|---|---|---|---|---|---|
| Tangerine Orange Juice | 8 fl oz | 110 | 25 | – | – |
| Tropics Orange Strawberry Banana | 8 fl oz | 110 | 27 | 23 | – |
| Tropics Orange Kiwi Passion | 8 fl oz | 100 | 26 | 23 | – |
| Tropics Orange Peach Mango | 8 fl oz | 110 | 28 | 24 | – |
| Tropics Orange Pineapple | 8 fl oz | 110 | 27 | 24 | – |
| Twister Apple Raspberry Blackberry | 1 bottle (10 fl oz) | 160 | 38 | – | – |
| Twister Citrus Punch | 1 bottle (10 oz) | 180 | 45 | – | – |
| Twister Cranberry Punch | 1 bottle (10 oz) | 170 | 43 | – | – |
| Twister Fruit Punch | 1 bottle (10 oz) | 170 | 43 | – | – |
| Twister Light Orange Strawberry Banana | 1 bottle (10 oz) | 45 | 11 | – | – |
| Twister Orange Cranberry | 1 bottle (10 fl oz) | 160 | 40 | – | – |
| Twister Orange Strawberry Banana | 1 bottle (10 oz) | 160 | 40 | – | – |
| Twister Ruby Red Tangerine | 1 bottle (10 oz) | 160 | 40 | – | – |
| Twister Strawberry Kiwi | 1 bottle (10 oz) | 160 | 42 | – | – |
| ***V8*** | | | | | |
| Splash Berry Blend | 8 oz | 110 | 28 | 26 | – |
| ***Wellfleet Farms*** | | | | | |
| Cranberry & Georgia Peach | 8 oz | 140 | 35 | 35 | 0 |
| Cranberry & Granny Smith Apple | 8 oz | 130 | 33 | 33 | 0 |
| Cranberry & Key Lime | 8 oz | 140 | 35 | 35 | 0 |
| **FRUIT MIXED** *(see also individual names)* | | | | | |
| **CANNED** | | | | | |
| ***Del Monte*** | | | | | |
| Cherry Mixed Light Syrup | ½ cup (4.4 oz) | 90 | 22 | 19 | 1 |
| Chunky Mixed in Heavy Syrup | ½ cup (4.5 oz) | 100 | 24 | 23 | 1 |
| Chunky Mixed Fruit Naturals | ½ cup (4.4 oz) | 60 | 15 | 14 | 1 |
| Chunky Mixed in Extra Light Syrup | ½ cup (4.4 oz) | 60 | 15 | 14 | 1 |

| FOOD | PORTION | CALS | CARB | SUGAR | FIBER |
|---|---|---|---|---|---|
| Citrus Salad | ½ cup (4.4 oz) | 80 | 20 | 17 | 0 |
| Fruit Cocktail Fruit Naturals | ½ cup (4.4 oz) | 60 | 15 | 14 | 1 |
| Fruit Cocktail in Extra Light Syrup | ½ cup (4.4 oz) | 60 | 15 | 14 | 1 |
| Fruit Cocktail in Heavy Syrup | ½ cup (4.5 oz) | 100 | 24 | 23 | 1 |
| Fruit Cup Fruit Naturals Mixed | 1 pkg (4 oz) | 50 | 13 | 12 | 1 |
| Fruit Cup Mixed in Extra Light Syrup | 1 pkg (4 oz) | 50 | 13 | 12 | 1 |
| Fruit Salad in Extra Light Syrup | ½ cup (4.5 oz) | 70 | 22 | 13 | 2 |
| Fruit To Go Fruit Combo | 1 pkg (4 oz) | 70 | 18 | 16 | 1 |
| Fruit To Go Wild Berry Jumble | 1 pkg (4 oz) | 80 | 20 | 17 | 1 |
| Fruitrageous Crazy Cherry Mixed | 1 pkg (4 oz) | 90 | 22 | 19 | 1 |
| Orchard Select California Mixed | ½ cup (4.5 oz) | 80 | 19 | 18 | 1 |
| Orchard Select Premium Mixed | ½ cup (4.4 oz) | 80 | 20 | 18 | tr |
| Snack Cups Mixed Fruit in Heavy Syrup | 1 serv (4 oz) | 80 | 20 | 19 | 1 |
| SunFresh Ambrosia Salad | ½ cup | 70 | 16 | 13 | 1 |
| Tropical Fruit Salad | ½ cup (4.3 oz) | 60 | 16 | 14 | 1 |
| Tropical Fruit Salad in Light Syrup | ½ cup (4.4 oz) | 80 | 21 | 20 | 1 |
| Very Cherry Mixed Fruit | ½ cup (4.4 oz) | 90 | 22 | 19 | 1 |
| ***Dole*** | | | | | |
| FruitBowls Tropical Fruit | 1 pkg (4 oz) | 60 | 16 | 14 | 2 |
| Tropical Fruit Salad | ½ cup (4.3 oz) | 80 | 20 | 18 | 1 |
| ***Mott's*** | | | | | |
| Fruitsations Banana | 1 pkg (4 oz) | 90 | 23 | – | – |
| Fruitsations Cherry | 1 pkg (4 oz) | 70 | 19 | – | – |
| Fruitsations Mango Peach | 1 pkg (4 oz) | 70 | 22 | – | – |
| Fruitsations Mixed Berry | 1 pkg (4 oz) | 90 | 22 | 20 | 1 |
| Fruitsations Pear | 1 pkg (4 oz) | 90 | 23 | – | – |
| Fruitsations Strawberry | 1 pkg (4 oz) | 80 | 19 | – | – |
| Fruitsations Tropical Fruit | 1 pkg (4 oz) | 70 | 19 | – | – |
| Healthy Harvest Peach Medley | 1 pkg (3.9 oz) | 50 | 13 | 11 | 1 |
| ***Ocean Spray*** | | | | | |
| Cran*Fruit Cranberry Raspberry | ¼ cup | 120 | 29 | 27 | 2 |

| FOOD | PORTION | CALS | CARB | SUGAR | FIBER |
|---|---|---|---|---|---|
| Cran*Fruit Cranberry Strawberry | ¼ cup | 120 | 29 | 27 | 2 |
| ***SunFresh*** | | | | | |
| Ambrosia Salad | ½ cup (4.5 oz) | 70 | 16 | 13 | 1 |
| Mixed Fruit in Light Syrup | ½ cup (4.6 oz) | 90 | 20 | 12 | 2 |
| Tropical Salad in Extra Light Syrup | ½ cup (4.5 oz) | 80 | 20 | 16 | 0 |
| ***White House*** | | | | | |
| Apple Banana Sauce | 1 pkg (4 oz) | 100 | 23 | 21 | 1 |
| Apple Mixed Berry Sauce | 1 pkg (4 oz) | 110 | 23 | 23 | 1 |
| Apple Peach Sauce | 1 pkg (4 oz) | 100 | 23 | 21 | 1 |
| **DRIED** | | | | | |
| mixed | 11 oz pkg | 712 | 188 | – | – |
| ***Paradise*** | | | | | |
| Old English Fruit & Peel Mix | 1 tbsp (0.8 oz) | 70 | 18 | 11 | 1 |
| ***Sun-Maid*** | | | | | |
| Tropical Medley | ¼ cup (1.4 oz) | 130 | 32 | 29 | 1 |
| **FROZEN** | | | | | |
| mixed fruit sweetened | 1 cup | 245 | 61 | – | – |
| ***Birds Eye*** | | | | | |
| Mixed Fruit | ½ cup | 90 | 23 | 21 | – |
| ***Tree Of Life*** | | | | | |
| Organic Mixed Berries | ¾ cup (5 oz) | 60 | 16 | 6 | 3 |

## FRUIT SNACKS

| FOOD | PORTION | CALS | CARB | SUGAR | FIBER |
|---|---|---|---|---|---|
| fruit leather | 1 bar (0.8 oz) | 81 | 18 | – | – |
| fruit leather pieces | 1 oz | 97 | 22 | – | – |
| fruit leather pieces | 1 pkg (0.9 oz) | 92 | 21 | – | – |
| fruit leather rolls | 1 sm (0.5 oz) | 49 | 12 | – | – |
| fruit leather rolls | 1 lg (0.7 oz) | 73 | 18 | – | – |
| ***Betty Crocker*** | | | | | |
| Fruit By The Foot All Flavors | 1 roll | 80 | 17 | 10 | – |
| ***CoolFruits*** | | | | | |
| Apple Grape | 1 bar (0.5 oz) | 51 | 12 | 9 | 1 |
| Apple Strawberry | 1 bar (0.5 oz) | 51 | 12 | 9 | 1 |
| Wild Blueberry | 1 bar (0.5 oz) | 51 | 12 | 9 | 1 |
| ***Health Valley*** | | | | | |
| Bakes Apple | 1 bar | 70 | 19 | 11 | 2 |
| Bakes Date | 1 bar | 70 | 19 | 11 | 2 |
| Bakes Raisin | 1 bar | 70 | 19 | 11 | 2 |

| FOOD | PORTION | CALS | CARB | SUGAR | FIBER |
|---|---|---|---|---|---|
| Fruit Bars Apple | 1 | 140 | 35 | 13 | 3 |
| Fruit Bars Apricot | 1 | 140 | 35 | 12 | 4 |
| Fruit Bars Date | 1 | 140 | 34 | 12 | 3 |
| Fruit Bars Raisin | 1 | 140 | 35 | 17 | 3 |
| ***Sunbelt*** | | | | | |
| Fruit Jammers | 1 pkg (1 oz) | 100 | 23 | 13 | 0 |
| 100% Fruit Roll All Flavors | 1 (0.5 oz) | 50 | 12 | 5 | 1 |
| ***Weight Watchers*** | | | | | |
| Apple & Cinnamon | 1 pkg (0.5 oz) | 50 | 13 | 9 | 2 |
| Apple Chips | 1 pkg (0.75 oz) | 70 | 18 | 13 | 3 |
| Peach & Strawberry | 1 pkg (0.5 oz) | 50 | 13 | 11 | 2 |
| **GARLIC** | | | | | |
| clove | 1 | 4 | 1 | – | – |
| fresh chopped | 1 tsp | 4 | tr | tr | 1 |
| powder | 1 tsp | 9 | 2 | – | – |
| ***Dorot*** | | | | | |
| Frozen Crushed Cubes | 1 cube (4 g) | 5 | 1 | 0 | 0 |
| ***McCormick*** | | | | | |
| Garlic Salt | ¼ tsp | 0 | 0 | 0 | 0 |
| **GEFILTE FISH** | | | | | |
| sweet | 1 piece (1.5 oz) | 35 | 3 | – | – |
| **GELATIN** | | | | | |
| **MIX** | | | | | |
| low calorie | ½ cup | 8 | 0 | 0 | 0 |
| mix as prep | ½ cup (4.7 oz) | 80 | 19 | 11 | – |
| mix not prep | 1 pkg (3 oz) | 324 | 77 | – | – |
| mix w/ fruit | ½ cup (3.7 oz) | 73 | 18 | – | – |
| **READY-TO-EAT** | | | | | |
| ***Hunt's*** | | | | | |
| Snack Pack Gels Cherry | 1 serv (3.5 oz) | 100 | 25 | 24 | 0 |
| Snack Pack Gels Raspberry Berry | 1 serv (3.5 oz) | 100 | 25 | 24 | 0 |
| Snack Pack Gels Strawberry | 1 serv (3.5 oz) | 100 | 25 | 24 | 0 |
| Snack Pack Gels Strawberry Orange | 1 serv (3.5 oz) | 100 | 25 | 24 | 0 |

| FOOD | PORTION | CALS | CARB | SUGAR | FIBER |
|---|---|---|---|---|---|
| ***Swiss Miss*** | | | | | |
| Gels Berry Strawberry | 1 pkg (3.5 oz) | 79 | 18 | 18 | 0 |
| Gels Berry Lemon | 1 pkg (3.5 oz) | 79 | 18 | 18 | 0 |
| Gels Raspberry Orange | 1 pkg (3.5 oz) | 79 | 18 | 18 | 0 |
| Gels Strawberry Raspberry | 1 pkg (3.5 oz) | 79 | 18 | 18 | 0 |
| **GIBLETS** | | | | | |
| capon simmered | 1 cup (5 oz) | 238 | 0 | 0 | 0 |
| chicken floured & fried | 1 cup (5 oz) | 402 | 6 | – | – |
| chicken simmered | 1 cup (5 oz) | 228 | 1 | – | – |
| turkey simmered | 1 cup (5 oz) | 243 | 3 | – | – |
| **GINGER** | | | | | |
| ground | 1 tsp (1.8 g) | 6 | 1 | – | – |
| pickled | 0.5 oz | 5 | 1 | – | tr |
| root fresh | ¼ cup | 17 | 4 | – | – |
| root fresh | 5 slices | 8 | 2 | – | – |
| root fresh sliced | ¼ cup | 17 | 4 | – | – |
| ***Eden*** | | | | | |
| Pickled w/ Shiso Leaves | 1 tbsp | 15 | 3 | 1 | 1 |
| ***McCormick*** | | | | | |
| Crystallized | ¼ tsp | 15 | 3 | – | – |
| **GINKGO NUTS** | | | | | |
| canned | 1 oz | 32 | 6 | – | – |
| dried | 1 oz | 99 | 21 | – | – |
| raw | 1 oz | 52 | 11 | – | – |
| **GINSENG** | | | | | |
| dried | 1 oz | 90 | 20 | – | 2 |
| fresh | 1 oz | 28 | 6 | – | tr |
| **GIZZARDS** | | | | | |
| chicken simmered | 1 cup (5 oz) | 222 | 2 | – | – |
| turkey simmered | 1 cup (5 oz) | 236 | 1 | – | – |
| **GNOCCHI** | | | | | |
| ***Bellino*** | | | | | |
| W/ Potato | 1 cup | 240 | 55 | 2 | 2 |
| **GOAT** | | | | | |
| roasted | 3 oz | 122 | 0 | 0 | 0 |

| FOOD | PORTION | CALS | CARB | SUGAR | FIBER |
|---|---|---|---|---|---|
| **GOOSE** | | | | | |
| w/ skin roasted | 6.6 oz | 574 | 0 | 0 | 0 |
| w/ skin roasted | ½ goose (1.7 lbs) | 2362 | 0 | 0 | 0 |
| w/o skin roasted | 5 oz | 340 | 0 | 0 | 0 |
| w/o skin roasted | ½ goose (1.3 lbs) | 1406 | 0 | 0 | 0 |
| **GOOSEBERRIES** | | | | | |
| canned in light syrup | ½ cup | 93 | 24 | – | – |
| fresh | 1 cup | 67 | 15 | – | – |
| **GRAPE JUICE** | | | | | |
| bottled | 1 cup | 155 | 38 | – | – |
| frzn sweetened as prep | 1 cup | 128 | 32 | – | – |
| frzn sweetened not prep | 6 oz | 386 | 96 | – | – |
| grape drink | 6 oz | 84 | 22 | – | – |
| ***Daily*** | | | | | |
| Drink | 8 oz | 110 | 27 | 27 | – |
| ***Hansen's*** | | | | | |
| White Grape 100% Juice | 1 box (4.23 oz) | 90 | 22 | 21 | – |
| ***Juicy Juice*** | | | | | |
| Drink | 1 box (8.45 oz) | 140 | 34 | 32 | 0 |
| Drink | 1 box (4.23 oz) | 70 | 17 | 16 | – |
| ***Keto*** | | | | | |
| Kooler | ½ tsp | 0 | 0 | 0 | 0 |
| ***Langers*** | | | | | |
| Cocktail | 8 oz | 160 | 40 | 36 | – |
| ***Mott's*** | | | | | |
| 100% Juice | 1 box (8 oz) | 130 | 33 | – | – |
| Grape Juice | 8 fl oz | 130 | 31 | – | – |
| ***Nantucket Nectars*** | | | | | |
| Grapeade | 8 oz | 130 | 33 | 29 | – |
| ***Squeezit*** | | | | | |
| Grumpy Grape | 1 bottle (7 oz) | 110 | 28 | 27 | 0 |
| ***Welch's*** | | | | | |
| 100% White | 8 oz | 160 | 39 | 37 | – |

| FOOD | PORTION | CALS | CARB | SUGAR | FIBER |
|---|---|---|---|---|---|
| **GRAPE LEAVES** | | | | | |
| canned | 1 (4 g) | 3 | tr | – | 0 |
| fresh raw | 1 (3 g) | 3 | 1 | – | tr |
| **TAKE-OUT** | | | | | |
| dolmas | 5 (4.2 oz) | 200 | 23 | 3 | 2 |
| **GRAPEFRUIT** | | | | | |
| **CANNED** | | | | | |
| juice pack | ½ cup | 46 | 11 | – | – |
| unsweetened | 1 cup | 93 | 22 | – | – |
| water pack | ½ cup | 44 | 11 | – | – |
| ***SunFresh*** | | | | | |
| Red & White | ½ cup (4.4 oz) | 45 | 9 | 8 | 2 |
| **FRESH** | | | | | |
| pink | ½ | 37 | 9 | – | 1 |
| pink sections | 1 cup | 69 | 18 | – | 1 |
| red | ½ | 37 | 9 | – | – |
| red sections | 1 cup | 69 | 18 | – | – |
| white | ½ | 39 | 10 | – | 1 |
| white sections | 1 cup | 76 | 19 | – | 1 |
| ***Ocean Spray*** | | | | | |
| Fresh | 2 oz | 50 | 14 | 31 | 0 |
| **GRAPEFRUIT JUICE** | | | | | |
| fresh | 1 cup | 96 | 23 | – | – |
| frzn as prep | 1 cup | 102 | 24 | – | – |
| frzn not prep | 6 oz | 302 | 72 | – | – |
| sweetened | 1 cup | 116 | 28 | – | – |
| ***Fresh Samantha*** | | | | | |
| Juice | 1 cup (8 oz) | 90 | 7 | – | 0 |
| ***Langers*** | | | | | |
| Diet Ruby Red | 8 oz | 40 | 9 | 9 | – |
| Ruby Red | 8 oz | 130 | 33 | 30 | – |
| ***Mott's*** | | | | | |
| 100% Juice | 8 fl oz | 110 | 27 | – | – |
| ***Nantucket Nectars*** | | | | | |
| 100% Juice | 8 oz | 100 | 23 | 16 | – |
| 100% Ruby Red | 8 oz | 100 | 25 | 20 | – |
| ***Ocean Spray*** | | | | | |
| 100% Juice | 8 oz | 100 | 24 | 23 | 0 |
| 100% Juice Pink | 8 oz | 110 | 28 | 28 | 0 |

| FOOD | PORTION | CALS | CARB | SUGAR | FIBER |
|---|---|---|---|---|---|
| Ruby Red Drink | 8 oz | 130 | 33 | 33 | 0 |
| ***Odwalla*** | | | | | |
| Juice | 8 fl oz | 90 | 20 | 16 | 0 |
| ***Tropicana*** | | | | | |
| Golden | 8 oz | 90 | 22 | – | – |
| Ruby Red | 8 oz | 90 | 22 | – | – |
| Season's Best | 8 oz | 90 | 22 | – | – |
| Twister Pink | 1 bottle (10 oz) | 140 | 34 | – | – |
| W/ Double Vitamin C | 8 fl oz | 110 | 27 | – | – |
| **GRAPES** | | | | | |
| fresh | 10 | 36 | 9 | – | tr |
| thompson seedless in heavy syrup | ½ cup | 94 | 25 | – | – |
| thompson seedless water pack | ½ cup | 48 | 13 | – | – |
| ***Chiquita*** | | | | | |
| Grapes | 1½ cups (4.8 oz) | 90 | 24 | 23 | 1 |
| **GRAVY** | | | | | |
| **CANNED** | | | | | |
| au jus | 1 cup | 38 | 6 | – | – |
| beef | 1 cup | 124 | 11 | – | – |
| beef | 1 can (10 oz) | 155 | 14 | – | – |
| chicken | 1 cup | 189 | 13 | – | – |
| mushroom | 1 cup | 120 | 13 | – | – |
| turkey | 1 cup | 122 | 12 | – | – |
| ***Campbell's*** | | | | | |
| Beef | ¼ cup | 29 | 4 | 1 | tr |
| Brown | ¼ cup | 46 | 4 | 1 | 1 |
| Chicken | ¼ cup | 42 | 4 | tr | 1 |
| Turkey | ¼ cup | 29 | 3 | tr | tr |
| **MIX** | | | | | |
| au jus as prep w/ water | 1 cup | 32 | 4 | – | – |
| brown as prep w/ water | 1 cup | 75 | 13 | – | – |
| chicken as prep | 1 cup | 83 | 14 | – | – |
| mushroom as prep | 1 cup | 70 | 14 | – | – |
| onion as prep w/ water | 1 cup | 77 | 16 | – | – |
| pork as prep | 1 cup | 76 | 13 | – | – |
| turkey as prep | 1 cup | 87 | 15 | – | – |

| FOOD | PORTION | CALS | CARB | SUGAR | FIBER |
|---|---|---|---|---|---|
| ***Bournvita*** | | | | | |
| Extract | 2 heaping tsp | 34 | 7 | – | – |
| ***Bovril*** | | | | | |
| Extract | 1 heaping tsp | 9 | tr | – | 0 |
| ***Durkee*** | | | | | |
| Au Jus as prep | ¼ cup | 5 | 1 | 0 | 0 |
| Brown as prep | ¼ cup | 10 | 3 | 0 | 0 |
| Brown Mushroom as prep | ¼ cup | 15 | 3 | 0 | 0 |
| Brown Onion as prep | ¼ cup | 15 | 4 | 0 | 0 |
| Chicken as prep | ¼ cup | 20 | 4 | 0 | 0 |
| Country as prep | ¼ cup | 35 | 5 | 1 | 0 |
| Homestyle as prep | ¼ cup | 15 | 3 | 0 | 0 |
| Onion as prep | ¼ cup | 10 | 3 | 0 | 0 |
| Pork as prep | ¼ cup | 10 | 3 | 0 | 0 |
| Sausage as prep | ¼ cup | 35 | 5 | 1 | 0 |
| Swiss Steak as prep | ¼ cup | 15 | 4 | 0 | 0 |
| Turkey as prep | ¼ cup | 20 | 4 | 1 | 0 |
| ***French's*** | | | | | |
| Au Jus as prep | ¼ cup | 5 | 1 | 0 | 0 |
| Brown as prep | ¼ cup | 10 | 3 | 0 | 0 |
| Chicken as prep | ¼ cup | 25 | 4 | 0 | 0 |
| Country as prep | ¼ cup | 35 | 5 | 1 | 0 |
| Herb Brown as prep | ¼ cup | 15 | 3 | 0 | 0 |
| Homestyle as prep | ¼ cup | 10 | 3 | 0 | 0 |
| Mushroom as prep | ¼ cup | 10 | 3 | 0 | 0 |
| Onion | ¼ cup | 15 | 4 | 0 | 0 |
| Pork as prep | ¼ cup | 10 | 3 | 0 | 0 |
| Turkey as prep | ¼ cup | 20 | 4 | 1 | 0 |
| ***Loma Linda*** | | | | | |
| Gravy Quik Brown | 1 tbsp (5 g) | 20 | 4 | 0 | 0 |
| Gravy Quik Chicken | 1 tbsp (5 g) | 20 | 3 | 0 | 0 |
| Quik Gravy Country | 1 tbsp (5 g) | 25 | 4 | 0 | 0 |
| Quik Gravy Mushroom | 1 tbsp (5 g) | 15 | 3 | 0 | tr |
| Quik Gravy Onion | 1 tbsp (5 g) | 20 | 3 | 0 | tr |
| ***Marmite*** | | | | | |
| Extract | 1 heaping tsp | 9 | tr | – | – |
| ***McCormick*** | | | | | |
| Au Jus Natural as prep | ¼ cup | 5 | 1 | – | – |
| Beef & Herb as prep | ¼ cup | 30 | 3 | 1 | – |
| Brown as prep | ¼ cup | 20 | 3 | – | – |

| FOOD | PORTION | CALS | CARB | SUGAR | FIBER |
|---|---|---|---|---|---|
| Chicken as prep | ¼ cup | 20 | 4 | 1 | – |
| Onion as prep | ¼ cup | 20 | 3 | – | – |
| Pork as prep | ¼ cup | 20 | 4 | 1 | – |
| Turkey as prep | ¼ cup | 20 | 3 | 1 | – |
| **GREAT NORTHERN BEANS** | | | | | |
| canned | 1 cup | 299 | 55 | – | 13 |
| dried cooked | 1 cup | 20921 | 37 | – | 12 |
| ***Eden*** | | | | | |
| Organic | ½ cup (4.6 oz) | 110 | 20 | 1 | 8 |
| **GREEN BEANS** | | | | | |
| **CANNED** | | | | | |
| green beans | ½ cup | 13 | 3 | – | 1 |
| italian | ½ cup | 13 | 3 | – | 1 |
| italian low sodium | ½ cup | 13 | 3 | – | 1 |
| low sodium | ½ cup | 13 | 3 | – | 1 |
| ***Del Monte*** | | | | | |
| Cut | ½ cup (4.2 oz) | 20 | 4 | 2 | 2 |
| Cut Italian | ½ cup (4.2 oz) | 30 | 6 | 2 | 3 |
| Cut No Salt Added | ½ cup (4.2 oz) | 20 | 4 | 2 | 2 |
| French Style | ½ cup (4.2 oz) | 20 | 4 | 2 | 2 |
| French Style No Salt Added | ½ cup (4.2 oz) | 20 | 4 | 2 | 2 |
| French Style Seasoned | ½ cup (4.2 oz) | 20 | 4 | 2 | 2 |
| Whole | ½ cup (4.2 oz) | 20 | 4 | 2 | 2 |
| ***S&W*** | | | | | |
| Blue Lake Cut | ½ cup (4.2 oz) | 20 | 4 | 2 | 2 |
| French Style | ½ cup (4.2 oz) | 20 | 4 | 2 | 2 |
| Whole Small | ½ cup (4.2 oz) | 20 | 4 | 2 | 2 |
| ***Veg-All*** | | | | | |
| French Style | ½ cup | 20 | 4 | 2 | 2 |
| **FRESH** | | | | | |
| cooked | ½ cup | 22 | 5 | – | – |
| raw | ½ cup | 17 | 4 | – | 1 |
| **FROZEN** | | | | | |
| cooked | ½ cup | 18 | 4 | – | – |
| italian cooked | ½ cup | 18 | 4 | – | – |
| ***Fresh Like*** | | | | | |
| Cut | 3.5 oz | 29 | 7 | – | 1 |
| French Cut | 3.5 oz | 29 | 7 | – | 1 |

| FOOD | PORTION | CALS | CARB | SUGAR | FIBER |
|---|---|---|---|---|---|
| ***Tree Of Life*** | | | | | |
| Cut | ⅔ cup (2.8 oz) | 25 | 4 | 2 | 2 |
| **GROUNDCHERRIES** | | | | | |
| fresh | ½ cup | 37 | 8 | – | – |
| **GROUPER** | | | | | |
| cooked | 3 oz | 100 | 0 | 0 | 0 |
| cooked | 1 fillet (7.1 oz) | 238 | 0 | 0 | 0 |
| **GUAR GUM** | | | | | |
| ***Bob's Red Mill*** | | | | | |
| Guar Gum | 1 tbsp | 20 | 6 | 0 | 6 |
| **GUAVA** | | | | | |
| fresh | 1 | 45 | 11 | – | – |
| guava sauce | ½ cup | 43 | 11 | – | – |
| **GUAVA JUICE** | | | | | |
| ***Nantucket Nectars*** | | | | | |
| Guava | 8 oz | 130 | 33 | 29 | 0 |
| **GUINEA HEN** | | | | | |
| w/ skin raw | ½ hen (12.1 oz) | 545 | 0 | 0 | 0 |
| w/o skin raw | ½ hen (9.3 oz) | 292 | 0 | 0 | 0 |
| **HADDOCK** | | | | | |
| fresh cooked | 1 fillet (5.3 oz) | 168 | 0 | 0 | 0 |
| fresh cooked | 3 oz | 95 | 0 | 0 | 0 |
| fresh raw | 3 oz | 74 | 0 | 0 | 0 |
| roe raw | 1 oz | 37 | tr | – | – |
| smoked | 1 oz | 33 | 0 | 0 | 0 |
| smoked | 3 oz | 99 | 0 | 0 | 0 |
| **TAKE-OUT** | | | | | |
| breaded & fried | 1 piece (3.5 oz) | 187 | 3 | 0 | tr |
| **HALIBUT** | | | | | |
| atlantic & pacific cooked | ½ fillet (5.6 oz) | 223 | 0 | 0 | 0 |
| atlantic & pacific cooked | 3 oz | 119 | 0 | 0 | 0 |
| atlantic & pacific raw | 3 oz | 93 | 0 | 0 | 0 |

| FOOD | PORTION | CALS | CARB | SUGAR | FIBER |
|---|---|---|---|---|---|
| greenland baked | 3 oz | 203 | 0 | 0 | 0 |
| greenland baked | 5.6 oz | 380 | 0 | 0 | 0 |
| **HALVA** *(see SESAME)* | | | | | |
| **HAM** | | | | | |
| canned extra lean roasted | 3 oz | 116 | tr | – | 0 |
| center slice country style lean roasted | 4 oz | 220 | tr | – | 0 |
| chopped canned | 1 oz | 68 | tr | – | – |
| ham & cheese loaf | 1 oz | 73 | 1 | – | – |
| ham & cheese spread | 1 tbsp | 37 | tr | – | – |
| ham salad spread | 1 tbsp | 32 | 2 | – | – |
| minced | 1 oz | 75 | 1 | – | – |
| patty cooked | 1 patty (2 oz) | 203 | 1 | – | 0 |
| prosciutto | 1 oz | 55 | tr | – | 0 |
| sliced extra lean 5% fat | 1 oz | 37 | tr | – | – |
| sliced regular 11% fat | 1 oz | 52 | 1 | – | – |
| steak boneless extra lean | 1 (2 oz) | 69 | 0 | 0 | 0 |
| westphalian smoked | 1 oz | 105 | 0 | 0 | 0 |
| ***Alpine Lace*** | | | | | |
| Boneless Cooked 98% Fat Free | 2 slices (2 oz) | 60 | 2 | 1 | 0 |
| Honey Ham 98% Fat Free | 2 slices (2 oz) | 60 | 2 | 1 | 0 |
| Smoked Virginia 98% Fat Free | 2 slices (2 oz) | 60 | 2 | 1 | 0 |
| ***Armour*** | | | | | |
| Chopped Ham canned | 2 oz | 130 | 1 | 1 | 0 |
| Deviled Ham Spread | 1 pkg (3 oz) | 210 | 0 | 0 | 0 |
| Lean Slices Brown Sugar | 1 pkg (2.5 oz) | 90 | 4 | 1 | – |
| ***Boar's Head*** | | | | | |
| Black Forest Smoked | 2 oz | 60 | 2 | 2 | 0 |
| Cappy | 2 oz | 60 | 3 | 2 | 0 |
| Deluxe | 2 oz | 60 | 2 | 2 | 0 |
| Deluxe Lowered Sodium | 2 oz | 50 | tr | 0 | 0 |
| Maple Glazed Honey | 2 oz | 60 | 3 | 3 | 0 |
| Pepper | 2 oz | 60 | 2 | 1 | 0 |
| Rosemary & Sundried Tomato | 2 oz | 70 | 2 | 0 | 0 |
| Sweet Slice Smoked | 3 oz | 100 | 1 | 0 | 0 |
| Virginia | 2 oz | 60 | 3 | 3 | 0 |
| Virginia Smoked | 2 oz | 60 | 2 | 2 | 0 |
| ***Carl Buddig*** | | | | | |
| Ham Sliced w/ Natural Juices | 1 pkg (2.5 oz) | 120 | 1 | 1 | – |

| FOOD | PORTION | CALS | CARB | SUGAR | FIBER |
|---|---|---|---|---|---|
| Honey Ham Sliced w/ Natural Juice | 1 pkg (2.5 oz) | 120 | 3 | 3 | – |
| Lean Slices Oven Roasted Honey Ham | 1 pkg (2.5 oz) | 90 | 4 | 4 | – |
| Lean Slices Smoked | 1 pkg (2.5 oz) | 80 | 1 | 1 | – |
| ***Hillshire*** | | | | | |
| Deli Select Honey Ham | 6 slices (2 oz) | 60 | 2 | 2 | 0 |
| ***Oscar Mayer*** | | | | | |
| Lunchables Ham Bagels | 1 pkg | 410 | 64 | 27 | 2 |
| Lunchables Ham Wraps | 1 pkg | 430 | 64 | 25 | 2 |
| ***Wampler*** | | | | | |
| Black Forest | 2 oz | 60 | 2 | – | – |
| **HAM DISHES** | | | | | |
| **TAKE-OUT** | | | | | |
| croquettes | 1 (3.1 oz) | 217 | 11 | – | tr |
| salad | ½ cup | 287 | 5 | – | tr |
| **HAM SUBSTITUTES** | | | | | |
| ***Yves*** | | | | | |
| Veggie Ham Deli Slices | 1 serv (2.2 oz) | 80 | 6 | 2 | 1 |
| **HAMBURGER** | | | | | |
| ***Kid Cuisine*** | | | | | |
| Buckaroo Beef Patty Sandwich w/ Cheese | 1 meal (8.5 oz) | 410 | 58 | 27 | 4 |
| **TAKE-OUT** | | | | | |
| double patty w/ bun | 1 reg | 544 | 43 | – | – |
| double patty w/ cheese & bun | 1 reg | 457 | 22 | – | – |
| double patty w/ cheese & double bun | 1 reg | 461 | 44 | – | – |
| double patty w/ cheese ketchup mayonnaise onion pickle tomato & bun | 1 reg | 416 | 35 | – | – |
| double patty w/ ketchup mayonnaise onion pickle tomato & bun | 1 reg | 649 | 53 | – | – |
| double patty w/ ketchup cheese mayonnaise mustard pickle tomato & bun | 1 lg | 706 | 40 | – | – |
| double patty w/ ketchup mustard mayonnaise onion pickle tomato & bun | 1 lg | 540 | 40 | – | – |
| double patty w/ ketchup mustard onion pickle & bun | 1 reg | 576 | 39 | – | – |

| FOOD | PORTION | CALS | CARB | SUGAR | FIBER |
|---|---|---|---|---|---|
| single patty w/ bacon ketchup cheese mustard onion pickle & bun | 1 lg | 609 | 37 | – | – |
| single patty w/ bun | 1 reg | 275 | 31 | – | – |
| single patty w/ bun | 1 lg | 400 | 25 | – | – |
| single patty w/ cheese & bun | 1 reg | 320 | 32 | – | – |
| single patty w/ cheese & bun | 1 lg | 608 | 47 | – | – |
| single patty w/ ketchup cheese ham mayonnaise pickle tomato & bun | 1 lg | 745 | 38 | – | – |
| single patty w/ ketchup mustard mayonnaise onion pickle tomato & bun | 1 reg | 279 | 27 | – | – |
| triple patty w/ cheese & bun | 1 lg | 769 | 27 | – | – |
| triple patty w/ ketchup mustard pickle & bun | 1 lg | 693 | 29 | – | – |

## HAMBURGER SUBSTITUTES *(see also* MEAT SUBSTITUTES*)*

| FOOD | PORTION | CALS | CARB | SUGAR | FIBER |
|---|---|---|---|---|---|
| ***Amy's*** | | | | | |
| All American Burger | 1 (2.5 oz) | 120 | 15 | 2 | 3 |
| California Burger | 1 (2.5 oz) | 130 | 19 | 2 | 5 |
| Chicago Burger | 1 (2.5 oz) | 160 | 20 | 2 | 3 |
| ***Boca Burgers*** | | | | | |
| Flamed Grilled | 1 | 120 | 6 | 0 | 4 |
| ***Franklin Farms*** | | | | | |
| Veggiburger Portabella | 1 (3 oz) | 120 | 11 | 3 | 4 |
| ***Gardenburger*** | | | | | |
| Classic Greek | 1 (2.5 oz) | 120 | 17 | 2 | 2 |
| Fire Roasted Vegetable | 1 (2.5 oz) | 120 | 17 | 2 | 2 |
| ***Harmony Farms*** | | | | | |
| Soy Burger Onion | 1 (2.5 oz) | 90 | 7 | 1 | 3 |
| Soy Burgers Garlic | 1 (2.5 oz) | 110 | 10 | 1 | 23 |
| Soy Burgers Mushroom | 1 (2.5 oz) | 110 | 9 | 1 | 3 |
| Soy Burgers Original | 1 (2.5 oz) | 110 | 7 | 1 | 4 |
| ***Lightlife*** | | | | | |
| Barbecue Grilles | 1 patty (2.7 oz) | 120 | 11 | 3 | 0 |
| Lemon Grilles | 1 patty (2.7 oz) | 140 | 11 | 2 | 0 |
| Light Burgers | 1 (3 oz) | 130 | 12 | 2 | 2 |
| Tamari Grilles | 1 patty (2.7 oz) | 120 | 9 | 2 | 0 |

| FOOD | PORTION | CALS | CARB | SUGAR | FIBER |
|---|---|---|---|---|---|
| ***Loma Linda*** | | | | | |
| Patty Mix not prep | ⅓ cup (0.9 oz) | 90 | 7 | 0 | 5 |
| Redi-Burger | ⅝ in slice (3 oz) | 120 | 7 | 1 | 4 |
| Vege-Burger | ¼ cup (1.9 oz) | 70 | 2 | 0 | 2 |
| ***Morningstar Farms*** | | | | | |
| Better'n Burger | 1 (2.7 oz) | 80 | 8 | tr | 3 |
| Garden Grille | 1 patty (2.5 oz) | 120 | 18 | 1 | 4 |
| Garden Veggie Patties | 1 patty (2.4 oz) | 100 | 9 | 1 | 4 |
| Hard Rock Cafe Veggie Burger | 1 (3 oz) | 170 | 18 | 3 | 3 |
| Harvest Burger Italian Style | 1 patty (3.2 oz) | 140 | 8 | tr | 5 |
| Harvest Burger Original | 1 (3.2 oz) | 140 | 8 | tr | 5 |
| Harvest Burger Southwestern | 1 (3.2 oz) | 140 | 9 | 1 | 5 |
| Spicy Black Bean Burger | 1 (2.7 oz) | 110 | 16 | 2 | 5 |
| ***Natural Touch*** | | | | | |
| Garden Veggie Pattie | 1 (2.4 oz) | 110 | 8 | 0 | 3 |
| Okara Pattie | 1 (2.2 oz) | 110 | 4 | 0 | 3 |
| Original Veggie Burger Kit not prep | ¼ pkg (0.8 oz) | 80 | 6 | 0 | 4 |
| Southwestern Veggie Burger Kit not prep | ¼ pkg (0.9 oz) | 90 | 9 | tr | 4 |
| Spicy Black Bean Burger | 1 (2.7 oz) | 100 | 15 | 2 | 5 |
| Vegan Burger | 1 (2.7 oz) | 70 | 6 | 0 | 3 |
| ***Superburgers*** | | | | | |
| Vegan Organic Original | 1 (3 oz) | 98 | 14 | 0 | 2 |
| Vegan Organic Smoked | 1 (3 oz) | 98 | 14 | 0 | 2 |
| Vegan Organic TexMex | 1 (3 oz) | 110 | 14 | 0 | 3 |
| ***V'dora*** | | | | | |
| Vegetable Burger Lites | 1 (3.3 oz) | 58 | 4 | 1 | 0 |
| ***Worthington*** | | | | | |
| Grainburger not prep | 3 tbsp (0.6 oz) | 60 | 3 | 0 | 2 |
| Prosage Patties | 1 (1.3 oz) | 80 | 3 | 0 | 2 |
| ***Yves*** | | | | | |
| Black Bean & Mushroom Burgers | 1 (3 oz) | 100 | 13 | 1 | 7 |
| Garden Vegetable Patties | 1 (3 oz) | 90 | 11 | 1 | 7 |
| Veggie Burger | 1 (3 oz) | 119 | 9 | 2 | 4 |

| FOOD | PORTION | CALS | CARB | SUGAR | FIBER |
|---|---|---|---|---|---|
| **HAZELNUTS** | | | | | |
| dried blanched | 1 oz | 191 | 5 | – | – |
| dried unblanched | 1 oz | 179 | 4 | – | – |
| dry roasted unblanched | 1 oz | 188 | 5 | – | – |
| oil roasted unblanched | 1 oz | 187 | 5 | – | 2 |
| ***Low Carb Creations*** | | | | | |
| Soft Hazelnut Brittle Brittle | 2 pieces (1 oz) | 160 | 16 | 1 | 1 |
| ***Torras*** | | | | | |
| Hazelnut Chocolate Spread | 1 tsp | 27 | 3 | 0 | 0 |
| ***Twist*** | | | | | |
| Sugar Free Chocolate Hazelnut Spread | 2 tbsp | 180 | 2 | 0 | 0 |
| **HEART** | | | | | |
| beef simmered | 3 oz | 148 | tr | – | – |
| chicken simmered | 1 cup (5 oz) | 268 | tr | – | – |
| lamb braised | 3 oz | 158 | 2 | – | – |
| pork braised | 1 cup | 215 | 1 | – | 0 |
| pork braised | 1 | 191 | 1 | – | 0 |
| turkey simmered | 1 cup (5 oz) | 257 | 3 | – | – |
| veal braised | 3 oz | 158 | tr | – | – |
| **HEARTS OF PALM** | | | | | |
| canned | 1 cup (5.1 oz) | 41 | 7 | – | – |
| canned | 1 (1.2 oz) | 9 | 2 | – | – |
| **HEMP** | | | | | |
| ***HempNut*** | | | | | |
| Shelled Hempseed | 1 oz | 162 | 3 | 1 | 2 |
| ***Nutiva*** | | | | | |
| Hempseed | 1½ tbsp (0.5 oz) | 70 | 3 | 0 | 2 |
| **HERBAL TEA** *(see TEA/HERBAL TEA)* | | | | | |
| **HERBS/SPICES** *(see also individual names)* | | | | | |
| chinese five spice | 1 tsp | 7 | 2 | – | tr |
| curry powder | 1 tsp | 6 | 1 | – | – |
| garam masala | 1 tsp | 8 | 1 | – | – |
| poultry seasoning | 1 tsp | 5 | 1 | – | – |
| pumpkin pie spice | 1 tsp | 6 | 1 | – | – |

| FOOD | PORTION | CALS | CARB | SUGAR | FIBER |
|---|---|---|---|---|---|
| ***Eden*** | | | | | |
| Furikake Seasoning | ½ tsp | 5 | 1 | 0 | 1 |
| ***Gringo Billy's*** | | | | | |
| Meat Rubs Chipotle | ¼ tsp | 0 | 0 | 0 | 0 |
| Meat Rubs Ultimate | ¼ tsp | 0 | 0 | 0 | 0 |
| Tuna Seasoning | 1 tsp | 5 | 1 | 0 | 1 |
| ***Instant India*** | | | | | |
| Curry Paste Cilantro Garlic | 2 tbsp (1 oz) | 110 | 4 | 2 | 0 |
| Curry Paste Ginger Garlic | 2 tbsp (1 oz) | 90 | 8 | 6 | 0 |
| ***McCormick*** | | | | | |
| Big'n Season Buffalo Wings | 1 tbsp (8 g) | 30 | 5 | 3 | – |
| Big'n Season Chicken | 1 tbsp (6 g) | 20 | 3 | – | – |
| Big'n Season Pot Roast | 1 tsp | 10 | 1 | – | – |
| Blends Bon Appetit | ¼ tsp | 0 | 0 | 0 | 0 |
| Cajun Seasoning | ¼ tsp | 0 | 0 | 0 | 0 |
| Greek Seasoning | ¼ tsp | 0 | 0 | 0 | 0 |
| Jamaican Jerk Seasoning | ¼ tsp | 0 | 0 | 0 | 0 |
| Meat Loaf Seasoning | 1 tsp (4 g) | 15 | 2 | 2 | – |
| Seafood Seasoning | ¼ tsp | 0 | 0 | 0 | 0 |
| ***Mrs. Dash*** | | | | | |
| Classic Italian | ¼ tsp | 0 | 0 | 0 | 0 |
| Extra Spicy | ¼ tsp | 0 | 0 | 0 | 0 |
| Garlic & Herb | ¼ tsp | 0 | 0 | 0 | 0 |
| Grilling Blend Mesquite | ¼ tsp | 0 | 0 | 0 | 0 |
| Grilling Blend Original Chicken | ¼ tsp | 0 | 0 | 0 | 0 |
| Grilling Blend Original Steak | ¼ tsp | 0 | 0 | 0 | 0 |
| Lemon Pepper | ¼ tsp | 0 | 0 | 0 | 0 |
| Minced Onion Medley | ¼ tsp | 0 | 0 | 0 | 0 |
| Original Blend | ¼ tsp | 0 | 0 | 0 | 0 |
| Table Blend | ¼ tsp | 0 | 0 | 0 | 0 |
| Tomato Basil Garlic | ¼ tsp | 0 | 0 | 0 | 0 |
| **HERRING** | | | | | |
| atlantic cooked | 3 oz | 172 | 0 | 0 | 0 |
| atlantic cooked | 1 fillet (5 oz) | 290 | 0 | 0 | 0 |
| atlantic raw | 3 oz | 134 | 0 | 0 | 0 |
| pacific baked | 3 oz | 213 | 0 | 0 | 0 |
| pacific fillet baked | 5.1 oz | 360 | 0 | 0 | 0 |
| roe canned | 1 oz | 34 | tr | – | – |
| roe raw | 1 oz | 37 | tr | – | – |

| FOOD | PORTION | CALS | CARB | SUGAR | FIBER |
|---|---|---|---|---|---|
| smoked | 3.5 oz | 210 | 0 | 0 | 0 |
| **TAKE-OUT** | | | | | |
| atlantic kippered | 1 fillet (1.4 oz) | 87 | 0 | 0 | 0 |
| atlantic pickled | ½ oz | 39 | 1 | – | – |
| fried | 1 serv (3.5 oz) | 233 | 2 | – | 0 |
| **HICKORY NUTS** | | | | | |
| dried | 1 oz | 187 | 5 | – | – |
| **HOMINY** | | | | | |
| **CANNED** | | | | | |
| white | 1 cup (5.6 oz) | 482 | 23 | – | 4 |
| ***Van Camp*** | | | | | |
| Golden | ½ cup (4.3 oz) | 80 | 17 | 0 | 1 |
| White | ½ cup (4.3 oz) | 80 | 16 | 0 | 1 |
| **HONEY** | | | | | |
| honey | 1 cup (11.9 oz) | 1031 | 279 | 270 | – |
| honey | 1 tbsp (0.7 oz) | 64 | 17 | 17 | – |
| orange blossom | 1 tbsp | 60 | 17 | 16 | 0 |
| wild honey | 1 tbsp | 60 | 17 | 16 | – |
| ***Steel's*** | | | | | |
| Sugar Free | 1 tbsp | 24 | 6 | 0 | 0 |
| ***SueBee*** | | | | | |
| Clover | 1 tbsp | 60 | 17 | 16 | – |
| **HONEYDEW** | | | | | |
| **FRESH** | | | | | |
| cubed | 1 cup | 60 | 16 | – | – |
| wedge | 1/10 | 46 | 12 | – | – |
| ***Chiquita*** | | | | | |
| Wedge | 1/10 melon (4.7 oz) | 50 | 13 | 12 | 1 |
| **HORSE** | | | | | |
| roasted | 3 oz | 149 | 0 | 0 | 0 |
| **HORSERADISH** | | | | | |
| japanese wasabi | ¼ tsp | 1 | tr | – | 0 |
| wasabi root raw | 1 (5.9 oz) | 184 | 40 | – | 12 |
| wasabi root raw sliced | 1 cup (4.6 oz) | 142 | 31 | – | 10 |

| FOOD | PORTION | CALS | CARB | SUGAR | FIBER |
|---|---|---|---|---|---|
| ***Boar's Head*** | | | | | |
| Horseradish | 1 tsp (5 g) | 5 | 0 | 0 | 0 |
| ***Eden*** | | | | | |
| Wasabi Powder | 1 tsp | 10 | 1 | 0 | 1 |
| **HOT COCOA** | | | | | |
| mix as prep w/ water | 7 oz | 103 | 23 | – | – |
| mix w/ equal as prep w/ water | 7 oz | 48 | 9 | – | – |
| ***Carnation*** | | | | | |
| Hot Cocoa 70 calorie | 1 pkg (0.7 oz) | 70 | 15 | 15 | tr |
| Hot Cocoa Double Chocolate Meltdown | 1 pkg (1.2 oz) | 150 | 27 | 24 | 1 |
| Hot Cocoa Fat Free Raspberry | 1 pkg (0.3 oz) | 30 | 4 | 3 | 1 |
| Hot Cocoa Fat Free w/ Marshmallows | 1 pkg (0.4 oz) | 45 | 10 | 7 | tr |
| Hot Cocoa Lactose Free | 1 pkg (1 oz) | 120 | 25 | 19 | 1 |
| Hot Cocoa Marshmallow Blizzard | 1 pkg (1.5 oz) | 180 | 39 | 33 | tr |
| Hot Cocoa Milk Chocolate | 3 tbsp (1 oz) | 110 | 24 | 20 | tr |
| Hot Cocoa Rich Chocolate | 3 tbsp (1 oz) | 110 | 24 | 21 | tr |
| Hot Cocoa Rich Chocolate Fat Free | 1 pkg (0.3 oz) | 25 | 4 | 3 | 1 |
| Hot Cocoa Rich Chocolate No Sugar Added | 3 tbsp (0.5 oz) | 50 | 8 | 7 | tr |
| Hot Cocoa Rich Chocolate w/ Marshmallows | 3 tbsp (1 oz) | 110 | 24 | 21 | tr |
| ***Keto*** | | | | | |
| Hot Cocoa | 1 tsp | 12 | 2 | 0 | 1 |
| ***Nestle*** | | | | | |
| Hot Cocoa Rich Chocolate | 1 pkg (1 oz) | 110 | 24 | 19 | tr |
| Hot Cocoa Rich w/ Marshmallows | 1 pkg (1 oz) | 110 | 24 | 19 | tr |
| ***Sipper Sweets*** | | | | | |
| Sugar Free Low Carb Mix | 1 serv | 50 | 3 | 0 | 0 |
| ***Swiss Miss*** | | | | | |
| Hot Cocoa And Cream | 1 serv | 153 | 25 | 21 | 1 |
| Hot Cocoa Chocolate Sensation | 1 serv | 148 | 27 | 23 | 1 |
| Hot Cocoa Diet | 1 serv | 22 | 4 | 2 | 1 |
| Hot Cocoa Fat Free | 1 serv | 52 | 9 | 7 | 1 |

| FOOD | PORTION | CALS | CARB | SUGAR | FIBER |
|---|---|---|---|---|---|
| Hot Cocoa Fat Free Marshmallow Lovers | 1 serv | 65 | 13 | 10 | 1 |
| Hot Cocoa Lite | 1 serv | 76 | 18 | 15 | 2 |
| Hot Cocoa Marshmallow Lovers | 1 serv | 142 | 27 | 22 | 1 |
| Hot Cocoa Milk Chocolate | 1 serv | 118 | 22 | 16 | 1 |
| Hot Cocoa Milk Chocolate No Sugar Added | 1 serv | 55 | 10 | 6 | 1 |
| Hot Cocoa Milk Chocolate w/ Marshmallows | 1 serv | 118 | 22 | 17 | 1 |
| Hot Cocoa Rich Chocolate | 1 serv | 110 | 23 | 21 | 1 |
| Hot Cocoa White Chocolate | 1 serv | 109 | 21 | 21 | tr |
| Hot Cocoa w/ Marshmallows No Sugar Added | 1 serv | 56 | 10 | 6 | 1 |
| Premiere Hot Cocoa Almond Mocha | 1 serv | 144 | 28 | 26 | 1 |
| Premiere Hot Cocoa English Toffee | 1 serv | 142 | 29 | 26 | 4 |
| Premiere Hot Cocoa Raspberry Truffle | 1 serv | 144 | 28 | 26 | 1 |
| Premiere Hot Cocoa Suisse Truffle | 1 serv | 142 | 28 | 26 | 1 |
| Rich Hot Cocoa No Sugar Added | 1 serv | 54 | 10 | 6 | 1 |
| Sidewalk Cafe Cappuccino | 1 serv | 119 | 18 | 17 | 1 |
| Sidewalk Cafe Cinnamon | 1 serv | 126 | 21 | 20 | 1 |
| Sidewalk Cafe French Vanilla | 1 serv | 121 | 19 | 15 | tr |
| Sidewalk Cafe Mocha | 1 serv | 120 | 20 | 19 | 1 |
| ***Weight Watchers*** | | | | | |
| Hot Cocoa Mix as prep | 1 pkg | 70 | 7 | 6 | 1 |
| **TAKE-OUT** | | | | | |
| hot cocoa | 1 cup | 218 | 26 | – | – |
| mexican hot chocolate | 1 cup | 173 | 20 | – | 1 |

## HOT DOG

| FOOD | PORTION | CALS | CARB | SUGAR | FIBER |
|---|---|---|---|---|---|
| beef | 1 (2 oz) | 180 | 1 | – | – |
| beef | 1 (1.5) | 142 | 1 | – | – |
| beef & pork | 1 (2 oz) | 183 | 1 | – | – |
| beef & pork | 1 (1.5 oz) | 144 | 1 | – | – |
| chicken | 1 (1.5 oz) | 116 | 3 | – | – |
| pork cheesefurter smokie | 1 (1.5 oz) | 141 | 1 | – | – |

| FOOD | PORTION | CALS | CARB | SUGAR | FIBER |
|---|---|---|---|---|---|
| turkey | 1 (1.5 oz) | 102 | 1 | – | – |
| ***Boar's Head*** | | | | | |
| Beef | 1 (2 oz) | 160 | 1 | 0 | 0 |
| Beef Lite | 1 (1.6 oz) | 90 | 0 | 0 | 0 |
| Pork & Beef | 1 (2 oz) | 150 | 0 | 0 | 0 |
| ***Health Is Wealth*** | | | | | |
| Uncured Beef | 1 (1.5 oz) | 80 | 1 | – | – |
| Uncured Chicken | 1 (1.5 oz) | 100 | 1 | – | – |
| ***Healthy Choice*** | | | | | |
| Beef Low Fat | 1 (1.8 oz) | 70 | 7 | 2 | 0 |
| Low Fat Turkey Pork Beef | 1 (1.4 oz) | 60 | 5 | 1 | – |
| ***Kid Cuisine*** | | | | | |
| Mystical Mini Corn Dogs | 4 pieces | 230 | 18 | 7 | 0 |
| ***Organic Valley*** | | | | | |
| All-Natural Beef | 1 (1.6 oz) | 90 | 1 | – | – |
| ***Oscar Mayer*** | | | | | |
| Fat Free Turkey & Beef | 1 (1.8 oz) | 40 | 3 | 1 | 0 |
| Light Beef | 1 (1.6 oz) | 90 | 2 | tr | – |
| ***Wampler*** | | | | | |
| Chicken | 1 (2 oz) | 120 | 0 | 0 | 1 |
| **TAKE-OUT** | | | | | |
| corndog | 1 | 460 | 56 | – | – |
| w/ bun chili | 1 | 297 | 31 | – | – |
| w/ bun plain | 1 | 242 | 18 | – | – |
| **HOT DOG SUBSTITUTES** | | | | | |
| ***Lightlife*** | | | | | |
| Smart Deli Jumbo's | 1 link (2.7 oz) | 80 | 4 | 1 | 1 |
| Smart Dogs | 1 (1.5 oz) | 45 | 2 | 0 | 0 |
| Tofu Pups | 1 (1.4 oz) | 60 | 2 | 0 | 0 |
| Wonder Dogs | 1 (1.5 oz) | 60 | 2 | 0 | 0 |
| ***Loma Linda*** | | | | | |
| Big Franks | 1 (1.8 oz) | 110 | 2 | 0 | 2 |
| Big Franks Low Fat | 1 (1.8 oz) | 80 | 3 | 0 | 2 |
| Corn Dogs | 1 (2.5 oz) | 150 | 22 | 4 | 3 |
| ***Morningstar Farms*** | | | | | |
| America's Original Veggie Dog | 1 (2 oz) | 80 | 6 | 2 | 1 |
| Meatfree Corn Dog | 1 (2.5 oz) | 150 | 22 | 4 | 3 |
| Meatfree Mini Corn Dog | 4 (2.7 oz) | 170 | 21 | 6 | 1 |

| FOOD | PORTION | CALS | CARB | SUGAR | FIBER |
|---|---|---|---|---|---|
| ***Natural Touch*** | | | | | |
| Vege Frank | 1 (1.6 oz) | 100 | 2 | 0 | 2 |
| ***Quorn*** | | | | | |
| Meat-Free Dogs | 1 (1.5 oz) | 70 | 3 | 0 | 2 |
| ***Yves*** | | | | | |
| Good Dog | 1 (1.8 oz) | 70 | 2 | 1 | 1 |
| Tofu Dogs | 1 (1.3 oz) | 45 | 2 | 0 | 0 |
| Veggie Dogs | 1 (1.6 oz) | 60 | 1 | 0 | 1 |
| Veggie Dogs Chili | 1 (1.6 oz) | 50 | 3 | 1 | 2 |
| Veggie Dogs Jumbo | 1 (2.7 oz) | 100 | 7 | 1 | 2 |
| Veggie Dogs Jumbo Hot N' Spicy | 1 (2.7 oz) | 106 | 4 | 2 | 2 |
| **HUMMUS** | | | | | |
| hummus | 1 cup | 420 | 50 | – | – |
| **TAKE-OUT** | | | | | |
| hummus | ⅓ cup | 140 | 17 | – | – |
| **HYACINTH BEANS** | | | | | |
| dried cooked | 1 cup | 228 | 40 | – | – |
| **ICE CREAM AND FROZEN DESSERTS** (*see also* ICES AND ICE POPS, PUDDING POPS, SHERBET, YOGURT FROZEN) | | | | | |
| chocolate | ½ cup (4 fl oz) | 143 | 19 | 13 | – |
| dixie cup chocolate | 1 (3.5 fl oz) | 125 | 16 | 11 | – |
| dixie cup strawberry | 1 (3.5 fl oz) | 112 | 16 | 9 | – |
| dixie cup vanilla | 1 (3.5 fl oz) | 116 | 14 | 9 | – |
| strawberry | ½ cup (4 fl oz) | 127 | 18 | 10 | – |
| vanilla | ½ cup (4 fl oz) | 132 | 16 | 10 | – |
| vanilla soft serve | ½ cup | 111 | 19 | – | – |
| ***Atkins*** | | | | | |
| Endulge Butter Pecan | ½ cup | 170 | 12 | 1 | 4 |
| Endulge Chocolate | ½ cup | 140 | 13 | 1 | 5 |
| Endulge Chocolate Peanut Butter Swirl | ½ cup | 170 | 14 | 1 | 5 |
| Endulge Vanilla | ½ cup | 140 | 13 | 1 | 4 |
| Endulge Vanilla Fudge | ½ cup | 140 | 14 | 1 | 4 |
| Endulge Bars Chocolate Fudge | 1 bar | 130 | 12 | 1 | 5 |

| FOOD | PORTION | CALS | CARB | SUGAR | FIBER |
|---|---|---|---|---|---|
| Endulge Bars Chocolate Fudge Swirl | 1 bar | 180 | 12 | 1 | 4 |
| Endulge Bars Peanut Butter Swirl | 1 bar | 180 | 12 | 1 | 4 |
| Endulge Bars Vanilla Fudge Swirl | 1 bar | 180 | 12 | 1 | 4 |
| ***Better Than Ice Creme*** | | | | | |
| Soy Vanilla as prep | ½ cup | 110 | 21 | 8 | 0 |
| ***Bon Bons*** | | | | | |
| Dark Chocolate | 5 pieces | 190 | 16 | 12 | 0 |
| Milk Chocolate | 5 pieces | 200 | 17 | 13 | 0 |
| ***Breyers*** | | | | | |
| Almond Joy | ½ cup | 140 | 20 | 16 | tr |
| Banana Fudge Chunk | ½ cup | 170 | 21 | 19 | tr |
| Butter Almond | ½ cup | 160 | 14 | 14 | tr |
| Butter Pecan | ½ cup | 170 | 14 | 14 | 0 |
| Butter Pecan Homemade | ½ cup | 170 | 18 | 13 | 0 |
| Butter Pecan No Sugar Added | ½ cup | 120 | 15 | 4 | tr |
| Caramel Praline Crunch | ½ cup | 180 | 22 | 19 | 0 |
| Caramel Toffee Crunch | ½ cup | 180 | 22 | 20 | 0 |
| CarbSmart Chocolate | ½ cup | 130 | 10 | 4 | 3 |
| CarbSmart Strawberry | ½ cup | 130 | 10 | 4 | 3 |
| CarbSmart Vanilla | ½ cup | 130 | 10 | 4 | 3 |
| Cherry Chocolate Chip | ½ cup | 150 | 18 | 17 | 0 |
| Cherry Vanilla | ½ cup | 140 | 16 | 16 | 0 |
| Chocolate | ½ cup | 150 | 17 | 16 | tr |
| Chocolate 98% Fat Free | ½ cup | 90 | 21 | 14 | 4 |
| Chocolate Caramel No Sugar Added | ½ cup | 110 | 16 | 4 | tr |
| Chocolate Chip | ½ cup | 160 | 17 | 17 | 0 |
| Chocolate Chip Cookie Dough | ½ cup | 170 | 20 | 17 | 0 |
| Chocolate Rainbow | ½ cup | 140 | 16 | 14 | 0 |
| Coffee | ½ cup | 140 | 15 | 15 | 0 |
| Cookies & Cream | ½ cup | 160 | 18 | 16 | tr |
| Creamsicle | ½ cup | 130 | 20 | 16 | 0 |
| Deep Chocolate Fudge | ½ cup | 200 | 21 | 19 | 1 |
| Dulce De Leche | ½ cup | 150 | 20 | 19 | 0 |
| French Vanilla | ½ cup | 150 | 15 | 15 | 0 |
| French Vanilla Light | ½ cup | 120 | 18 | 14 | 0 |
| French Vanilla No Sugar Added | ½ cup | 110 | 14 | 5 | 0 |

| FOOD | PORTION | CALS | CARB | SUGAR | FIBER |
|---|---|---|---|---|---|
| Fresa Banana | ½ cup | 140 | 20 | 16 | 0 |
| Heath English Toffee | ½ cup | 190 | 22 | 20 | 0 |
| Hershey w/ Almonds | ½ cup | 170 | 24 | 21 | tr |
| Ice Cream Cake Oreo | 1 slice | 190 | 21 | 17 | tr |
| Ice Cream Cake Vanilla | 1 slice | 190 | 19 | 16 | 0 |
| Klondike Sandwich | ½ cup | 160 | 21 | 15 | 0 |
| Mint Chocolate Chip | ½ cup | 160 | 17 | 17 | 0 |
| Mint Chocolate Chip Light | ½ cup | 130 | 20 | 18 | 0 |
| Mint Oreo | ½ cup | 170 | 23 | 17 | 0 |
| Mocha Almond Fudge | ½ cup | 170 | 18 | 15 | 2 |
| Oreo | ½ cup | 160 | 20 | 16 | 0 |
| Peach | ½ cup | 130 | 17 | 16 | 0 |
| Peanut Butter & Fudge | ½ cup | 170 | 17 | 15 | tr |
| Reese's Peanut Butter Cups | ½ cup | 180 | 22 | 18 | 0 |
| Rocky Road | ½ cup | 160 | 20 | 19 | tr |
| SpongeBob Cookie Dough | ½ cup | 160 | 21 | 17 | 0 |
| Strawberry | ½ cup | 120 | 15 | 15 | 0 |
| Strawberry Shortcake | ½ cup | 160 | 23 | 18 | 0 |
| Turtle Sundae | ½ cup | 190 | 20 | 17 | tr |
| Vanilla | ½ cup | 140 | 15 | 15 | 0 |
| Vanilla Calcium Rich | ½ cup | 130 | 14 | 14 | 0 |
| Vanilla Fudge Twirl | ½ cup | 140 | 18 | 15 | tr |
| Vanilla Homemade | ½ cup | 140 | 16 | 14 | 0 |
| Vanilla Lactose Free | ½ cup | 130 | 14 | 14 | 0 |
| Vanilla Light | ½ cup | 110 | 17 | 15 | 0 |
| Vanilla Light 2% Milk | ½ cup | 130 | 18 | 15 | 0 |
| Vanilla No Sugar Added | ½ cup | 100 | 15 | 4 | 0 |
| Vanilla Caramel Brownie | ½ cup | 170 | 20 | 17 | 0 |
| Vanilla Fudge Brownie | ½ cup | 180 | 19 | 16 | tr |
| Vanilla Fudge Twirl No Sugar Added | ½ cup | 110 | 19 | 4 | tr |
| Wild Berry Swirl | ½ cup | 140 | 16 | 16 | 0 |
| ***Butterfinger*** | | | | | |
| Bar | 1 (2.5 oz) | 190 | 16 | 14 | 0 |
| ***Carnation*** | | | | | |
| Cup Chocolate | 1 (3 oz) | 140 | 16 | 14 | 0 |
| Cup Chocolate Malt | 1 (12 oz) | 270 | 48 | 36 | 1 |
| Cup Strawberry | 1 (3 oz) | 100 | 12 | 10 | 0 |
| Cup Vanilla | 1 (3 oz) | 100 | 11 | 9 | 0 |
| Cup Vanilla | 1 (5 oz) | 170 | 19 | 16 | 0 |

| FOOD | PORTION | CALS | CARB | SUGAR | FIBER |
|---|---|---|---|---|---|
| Cup Vanilla Malt | 1 (12 oz) | 260 | 48 | 37 | 0 |
| Sundae Cup Strawberry | 1 (5 oz) | 200 | 29 | 23 | 0 |
| Sunday Cup Chocolate | 1 (5 oz) | 210 | 30 | 22 | 1 |
| ***Cool Creations*** | | | | | |
| Cookies & Cream Sandwich | 1 (3.5 oz) | 240 | 34 | 18 | 1 |
| Mickey Mouse Bar | 1 (2.5 oz) | 120 | 10 | 9 | 0 |
| Mini Sandwich | 1 (2.3 oz) | 110 | 16 | 8 | 0 |
| ***Dippin' Dots*** | | | | | |
| Dipping Dots Chocolate | ⅝ cup (3 oz) | 190 | 22 | 22 | 0 |
| ***Drumstick*** | | | | | |
| Cone Chocolate | 1 (4.6 oz) | 320 | 36 | 20 | 2 |
| Cone Chocolate Dipped | 1 (4.6 oz) | 320 | 40 | 20 | 1 |
| Cone Vanilla | 1 (4.6 oz) | 340 | 35 | 20 | 2 |
| Cone Vanilla Caramel | 1 (4.6 oz) | 360 | 38 | 24 | 2 |
| Cone Vanilla Fudge | 1 (4.6 oz) | 360 | 39 | 25 | 2 |
| ***Edy's*** | | | | | |
| 3 Musketeers | ½ cup | 160 | 22 | 19 | – |
| Dreamery Banana Split | ½ cup | 240 | 31 | 27 | 1 |
| Dreamery Black Raspberry Avalanche | ½ cup | 270 | 27 | 23 | 1 |
| Dreamery Caramel Toffee Bar Heaven | ½ cup | 290 | 32 | 29 | 0 |
| Dreamery Cashew Praline Parfait | ½ cup | 280 | 30 | 26 | 0 |
| Dreamery Chocolate Truffle Explosion | ½ cup | 280 | 31 | 27 | 1 |
| Dreamery Chocolate Peanut Butter Chunk | ½ cup | 310 | 29 | 25 | 2 |
| Dreamery Coney Island Waffle Cone | ½ cup | 310 | 32 | 28 | 1 |
| Dreamery Cool Mint | ½ cup | 300 | 32 | 29 | 1 |
| Dreamery Deep Dish Apple Pie | ½ cup | 280 | 34 | 28 | 0 |
| Dreamery Dulce De Leche | ½ cup | 270 | 32 | 30 | 0 |
| Dreamery Grandma's Cookie Dough | ½ cup | 300 | 32 | 25 | 0 |
| Dreamery Harvest Peach | ½ cup | 230 | 25 | 22 | 0 |
| Dreamery New York Strawberry Cheesecake | ½ cup | 260 | 27 | 23 | 0 |
| Dreamery Nothing But Chocolate | ½ cup | 280 | 34 | 28 | 1 |

| FOOD | PORTION | CALS | CARB | SUGAR | FIBER |
|---|---|---|---|---|---|
| Dreamery Nuts About Malt | ½ cup | 290 | 29 | 24 | 1 |
| Dreamery Raspberry Brownie A La Mode | ½ cup | 270 | 34 | 27 | 1 |
| Dreamery Raspberry Brownie A La Mode | ½ cup | 130 | 34 | 27 | 1 |
| Dreamery Strawberry Fields | ½ cup | 220 | 26 | 23 | 1 |
| Dreamery Tiramisu | ½ cup | 260 | 31 | 25 | 0 |
| Dreamery Vanilla | ½ cup | 260 | 25 | 24 | 0 |
| Grand Black Cherry Vanilla | ½ cup | 140 | 17 | 15 | – |
| Grand Blue Ribbon Chocolate Cake | ½ cup | 180 | 20 | 15 | – |
| Grand Butter Pecan | ½ cup | 170 | 16 | 13 | – |
| Grand Cherry Chocolate Chip | ½ cup | 160 | 19 | 16 | – |
| Grand Chocolate | ½ cup | 150 | 16 | 15 | – |
| Grand Chocolate Caramel Swirl | ½ cup | 170 | 19 | 16 | – |
| Grand Chocolate Chips | ½ cup | 170 | 18 | 15 | – |
| Grand Chocolate Fudge Mousse | ½ cup | 160 | 19 | 15 | – |
| Grand Chocolate Fudge Sundae | ½ cup | 170 | 20 | 16 | – |
| Grand Coffee | ½ cup | 140 | 15 | 13 | – |
| Grand Cookie Dough | ½ cup | 180 | 21 | 15 | – |
| Grand Cookies'N Cream | ½ cup | 160 | 19 | 14 | – |
| Grand Double Fudge Brownie | ½ cup | 170 | 19 | 15 | – |
| Grand Espresso Chip | ½ cup | 150 | 17 | 14 | – |
| Grand French Vanilla | ½ cup | 160 | 17 | 11 | – |
| Grand French Vanilla Fudge Pie | ½ cup | 160 | 20 | 14 | – |
| Grand Mint Chocolate Chips | ½ cup | 170 | 18 | 15 | – |
| Grand Neapolitan | ½ cup | 140 | 16 | 14 | – |
| Grand Nutty Cone Crunch | ½ cup | 180 | 19 | 15 | – |
| Grand Real Strawberry | ½ cup | 130 | 16 | 15 | – |
| Grand Rocky Road | ½ cup | 170 | 17 | 13 | – |
| Grand Spumoni | ½ cup | 150 | 16 | 13 | – |
| Grand Strawberry Cupcake | ½ cup | 140 | 19 | 15 | – |
| Grand Tin Roof Sundae | ½ cup | 170 | 18 | 15 | – |
| Grand Utimate Caramel Cup | ½ cup | 170 | 22 | 19 | – |
| Grand Vanilla | ½ cup | 140 | 15 | 13 | – |
| Grand Vanillaberry Bar | ½ cup | 130 | 19 | 16 | – |
| Grand Light Butter Pecan | ½ cup | 120 | 16 | 12 | – |
| Grand Light Chocolate Raspberry Escape | ½ cup | 130 | 19 | 14 | – |

| FOOD | PORTION | CALS | CARB | SUGAR | FIBER |
|---|---|---|---|---|---|
| Grand Light Chocolate Fudge Mousse | ½ cup | 120 | 17 | 13 | – |
| Grand Light Cookie Dough | ½ cup | 130 | 19 | 13 | – |
| Grand Light Cookies'N Cream | ½ cup | 120 | 18 | 12 | – |
| Grand Light Crazy For Caramel | ½ cup | 120 | 19 | 15 | – |
| Grand Light French Silk | ½ cup | 130 | 19 | 14 | – |
| Grand Light Mint Chocolate Chips | ½ cup | 120 | 17 | 13 | – |
| Grand Light Peanut Butter Cups | ½ cup | 120 | 17 | 13 | – |
| Grand Light Rocky Road | ½ cup | 120 | 17 | 12 | – |
| Grand Light S'Mores & More | ½ cup | 130 | 22 | 13 | – |
| Grand Light Strawberry Shortcake | ½ cup | 110 | 18 | 14 | – |
| Grand Light Vanilla | ½ cup | 100 | 15 | 11 | – |
| Homemade All Natural Vanilla | ½ cup | 130 | 14 | 14 | – |
| Homemade Brownie A La Mode | ½ cup | 150 | 18 | 16 | – |
| Homemade Chocolate Chip Cookie Jar | ½ cup | 180 | 19 | 16 | – |
| Homemade Chocolate Chip Mousse | ½ cup | 170 | 19 | 18 | – |
| Homemade Double Chocolate Chunk | ½ cup | 170 | 19 | 18 | – |
| Homemade Mint Chocolate Chunk | ½ cup | 170 | 18 | 17 | – |
| Homemade Old Fashioned Butter Pecan | ½ cup | 160 | 15 | 14 | – |
| Homemade Strawberries & Cream | ½ cup | 120 | 15 | 15 | – |
| Homemade Vanilla Custard | ½ cup | 150 | 15 | 15 | – |
| M&M's Almond | ½ cup | 180 | 21 | 17 | – |
| M&M's Chocolate Brownie Sundae | ½ cup | 180 | 22 | 18 | – |
| M&M's Mint | ½ cup | 200 | 21 | 19 | – |
| M&M's Vanilla | ½ cup | 180 | 22 | 18 | – |
| Milky Way | ½ cup | 160 | 21 | 17 | – |
| Snickers | ½ cup | 180 | 21 | 15 | – |
| Snickers Cruncher | ½ cup | 190 | 21 | 17 | – |
| Twix | ½ cup | 190 | 23 | 18 | – |
| Twix Peanut Butter | ½ cup | 190 | 20 | 15 | – |

| FOOD | PORTION | CALS | CARB | SUGAR | FIBER |
|---|---|---|---|---|---|
| ***Flintstones*** | | | | | |
| Cool Cream | 1 (2.75 oz) | 90 | 18 | 14 | 0 |
| Push-Up Pebbles Treats | 1 (2.75 oz) | 120 | 15 | 14 | 0 |
| ***Good Humor*** | | | | | |
| Bar Oreo | 1 (4 oz) | 250 | 28 | 18 | tr |
| Bar Reese's Peanut Butter | 1 (4 oz) | 310 | 27 | 23 | tr |
| Bar Toasted Almond | 1 (3 oz) | 180 | 22 | 16 | tr |
| Bar Vanilla Dark Chocolate | 1 (3 oz) | 190 | 15 | 12 | tr |
| Bar Vanilla Milk Chocolate | 1 (3 oz) | 180 | 15 | 12 | 0 |
| Bar Candy Center Crunch | 1 (4 oz) | 310 | 24 | 19 | tr |
| Bar Strawberry Shortcake | 1 (4 oz) | 230 | 30 | 17 | tr |
| Chocolate Eclair Bar | 1 (4 oz) | 220 | 30 | 16 | tr |
| Cone Premium Sundae | 1 (4.3 oz) | 270 | 29 | 18 | tr |
| Cone Strawberry Shortcake | 1 (4.3 oz) | 230 | 34 | 19 | tr |
| Giant Sandwich Neapolitan | 1 (6 oz) | 250 | 37 | 20 | tr |
| Giant Sandwich Vanilla | 1 (6 oz) | 250 | 36 | 20 | 0 |
| King Cone | 1 (4.6 fl oz) | 250 | 30 | 19 | tr |
| King Cone Giant | 1 (8 oz) | 190 | 44 | 30 | tr |
| Number 1 Bar | 1 (4 oz) | 200 | 21 | 15 | tr |
| Sandwich Chocolate Chip Cookie | 1 (4.5 oz) | 290 | 41 | 24 | 1 |
| Sandwich Vanilla | 1 (3.5 oz) | 160 | 25 | 12 | 0 |
| Sundae Twist Cup | 1 (6 oz) | 160 | 33 | 29 | 0 |
| ***Häagen-Dazs*** | | | | | |
| Bars Chocolate & Almonds | 1 (3.7 oz) | 380 | 27 | 24 | 2 |
| Bars Chocolate & Dark Chocolate | 1 (3.6 oz) | 350 | 28 | 24 | 2 |
| Bars Chocolate Peanut Butter Swirl | 1 (3 oz) | 320 | 21 | 19 | 2 |
| Bars Coffee & Almond Crunch | 1 (3.7 oz) | 370 | 27 | 26 | tr |
| Bars Cookies & Cream Crunch | 1 (3.6 oz) | 370 | 30 | 26 | tr |
| Bars Dulce De Leche Caramel | 1 (3.7 oz) | 370 | 34 | 33 | 0 |
| Bars Tropical Coconut | 1 (3.5 oz) | 340 | 25 | 25 | 0 |
| Bars Vanilla & Almonds | 1 (3.7 oz) | 380 | 26 | 24 | 1 |
| Bars Vanilla & Dark Chocolate | 1 (3.6 oz) | 350 | 27 | 24 | 1 |
| Bars Vanilla & Milk Chocolate | 1 (3.5 oz) | 340 | 25 | 24 | tr |
| Butter Pecan | ½ cup | 310 | 21 | 18 | tr |
| Cappuccino Commotion | ½ cup | 310 | 25 | 23 | 1 |
| Cherry Vanilla | ½ cup | 240 | 23 | 22 | 0 |
| Chocolate | ½ cup | 270 | 22 | 21 | 1 |

| FOOD | PORTION | CALS | CARB | SUGAR | FIBER |
|---|---|---|---|---|---|
| Chocolate Brownie w/ Walnuts | ½ cup | 290 | 25 | 20 | 1 |
| Chocolate Chocolate Fudge | ½ cup | 290 | 27 | 24 | tr |
| Chocolate Chocolate Chip | ½ cup | 300 | 26 | 24 | 2 |
| Chocolate Swiss Almond | ½ cup | 300 | 24 | 21 | 2 |
| Cinnamon | ½ cup | 250 | 20 | 20 | 0 |
| Coffee | ½ cup | 270 | 21 | 21 | 0 |
| Coffee Mocha Chip | ½ cup | 290 | 25 | 22 | tr |
| Cookie Dough Chip | ½ cup | 310 | 29 | 24 | 0 |
| Cookies & Cream | ½ cup | 270 | 23 | 21 | 0 |
| Creme Caramel Pecan | ½ cup | 320 | 29 | 26 | 0 |
| Dulce De Leche Caramel | ½ cup | 290 | 28 | 26 | 0 |
| Low Fat Chocolate | ½ cup | 170 | 29 | 15 | tr |
| Low Fat Coffee Fudge | ½ cup | 170 | 32 | 22 | 0 |
| Low Fat Strawberry | ½ cup | 150 | 28 | 18 | 0 |
| Low Fat Vanilla | ½ cup | 170 | 29 | 15 | 0 |
| Macadamia Brittle | ½ cup | 300 | 25 | 24 | 0 |
| Mango | ½ cup | 250 | 28 | 27 | tr |
| Mint Chip | ½ cup | 300 | 26 | 23 | tr |
| Pineapple Coconut | ½ cup | 230 | 25 | 24 | 0 |
| Pistachio | ½ cup | 290 | 22 | 19 | tr |
| Rum Raisin | ½ cup | 270 | 22 | 21 | 0 |
| Strawberry | ½ cup | 250 | 23 | 22 | tr |
| Vanilla | ½ cup | 270 | 21 | 21 | 0 |
| Vanilla Chocolate Chip | ½ cup | 310 | 26 | 22 | tr |
| Vanilla Fudge | ½ cup | 290 | 25 | 24 | 0 |
| Vanilla Swiss Almond | ½ cup | 300 | 24 | 21 | tr |
| ***Healthy Choice*** | | | | | |
| Butter Pecan Crunch | ½ cup | 120 | 22 | 21 | tr |
| Cappuccino Chocolate Chunk | ½ cup | 120 | 22 | 19 | 1 |
| Cappuccino Mocha Crunch | ½ cup | 120 | 22 | 19 | tr |
| Cherry Chocolate Chunk | ½ cup | 110 | 19 | 19 | tr |
| Chocolate Chocolate Chunk | ½ cup | 120 | 21 | 18 | 2 |
| Coconut Cream Pie | ½ cup | 120 | 23 | 17 | 1 |
| Cookies 'N Cream | ½ cup | 120 | 21 | 19 | tr |
| Cookies Creme De Mint | ½ cup | 130 | 24 | 20 | tr |
| Fudge Brownie | ½ cup | 120 | 22 | 20 | tr |
| Mint Chocolate Chip | ½ cup | 120 | 21 | 20 | tr |
| Old Fashioned Blueberry Hill | ½ cup | 120 | 23 | 17 | 1 |
| Old Fashioned Butterscotch Blonde | ½ cup | 140 | 26 | 22 | tr |

| FOOD | PORTION | CALS | CARB | SUGAR | FIBER |
|---|---|---|---|---|---|
| Old Fashioned Cherry Vanilla | ½ cup | 120 | 22 | 17 | tr |
| Old Fashioned Strawberry | ½ cup | 110 | 20 | 17 | 1 |
| Peanut Butter Cup | ½ cup | 110 | 19 | 18 | tr |
| Praline & Caramel | ½ cup | 130 | 25 | 24 | tr |
| Praline Caramel Cluster | ½ cup | 130 | 25 | 24 | tr |
| Rocky Road | ½ cup | 140 | 28 | 19 | tr |
| Turtle Fudge Cake | ½ cup | 130 | 25 | 23 | 2 |
| Vanilla | ½ cup | 100 | 18 | 17 | tr |
| Vanilla Bean | ½ cup | 110 | 19 | 18 | tr |
| Wild Raspberry Truffle | ½ cup | 120 | 22 | 15 | tr |
| ***Klondike*** | | | | | |
| Bar Almond | 1 | 300 | 24 | 21 | 0 |
| Bar Cappuccino | 1 | 280 | 24 | 21 | 0 |
| Bar Caramel & Peanut | 1 | 290 | 25 | 21 | tr |
| Bar Caramel & Peanut | 1 | 300 | 28 | 24 | 1 |
| Bar Caramel Crunch | 1 | 270 | 26 | 24 | 0 |
| Bar Chocolate | 1 | 280 | 23 | 21 | tr |
| Bar Dark Chocolate | 1 | 280 | 24 | 20 | tr |
| Bar Heath | 1 | 300 | 26 | 24 | 0 |
| Bar Krunch | 1 | 260 | 24 | 20 | 0 |
| Bar Krunch | 1 | 280 | 25 | 21 | 0 |
| Bar Original | 1 | 280 | 24 | 22 | 0 |
| Bar Peppermint Patty | 1 | 280 | 24 | 20 | tr |
| Bar Reese's | 1 | 220 | 20 | 17 | tr |
| Big Bear Sandwich Neapolitan | 1 | 300 | 42 | 25 | 1 |
| Big Bear Sandwich Vanilla | 1 | 300 | 42 | 25 | tr |
| Big Bear Cone Vanilla | 1 | 330 | 33 | 23 | 1 |
| Big Bear Cone Vanilla Caramel | 1 | 360 | 36 | 27 | 1 |
| Big Bear Cone Vanilla Fudge | 1 | 380 | 38 | 28 | 1 |
| CarbSmart Fudge Bar | 1 bar | 60 | 9 | 3 | 1 |
| CarbSmart Ice Cream Bar | 1 bar | 130 | 9 | 5 | 2 |
| Choco Taco | 1 | 290 | 35 | 24 | 1 |
| Cone Oreo | 1 | 250 | 32 | 21 | 1 |
| Cone Reese's | 1 | 290 | 33 | 24 | tr |
| Cookie Sandwich Chips | 1 | 470 | 66 | 38 | 2 |
| Cookie Sandwich Oreo | 1 | 230 | 34 | 18 | 2 |
| Minis | 2 pieces | 170 | 15 | 13 | 0 |
| Slim-A-Bear 98% Fat Free Sandwich Vanilla | 1 | 130 | 28 | 14 | 3 |

| FOOD | PORTION | CALS | CARB | SUGAR | FIBER |
|---|---|---|---|---|---|
| Slim-A-Bear No Sugar Added Cone Vanilla | 1 | 270 | 31 | 6 | 4 |
| Slim-A-Bear No Sugar Added Fudge Bar | 1 | 90 | 22 | 5 | 4 |
| Slim-A-Bear No Sugar Added Reduced Fat Bar Vanilla | 1 | 160 | 21 | 6 | 4 |
| Slim-A-Bear No Sugar Added Sandwich Vanilla | 1 | 120 | 25 | 3 | 2 |
| Sundae Cup | 1 | 280 | 26 | 22 | tr |
| ***Nestle Crunch*** | | | | | |
| Chocolate | 1 bar (3 oz) | 200 | 17 | 14 | 0 |
| Crunch King | 1 (4 oz) | 270 | 21 | 16 | 0 |
| Nuggets | 8 pieces | 310 | 25 | 19 | 0 |
| Reduced Fat | 1 (2.5 oz) | 130 | 14 | 6 | 0 |
| Vanilla | 1 bar (3 oz) | 200 | 16 | 13 | 0 |
| ***NutraShake*** | | | | | |
| High Calorie High Protein All Flavors | 1 serv (4 oz) | 200 | 24 | – | – |
| ***Popsicle*** | | | | | |
| Bar Col Crunch Chocolate Eclair | 1 (3 oz) | 160 | 20 | 12 | tr |
| Bar Col Crunch Strawberry Shortcake | 1 (3 oz) | 170 | 21 | 12 | 0 |
| Bar Snoopy | 1 (3.5 oz) | 150 | 16 | 13 | 0 |
| Bar Sprinklers | 1 (2.1 oz) | 130 | 18 | 14 | 0 |
| Cone Crispy | 1 (2.5 oz) | 150 | 20 | 12 | 0 |
| Creamsicle Pop | 1 (1.75 oz) | 70 | 13 | 10 | 0 |
| Cup Cookies & Cream | 1 (10 oz) | 310 | 45 | 29 | 1 |
| Fruit Juicee Cups | 1 (4 oz) | 80 | 20 | 19 | – |
| Ice Cream Bar Vanilla | 1 (3 oz) | 160 | 15 | 15 | 1 |
| Ice Cream Pops Minis | 2 (2.8 oz) | 190 | 18 | 15 | 0 |
| Sandwich Cookie Rugrats | 1 (2.5 oz) | 140 | 20 | 10 | tr |
| Sandwiches Minis | 1 (2 oz) | 100 | 15 | 7 | 0 |
| Scribblers Ice Cream Pops | 2 (2.4 oz) | 130 | 17 | 13 | 0 |
| Swirl Bar Bubble Gum | 1 (2.6 oz) | 60 | 13 | 10 | – |
| WWE Bar | 1 (3.6 oz) | 180 | 23 | 13 | tr |
| X-Men Wolverine Bar | 1 (4 oz) | 100 | 25 | 20 | – |
| ***Rice Dream*** | | | | | |
| Cappuccino | ½ cup (3.2 oz) | 150 | 23 | 17 | 1 |
| Carob | ½ cup (3.2 oz) | 150 | 24 | 17 | 2 |

| FOOD | PORTION | CALS | CARB | SUGAR | FIBER |
|---|---|---|---|---|---|
| Carob Almond | ½ cup (3.2 oz) | 170 | 24 | 17 | 2 |
| Cherry Vanilla | ½ cup (3.2 oz) | 150 | 24 | 18 | 1 |
| Cocoa Marble Fudge | ½ cup (3.2 oz) | 150 | 25 | 15 | 2 |
| Cookies N' Dream | ½ cup (3.2 oz) | 170 | 26 | 17 | 1 |
| Mint Chocolate Chip | ½ cup (3.2 oz) | 170 | 26 | 19 | 1 |
| Neapolitan | ½ cup (3.2 oz) | 150 | 24 | 18 | 2 |
| Orange Vanilla Swirl | ½ cup (3.2 oz) | 250 | 23 | 17 | 1 |
| Strawberry | ½ cup (3.2 oz) | 140 | 24 | 19 | 1 |
| Vanilla Swiss Almond | ½ cup (3.2 oz) | 180 | 25 | 18 | 1 |
| ***Rice Dream Supreme*** | | | | | |
| Cappuccino Almond Fudge | ½ cup (3.2 oz) | 170 | 24 | 15 | 2 |
| Cherry Chocolate Chunk | ½ cup (3.2 oz) | 170 | 27 | 19 | 1 |
| Chocolate Almond Chunk | ½ cup (3.2 oz) | 170 | 25 | 18 | 2 |
| Chocolate Fudge Brownie | ½ cup (3.2 oz) | 170 | 28 | 16 | 2 |
| Double Espresso Bean | ½ cup (3.2 oz) | 160 | 24 | 17 | 1 |
| Mint Chocolate Cookie | ½ cup (3.2 oz) | 170 | 26 | 18 | 1 |
| Peanut Butter Cup | ½ cup (3.2 oz) | 180 | 25 | 18 | 2 |
| Pralines N' Dream | ½ cup (3.2 oz) | 180 | 25 | 16 | 1 |
| ***Silhouette*** | | | | | |
| The Skinny Cow Low Fat Ice Cream Sandwich Vanilla | 1 | 130 | 23 | 22 | 2 |
| ***Slim-Fast*** | | | | | |
| Chocolate Fudge Bar | 1 bar | 110 | 22 | 17 | tr |
| Ice Cream Sandwich Chocolate | 1 | 130 | 27 | 14 | tr |
| Ice Cream Sandwich Vanilla | 1 | 130 | 27 | 14 | tr |
| ***Starbucks*** | | | | | |
| Caramel Cappuccino Swirl | ½ cup | 240 | 30 | 28 | 0 |
| Classic Coffee | ½ cup | 230 | 26 | 24 | 0 |
| Coffee Almond Fudge | ½ cup | 250 | 29 | 25 | 1 |
| Frappuccino Bar Java Fudge | 1 bar | 130 | 25 | 16 | 4 |
| Frappuccino Bar Mocha | 1 bar | 120 | 22 | 15 | 3 |
| Java Chip | ½ cup | 250 | 29 | 26 | 0 |
| Low Fat Latte | ½ cup | 170 | 30 | 23 | 0 |
| Mud Pie | ½ cup | 240 | 32 | 27 | 1 |
| White Chocolate Latte | ½ cup | 280 | 31 | 29 | 0 |
| ***Tofutti*** | | | | | |
| Cuties Chocolate | 1 (1.4 oz) | 130 | 16 | 9 | 0 |
| Monkey Bars Peanut Butter | 1 bar (2.5 oz) | 220 | 22 | 18 | tr |
| ***Turkey Hill*** | | | | | |
| Black Cherry | ½ cup | 140 | 18 | 16 | 0 |

| FOOD | PORTION | CALS | CARB | SUGAR | FIBER |
|---|---|---|---|---|---|
| Black Raspberry | ½ cup | 140 | 18 | – | – |
| Butter Pecan | ½ cup | 170 | 16 | 15 | 0 |
| Chocolate Marshmallow | ½ cup | 160 | 24 | – | – |
| Chocolate Mint Chip | ½ cup | 180 | 18 | – | – |
| Chocolate Peanut Butter Cup | ½ cup | 180 | 18 | – | – |
| Colombian Coffee | ½ cup | 140 | 16 | – | – |
| Cookies 'N Cream | ½ cup | 160 | 19 | 17 | 0 |
| Death By Chocolate | ½ cup | 160 | 21 | – | – |
| Dutch Chocolate | ½ cup | 150 | 19 | – | – |
| Egg Nog | ½ cup | 150 | 17 | – | – |
| Fat Free No Sugar Added Caramel Fudge Decadence | ½ cup | 100 | 23 | – | – |
| Fat Free No Sugar Added Cherry Vanilla Fudge | ½ cup | 90 | 20 | – | – |
| Fat Free No Sugar Added Dutch Chocolate | ½ cup | 90 | 20 | – | – |
| Fat Free No Sugar Added Vanilla Bean | ½ cup | 90 | 20 | – | – |
| Fudge Ripple | ½ cup | 140 | 20 | – | – |
| Light Butter Pecan | ½ cup | 130 | 17 | 16 | 0 |
| Light Choco Mint Chip | ½ cup | 140 | 19 | 18 | 0 |
| Light Tin Lissie Sundae | ½ cup | 140 | 21 | – | – |
| Light Vanilla & Chocolate | ½ cup | 110 | 18 | 18 | 0 |
| Light Vanilla Bean | ½ cup | 110 | 18 | 17 | 0 |
| Neapolitan | ½ cup | 150 | 18 | 17 | 0 |
| Orange Swirl | ½ cup | 140 | 19 | – | – |
| Original Vanilla | ½ cup | 140 | 16 | – | – |
| Peanut Butter Ripple | ½ cup | 170 | 16 | – | – |
| Philadelphia Style Butter Almond | ½ cup | 180 | 15 | – | – |
| Philadelphia Style Chocolate | ½ cup | 170 | 18 | – | – |
| Philadelphia Style Mint Chocolate Chip | ½ cup | 180 | 18 | – | – |
| Philadelphia Style Sweet Cherry Vanilla | ½ cup | 160 | 18 | – | – |
| Philadelphia Style Vanilla Bean | ½ cup | 170 | 16 | – | – |
| Rocky Road | ½ cup | 170 | 23 | 19 | 0 |
| Rum Raisin | ½ cup | 150 | 19 | – | – |
| Sandwich Choco Mint Chip | 1 | 200 | 27 | – | – |
| Sandwiches Vanilla | 1 | 190 | 26 | – | – |

| FOOD | PORTION | CALS | CARB | SUGAR | FIBER |
|---|---|---|---|---|---|
| Strawberries 'N Cream | ½ cup | 140 | 19 | – | – |
| Sundae Cones Rocky Road | 1 | 340 | 37 | – | – |
| Sundae Cones Tin Roof Sundae | 1 | 290 | 30 | – | – |
| Tin Roof Sundae | ½ cup | 160 | 19 | 18 | 0 |
| Vanilla & Chocolate | ½ cup | 150 | 17 | 16 | 0 |
| Vanilla Bean | ½ cup | 140 | 16 | 16 | 0 |
| ***Weight Watchers*** | | | | | |
| Chocolate Chip Cookie Dough Sundae | 1 (2.64 oz) | 190 | 35 | 15 | 1 |
| Chocolate Mousse | 1 bar | 40 | 9 | 3 | 1 |
| Chocolate Treat | 1 bar | 100 | 20 | 17 | 1 |
| Orange Vanilla Treat | 1 bar | 40 | 10 | 3 | 0 |
| Vanilla Sandwich | 1 bar | 150 | 28 | 14 | 1 |
| **TAKE-OUT** | | | | | |
| cone vanilla light soft serve | 1 (4.6 oz) | 164 | 24 | – | – |
| gelato chocolate hazelnut | ½ cup (5.3 oz) | 370 | 26 | 21 | 2 |
| gelato vanilla | ½ cup (3 oz) | 211 | 18 | 18 | 0 |
| sundae caramel | 1 (5.4 oz) | 303 | 49 | – | – |
| sundae hot fudge | 1 (5.4 oz) | 284 | 48 | – | – |
| sundae strawberry | 1 (5.4 oz) | 269 | 45 | – | – |
| **ICE CREAM CONES AND CUPS** | | | | | |
| sugar cone | 1 | 40 | 8 | – | tr |
| wafer cone | 1 | 17 | 3 | – | tr |
| ***Dutch Mill*** | | | | | |
| Chocolate Covered Wafer Cups | 1 (0.5 oz) | 80 | 8 | 6 | 0 |
| ***Frookie*** | | | | | |
| Chocolate Crunch | 1 (0.4 oz) | 50 | 10 | 4 | tr |
| Honey Crunch | 1 (0.4 oz) | 45 | 9 | 1 | tr |
| ***Keebler*** | | | | | |
| Chocolatey Cone | 1 (0.4 oz) | 50 | 10 | 4 | 0 |
| Fudge Dipped Cup | 1 (0.3 oz) | 35 | 6 | 2 | 0 |
| Ice Creme Cup | 1 (0.2 oz) | 15 | 4 | 0 | 0 |
| Sugar Cone | 1 (0.4 oz) | 50 | 10 | 4 | 0 |
| Waffle Bowl | 1 (0.4 oz) | 50 | 10 | 4 | 0 |
| Waffle Cone | 1 (0.4 oz) | 50 | 10 | 4 | 0 |
| **ICE CREAM TOPPINGS** | | | | | |
| butterscotch | 2 tbsp (1.4 oz) | 103 | 27 | – | – |
| caramel | 2 tbsp (1.4 oz) | 103 | 27 | – | – |
| marshmallow cream | 1 jar (7 oz) | 615 | 157 | – | – |

| FOOD | PORTION | CALS | CARB | SUGAR | FIBER |
|---|---|---|---|---|---|
| marshmallow cream | 1 oz | 88 | 23 | – | – |
| pineapple | 1 cup (11.5 oz) | 861 | 226 | – | – |
| pineapple | 2 tbsp (1.5 oz) | 106 | 28 | – | – |
| strawberry | 2 tbsp (1.5 oz) | 107 | 28 | – | – |
| strawberry | 1 cup (11.5 oz) | 863 | 225 | – | – |
| walnuts in syrup | 2 tbsp (1.4 oz) | 167 | 22 | – | – |
| ***Colac*** | | | | | |
| Passion Fruit | 1 tbsp | 31 | 13 | 0 | 0 |
| Strawberry | 1 tbsp | 31 | 13 | 0 | 0 |
| ***Hershey*** | | | | | |
| Chocolate Shop Double Chocolate | 1 tbsp (0.7 oz) | 50 | 13 | – | – |
| Chocolate Shoppe Apple Pie A La Mode | 2 tbsp (1.3 oz) | 100 | 25 | – | – |
| Chocolate Shoppe Butterscotch Caramel | 1 tbsp (0.7 oz) | 70 | 14 | – | – |
| Chocolate Shoppe Caramel | 2 tbsp (1.3 oz) | 100 | 25 | – | – |
| Chocolate Shoppe Chocolate Mini | 1 tbsp (0.7 oz) | 50 | 13 | – | – |
| Chocolate Shoppe Double Chocolate | 1 tbsp (0.6 oz) | 60 | 12 | – | – |
| Chocolate Shoppe Hot Fudge | 1 tbsp (0.7 oz) | 70 | 10 | – | – |
| Chocolate Shoppe Hot Fudge Fat Free | 2 tbsp (1.4 oz) | 100 | 23 | – | – |
| Chocolate Shoppe Sprinkles Milk Chocolate | 1 tbsp (0.5 oz) | 70 | 10 | – | – |
| Chocolate Shoppe Sprinkles Reeses | 1 tbsp (0.5 oz) | 70 | 10 | – | – |
| Chocolate Shoppe Sprinkles York | 1 tbsp (0.6 oz) | 80 | 11 | – | – |
| ***Smucker's*** | | | | | |
| Plate Scapers Caramel | 2 tbsp | 100 | 25 | 18 | – |
| ***Steel's*** | | | | | |
| Sugar Free Butterscotch | 2 tbsp | 60 | 21 | 0 | 0 |
| Sugar Free Chocolate Fudge | 2 tbsp | 45 | 5 | 0 | 2 |
| Sugar Free Hot Fudge | 2 tbsp | 65 | 18 | 0 | 1 |
| Sugar Free Peanut Butter Fudge | 2 tbsp | 75 | 5 | 0 | 2 |

| FOOD | PORTION | CALS | CARB | SUGAR | FIBER |
|---|---|---|---|---|---|
| **ICED TEA** | | | | | |
| **MIX** | | | | | |
| instant artificially sweetened lemon flavored as prep w/ water | 8 oz | 5 | 1 | – | – |
| instant sweetened lemon flavor as prep w/ water | 9 oz | 87 | 22 | – | – |
| instant unsweetened lemon flavor as prep w/ water | 8 oz | 4 | 0 | 0 | 0 |
| ***Atkins*** | | | | | |
| Sugar Free Lemon not prep | 2 tbsp | 0 | 0 | 0 | 0 |
| ***Carb Options*** | | | | | |
| Lemon as prep | 1 serv | 0 | 0 | 0 | 0 |
| ***Nestea*** | | | | | |
| 100% Tea | 2 tsp (1 g) | 0 | tr | 0 | 0 |
| 100% Tea Decafe | 2 tsp (1 g) | 0 | tr | 0 | 0 |
| Ice Teasers Lemon | 1 serv (0.5 oz) | 5 | 1 | 0 | 0 |
| Ice Teasers Orange | 1 serv (0.5 oz) | 5 | 1 | 0 | 0 |
| Ice Teasers Wild Cherry | 1 serv (0.5 oz) | 5 | 1 | 0 | 0 |
| Lemon | 2 tsp (1 g) | 5 | 1 | 0 | 0 |
| Lemon & Sugar | 2 tbsp (0.7 oz) | 80 | 19 | 19 | 0 |
| Lemonade Tea | 2 tbsp (0.7 oz) | 80 | 19 | 17 | 0 |
| Sugar Free | 2 tbsp (0.7 oz) | 5 | 1 | 0 | 0 |
| Sugar Free Decafe | 1 tbsp (0.7 oz) | 5 | 1 | 0 | 0 |
| Sun Tea | 1 tsp (1 g) | 0 | tr | 0 | 0 |
| **READY-TO-DRINK** | | | | | |
| ***Apple & Eve*** | | | | | |
| Lemon Fruit | 8 fl oz | 100 | 25 | 22 | – |
| Peach Fruit | 8 fl oz | 100 | 25 | 22 | – |
| Raspberry Fruit | 8 fl oz | 100 | 25 | 22 | – |
| Tangerine Fruit | 8 fl oz | 100 | 25 | 22 | – |
| ***Fuze*** | | | | | |
| Vitamin Tea Diet Peach | 8 oz | 5 | 1 | 0 | 0 |
| Vitamin Tea Green Tea w/ Ginseng | 8 oz | 60 | 16 | 16 | – |
| White Tea | 8 oz | 60 | 15 | 15 | – |
| ***Hansen's*** | | | | | |
| Chai | 8 oz | 150 | 38 | 32 | – |
| China Black | 8 oz | 90 | 25 | 24 | – |
| Green | 8 oz | 70 | 18 | 18 | – |
| Green Diet Lemon | 8 oz | 0 | 0 | 0 | – |

| FOOD | PORTION | CALS | CARB | SUGAR | FIBER |
|---|---|---|---|---|---|
| Green Diet Peach | 8 oz | 0 | 0 | 0 | – |
| Green Lemon | 8 oz | 70 | 18 | 17 | – |
| Green Peach | 8 oz | 70 | 18 | 17 | – |
| Oolong | 8 oz | 70 | 25 | 24 | – |
| Spice | 8 oz | 90 | 24 | – | – |
| ***Honest Tea*** | | | | | |
| Black Forest Berry | 8 oz | 17 | 5 | 5 | – |
| Gold Rush Herbal Cinnamon | 8 fl oz | 9 | 3 | 2 | – |
| Kashmiri Chai | 8 oz | 17 | 6 | 5 | – |
| Lori's Lemon | 8 oz | 30 | 9 | 9 | – |
| Moroccan Mint | 8 oz | 17 | 5 | 5 | – |
| Peach Oo-La-Long | 8 oz | 30 | 9 | 9 | – |
| ***Inko's*** | | | | | |
| White Tea | 1 bottle (16 oz) | 56 | 14 | 14 | – |
| White Tea Hint O'Mint | 1 bottle | 0 | 0 | 0 | – |
| ***Mad River*** | | | | | |
| Red Tea w/ Guarana | 8 oz | 90 | 24 | 23 | – |
| ***Nantucket Nectars*** | | | | | |
| Diet | 8 oz | 5 | 1 | 0 | – |
| Diet Green Tea | 8 oz | 5 | 1 | 0 | – |
| Half & Half | 8 oz | 90 | 23 | 21 | – |
| Iced Tea | 8 oz | 80 | 20 | 19 | – |
| Matt Fee | 8 oz | 80 | 20 | 18 | – |
| Raspberry | 8 oz | 90 | 23 | 22 | – |
| Savannah | 8 oz | 80 | 20 | 18 | – |
| ***Oregon Chai*** | | | | | |
| Original Latte | 1 bottle (9.5 oz) | 150 | 26 | 25 | 0 |
| ***Republic Of Tea*** | | | | | |
| No Carb Unsweetened All Flavors | 1 bottle (12 oz) | 0 | 0 | 0 | 0 |
| ***Snapple*** | | | | | |
| Diet Lemon | 8 fl oz | 0 | 1 | 0 | – |
| Diet Peach | 8 fl oz | 0 | 1 | 0 | – |
| Diet Raspberry | 8 fl oz | 0 | 1 | 0 | – |
| Ginseng Tea | 8 fl oz | 80 | 20 | 18 | – |
| Green Tea w/ Lemon | 8 fl oz | 100 | 25 | 24 | – |
| Lemon | 8 fl oz | 100 | 25 | 23 | – |
| Lemonade Ice Tea | 8 fl oz | 110 | 28 | 28 | – |

| FOOD | PORTION | CALS | CARB | SUGAR | FIBER |
|---|---|---|---|---|---|
| Peach | 8 fl oz | 100 | 26 | 24 | – |
| Raspberry | 8 fl oz | 100 | 26 | 25 | – |
| ***SoBe*** | | | | | |
| Lemon | 8 oz | 90 | 25 | 24 | – |
| ***Turkey Hill*** | | | | | |
| Blueberry Oolong w/ Vitamins C & E | 1 cup | 100 | 24 | 24 | – |
| Decaffeinated | 1 cup | 80 | 20 | 20 | – |
| Decaffeinated Orange | 1 cup | 10 | 2 | 2 | – |
| Diet | 1 cup | 0 | 0 | 0 | – |
| Diet Decaffeinated | 1 cup | 0 | 0 | 0 | – |
| Diet Green Tea w/ Ginseng & Honey | 1 cup | 5 | tr | tr | – |
| Green Tea w/ Ginseng & Honey | 1 cup | 70 | 17 | – | – |
| Lemon | 1 cup | 100 | 24 | 24 | – |
| Mint Tea w/ Chamomile | 1 cup | 90 | 21 | 21 | – |
| Oolong w/ Ginkgo Biloba & Ginseng | 1 cup | 100 | 25 | 25 | – |
| Orange | 1 cup | 100 | 25 | 25 | – |
| Peach | 1 cup | 110 | 28 | 28 | – |
| Raspberry Tea | 1 cup | 110 | 28 | 28 | – |
| Regular | 1 cup | 90 | 22 | 22 | – |

## ICES AND ICE POPS

| FOOD | PORTION | CALS | CARB | SUGAR | FIBER |
|---|---|---|---|---|---|
| fruit & juice bar | 1 (3 fl oz) | 75 | 19 | 17 | – |
| gelatin pop | 1 (1.5 oz) | 31 | 7 | 7 | – |
| ice coconut pineapple | ½ cup (4 fl oz) | 109 | 23 | – | – |
| ice fruit w/ Equal | 1 bar (1.7 oz) | 12 | 3 | – | – |
| ice lime | ½ cup (4 fl oz) | 75 | 31 | – | – |
| ice pop | 1 (2 fl oz) | 42 | 11 | – | – |
| ***Breyers*** | | | | | |
| Fruit Bars No Sugar Added | 1 (1.75 oz) | 25 | 5 | 2 | 0 |
| Juice Bar Strawberry | 1 (3.75 oz) | 120 | 30 | 23 | tr |
| Soft Frozen Cup Lemonade | 1 pkg (12 oz) | 290 | 74 | 56 | – |
| Soft Frozen Cup Strawberry | 1 pkg (12 oz) | 260 | 66 | 51 | – |
| ***Carnation*** | | | | | |
| Cup Orange Sherbet | 1 (5 oz) | 150 | 32 | 28 | 0 |
| Cup Orange Sherbet | 1 (3 oz) | 90 | 19 | 17 | 0 |
| ***Cold Fusion*** | | | | | |
| Protein Juice Bar All Flavors | 1 bar (3.8 oz) | 130 | 23 | 23 | 0 |

| FOOD | PORTION | CALS | CARB | SUGAR | FIBER |
|---|---|---|---|---|---|
| ***Cool Creations*** | | | | | |
| Ice Pop | 1 pop (2 oz) | 50 | 13 | 13 | 0 |
| Mickey Mouse Bar | 1 (4 oz) | 170 | 17 | 10 | 0 |
| Surprise Pops | 1 (2 oz) | 60 | 14 | 13 | 0 |
| ***CoolFruits*** | | | | | |
| Fruite Juice Freezer Pops Grape & Cherry | 3 pops (3 oz) | 70 | 18 | 18 | 0 |
| ***Dole*** | | | | | |
| Fruit'n Juice Coconut | 1 bar (4 oz) | 210 | 33 | 30 | 0 |
| Fruit'n Juice Lemonade | 1 bar (4 oz) | 120 | 28 | 24 | 0 |
| Fruit'n Juice Lime | 1 bar (4 oz) | 110 | 28 | 24 | 0 |
| Fruit'n Juice Peach Passion | 1 bar (2.5 oz) | 70 | 17 | 15 | 0 |
| Fruit'n Juice Pineapple Coconut | 1 bar (4 oz) | 150 | 27 | 24 | 0 |
| Fruit'n Juice Pineapple Orange Banana | 1 bar (2.5 oz) | 70 | 16 | 15 | 0 |
| Fruit'n Juice Pineapple Orange Banana | 1 bar (4 oz) | 110 | 26 | 24 | 0 |
| Fruit'n Juice Raspberry | 1 bar (2.5 oz) | 70 | 16 | 13 | 0 |
| Fruit'n Juice Strawberry | 1 bar (2.5 oz) | 70 | 17 | 15 | 0 |
| Fruit'n Juice Strawberry | 1 bar (4 oz) | 110 | 26 | 24 | 0 |
| Grape No Sugar Added | 1 bar (1.75 oz) | 25 | 6 | 3 | 0 |
| Raspberry | 1 bar (1.75 oz) | 45 | 11 | 10 | 0 |
| Raspberry No Sugar Added | 1 bar (1.75 oz) | 25 | 6 | 3 | 0 |
| Strawberry | 1 bar (1.75 oz) | 45 | 11 | 10 | 0 |
| Strawberry No Sugar | 1 bar (1.75 oz) | 25 | 6 | 3 | 0 |
| ***Edy's*** | | | | | |
| Fruit Bars Strawberry | 1 (3 oz) | 80 | 21 | 20 | 0 |
| Sherbet Berry Rainbow | ½ cup | 130 | 29 | 23 | – |
| Sherbet Lime | ½ cup | 130 | 28 | 23 | – |
| Sherbet Orange Cream | ½ cup | 120 | 23 | 19 | – |
| Sherbet Raspberry | ½ cup | 130 | 28 | 22 | – |
| Sherbet Starburst Orange & Cherry | ½ cup | 150 | 33 | 25 | – |
| Sherbet Starburst Strawberry | ½ cup | 160 | 33 | 25 | – |
| Sherbet Swiss Orange | ½ cup | 150 | 30 | 25 | – |
| Sherbet Tropical Rainbow | ½ cup | 130 | 29 | 24 | – |
| Sorbet Coconut | ½ cup | 140 | 28 | 21 | 0 |
| Sorbet Lemon | ½ cup | 140 | 35 | 25 | 0 |
| Sorbet Mandarin Orange | ½ cup | 130 | 32 | 24 | 0 |
| Sorbet Peach | ½ cup | 130 | 32 | 28 | 1 |

| FOOD | PORTION | CALS | CARB | SUGAR | FIBER |
|---|---|---|---|---|---|
| Sorbet Raspberry | ½ cup | 130 | 33 | 23 | 1 |
| Sorbet Strawberry | ½ cup | 120 | 31 | 27 | 0 |
| Whole Fruit Bars Creamy Coconut | 1 bar | 120 | 21 | 16 | – |
| Whole Fruit Bars Lemonade | 1 bar | 80 | 20 | 19 | – |
| Whole Fruit Bars Lime | 1 bar | 80 | 20 | 19 | – |
| Whole Fruit Bars Tangerine | 1 bar | 80 | 20 | 19 | – |
| Whole Fruit Bars Wild Berry | 1 bar | 80 | 21 | 20 | – |
| ***Flintstones*** | | | | | |
| Push-Up Sherbet Treats | 1 (2.75 oz) | 100 | 20 | 14 | 0 |
| ***Good Humor*** | | | | | |
| Great White | 1 (3 oz) | 70 | 18 | 14 | – |
| Hyper Stripe | 1 (2.7 oz) | 80 | 19 | 15 | – |
| ***Häagen-Dazs*** | | | | | |
| Sorbet Chocolate | ½ cup | 120 | 28 | 20 | 2 |
| Sorbet Mango | ½ cup | 120 | 31 | 29 | tr |
| Sorbet Orange | ½ cup | 120 | 30 | 24 | tr |
| Sorbet Orchard Peach | ½ cup | 130 | 33 | 29 | tr |
| Sorbet Raspberry | ½ cup | 120 | 30 | 26 | 2 |
| Sorbet Strawberry | ½ cup | 120 | 30 | 27 | 1 |
| Sorbet Zesty Lemon | ½ cup | 120 | 31 | 27 | tr |
| Sorbet Bar Chocolate | 1 (2.7 oz) | 80 | 20 | 14 | 1 |
| Sorbet Bars Raspberry & Vanilla Yogurt | 1 (2.5 oz) | 90 | 21 | 15 | tr |
| Sorbet Bars Strawberry & Vanilla Ice Cream | 1 (2.5 oz) | 110 | 15 | 14 | 0 |
| ***Natural Choice*** | | | | | |
| Organic Banana | ½ cup (3.6 oz) | 110 | 28 | 27 | tr |
| Organic Blueberry | ½ cup (3.6 oz) | 100 | 27 | 25 | tr |
| Organic Kiwi | ½ cup (3.6 oz) | 110 | 28 | 27 | tr |
| Organic Lemon | ½ cup (3.6 oz) | 110 | 28 | 27 | tr |
| Organic Mango | ½ cup (3.6 oz) | 110 | 28 | 27 | tr |
| Organic Strawberry | ½ cup (3.6 oz) | 110 | 28 | 27 | tr |
| Organic Strawberry Kiwi | ½ cup (3.6 oz) | 110 | 28 | 27 | tr |
| ***Popsicle*** | | | | | |
| All Natural Ice Pops | 1 (1.75 oz) | 50 | 12 | 9 | – |
| Bar Bart Simpson | 1 (4 oz) | 110 | 26 | 20 | – |
| Bar Dora The Explorer | 1 (4 oz) | 100 | 25 | 20 | – |
| Bar Fruti Holanda Lemon Lime | 1 (3 oz) | 90 | 23 | 18 | – |
| Bar Fruti Holanda Strawberry | 1 (3 oz) | 90 | 23 | 19 | – |

| FOOD | PORTION | CALS | CARB | SUGAR | FIBER |
|---|---|---|---|---|---|
| Bar Incredible Hulk | 1 (4 oz) | 100 | 25 | 20 | – |
| Bar Jimmy Neutron | 1 (4 oz) | 100 | 25 | 19 | – |
| Bar Mega Warheads | 1 (4 oz) | 110 | 26 | 20 | 0 |
| Bar Power Ranger | 1 (4 oz) | 100 | 23 | 18 | – |
| Bar Spider Man | 1 (4 oz) | 100 | 25 | 20 | – |
| Bar SpongeBob | 1 (4 oz) | 100 | 25 | 20 | – |
| Big Stick Pops Big Redds | 1 (3.5 oz) | 70 | 17 | 12 | – |
| Big Stick Pops Cherry Pineapple | 1 (3.5 oz) | 50 | 12 | 10 | 0 |
| Bubble Play | 1 (4 oz) | 100 | 28 | 21 | – |
| Creamsicle Bar | 1 (2.5 oz) | 100 | 18 | 14 | 0 |
| Creamsicle Sugar Free | 2 (3.3 oz) | 40 | 10 | 0 | 6 |
| Creamsicle Pop No Sugar Added | 1 (1.75 oz) | 25 | 6 | 1 | 0 |
| Cup Cherry | 1 (12 oz) | 240 | 62 | 59 | – |
| Cup Frostee Fudge | 1 (10 oz) | 280 | 41 | 33 | 2 |
| Cup Lemon | 1 (12 oz) | 230 | 60 | 59 | – |
| Cup Screwball | 1 (3.75 oz) | 110 | 27 | 22 | – |
| Firecracker | 1 (1.6 oz) | 35 | 9 | 7 | – |
| Fruita Holanda Coconut Bar | 1 (3 oz) | 120 | 25 | 21 | tr |
| Fudgsicle Bar | 1 (2.5 oz) | 90 | 16 | 13 | tr |
| Fudgsicle Bar Fat Free | 1 (1.75 oz) | 60 | 13 | 10 | tr |
| Fudgsicle Pop | 1 (1.75 oz) | 60 | 11 | 9 | tr |
| Fudgsicle Pops No Sugar Added | 2 (1.75 oz) | 90 | 19 | 3 | 1 |
| Minis Fudge Bar | 2 (2.4 oz) | 80 | 16 | 13 | tr |
| Pop Lick-A-Color | 1 (2 oz) | 50 | 13 | 12 | – |
| Pop Sherbet Cyclone | 1 (1.8 oz) | 50 | 11 | 10 | 0 |
| Pop Towering Tornado | 1 (3.5 oz) | 90 | 21 | 10 | – |
| Pop Ups Orange Burst | 1 (2.75 oz) | 80 | 19 | 15 | 0 |
| Pop Ups Reckless Rainbow | 1 (2.75 oz) | 90 | 19 | 15 | 0 |
| Pop Ups SpongeBob | 1 (2.75 oz) | 90 | 17 | 13 | 0 |
| Pops Tropical Sugar Free | 1 (1.75 oz) | 15 | 3 | 0 | – |
| Pops Wild Bunch | 2 (2.2 oz) | 60 | 14 | 11 | – |
| Rainbow Floats | 1 (1.75 oz) | 60 | 11 | 8 | 0 |
| Rainbow Pops | 1 (1.75 oz) | 45 | 11 | 11 | – |
| Scribblers Juice Pops | 2 (2.4 oz) | 60 | 16 | 15 | – |
| Shots | 1 serv (1.7 oz) | 40 | 9 | 9 | – |
| Snow Cone | 1 (7 oz) | 30 | 7 | 5 | – |
| Sugar Free Pops Orange Cherry Grape | 1 (1.75 oz) | 15 | 3 | 0 | – |
| Super Mario Bros Bar | 1 (4 oz) | 100 | 25 | 20 | – |

| FOOD | PORTION | CALS | CARB | SUGAR | FIBER |
|---|---|---|---|---|---|
| Swirl Bar Cotton Candy | 1 (2.6 oz) | 60 | 13 | 10 | – |
| Tingle Twister Ice Pops | 1 (1.75 oz) | 45 | 11 | 9 | – |
| Torpedo Pop Cherry | 1 (1.75 oz) | 35 | 8 | 6 | – |
| **JACKFRUIT** | | | | | |
| fresh | 3.5 oz | 70 | 4 | – | – |
| **JALAPEÑO** *(see* PEPPERS*)* | | | | | |
| **JAM/JELLY/PRESERVES** | | | | | |
| all flavors jam | 1 tbsp (0.7 oz) | 48 | 13 | 10 | tr |
| all flavors jam | 1 pkg (0.5 oz) | 34 | 9 | 7 | tr |
| all flavors jelly | 1 pkg (0.5 oz) | 38 | 10 | 9 | tr |
| all flavors jelly | 1 tbsp (0.7 oz) | 52 | 14 | 12 | tr |
| all flavors preserve | 1 pkg (0.5 oz) | 34 | 9 | 7 | tr |
| all flavors preserve | 1 tbsp (0.7 oz) | 48 | 13 | 10 | tr |
| apple butter | 1 cup (9.9 oz) | 519 | 135 | – | – |
| apple butter | 1 tbsp (0.6 oz) | 33 | 9 | – | – |
| apple jelly | 1 pkg (0.5 oz) | 38 | 10 | 9 | tr |
| apple jelly | 1 tbsp (0.7 oz) | 52 | 14 | 12 | tr |
| apricot jam | 0.5 oz | 36 | 9 | – | – |
| blackberry jam | 0.5 oz | 34 | 8 | – | – |
| cherry jam | 0.5 oz | 36 | 9 | – | – |
| linganberry jam | 0.5 oz | 23 | 6 | 4 | tr |
| orange jam | 0.5 oz | 35 | 9 | – | – |
| orange marmalade | 1 tbsp (0.7 oz) | 49 | 13 | – | – |
| orange marmalade | 1 pkg (0.5 oz) | 34 | 9 | – | – |
| plum jam | 0.5 oz (0.5 oz) | 34 | 9 | – | – |
| quince jam | 0.5 oz | 43 | 8 | – | – |
| raspberry jam | 0.5 oz | 35 | 9 | – | – |
| raspberry jelly | 0.5 oz | 37 | 9 | – | – |
| red currant jam | 0.5 oz | 34 | 8 | – | – |
| red currant jelly | 0.5 oz | 38 | 9 | – | – |
| rose hip jam | 0.5 oz | 36 | 9 | – | – |
| strawberry jam | 1 pkg (0.5 oz) | 34 | 9 | 7 | tr |
| strawberry jam | 1 tbsp (0.7 oz) | 48 | 13 | 10 | tr |
| strawberry preserve | 1 pkg (0.5 oz) | 34 | 9 | 7 | tr |
| strawberry preserve | 1 tbsp (0.7 oz) | 48 | 13 | 10 | tr |
| ***Eden*** | | | | | |
| Cherry Butter | 1 tbsp | 35 | 9 | 8 | 1 |
| Organic Apple Butter | 1 tbsp | 20 | 5 | 4 | 0 |

| FOOD | PORTION | CALS | CARB | SUGAR | FIBER |
|---|---|---|---|---|---|
| ***Estee*** | | | | | |
| Fruit Spread Apple Spice | 1 tbsp | 16 | 4 | 4 | 0 |
| Fruit Spread Apricot | 1 tbsp | 16 | 4 | 4 | 0 |
| Fruit Spread Grape | 1 tbsp | 16 | 4 | 4 | 0 |
| Fruit Spread Peach | 1 tbsp | 16 | 4 | 4 | 0 |
| Fruit Spread Red Raspberry | 1 tbsp | 16 | 4 | 4 | 0 |
| Fruit Spread Strawberry | 1 tbsp | 16 | 4 | 4 | 0 |
| ***Polaner*** | | | | | |
| All Fruit Peach | 1 tbsp | 40 | 8 | – | – |
| All Fruit Raspberry | 1 tbsp | 40 | 10 | 9 | – |
| ***Sarabeth's*** | | | | | |
| Spreadable Fruit Peach Apricot | 1 tbsp | 40 | 96 | 6 | 1 |
| Spreadable Fruit Strawberry Raspberry | 1 tbsp | 40 | 10 | 9 | tr |
| ***Smucker's*** | | | | | |
| Concord Grape Jelly | 1 tbsp | 50 | 13 | 12 | – |
| Peach Preserves | 1 tbsp | 50 | 13 | 12 | – |
| Simply Fruit Red Raspberry | 1 tbsp | 40 | 10 | 8 | – |
| ***Welch's*** | | | | | |
| Grape Jam | 1 tbsp | 50 | 13 | 13 | – |
| ***White House*** | | | | | |
| Apple Butter | 1 tbsp (0.6 oz) | 35 | 9 | 7 | – |
| ***Wild Thyme Farms*** | | | | | |
| Fruit Spreads Blackberry Currant Ginger | 1 tsp | 8 | 2 | 2 | – |
| Fruit Spreads Mango Apricot | 1 tsp | 7 | 2 | 2 | – |

**JAPANESE FOOD** *(see* ASIAN FOOD, SUSHI*)*

**JAVA PLUM**

| FOOD | PORTION | CALS | CARB | SUGAR | FIBER |
|---|---|---|---|---|---|
| fresh | 1 cup | 82 | 21 | – | – |
| fresh | 3 | 5 | 1 | – | – |

**JELLY** *(see* JAM/JELLY/PRESERVE*)*

**JUTE**

| FOOD | PORTION | CALS | CARB | SUGAR | FIBER |
|---|---|---|---|---|---|
| cooked | 1 cup | 32 | 6 | 1 | 2 |

**KALE**

| FOOD | PORTION | CALS | CARB | SUGAR | FIBER |
|---|---|---|---|---|---|
| chopped cooked | ½ cup | 21 | 4 | – | – |
| frzn chopped cooked | ½ cup | 20 | 4 | – | – |
| scotch chopped cooked | ½ cup | 18 | 4 | – | – |

| FOOD | PORTION | CALS | CARB | SUGAR | FIBER |
|---|---|---|---|---|---|
| **KEFIR** | | | | | |
| kefir | 7 oz | 132 | 10 | – | – |
| **KETCHUP** | | | | | |
| banana | 1 tsp | 10 | 2 | 2 | 0 |
| ketchup | 1 tbsp | 16 | 4 | – | tr |
| ketchup | 1 pkg (0.2 oz) | 6 | 2 | – | tr |
| low sodium | 1 tbsp | 16 | 4 | – | tr |
| ***Atkins*** | | | | | |
| Ketch-A-Tomato | 1 tbsp | 10 | 2 | 0 | 1 |
| ***Del Monte*** | | | | | |
| Ketchup | 1 tbsp (0.5 oz) | 15 | 4 | 4 | 0 |
| ***Estee*** | | | | | |
| Ketchup | 1 tbsp | 15 | 5 | 1 | 0 |
| ***Healthy Choice*** | | | | | |
| Ketchup | 1 tbsp (0.5 oz) | 9 | 2 | 2 | tr |
| ***Heinz*** | | | | | |
| Ketchup | 1 tbsp (0.6 oz) | 15 | 4 | 4 | 0 |
| ***Hunt's*** | | | | | |
| Ketchup | 1 tbsp (0.6 oz) | 16 | 3 | 4 | 0 |
| No Salt Added | 1 tbsp (0.6 oz) | 16 | 3 | 4 | 0 |
| ***Keto*** | | | | | |
| Ketchup | 1 tbsp | 4 | 1 | 0 | 0 |
| ***Muir Glen*** | | | | | |
| Organic | 1 tbsp (0.6 oz) | 15 | 3 | 3 | 0 |
| ***Smucker's*** | | | | | |
| Tomato | 1 tbsp | 25 | 7 | 6 | – |
| ***Steel's*** | | | | | |
| Sugar Free | 1 tbsp | 10 | 0 | 0 | 0 |
| ***Stokelys*** | | | | | |
| Tomato | 1 tbsp | 15 | 4 | 4 | – |
| ***Tree Of Life*** | | | | | |
| Ketchup | 1 tbsp (0.5 oz) | 10 | 3 | 3 | – |
| ***Walden Farms*** | | | | | |
| Calorie Free | 1 tbsp | 0 | 0 | 0 | 0 |
| **KIDNEY** | | | | | |
| beef simmered | 3 oz | 122 | 0 | 0 | 0 |
| lamb braised | 3 oz | 117 | 1 | – | – |
| pork cooked | 3 oz | 128 | 0 | 0 | 0 |
| pork cooked | 1 cup | 211 | 0 | 0 | 0 |

| FOOD | PORTION | CALS | CARB | SUGAR | FIBER |
|---|---|---|---|---|---|
| veal braised | 3 oz | 139 | 0 | 0 | 0 |
| **KIDNEY BEANS** | | | | | |
| canned | 1 cup | 207 | 38 | – | 9 |
| dried cooked | 1 cup | 225 | 40 | – | 11 |
| ***Eden*** | | | | | |
| Organic Cannellini | ½ cup (4.6 oz) | 100 | 17 | 1 | 5 |
| ***Hunt's*** | | | | | |
| Kidney Beans | ½ cup (4.5 oz) | 94 | 20 | 6 | 5 |
| ***Progresso*** | | | | | |
| Dark Red | ½ cup (4.5 oz) | 110 | 20 | 2 | 6 |
| Red | ½ cup (4.6 oz) | 110 | 20 | 0 | 8 |
| ***S&W*** | | | | | |
| Dark Red Premium | ½ cup (4.6 oz) | 100 | 23 | 7 | 6 |
| ***Van Camp*** | | | | | |
| Dark Red | ½ cup (4.6 oz) | 90 | 20 | 2 | 6 |
| Light Red | ½ cup (4.6 oz) | 90 | 20 | 3 | 6 |
| **KIWIS** | | | | | |
| fresh | 1 med | 46 | 11 | – | 3 |
| ***Chiquita*** | | | | | |
| Fresh | 2 med (5.2 oz) | 100 | 24 | 16 | 4 |
| **KNISH** | | | | | |
| **TAKE-OUT** | | | | | |
| cheese & blueberry | 1 (7 oz) | 378 | 40 | – | – |
| cheese & cherry | 1 (7 oz) | 378 | 40 | – | – |
| everything | 1 (7 oz) | 221 | 34 | – | – |
| kashe | 1 (7 oz) | 270 | 45 | – | – |
| potato | 1 lg (7 oz) | 332 | 49 | 5 | 1 |
| potato | 1 med (3.5 oz) | 166 | 25 | 2 | tr |
| potato w/ broccoli & cheese | 1 (7 oz) | 312 | 33 | – | – |
| potato w/ spinach & mushroom | 1 (7 oz) | 214 | 32 | – | – |
| **KOHLRABI** | | | | | |
| raw sliced | ½ cup | 19 | 4 | – | – |
| sliced cooked | ½ cup | 24 | 5 | – | – |
| **KRILL** | | | | | |
| fresh | 1 oz | 22 | tr | – | 0 |

| FOOD | PORTION | CALS | CARB | SUGAR | FIBER |
|---|---|---|---|---|---|
| **KUMQUATS** | | | | | |
| fresh | 1 | 12 | 3 | – | – |
| **LAMB** | | | | | |
| cubed lean only braised | 3 oz | 190 | 0 | 0 | 0 |
| cubed lean only broiled | 3 oz | 158 | 0 | 0 | 0 |
| ground broiled | 3 oz | 240 | 0 | 0 | 0 |
| leg lean & fat Choice roasted | 3 oz | 219 | 14 | – | – |
| loin chop w/ bone lean & fat Choice broiled | 1 chop (2.3 oz) | 201 | 0 | 0 | 0 |
| loin chop w/ bone lean only Choice broiled | 1 chop (1.6 oz) | 100 | 0 | 0 | 0 |
| new zealand lean & fat cooked | 3 oz | 259 | 0 | 0 | 0 |
| new zealand lean only cooked | 3 oz | 175 | 0 | 0 | 0 |
| rib chop lean & fat Choice broiled | 3 oz | 307 | 0 | 0 | 0 |
| rib chop lean only Choice broiled | 3 oz | 200 | 0 | 0 | 0 |
| shank lean & fat Choice braised | 3 oz | 206 | 0 | 0 | 0 |
| shank lean & fat Choice roasted | 3 oz | 191 | 0 | 0 | 0 |
| shoulder chop w/ bone lean & fat Choice braised | 1 chop (2.5 oz) | 244 | 0 | 0 | 0 |
| shoulder chop w/ bone lean only Choice braised | 1 chop (1.9 oz) | 152 | 0 | 0 | 0 |
| sirloin lean & fat Choice roasted | 3 oz | 248 | 0 | 0 | 0 |
| **LAMB DISHES** | | | | | |
| **TAKE-OUT** | | | | | |
| curry | ¾ cup | 345 | 22 | – | – |
| moussaka | 5.6 oz | 312 | 16 | – | 1 |
| stew | ¾ cup | 124 | 11 | – | 2 |
| **LAMBSQUARTERS** | | | | | |
| chopped cooked | ½ cup | 29 | 5 | – | – |
| **LEEKS** | | | | | |
| chopped cooked | ¼ cup | 8 | 2 | – | – |
| cooked | 1 (4.4 oz) | 38 | 9 | – | – |
| freeze dried | 1 tbsp | 1 | tr | – | – |

| FOOD | PORTION | CALS | CARB | SUGAR | FIBER |
|---|---|---|---|---|---|
| raw | 1 (4.4 oz) | 76 | 18 | – | – |
| raw chopped | ¼ cup | 16 | 4 | – | – |
| **LEMON** | | | | | |
| fresh | 1 med | 22 | 12 | – | – |
| peel | 1 tbsp | 0 | 1 | – | – |
| wedge | 1 | 5 | 3 | – | – |
| **LEMON CURD** | | | | | |
| lemon curd made w/ egg | 2 tsp | 29 | 4 | – | 0 |
| lemon curd made w/ starch | 2 tsp | 28 | 6 | – | 0 |
| **LEMON GRASS** | | | | | |
| fresh | 1 cup (2.4 oz) | 66 | 17 | – | 0 |
| fresh | 1 tbsp (5 g) | 5 | 1 | – | 0 |
| **LEMON JUICE** | | | | | |
| bottled | 1 tbsp | 3 | 1 | – | – |
| fresh | 1 tbsp | 4 | 1 | – | – |
| frzn | 1 tbsp | 3 | 1 | – | – |
| ***Canarino*** | | | | | |
| Italian Hot Lemon Beverage | 1 cup oz) | 0 | 0 | 0 | 0 |
| ***Realemon*** | | | | | |
| Juice | 1 tsp (5 ml) | 0 | 0 | – | – |
| **FROZEN** | | | | | |
| as prep w/ water | 1 cup | 100 | 26 | – | – |
| not prep | 1 can (6 oz) | 397 | 103 | – | – |
| **MIX** | | | | | |
| powder as prep w/ water | 9 fl oz | 113 | 29 | – | – |
| powder w/ equal | 1 pitcher (67 oz) | 40 | 10 | – | – |
| ***Keto*** | | | | | |
| Kooler Pink | ½ tsp | 0 | 0 | 0 | 0 |
| ***Sipper Sweets*** | | | | | |
| Sugar Free Low Carb | 1 serv | 8 | 1 | 0 | 0 |
| **READY-TO-DRINK** | | | | | |
| ***Hansen's*** | | | | | |
| Sparkling | 8 fl oz | 100 | 25 | 25 | – |
| Sparkling Pink | 8 fl oz | 120 | 31 | 31 | – |
| ***Langers*** | | | | | |
| Raspberry Lemonade | 8 oz | 120 | 29 | 26 | – |

| FOOD | PORTION | CALS | CARB | SUGAR | FIBER |
|---|---|---|---|---|---|
| White Cranberry Lemonade | 8 oz | 120 | 30 | 28 | – |
| ***Minute Maid*** | | | | | |
| Chilled | 8 fl oz | 110 | 28 | 26 | – |
| ***Nantucket Nectars*** | | | | | |
| Authentic | 8 oz | 120 | 30 | 28 | – |
| Pink | 8 oz | 120 | 30 | 27 | – |
| ***Odwalla*** | | | | | |
| Pure Squeezed | 8 fl oz | 96 | 24 | 18 | 0 |
| Strawberry Quencher | 8 fl oz | 110 | 28 | 25 | 0 |
| ***Snapple*** | | | | | |
| Diet Pink | 8 fl oz | 20 | 4 | 4 | – |
| Lemonade | 8 fl oz | 120 | 30 | 28 | – |
| Pink | 8 fl oz | 120 | 29 | 28 | – |
| ***Turkey Hill*** | | | | | |
| Lemonade | 1 cup | 120 | 29 | 29 | – |
| Raspberry | 1 cup | 120 | 29 | 29 | – |
| Strawberry Kiwi | 1 cup | 120 | 29 | 29 | – |
| **LENTILS** | | | | | |
| dried cooked | 1 cup | 231 | 40 | – | – |
| ***Natural Touch*** | | | | | |
| Lentil Rice Loaf | 1 in slice (3.2 oz) | 170 | 14 | tr | 4 |
| ***Shiloh Farms*** | | | | | |
| Organic Green not prep | ¼ cup (1.6 oz) | 150 | 27 | 2 | 7 |
| ***TastyBite*** | | | | | |
| Bengal Lentils | ½ pkg (5 oz) | 190 | 30 | 2 | 1 |
| Jodhpur Lentils | ½ pkg (5 oz) | 190 | 22 | 0 | 2 |
| Madras Lentils | ½ pkg (5 oz) | 130 | 12 | 2 | 5 |
| **TAKE-OUT** | | | | | |
| indian sambar | 1 serv | 236 | 37 | – | 9 |
| yemiser selatta ethiopian lentil salad | 1 serv (3 oz) | 115 | 11 | 1 | 2 |
| **LETTUCE** *(see also* SALAD*)* | | | | | |
| arugula | ½ cup (0.4 oz) | 3 | tr | – | tr |
| bibb | 1 head (6 oz) | 21 | 4 | – | 2 |
| boston | 1 head (6 oz) | 21 | 4 | – | 2 |
| boston | 2 leaves | 2 | tr | – | tr |
| cornsalad field salad | 1 cup (1.9 oz) | 7 | 1 | – | 1 |
| iceberg | 1 leaf | 3 | tr | – | tr |

| FOOD | PORTION | CALS | CARB | SUGAR | FIBER |
|---|---|---|---|---|---|
| iceberg | 1 head (19 oz) | 70 | 11 | – | 5 |
| looseleaf shredded | ½ cup | 5 | 1 | – | – |
| romaine shredded | ½ cup | 4 | 1 | – | tr |
| ***Dole*** | | | | | |
| Iceberg | 1 cup (3 oz) | 15 | 3 | 2 | 1 |
| Romaine | 1½ cups (3 oz) | 15 | 2 | 2 | 2 |
| Shredded | 1½ cup (3 oz) | 15 | 3 | 2 | 1 |
| ***Earthbound Farm*** | | | | | |
| Romaine Salad Organic | 1½ cups (2.9 oz) | 15 | 3 | 2 | 1 |
| **LILY ROOT** | | | | | |
| dried | 1 oz | 89 | 21 | – | tr |
| fresh | 1 oz | 32 | 8 | – | tr |
| **LIMA BEANS** | | | | | |
| **CANNED** | | | | | |
| large | 1 cup | 191 | 36 | – | – |
| lima beans | ½ cup | 88 | 17 | – | 5 |
| ***Del Monte*** | | | | | |
| Green | ½ cup (4.4 oz) | 80 | 15 | 0 | 4 |
| ***Eden*** | | | | | |
| Organic Baby | ½ cup (4.6 oz) | 100 | 17 | – | 4 |
| ***S&W*** | | | | | |
| Small Green | ½ cup (4.4 oz) | 80 | 15 | 0 | 4 |
| ***Veg-All*** | | | | | |
| Baby Green | ½ cup | 90 | 15 | 1 | 3 |
| **DRIED** | | | | | |
| baby cooked | 1 cup | 229 | 42 | – | 17 |
| cooked | ½ cup | 104 | 20 | – | – |
| large cooked | 1 cup | 217 | 39 | – | 14 |
| **FROZEN** | | | | | |
| cooked | ½ cup | 94 | 18 | – | – |
| fordhook cooked | ½ cup | 85 | 16 | – | – |
| ***Birds Eye*** | | | | | |
| Baby | ½ cup | 130 | 24 | 2 | 6 |
| Fordhook | ½ cup | 100 | 19 | 3 | 5 |
| ***Fresh Like*** | | | | | |
| Baby | 3.5 oz | 138 | 25 | – | 2 |

| FOOD | PORTION | CALS | CARB | SUGAR | FIBER |
|---|---|---|---|---|---|
| **LIME** | | | | | |
| fresh | 1 | 20 | 7 | – | – |
| **LIME JUICE** | | | | | |
| bottled | 1 tbsp | 3 | 1 | – | – |
| fresh | 1 tbsp | 4 | 1 | – | – |
| ***Odwalla*** | | | | | |
| Summertime Lime | 8 fl oz | 90 | 23 | 21 | 0 |
| ***Realime*** | | | | | |
| Juice | 1 tsp (5 ml) | 0 | 0 | – | – |
| **LING** | | | | | |
| blue raw | 3.5 oz | 83 | 0 | 0 | 0 |
| fresh baked | 3 oz | 95 | 0 | 0 | 0 |
| fresh fillet baked | 5.3 oz | 168 | 0 | 0 | 0 |
| **LINGCOD** | | | | | |
| baked | 3 oz | 93 | 0 | 0 | 0 |
| fillet baked | 5.3 oz | 164 | 0 | 0 | 0 |
| **LIQUOR/LIQUEUR** *(see also* BEER AND ALE, CHAMPAGNE, WINE*)* | | | | | |
| 7&7 | 1 serv | 178 | 19 | – | 0 |
| B 52 | 1 serv | 247 | 25 | – | 0 |
| alabama slammer | 1 serv | 103 | 7 | – | tr |
| amaretto sour | 1 serv | 295 | 57 | – | 4 |
| angel's kiss | 1 serv | 85 | 5 | – | 0 |
| anisette | 1 oz | 111 | 11 | – | 0 |
| antifreeze | 1 serv | 177 | 31 | – | tr |
| apricot brandy | 1 oz | 96 | 9 | – | 0 |
| apricot sour | 1 serv | 164 | 8 | – | tr |
| aquavit | 1 oz | 65 | 0 | 0 | 0 |
| b&b | 1 serv | 75 | 0 | 0 | 0 |
| bahama breeze | 1 serv | 70 | 9 | – | tr |
| bahama mama | 1 serv | 153 | 23 | – | tr |
| bailey's & amaretto | 1 serv | 184 | 16 | – | 0 |
| banana colada | 1 serv | 376 | 64 | – | 3 |
| bay breeze | 1 serv | 173 | 18 | – | tr |
| bend me over | 1 serv | 242 | 32 | – | tr |
| benedictine | 1 oz | 104 | 11 | – | 0 |
| betsy ross | 1 serv | 206 | 5 | – | 0 |
| black devil | 1 serv | 220 | 1 | – | tr |
| black russian | 1 serv | 184 | 12 | – | 0 |

| FOOD | PORTION | CALS | CARB | SUGAR | FIBER |
|---|---|---|---|---|---|
| bloody mary | 1 serv | 150 | 5 | – | 1 |
| blue whale | 1 serv | 222 | 23 | – | 0 |
| bourbon & soda | 1 serv (4 oz) | 105 | 0 | 0 | 0 |
| bourbon sour | 1 serv | 166 | 8 | – | tr |
| brandy alexander | 1 serv | 266 | 12 | – | 0 |
| brandy sour | 1 serv | 164 | 8 | – | tr |
| bushwacher | 1 serv | 286 | 27 | – | tr |
| coffee liqueur | 1 serv (1.5 oz) | 175 | 24 | – | 0 |
| coffee w/ cream liqueur | 1 serv (1.5 oz) | 154 | 10 | – | 0 |
| cognac | 1 oz | 67 | tr | 0 | 0 |
| cosmopolitan martini | 1 serv | 126 | 7 | – | tr |
| creme de menthe | 1 serv (1.5 oz) | 186 | 21 | – | 0 |
| curacao liqueur | 1 oz | 81 | 9 | – | 0 |
| daiquiri | 1 serv | 187 | 15 | – | 0 |
| daiquiri banana | 1 serv | 277 | 32 | – | 1 |
| dark & stormy | 1 serv | 64 | 0 | 0 | 0 |
| doctor pepper | 1 serv | 95 | 12 | – | 0 |
| frozen daiquiri pineapple | 1 serv | 186 | 28 | – | 2 |
| frozen tequila screwdriver | 1 serv | 159 | 17 | – | 1 |
| fuzzy navel | 1 serv | 247 | 10 | – | tr |
| gimlet vodka | 1 serv | 150 | 6 | – | 1 |
| gin | 1 serv (1.5 oz) | 110 | 0 | 0 | 0 |
| gin & tonic | 1 serv (7.5 oz) | 171 | 16 | – | – |
| gin ricky | 1 serv | 114 | 1 | – | tr |
| grasshopper | 1 serv | 275 | 26 | – | 0 |
| happy hawaiian | 1 serv | 434 | 60 | – | tr |
| harvey wallbanger | 1 serv | 198 | 16 | – | tr |
| head banger | 1 serv | 165 | 4 | – | 0 |
| hot buttered rum | 1 serv | 219 | 15 | – | 4 |
| hot toddy | 1 serv | 188 | 13 | – | 5 |
| hurricane | 1 serv | 205 | 19 | – | tr |
| kamikaze | 1 serv | 136 | 2 | – | 0 |
| long island iced tea | 1 serv | 292 | 7 | – | 0 |
| lynchburg lemonade | 1 serv | 465 | 85 | – | 1 |
| mai tai | 1 serv | 165 | 17 | – | tr |
| manhattan | 1 serv | 171 | 3 | – | tr |
| margarita | 1 serv | 173 | 11 | – | 0 |
| margarita strawberry | 1 serv | 106 | 11 | – | 1 |
| martini apple | 1 serv | 147 | 4 | – | tr |
| martini rum | 1 serv | 131 | tr | – | tr |

| FOOD | PORTION | CALS | CARB | SUGAR | FIBER |
|---|---|---|---|---|---|
| martini vodka | 1 serv | 135 | 1 | – | tr |
| mellow yellow | 1 serv | 95 | 4 | – | 0 |
| mexican grasshopper | 1 serv | 638 | 52 | – | 0 |
| mint julep | 1 serv | 136 | 17 | – | tr |
| mississippi mud | 1 serv | 496 | 46 | – | 0 |
| mudslide | 1 serv | 566 | 46 | – | 0 |
| narragansett | 1 serv | 168 | 2 | – | 0 |
| nutcracker | 1 serv | 730 | 64 | – | 0 |
| old fashioned | 1 serv | 223 | 4 | – | tr |
| orange crush | 1 serv | 461 | 65 | – | tr |
| pain killer | 1 serv | 277 | 20 | – | tr |
| peppermint pattie | 1 serv | 344 | 37 | – | 0 |
| pina colada | 1 serv (4.5 oz) | 262 | 40 | – | tr |
| planter's cocktail | 1 serv | 105 | 3 | – | tr |
| planter's punch | 1 serv | 233 | 34 | – | 4 |
| presbyterian | 1 serv | 170 | 8 | – | tr |
| purple passion | 1 serv | 215 | 22 | – | 0 |
| rob roy | 1 serv | 171 | 3 | – | tr |
| rum | 1 serv (1.5 oz) | 97 | 0 | 0 | 0 |
| rum cola | 1 serv | 209 | 21 | – | tr |
| rum highball | 1 serv | 170 | 11 | – | 0 |
| rum punch | 1 serv | 448 | 88 | – | 1 |
| rusty nail | 1 serv | 159 | 6 | – | 0 |
| salty dog | 1 serv | 210 | 19 | – | tr |
| scotch & soda | 1 serv | 104 | tr | – | tr |
| screwdriver rum | 1 serv | 166 | 16 | – | tr |
| sea breeze | 1 serv | 207 | 19 | – | tr |
| sex on the beach | 1 serv | 190 | 18 | – | tr |
| slippery nipple | 1 serv | 142 | 11 | – | 0 |
| sloe gin fizz | 1 serv (2.5 oz) | 132 | 4 | – | 0 |
| snake bite | 1 serv | 362 | 22 | – | 0 |
| sour rum | 1 serv | 156 | 8 | – | tr |
| swizzle rum | 1 serv | 187 | 15 | – | 0 |
| tequila gimlet | 1 serv | 150 | 6 | – | 1 |
| tequila sour | 1 serv | 156 | 8 | – | tr |
| tequila stinger | 1 serv | 221 | 14 | – | 0 |
| tequila sunrise | 1 serv (6.8 oz) | 232 | 24 | – | 0 |
| tom collins | 1 serv (7.5 oz) | 121 | 3 | – | – |
| vermouth cassis | 1 serv | 97 | 5 | – | tr |
| vodka | 1 serv (1.5 oz) | 97 | 0 | 0 | 0 |

| FOOD | PORTION | CALS | CARB | SUGAR | FIBER |
|---|---|---|---|---|---|
| vodka sour | 1 serv | 138 | 3 | – | tr |
| vodka stinger | 1 serv | 378 | 28 | – | 0 |
| whiskey | 1 serv (1.5 oz) | 105 | tr | – | 0 |
| whiskey sour | 1 serv | 159 | 6 | – | tr |
| white russian | 1 serv | 290 | 17 | – | 0 |
| zombie | 1 serv | 235 | 10 | – | tr |
| **LIVER** *(see also PÂTÉ)* | | | | | |
| beef braised | 3 oz | 137 | 3 | – | – |
| beef pan-fried | 3 oz | 184 | 7 | – | – |
| chicken stewed | 1 cup (5 oz) | 219 | 1 | – | – |
| duck raw | 1 (1.5 oz) | 60 | 2 | – | – |
| goose raw | 1 (3.3 oz) | 125 | 6 | – | – |
| lamb braised | 3 oz | 187 | 2 | – | – |
| lamb fried | 3 oz | 202 | 3 | – | – |
| pork braised | 3 oz | 140 | 3 | – | 0 |
| sheep raw | 3.5 oz | 131 | 0 | 0 | 0 |
| turkey simmered | 1 cup (5 oz) | 237 | 5 | – | – |
| veal braised | 3 oz | 140 | 2 | – | – |
| veal fried | 3 oz | 208 | 3 | – | – |
| **LOBSTER** | | | | | |
| northern cooked | 3 oz | 83 | 1 | – | – |
| northern cooked | 1 cup | 142 | 2 | – | – |
| northern raw | 3 oz | 77 | tr | – | – |
| northern raw | 1 lobster (5.3 oz) | 136 | 1 | – | – |
| spiny steamed | 1 (5.7 oz) | 233 | 5 | – | – |
| spiny steamed | 3 oz | 122 | 3 | – | – |
| ***Progresso*** | | | | | |
| Lobster Sauce | ½ cup (4.3 oz) | 100 | 6 | 3 | 2 |
| **TAKE-OUT** | | | | | |
| newburg | 1 cup | 485 | 13 | – | – |
| **LOGANBERRIES** | | | | | |
| frzn | 1 cup | 80 | 19 | – | – |
| **LONGANS** | | | | | |
| fresh | 1 | 2 | tr | – | – |
| **LOQUATS** | | | | | |
| fresh | 1 | 5 | 1 | – | – |

| FOOD | PORTION | CALS | CARB | SUGAR | FIBER |
|---|---|---|---|---|---|
| **LOTUS** | | | | | |
| root raw sliced | 10 slices | 45 | 14 | – | – |
| root sliced cooked | 10 slices | 59 | 14 | – | – |
| seeds dried | 1 oz | 94 | 18 | – | – |
| ***Eden*** | | | | | |
| Root | 1 serv (0.3 oz) | 35 | 8 | 1 | 2 |
| **LOX** *(see* SALMON*)* | | | | | |
| **LUPINES** | | | | | |
| dried cooked | 1 cup | 197 | 16 | – | – |
| **LYCHEES** | | | | | |
| fresh | 1 | 6 | 2 | – | – |
| **MACADAMIA NUTS** | | | | | |
| dry roasted w/ salt | 10-12 nuts (1 oz) | 200 | 4 | 2 | 1 |
| oil roasted | 1 oz | 204 | 4 | – | – |
| ***Hawaiian Host*** | | | | | |
| Chocolate Covered | 1 piece (0.5 oz) | 53 | 8 | 7 | tr |
| ***Keto*** | | | | | |
| Chocolately Covered | 1 oz | 171 | 6 | 0 | 4 |
| ***Maranatha*** | | | | | |
| Macadamia Butter | 2 tbsp | 230 | 5 | 1 | 3 |
| **MACE** | | | | | |
| ground | 1 tsp | 8 | 1 | – | – |
| **MACKEREL** | | | | | |
| **CANNED** | | | | | |
| jack | 1 cup | 296 | 0 | 0 | 0 |
| jack | 1 can (12.7 oz) | 563 | 0 | 0 | 0 |
| **DRIED** | | | | | |
| ***Eden*** | | | | | |
| Bonito Flakes | 2 tbsp | 4 | 0 | 0 | 0 |
| **FRESH** | | | | | |
| atlantic cooked | 3 oz | 223 | 0 | 0 | 0 |
| atlantic raw | 3 oz | 174 | 0 | 0 | 0 |
| jack baked | 3 oz | 171 | 0 | 0 | 0 |
| jack fillet baked | 6.2 oz | 354 | 0 | 0 | 0 |

| FOOD | PORTION | CALS | CARB | SUGAR | FIBER |
|---|---|---|---|---|---|
| king baked | 3 oz | 114 | 0 | 0 | 0 |
| king fillet baked | 5.4 oz | 207 | 0 | 0 | 0 |
| pacific baked | 3 oz | 171 | 0 | 0 | 0 |
| pacific fillet baked | 6.2 oz | 354 | 0 | 0 | 0 |
| spanish cooked | 1 fillet (5.1 oz) | 230 | 0 | 0 | 0 |
| spanish cooked | 3 oz | 134 | 0 | 0 | 0 |
| spanish raw | 3 oz | 118 | 0 | 0 | 0 |
| **SMOKED** | | | | | |
| atlantic | 3.5 oz | 296 | 0 | 0 | 0 |
| **MALANGA** | | | | | |
| fresh | ½ cup | 137 | 32 | – | – |
| **MALT** | | | | | |
| nonalcoholic | 12 fl oz | 32 | 5 | – | – |
| ***Skyy*** | | | | | |
| Blue | 1 bottle | 235 | 35 | – | – |
| Sport | 1 bottle | 160 | 15 | – | – |
| **MALTED MILK** | | | | | |
| chocolate as prep w/ milk | 1 cup | 229 | 30 | – | – |
| chocolate flavor powder | 3 heaping tsp (¾ oz) | 79 | 18 | – | – |
| natural flavor as prep w/ milk | 1 cup | 237 | 27 | – | – |
| natural flavor powder | 3 heaping tsp (¾ oz) | 87 | 19 | – | – |
| **MAMMY-APPLE** | | | | | |
| fresh | 1 | 431 | 106 | – | – |
| **MANGO** | | | | | |
| fresh | 1 | 135 | 35 | – | – |
| ***Del Monte*** | | | | | |
| In Extra Light Syrup | ½ cup (4.4 oz) | 100 | 25 | 20 | 0 |
| **MANGO JUICE** | | | | | |
| ***Fresh Samantha*** | | | | | |
| Mango Mama | 1 cup (8 oz) | 120 | 10 | – | 8 |
| ***Guzzler*** | | | | | |
| Mango Passion | 8 fl oz | 140 | 22 | 0 | – |
| ***Langers*** | | | | | |
| Mongo Mango | 8 oz | 120 | 30 | 27 | – |

| FOOD | PORTION | CALS | CARB | SUGAR | FIBER |
| --- | --- | --- | --- | --- | --- |
| ***Ocean Spray*** | | | | | |
| Mango Mango | 8 oz | 130 | 33 | 33 | 0 |
| ***Snapple*** | | | | | |
| Mango Madness | 8 fl oz | 110 | 29 | 27 | – |
| **MARGARINE** | | | | | |
| squeeze | 1 tsp | 34 | 0 | 0 | 0 |
| stick corn | 1 tsp | 34 | 0 | 0 | 0 |
| stick corn | 1 stick (4 oz) | 815 | 1 | – | – |
| tub corn | 1 tsp | 34 | 0 | 0 | 0 |
| tub diet | 1 tsp | 17 | 0 | 0 | 0 |
| ***Brummel & Brown*** | | | | | |
| Spread Make With Yogurt | 1 tbsp (0.5 oz) | 45 | 0 | 0 | 0 |
| ***I Can't Believe Its Not Butter*** | | | | | |
| Spray | 5 sprays | 0 | 0 | 0 | 0 |
| ***Take Control*** | | | | | |
| Light | 1 tbsp | 45 | 0 | 0 | – |
| Spread | 1 tbsp (0.5 oz) | 80 | 0 | 0 | 0 |
| ***Weight Watchers*** | | | | | |
| Light | 1 tbsp | 45 | 2 | 0 | 0 |
| Light Sodium Free | 1 tbsp | 45 | 2 | 0 | 0 |
| **MARINADE** *(see* SAUCE*)* | | | | | |
| **MARJORAM** | | | | | |
| dried | 1 tsp | 2 | tr | – | – |
| **MARSHMALLOW** | | | | | |
| marshmallow | 1 reg (0.3 oz) | 23 | 6 | – | – |
| marshmallow | 1 cup (1.6 oz) | 146 | 37 | – | – |
| ***Gol D Lite*** | | | | | |
| Sugar Free | ⅓ pkg (0.9 oz) | 51 | 19 | 0 | 0 |
| **MATZO** | | | | | |
| egg | 1 (1 oz) | 111 | 22 | – | 1 |
| egg & onion | 1 (1 oz) | 111 | 22 | – | 1 |
| plain | 1 (1 oz) | 112 | 24 | – | 1 |
| whole wheat | 1 (1 oz) | 99 | 22 | – | 3 |
| ***Manischewitz*** | | | | | |
| Matzo Meal | ¼ cup (1 oz) | 130 | 23 | 1 | 1 |
| **MAYONNAISE** | | | | | |
| mayonnaise | 1 cup | 1577 | 6 | – | – |

| FOOD | PORTION | CALS | CARB | SUGAR | FIBER |
|---|---|---|---|---|---|
| mayonnaise | 1 tbsp | 99 | tr | – | – |
| reduced calorie | 1 tbsp | 34 | 2 | – | – |
| reduced calorie | 1 cup | 556 | 38 | – | – |
| sandwich spread | 1 tbsp | 60 | 3 | – | – |
| ***Blue Plate*** | | | | | |
| Squeeze | 1 tbsp | 100 | 0 | 0 | 0 |
| ***Hellman's*** | | | | | |
| Mayonnaise | 1 tbsp | 100 | 0 | – | – |
| ***Weight Watchers*** | | | | | |
| Fat Free | 1 tbsp | 10 | 3 | 2 | 0 |
| Light | 1 tbsp | 25 | 1 | 1 | 0 |
| Light Low Sodium | 1 tbsp | 25 | 1 | 0 | 0 |

## MAYONNAISE TYPE SALAD DRESSING

| FOOD | PORTION | CALS | CARB | SUGAR | FIBER |
|---|---|---|---|---|---|
| mayonnaise type salad dressing | 1 cup | 916 | 56 | – | – |
| mayonnaise type salad dressing | 1 tbsp | 57 | 4 | – | – |
| reduced calorie w/o cholesterol | 1 tbsp | 68 | 2 | – | – |
| reduced calorie w/o cholesterol | 1 cup | 1084 | 36 | – | – |
| ***Carb Options*** | | | | | |
| Whipped Dressing | 1 tbsp | 50 | 0 | 0 | 0 |
| ***Nasoya*** | | | | | |
| Nayonaise | 1 tbsp | 35 | 1 | tr | 0 |
| Nayonaise Dijon | 1 tbsp | 30 | 1 | 0 | 0 |
| ***Weight Watchers*** | | | | | |
| Fat Free Whipped Dressing | 1 tbsp | 15 | 3 | 2 | 0 |

## MEAT STICKS

| FOOD | PORTION | CALS | CARB | SUGAR | FIBER |
|---|---|---|---|---|---|
| jerky beef | 1 oz | 96 | 4 | – | – |
| jerky beef | 1 lg piece (0.7 oz) | 67 | 3 | – | – |
| smoked | 1 (0.7 oz) | 109 | 1 | – | – |
| smoked | 1 oz | 156 | 2 | – | – |
| ***Big Ones*** | | | | | |
| BBQ | 1 (1 oz) | 130 | 1 | 1 | 0 |
| Hot n'Spicy | 1 (1 oz) | 130 | 1 | 1 | 0 |
| Original | 1 (1 oz) | 130 | 1 | 1 | 0 |
| Teriyaki | 1 (1 oz) | 130 | 2 | 2 | 0 |

| FOOD | PORTION | CALS | CARB | SUGAR | FIBER |
|---|---|---|---|---|---|
| ***Jack Link's*** | | | | | |
| Kippered Beefsteak Teriyaki | 1 oz | 80 | 5 | 4 | 0 |
| ***Lance*** | | | | | |
| Beef & Cheese | 1 pkg (1.5 oz) | 150 | 3 | 0 | 0 |
| Beef Jerky | 1 piece (0.25 oz) | 30 | tr | 0 | 0 |
| Beef Snack | 1 piece (0.63 oz) | 100 | 1 | 0 | 0 |
| Hot Sausage | 1 piece (0.9 oz) | 60 | 1 | 1 | 0 |
| ***Lowrey's*** | | | | | |
| Smokehouse Tender Hickory Smoked | 1 pkg (1 oz) | 80 | 5 | 4 | 0 |
| Smokehouse Tender Original | 1 pkg (1 oz) | 60 | 2 | 1 | 1 |
| Smokehouse Tender Peppered | 1 pkg (1 oz) | 60 | 2 | 1 | 1 |
| ***Oberto*** | | | | | |
| Beef Jerky | 1 pkg (1.3 oz) | 100 | 8 | 9 | – |
| ***Rustlers Roundup*** | | | | | |
| Beef Jerky | 1 serv (5 g) | 20 | tr | 0 | tr |
| Flamin' Hot | 1 serv (8 g) | 40 | 1 | tr | tr |
| Smoky Steak | 1 serv (0.8 oz) | 60 | 1 | tr | 0 |
| Spicy | 1 serv (0.5 oz) | 70 | 1 | 0 | tr |

**MEAT SUBSTITUTES** *(see also* BACON SUBSTITUTES, CANADIAN BACON SUBSTITUTES, CHICKEN SUBSTITUTES, HAMBURGER SUBSTITUTES, SAUSAGE SUBSTITUTES, TURKEY SUBSTITUTES*)*

| FOOD | PORTION | CALS | CARB | SUGAR | FIBER |
|---|---|---|---|---|---|
| simulated meat product | 1 oz | 88 | 11 | – | – |
| ***Frieda's*** | | | | | |
| SoyTaco | 1 oz | 50 | 3 | 0 | 2 |
| Soyrizo | 4 tbsp (1.9 oz) | 120 | 5 | 2 | 3 |
| ***Ken & Robert's*** | | | | | |
| Veggie Pockets | 1 (4.5 oz) | 250 | 40 | 3 | 5 |
| Veggie Pockets Bar B Que | 1 (4.5 oz) | 290 | 45 | 2 | 5 |
| Veggie Pockets Broccoli & Cheddar | 1 (4.5 oz) | 250 | 38 | 2 | 4 |
| Veggie Pockets Greek | 1 (4.5 oz) | 250 | 37 | 2 | 4 |
| Veggie Pockets Indian | 1 (4.5 oz) | 260 | 40 | 2 | 5 |
| Veggie Pockets Pizza | 1 (4.5 oz) | 270 | 41 | 2 | 4 |
| Veggie Pockets Pot Pie | 1 (4.5 oz) | 250 | 38 | 2 | 2 |

| FOOD | PORTION | CALS | CARB | SUGAR | FIBER |
|---|---|---|---|---|---|
| Veggie Pockets Potato & Cheddar | 1 (4.5 oz) | 260 | 42 | 2 | 2 |
| Veggie Pockets Santa Fe | 1 (4.5 oz) | 250 | 39 | 2 | 5 |
| Veggie Pockets Tex Mex | 1 (4.5 oz) | 260 | 46 | 2 | 6 |
| ***Lightlife*** | | | | | |
| Foney Baloney | 3 slices (1.5 oz) | 60 | 2 | 0 | 0 |
| Gimme Lean Beef | 2 oz | 70 | 8 | 1 | 1 |
| Smart Deli Bologna | 3 slices (1.5 oz) | 50 | 2 | 0 | 0 |
| Smart Deli Ham | 3 slices (1.5 oz) | 50 | 2 | 0 | 0 |
| Smart Deli Peppercorn | 3 slices (1.5 oz) | 45 | 1 | 0 | 0 |
| Smart Deli Sticks Soylami | 1 oz | 40 | 1 | 0 | 0 |
| Smart Deli Sticks Pepperoni | 1 oz | 45 | 2 | 1 | 0 |
| Smart Ground Original | ⅓ cup (1.9 oz) | 70 | 5 | 1 | 3 |
| Smart Ground Taco | ⅓ cup (2 oz) | 60 | 6 | 0 | 3 |
| ***Loma Linda*** | | | | | |
| Dinner Cuts | 2 slices (3.2 oz) | 90 | 3 | 0 | 2 |
| Nuteena | ⅜ in slice (1.9 oz) | 160 | 6 | tr | 2 |
| Sandwich Spread | ¼ cup (1.9 oz) | 80 | 7 | tr | 3 |
| Savory Dinner Loaf Mix not prep | ⅓ cup (0.9 oz) | 90 | 7 | 0 | 5 |
| Swiss Stake | 1 piece (3.2 oz) | 120 | 8 | tr | 4 |
| Tender Bits | 6 pieces (3 oz) | 110 | 7 | 0 | 3 |
| Tender Rounds | 6 pieces (2.8 oz) | 120 | 5 | tr | 3 |
| Vita Burger Chunks not prep | ¼ cup (0.7 oz) | 70 | 6 | 1 | 3 |
| Vita Burger Granules | 3 tbsp (0.7 oz) | 70 | 6 | 1 | 3 |
| ***Morningstar Farms*** | | | | | |
| Burger Style Recipe Crumbles | ⅔ cup (1.9 oz) | 80 | 4 | tr | 2 |
| Ground Meatless | ½ cup (1.9 oz) | 60 | 4 | 0 | 2 |
| Harvest Burger Recipe Crumbles | ½ cup (2 oz) | 70 | 5 | 0 | 3 |

| FOOD | PORTION | CALS | CARB | SUGAR | FIBER |
|---|---|---|---|---|---|
| Quarter Prime | 1 patty (3.4 oz) | 140 | 6 | 1 | 3 |
| ***Natural Touch*** | | | | | |
| Dinner Entree | 1 patty (3 oz) | 220 | 2 | 0 | 2 |
| Loaf Mix not prep | 4 tbsp (1 oz) | 100 | 10 | tr | 7 |
| Stroganoff Mix not prep | 4 tbsp (0.8 oz) | 90 | 10 | 1 | 3 |
| Taco Mix not prep | 3 tbsp (0.6 oz) | 60 | 5 | tr | 3 |
| Vegan Burger Crumbles | ½ cup (1.9 oz) | 60 | 4 | 0 | 2 |
| ***Quorn*** | | | | | |
| Grounds | ⅔ cup (3 oz) | 80 | 5 | 1 | 4 |
| ***Soy7*** | | | | | |
| Burger Bits as prep | ½ cup | 60 | 5 | tr | 2 |
| Burger Mix as prep | 1 serv (3.2 oz) | 120 | 9 | tr | 3 |
| Recipe Strips as prep | ¾ cup | 70 | 7 | tr | 3 |
| Taco Mix as prep | ¼ cup | 70 | 6 | 1 | 3 |
| ***Worthington*** | | | | | |
| Beef Style Meatless | ⅜ in slice (1.9 oz) | 110 | 4 | tr | 3 |
| Bologna | 3 slices (2 oz) | 80 | 2 | 0 | 2 |
| Choplets | 2 slices (3.2 oz) | 90 | 3 | 0 | 2 |
| Corned Beef Meatless | 4 slices (2 oz) | 140 | 5 | tr | 2 |
| Country Stew | 1 cup (8.4 oz) | 210 | 20 | 2 | 5 |
| Dinner Roast | ¾ in slice (3 oz) | 180 | 5 | 1 | 3 |
| FriPats | 1 patty (2.2 oz) | 130 | 4 | 0 | 3 |
| Multigrain Cutlets | 2 slices (3.2 oz) | 100 | 5 | 0 | 4 |
| Numete | ⅜ in slice (1.9 oz) | 130 | 5 | tr | 3 |
| Prime Stakes | 1 piece (3.2 oz) | 120 | 4 | 0 | 4 |
| Prosage Roll | ⅝ in slice (1.9 oz) | 140 | 2 | 0 | 2 |
| Protose | ⅜ in slice (1.9 oz) | 130 | 5 | tr | 3 |

| FOOD | PORTION | CALS | CARB | SUGAR | FIBER |
|---|---|---|---|---|---|
| ***Yves*** | | | | | |
| Veggie Bologna | 4 slices (2.2 oz) | 70 | 2 | 1 | 0 |
| Veggie Ground Italian | ⅓ cup (2 oz) | 60 | 4 | 0 | 3 |
| Veggie Ground Round Italian | ⅓ cup (1.9 oz) | 60 | 4 | 0 | 3 |
| Veggie Ground Round Original | 2 oz | 60 | 4 | 0 | 3 |
| Veggie Pizza Pepperoni Slices | 1 serv (1.7 oz) | 70 | 4 | 0 | 3 |
| Veggie Salami Deli Slices | 1 serv (2.2 oz) | 90 | 5 | 1 | 1 |
| **MELON** | | | | | |
| melon balls frzn | 1 cup | 55 | 14 | – | – |
| ***SunFresh*** | | | | | |
| Melon Salad In Extra Light Syrup | ½ cup (4.5 oz) | 45 | 10 | 8 | 2 |
| **MELON JUICE** | | | | | |
| ***Ocean Spray*** | | | | | |
| Mega Melon | 8 oz | 130 | 33 | 33 | 0 |
| **MEXICAN FOOD** *(see* SALSA, SPANISH FOOD, TORTILLA*)* | | | | | |
| **MILK** | | | | | |
| **CANNED** | | | | | |
| condensed sweetened | 1 oz | 123 | 21 | – | – |
| condensed sweetened | 1 cup | 982 | 166 | – | – |
| evaporated | ½ cup | 169 | 13 | – | – |
| evaporated skim | ½ cup | 99 | 14 | – | – |
| ***Carnation*** | | | | | |
| Evaporated | 2 tbsp | 40 | 3 | 3 | – |
| Evaporated Fat Free | 2 tbsp | 25 | 4 | 4 | – |
| Sweetened Condensed | ⅓ cup | 330 | 22 | 22 | 0 |
| ***Pet*** | | | | | |
| Evaporated | 2 tbsp | 40 | 3 | 3 | – |
| **DRIED** | | | | | |
| buttermilk | 1 tbsp | 25 | 3 | – | – |
| nonfat instantized | 1 pkg (3.2 oz) | 244 | 47 | – | – |
| ***Carnation*** | | | | | |
| Nonfat | ⅓ cup | 80 | 12 | 12 | 0 |
| ***Sanalac*** | | | | | |
| Powder | ¼ cup (0.8 oz) | 85 | 13 | 12 | 0 |
| **REFRIGERATED** | | | | | |
| 1% | 1 cup | 102 | 12 | – | – |

| FOOD | PORTION | CALS | CARB | SUGAR | FIBER |
|---|---|---|---|---|---|
| 1% | 1 qt | 409 | 47 | – | – |
| 1% protein fortified | 1 qt | 477 | 54 | – | – |
| 1% protein fortified | 1 cup | 119 | 14 | – | – |
| 2% | 1 cup | 121 | 12 | – | – |
| 2% | 1 qt | 485 | 47 | – | – |
| buffalo | 7 oz | 224 | 10 | – | – |
| buttermilk | 1 cup | 99 | 12 | – | – |
| buttermilk | 1 qt | 396 | 47 | – | – |
| camel | 7 oz | 160 | 10 | – | – |
| donkey | 7 oz | 86 | 12 | – | – |
| goat | 1 cup | 168 | 11 | – | – |
| goat | 1 qt | 672 | 43 | – | – |
| human | 1 cup | 171 | 17 | – | – |
| indian buffalo | 1 cup | 236 | 13 | – | – |
| low sodium | 1 cup | 149 | 11 | – | – |
| mare | 7 oz | 98 | 12 | – | – |
| nonfat | 1 cup | 86 | 12 | – | – |
| nonfat | 1 qt | 342 | 48 | – | – |
| nonfat protein fortified | 1 qt | 400 | 55 | – | – |
| nonfat protein fortified | 1 cup | 100 | 14 | – | – |
| sheep | 1 cup | 264 | 13 | – | – |
| whole | 1 cup | 150 | 11 | – | – |
| ***Horizon Organic*** | | | | | |
| Fat Free | 1 cup (8 oz) | 80 | 12 | 11 | 0 |
| ***Land O Lakes*** | | | | | |
| 1% Lowfat | 1 carton (10 oz) | 120 | 13 | 13 | – |
| Fat Free | 1 carton (10 oz) | 100 | 13 | 13 | – |
| Whole | 1 carton (10 oz) | 180 | 13 | 13 | – |
| ***NutraBalance*** | | | | | |
| LactaCare | 1 pkg (8 oz) | 500 | 64 | – | – |
| ***Organic Valley*** | | | | | |
| Low Fat | 1 cup | 100 | 12 | 12 | 0 |
| Nonfat | 1 cup | 80 | 13 | 12 | 0 |
| Reduced Fat | 1 cup | 130 | 12 | 11 | 0 |
| Whole | 1 cup | 150 | 12 | 11 | 0 |
| ***Stonyfield Farm*** | | | | | |
| Organic Whole Milk | 1 cup (8 oz) | 180 | 12 | 12 | 0 |

| FOOD | PORTION | CALS | CARB | SUGAR | FIBER |
|---|---|---|---|---|---|
| Organic Whole Milk Vanilla | 1 cup (8 oz) | 230 | 30 | 30 | 0 |
| ***Turkey Hill*** | | | | | |
| Cool Moos 2% Reduced Fat | 1 cup | 130 | 12 | 11 | – |
| Cool Moos Whole Milk | 1 cup | 160 | 12 | 11 | – |
| **MILK DRINKS** | | | | | |
| chocolate milk | 1 cup | 208 | 26 | – | – |
| chocolate milk | 1 qt | 833 | 103 | – | – |
| chocolate milk 1% | 1 cup | 158 | 26 | – | – |
| chocolate milk 1% | 1 qt | 630 | 104 | – | – |
| chocolate milk 2% | 1 cup | 179 | 26 | – | – |
| strawberry flavor mix as prep w/ whole milk | 9 oz | 234 | 33 | – | – |
| ***Cocio*** | | | | | |
| Chocolate Milk | 1 bottle | 225 | 32 | 28 | tr |
| ***Garelick*** | | | | | |
| Colossal Coffee | 1 cup | 145 | 23 | 22 | 0 |
| Ultimate Chocolate | 1 cup | 150 | 29 | 27 | 1 |
| ***Horizon Organic*** | | | | | |
| Lowfat Chocolate Milk | 1 cup (8 oz) | 160 | 26 | 24 | 1 |
| ***Keto*** | | | | | |
| Chocolate Milk Mix | 1 scoop | 36 | 3 | 0 | 1 |
| ***Land O Lakes*** | | | | | |
| Chocolate | 1 cup (8.4 oz) | 200 | 27 | 26 | 0 |
| ***Organic Valley*** | | | | | |
| Chocolate Milk Reduced Fat | 1 cup | 180 | 26 | 25 | 0 |
| ***Quik*** | | | | | |
| Banana Lowfat | 1 cup (8.4 oz) | 200 | 31 | 30 | 0 |
| Banana Powder | 2 tbsp (0.8 oz) | 90 | 27 | 20 | 0 |
| Chocolate | 1 cup (8.4 oz) | 230 | 33 | 30 | 1 |
| Chocolate Lowfat | 1 carton (8.4 oz) | 200 | 30 | 29 | 0 |
| Cookies n Cream Powder | 2 tbsp (0.8 oz) | 100 | 21 | 14 | 1 |
| Strawberry | 1 cup (8.4 oz) | 230 | 33 | 30 | 0 |
| Strawberry Lowfat | 1 carton (8.4 oz) | 210 | 35 | 35 | 0 |
| Strawberry Powder | 2 tbsp (0.8 oz) | 90 | 22 | 21 | 0 |
| ***Turkey Hill*** | | | | | |
| Cool Moos Chocolate 1% Lowfat | 1 cup | 180 | 32 | 30 | – |

| FOOD | PORTION | CALS | CARB | SUGAR | FIBER |
|---|---|---|---|---|---|
| Cool Moos Orange Cream 1% Lowfat | 1 cup | 190 | 33 | 32 | – |
| Cool Moos Strawberry 1% Lowfat | 1 cup | 160 | 27 | 27 | – |
| Cool Moos Vanilla 1% Lowfat | 1 cup | 160 | 26 | 25 | – |
| **MILK SUBSTITUTES** | | | | | |
| imitation milk | 1 cup | 150 | 15 | – | – |
| imitation milk | 1 qt | 600 | 60 | – | – |
| ***8th Continent*** | | | | | |
| Soymilk Low Fat Chocolate | 1 bottle (8 oz) | 140 | 23 | 21 | 1 |
| Soymilk Low Fat Original | 1 bottle (8 oz) | 80 | 8 | 6 | tr |
| Soymilk Low Fat Vanilla | 1 bottle (8 oz) | 90 | 11 | 10 | tr |
| ***Better Than Milk*** | | | | | |
| Rice Original | 2 tbsp (0.66 oz) | 78 | 15 | 4 | 1 |
| Rice Original Light | 2 tbsp (0.66 oz) | 66 | 17 | 4 | 1 |
| Rice Vanilla | 2 tbsp (0.66 oz) | 78 | 15 | 5 | 1 |
| Rice Vanilla Light | 2 tbsp (0.66 oz) | 66 | 17 | 5 | 1 |
| Soy Carob | 2 tbsp (1 oz) | 90 | 18 | 9 | 2 |
| Soy Chocolate | 2 tbsp (1.1 oz) | 112 | 21 | 19 | 1 |
| Soy Light | 2 tbsp (0.66 oz) | 73 | 8 | 5 | 1 |
| Soy Original | 2 tbsp (0.8 oz) | 100 | 16 | 5 | 0 |
| Soy Vanilla | 2 tbsp (0.7 oz) | 77 | 8 | 6 | 1 |
| ***Blue Diamond*** | | | | | |
| Almond Breeze Chocolate | 8 oz | 120 | 21 | 20 | 1 |
| Almond Breeze Original | 8 oz | 60 | 8 | 7 | 1 |
| Almond Breeze Vanilla | 8 oz | 90 | 15 | 15 | 1 |
| ***EdenBlend*** | | | | | |
| Organic | 8 oz | 120 | 18 | 8 | 0 |
| ***Edensoy*** | | | | | |
| Organic Light | 8 oz | 93 | 14 | 5 | 0 |
| Organic Light Vanilla | 8 oz | 120 | 21 | 10 | 0 |

| FOOD | PORTION | CALS | CARB | SUGAR | FIBER |
|---|---|---|---|---|---|
| ***Galaxy*** | | | | | |
| Veggi Milk Chocolate | 1 cup (8 oz) | 150 | 26 | 20 | 1 |
| Veggie Milk Original | 1 cup (8 oz) | 110 | 13 | 8 | 2 |
| ***Hansen's*** | | | | | |
| Soy Smoothie Lemon Chiffon | 8 oz | 150 | 33 | 32 | tr |
| Soy Smoothie Orange Dream | 8 oz | 150 | 31 | 31 | tr |
| ***Harmony Farms*** | | | | | |
| Original Rice Beverage | 1 cup (8 oz) | 90 | 21 | 14 | 0 |
| ***Harmony House*** | | | | | |
| Enriched Rice Beverage | 1 cup (8 oz) | 90 | 21 | 14 | 0 |
| Enriched Soy Beverage | 1 cup (8 oz) | 90 | 21 | 14 | 0 |
| Original Soy Beverage | 1 cup (8 oz) | 90 | 21 | 14 | 0 |
| ***Health Valley*** | | | | | |
| Soo Moo | 1 cup | 110 | 22 | 17 | 1 |
| ***Keto*** | | | | | |
| Low Carb Mix | 1 scoop | 54 | 1 | – | – |
| ***NutraBalance*** | | | | | |
| NuTaste | 1 pkg (8 oz) | 80 | 7 | – | 8 |
| ***Rice Dream*** | | | | | |
| Carob | 1 box (8 oz) | 150 | 32 | 24 | 0 |
| Chocolate | 1 box (8 oz) | 170 | 36 | 25 | 2 |
| Chocolate Enriched | 1 box (8 oz) | 170 | 36 | 25 | 0 |
| Organic Original | 1 box (8 oz) | 120 | 25 | 11 | 0 |
| Organic Original Enriched | 1 box (8 oz) | 120 | 25 | 11 | 0 |
| Vanilla | 1 box (8 oz) | 130 | 28 | 12 | 0 |
| Vanilla Enriched | 1 box (8 oz) | 130 | 28 | 12 | 0 |
| ***Silk*** | | | | | |
| Chocolate | 1 cup | 140 | 23 | 19 | 0 |
| Organic Plain | 1 cup | 100 | 8 | 4 | 0 |
| Vanilla | 1 bottle (11 oz) | 140 | 14 | 8 | 0 |
| ***Soy Dream*** | | | | | |
| Carob | 8 oz | 210 | 36 | 22 | – |
| Chocolate Enriched | 8 oz | 210 | 35 | 22 | – |
| Original | 8 oz | 140 | 14 | 8 | – |
| Original Enriched | 8 oz | 140 | 14 | 8 | – |
| Vanilla | 8 oz | 170 | 23 | 18 | – |
| Vanilla Enriched | 8 oz | 140 | 23 | 18 | – |
| ***Tree Of Life*** | | | | | |
| Original Rice Beverage | 1 cup | 90 | 21 | 14 | 0 |

| FOOD | PORTION | CALS | CARB | SUGAR | FIBER |
|---|---|---|---|---|---|
| ***Vitamite*** | | | | | |
| Non-Dairy | 1 cup (8 oz) | 110 | 14 | 4 | 0 |
| ***Vitasoy*** | | | | | |
| 1% Low Fat Vanilla Delight | 8 oz | 90 | 13 | 9 | 0 |
| Carob Supreme | 8 fl oz | 150 | 20 | 12 | tr |
| Creamy Unsweetened | 8 oz | 80 | 5 | 1 | 0 |
| Creamy Original | 8 fl oz | 110 | 9 | 4 | 1 |
| Enriched Light Original | 8 fl oz | 60 | 7 | 4 | 0 |
| Enriched Light Vanilla | 8 fl oz | 90 | 13 | 10 | 0 |
| Green Tea Soymilk | 8 oz | 130 | 16 | 7 | 1 |
| Original Creamy | 8 fl oz | 110 | 12 | 5 | 1 |
| Original Light | 8 fl oz | 60 | 7 | 4 | 0 |
| Rich Chocolate | 8 fl oz | 160 | 24 | 16 | 1 |
| Rich Cocoa | 8 fl oz | 150 | 21 | 10 | 1 |
| Vanilla Light | 8 fl oz | 90 | 14 | 10 | 0 |
| Vanilla Delite | 8 fl oz | 120 | 14 | 9 | 1 |
| ***White Wave*** | | | | | |
| Mocha | 1 cup | 140 | 20 | 15 | 1 |
| **MILKFISH** | | | | | |
| baked | 3 oz | 162 | 0 | 0 | 0 |
| **MILKSHAKE** | | | | | |
| chocolate | 10 oz | 360 | 58 | – | – |
| strawberry | 10 oz | 319 | 53 | – | – |
| thick shake chocolate | 10.6 oz | 356 | 63 | – | – |
| thick shake vanilla | 11 oz | 350 | 56 | – | – |
| vanilla | 10 oz | 314 | 51 | – | – |
| ***Breyers*** | | | | | |
| Quick Vanilla | 1 serv (10 oz) | 320 | 37 | 36 | 0 |
| ***Carb Options*** | | | | | |
| Chocolate Delite | 1 can (11 oz) | 190 | 6 | 1 | 4 |
| Creamy Vanilla | 1 can (11 oz) | 190 | 6 | 1 | 4 |
| **MILLET** | | | | | |
| cooked | 1 cup (6.1 oz) | 207 | 41 | – | 2 |
| **MINERAL WATER** *(see* WATER) | | | | | |
| **MISO** | | | | | |
| dried | 1 oz | 86 | 10 | – | 1 |
| miso | ½ cup | 284 | 39 | – | 7 |

| FOOD | PORTION | CALS | CARB | SUGAR | FIBER |
|---|---|---|---|---|---|
| ***Eden*** | | | | | |
| Organic Genmai | 1 tbsp | 25 | 3 | 1 | tr |
| Tekka | 1 tsp | 5 | tr | 0 | 0 |
| **MOLASSES** | | | | | |
| blackstrap | 1 tbsp (0.7 oz) | 47 | 12 | – | – |
| blackstrap | 1 cup (11.5 oz) | 771 | 199 | – | – |
| molasses | 1 tbsp (0.7 oz) | 53 | 14 | 12 | – |
| molasses | 1 cup (11.5 oz) | 873 | 226 | 195 | – |
| ***Brer Rabbit*** | | | | | |
| Dark | 1 tbsp | 60 | 16 | 13 | – |
| ***Mott's*** | | | | | |
| Sulphured | 1 tbsp | 50 | 12 | – | – |
| Unsulphured | 1 tbsp | 50 | 14 | – | – |
| **MONKFISH** | | | | | |
| baked | 3 oz | 82 | 0 | 0 | 0 |
| **MOOSE** | | | | | |
| roasted | 3 oz | 114 | 0 | 0 | 0 |
| **MOTH BEANS** | | | | | |
| dried cooked | 1 cup | 207 | 37 | – | – |
| **MOUSSE** | | | | | |
| **FROZEN** | | | | | |
| ***Sara Lee*** | | | | | |
| Chocolate | ⅕ pkg (4.3 oz) | 400 | 37 | 27 | 2 |
| ***Weight Watchers*** | | | | | |
| Chocolate Mousse | 1 (2.75 oz) | 190 | 31 | 14 | 3 |
| **TAKE-OUT** | | | | | |
| chocolate | ½ cup (7.1 oz) | 447 | 33 | – | – |
| orange | ½ cup | 87 | 19 | – | – |
| **MUFFIN** | | | | | |
| **FROZEN** | | | | | |
| ***Pepperidge Farm*** | | | | | |
| Blueberry | 1 (2 oz) | 180 | 28 | 12 | 0 |
| Bran w/ Raisins | 1 (2 oz) | 180 | 30 | 17 | 0 |
| Corn | 1 (2 oz) | 190 | 28 | 8 | 0 |
| Orange Cranberry | 1 (2 oz) | 180 | 29 | 12 | 0 |

| FOOD | PORTION | CALS | CARB | SUGAR | FIBER |
|---|---|---|---|---|---|
| ***Sara Lee*** | | | | | |
| Blueberry | 1 (2.2 oz) | 220 | 27 | 12 | tr |
| Corn | 1 (2.2 oz) | 260 | 30 | 14 | 1 |
| ***Weight Watchers*** | | | | | |
| Chocolate Chocolate Chip | 1 (2.5 oz) | 190 | 39 | 14 | 4 |
| Fat Free Banana | 1 (2.5 oz) | 170 | 41 | 17 | 3 |
| Fat Free Blueberry | 1 (2.5 oz) | 160 | 38 | 15 | 2 |
| **MIX** | | | | | |
| blueberry | 1 (1¾ oz) | 149 | 24 | – | – |
| corn | 1 (1.75 oz) | 160 | 25 | – | – |
| wheat bran as prep | 1 (1¾ oz) | 138 | 23 | – | – |
| ***Betty Crocker*** | | | | | |
| Apple Cinnamon as prep | 1 | 170 | 23 | 11 | – |
| Apple Streusel as prep | 1 | 210 | 33 | 18 | – |
| Banana Nut as prep | 1 | 170 | 27 | 12 | 1 |
| Cranberry Orange as prep | 1 | 150 | 25 | 12 | – |
| Double Chocolate as prep | 1 | 220 | 30 | 26 | – |
| Golden Corn as prep | 1 | 160 | 24 | 6 | – |
| Lemon Poppyseed as prep | 1 | 180 | 24 | 13 | – |
| Sunkist Lemon Poppyseed as prep | 1 | 190 | 29 | 14 | – |
| Twice The Blueberries as prep | 1 | 140 | 25 | 12 | 1 |
| Wild Blueberry as prep | 1 | 170 | 28 | 14 | tr |
| ***Carbsense*** | | | | | |
| Honey Bran not prep | 1 serv (1.3 oz) | 120 | 16 | 0 | 12 |
| ***Gold Medal*** | | | | | |
| Corn | 1 | 160 | 25 | 8 | 0 |
| ***Hodgson Mill*** | | | | | |
| Bran | ¼ cup (1.3 oz) | 130 | 27 | 5 | 3 |
| Cornbread | ¼ cup (1.3 oz) | 130 | 28 | 3 | 3 |
| Whole Wheat | ¼ cup (1.3 oz) | 130 | 27 | 6 | 3 |
| ***Ketogenics*** | | | | | |
| Apple Cinnamon Bran as prep | 1 | 190 | 10 | 0 | 7 |
| Chocolate Chip as prep | 1 | 215 | 10 | 0 | 5 |
| Wild Blueberry as prep | 1 | 190 | 10 | 0 | 4 |
| ***MiniCarb*** | | | | | |
| Apple Cinnamon as prep | 1 | 225 | 7 | 2 | 4 |
| Sweet Corn as prep | 1 | 225 | 80 | 1 | 6 |
| ***Robin Hood*** | | | | | |
| Apple Cinnamon | 1 | 170 | 23 | 11 | 0 |

| FOOD | PORTION | CALS | CARB | SUGAR | FIBER |
|---|---|---|---|---|---|
| Banana Nut | 1 | 170 | 21 | 9 | 0 |
| Blueberry | 1 | 160 | 24 | 12 | 0 |
| Caramel Nut | 1 | 170 | 24 | 11 | 0 |
| ***Sweet Rewards*** | | | | | |
| Low Fat Apple Cinnamon as prep | 1 | 140 | 26 | 15 | – |
| **READY-TO-EAT** | | | | | |
| blueberry | 1 (2 oz) | 158 | 27 | – | 2 |
| corn | 1 (2 oz) | 174 | 29 | – | – |
| oat bran wheat free | 1 (2 oz) | 154 | 28 | – | 4 |
| toaster type blueberry | 1 | 103 | 18 | – | – |
| toaster type corn | 1 | 114 | 19 | – | – |
| toaster type wheat bran w/ raisins | 1 (1.3 oz) | 106 | 19 | – | – |
| ***Dolly Madison*** | | | | | |
| Blueberry | 1 (1.75 oz) | 170 | 26 | 8 | 0 |
| Mega Banana Nut | 1 (5.9 oz) | 620 | 78 | 39 | 2 |
| Mega Blueberry | 1 (5.9 oz) | 590 | 78 | 41 | 1 |
| Mega Chocolate Chip | 1 (5.9 oz) | 620 | 78 | 41 | 2 |
| Mega Cranberry Orange | 1 (5.9 oz) | 590 | 79 | 41 | 1 |
| Mega Cream Cheese | 1 (5.9 oz) | 620 | 73 | 41 | 1 |
| ***Dutch Mill*** | | | | | |
| Apple Oat Bran | 1 (2 oz) | 180 | 31 | 5 | 1 |
| Banana Walnut | 1 (2 oz) | 220 | 33 | 15 | 1 |
| Carrot | 1 (2 oz) | 190 | 31 | 19 | 1 |
| Corn | 1 (2 oz) | 190 | 31 | 14 | 1 |
| Cranberry Orange | 1 (2 oz) | 170 | 26 | 14 | 1 |
| Raisin Bran | 1 (2 oz) | 230 | 37 | 12 | 3 |
| ***Hostess*** | | | | | |
| Banana Bran Low Fat | 1 (2.7 oz) | 240 | 47 | 24 | 2 |
| Blueberry Low Fat | 1 (2.7 oz) | 230 | 47 | 23 | 1 |
| Hearty Banana Nut | 1 (5.9 oz) | 620 | 78 | 39 | 2 |
| Hearty Blueberry | 1 (5.9 oz) | 590 | 78 | 41 | 1 |
| Hearty Chocolate Chip | 1 (5.9 oz) | 620 | 78 | 41 | 2 |
| Hearty Cranberry Orange | 1 (5.9 oz) | 590 | 79 | 41 | 1 |
| Hearty Cream Cheese | 1 (5.9 oz) | 620 | 73 | 41 | 1 |
| Mini Banana Walnut | 3 (1.2 oz) | 160 | 16 | 8 | 0 |
| Mini Blueberry | 3 (1.2 oz) | 150 | 18 | 8 | 0 |
| Mini Chocolate Chip | 3 (1.2 oz) | 160 | 17 | 9 | 0 |
| Mini Cinnamon Apple | 3 (1.2 oz) | 160 | 16 | 8 | 0 |

| FOOD | PORTION | CALS | CARB | SUGAR | FIBER |
|---|---|---|---|---|---|
| Mini Cinnamon Bites | 3 (1.1 oz) | 130 | 18 | 8 | 0 |
| Mini Rocky Road | 3 (1.2 oz) | 160 | 17 | 9 | 0 |
| Muffin Loaf Apple Spice | 1 (3.7 oz) | 430 | 61 | 41 | 1 |
| Muffin Loaf Banana Nut | 1 (3.8 oz) | 460 | 63 | 29 | 0 |
| Muffin Loaf Blueberry | 1 (3.8 oz) | 440 | 62 | 34 | 2 |
| Muffin Loaf Chocolate Chocolate Chip | 1 (3.8 oz) | 400 | 58 | 32 | 2 |
| Muffin Loaf Raspberry | 1 (3.8 oz) | 440 | 62 | 34 | 2 |
| Oat Bran | 1 (1.5 oz) | 160 | 21 | 9 | 1 |
| ***Otis Spunkmeyer*** | | | | | |
| Apple Cinnamon | 1 (2 oz) | 220 | 27 | 16 | tr |
| Low Fat Wild Blueberry | 1 (2.25 oz) | 200 | 38 | 24 | tr |
| Mayport Almond Poppy Seed | ½ muffin (2 oz) | 210 | 23 | 17 | tr |
| Mayport Banana Nut | 1 (2.25 oz) | 270 | 33 | 20 | tr |
| Mayport Cheese Streusel | ½ muffin (2 oz) | 220 | 30 | 18 | tr |
| Mayport Chocolate Chocolate Chip | 1 (2.25 oz) | 260 | 33 | 22 | 1 |
| Mayport Chocolate Chip | ½ muffin (2 oz) | 240 | 28 | 18 | tr |
| Mayport Cinnamon Spice | ½ muffin (2 oz) | 230 | 26 | 16 | 1 |
| Mayport Corn | ½ muffin (2 oz) | 230 | 26 | 14 | 0 |
| Mayport Harvest Bran | 1 (2.25 oz) | 240 | 34 | 20 | 3 |
| Mayport Lemon | ½ muffin (2 oz) | 230 | 27 | 15 | 1 |
| Mayport Orange | ½ muffin (2 oz) | 230 | 27 | 16 | tr |
| Mayport Pineapple | ½ muffin (2 oz) | 210 | 25 | 17 | 1 |
| Mayport Wild Blueberry | 1 (2.25 oz) | 230 | 27 | 20 | 1 |
| Mayport Low Fat Apple Cinnamon | 1 (4 oz) | 380 | 75 | 50 | 1 |
| Mayport Low Fat Banana Nut | 1 (4 oz) | 350 | 70 | 45 | 1 |
| Mayport Low Fat Chocolate Chocolate Chip | 1 (4 oz) | 370 | 73 | 47 | 2 |
| ***Uncle Wally's*** | | | | | |
| Chocolate Passion | 1 (2 oz) | 130 | 30 | 18 | 1 |

| FOOD | PORTION | CALS | CARB | SUGAR | FIBER |
|---|---|---|---|---|---|
| Cranberry Orange Supreme | 1 (2 oz) | 130 | 25 | 12 | 1 |
| Fat Free Apple Cinnamon Delight | 1 (2 oz) | 110 | 28 | 13 | 1 |
| Fat Free Wild Blueberry Bliss | 1 (2 oz) | 120 | 25 | 12 | 1 |
| Golden Waves Of Corn | 1 (2 oz) | 120 | 28 | 12 | 1 |
| Honey Raisin Bran | 1 (2 oz) | 130 | 29 | 15 | 1 |
| No Nut Banana | 1 (2 oz) | 130 | 27 | 15 | 1 |
| ***VitaMuffin*** | | | | | |
| Blue Bran | 1 (2 oz) | 100 | 24 | 13 | 4 |
| Cran Bran | 1 (2 oz) | 100 | 24 | 13 | 4 |
| Deep Chocolate | 1 (4 oz) | 200 | 50 | 24 | 12 |
| Multi Bran | 1 (2 oz) | 100 | 24 | 13 | 4 |
| VitaTops Apple Berry Bran | 1 (2 oz) | 100 | 25 | 10 | 5 |
| VitaTops Blue Bran | 1 (2 oz) | 100 | 24 | 13 | 4 |
| VitaTops Cran Bran | 1 (2 oz) | 100 | 24 | 13 | 4 |
| VitaTops Deep Chocolate | 1 (2 oz) | 100 | 25 | 12 | 6 |
| VitaTops MultiBran | 1 (2 oz) | 100 | 24 | 13 | 4 |
| ***Weight Watchers*** | | | | | |
| Fat Free Apple Crisp | 1 (2.5 oz) | 160 | 37 | 16 | 1 |
| Fat Free Cranberry Orange | 1 (2.5 oz) | 160 | 38 | 14 | 1 |
| Fat Free Double Chocolate | 1 (2.5 oz) | 180 | 40 | 26 | 2 |
| Fat Free Wild Blueberry | 1 (2.5 oz) | 160 | 36 | 15 | 1 |
| Low Fat Apple Cinnamon | 1 (2.5 oz) | 170 | 35 | 20 | 2 |
| Low Fat Blueberry | 1 (2.5 oz) | 180 | 37 | 20 | 2 |
| Low Fat Carrot | 1 (2.5 oz) | 160 | 34 | 16 | 2 |
| Low Fat Chocolate Chip | 1 (2.5 oz) | 180 | 38 | 21 | 2 |
| Low Fat Cranberry Orange | 1 (2.5 oz) | 180 | 38 | 20 | 2 |
| Low Fat Lemon Poppy | 1 (2.5 oz) | 190 | 38 | 20 | 2 |
| **TAKE-OUT** | | | | | |
| raisin bran lowfat | 1 (4 oz) | 270 | 61 | 35 | 5 |
| **MULBERRIES** | | | | | |
| fresh | 1 cup | 61 | 14 | – | – |
| **MULLET** | | | | | |
| striped cooked | 3 oz | 127 | 0 | 0 | 0 |
| striped raw | 3 oz | 99 | 0 | 0 | 0 |
| **MUNG BEANS** | | | | | |
| dried cooked | 1 cup | 213 | 39 | – | – |

| FOOD | PORTION | CALS | CARB | SUGAR | FIBER |
|---|---|---|---|---|---|
| **MUNGO BEANS** | | | | | |
| dried cooked | 1 cup | 190 | 33 | – | – |
| **MUSHROOMS** | | | | | |
| **CANNED** | | | | | |
| chanterelle | 3.5 oz | 12 | tr | – | 6 |
| pieces | ½ cup | 19 | 4 | – | – |
| straw | 1 cup (6.4 oz) | 58 | 8 | – | 5 |
| whole | 1 (0.4 oz) | 3 | 1 | – | – |
| **DRIED** | | | | | |
| chanterelle | 1 oz | 25 | tr | – | 17 |
| cloud ear | 1 (5 g) | 13 | 3 | – | 3 |
| cloud ears | 1 cup (1 oz) | 80 | 20 | – | 20 |
| shiitake | 4 (½ oz) | 44 | 11 | – | – |
| straw | 1 piece (6 g) | 2 | tr | – | tr |
| tree ear | ½ cup (0.4 oz) | 36 | 10 | – | – |
| wood ear mok yee | ½ cup (0.4 oz) | 25 | 8 | – | 4 |
| ***Eden*** | | | | | |
| Shitake | 6 (0.4 oz) | 35 | 7 | 2 | 5 |
| **FRESH** | | | | | |
| chanterelle | 3.5 oz | 11 | tr | – | 6 |
| enoki raw | 1 (4 in) | 2 | tr | – | – |
| morel | 3.5 oz | 9 | 0 | – | 7 |
| oyster raw | 1 lg (5.2 oz) | 55 | 9 | – | 4 |
| oyster raw | 1 sm (0.5 oz) | 6 | 1 | – | tr |
| portabella | 1 serv (2 oz) | 14 | 3 | – | – |
| raw | 1 (½ oz) | 5 | 1 | – | tr |
| raw sliced | ½ cup | 9 | 2 | – | tr |
| shitake cooked | 4 (2.5 oz) | 40 | 10 | – | – |
| sliced cooked | ½ cup | 21 | 4 | – | 1 |
| whole cooked | 1 (0.4 oz) | 3 | 1 | – | – |
| **MUSKRAT** | | | | | |
| roasted | 3 oz | 199 | 0 | 0 | 0 |
| **MUSSELS** | | | | | |
| blue raw | 3 oz | 73 | 3 | – | – |
| blue raw | 1 cup | 129 | 6 | – | – |
| fresh blue cooked | 3 oz | 147 | 6 | – | – |
| **MUSTARD** | | | | | |
| dry mustard | 1 tsp | 15 | 1 | – | – |

| FOOD | PORTION | CALS | CARB | SUGAR | FIBER |
|---|---|---|---|---|---|
| yellow ready to use | 1 tsp | 5 | tr | – | – |
| ***Boar's Head*** | | | | | |
| Delicatessen Style | 1 tsp (5 g) | 0 | 0 | 0 | 0 |
| Honey | 1 tsp (5 g) | 10 | 2 | 1 | 0 |
| ***Country Cupboard*** | | | | | |
| Smokey Garlic or Horseradish | 1 tsp | 10 | 2 | 1 | 0 |
| ***Eden*** | | | | | |
| Organic Stone Ground | 1 tsp | 0 | 1 | 0 | 0 |
| ***French's*** | | | | | |
| Classic Yellow | 1 tsp | 0 | 0 | 0 | 0 |
| ***Gulden's*** | | | | | |
| Spicy Brown | 1 tsp | 5 | 0 | – | – |
| ***Hunt's*** | | | | | |
| Mustard | 1 tsp (5 g) | 3 | tr | tr | tr |
| ***Kosciuszko*** | | | | | |
| Spicy Brown | 1 tsp | 5 | tr | – | – |
| ***Luzianne*** | | | | | |
| Creole Mustard | 1 tbsp | 10 | 2 | 0 | 0 |
| ***Tree Of Life*** | | | | | |
| Dijon | 1 tsp (5 g) | 0 | 0 | – | – |
| Dijon Imported | 1 tsp (5 g) | 5 | tr | – | – |
| Stone Ground | 1 tsp (5 g) | 0 | 0 | – | – |
| Yellow | 1 tsp (5 g) | 0 | 0 | – | – |
| ***Wild Thyme Farms*** | | | | | |
| Chili Pepper Garlic | 1 tsp | 5 | 1 | – | – |
| Dill Horseradish | 1 tsp | 5 | 1 | – | – |
| **MUSTARD GREENS** | | | | | |
| fresh chopped cooked | ½ cup | 11 | 1 | – | – |
| fresh raw chopped | ½ cup | 7 | 1 | – | – |
| frozen chopped cooked | ½ cup | 14 | 2 | – | – |
| ***Birds Eye*** | | | | | |
| Chopped | 1 cup | 30 | 2 | 1 | 2 |
| **NATTO** | | | | | |
| natto | ½ cup | 187 | 13 | – | – |
| **NAVY BEANS** | | | | | |
| **CANNED** | | | | | |
| navy | 1 cup | 296 | 54 | – | – |

| FOOD | PORTION | CALS | CARB | SUGAR | FIBER |
|---|---|---|---|---|---|
| **DRIED** | | | | | |
| cooked | 1 cup | 259 | 48 | – | – |
| **NECTARINE** | | | | | |
| fresh | 1 | 67 | 16 | – | 2 |
| ***Chiquita*** | | | | | |
| Fresh | 1 med (4.9 oz) | 70 | 16 | 12 | 2 |
| **NEUFCHATEL** | | | | | |
| neufchatel | 1 oz | 74 | 1 | – | – |
| neufchatel | 1 pkg (3 oz) | 221 | 3 | – | – |
| ***Horizon Organic*** | | | | | |
| Neufchatel | 2 tbsp | 70 | tr | tr | 0 |
| ***Organic Valley*** | | | | | |
| Neufchatel | 1 oz | 70 | 1 | tr | 0 |
| **NOODLE DISHES** *(see also* PASTA DINNERS*)* | | | | | |
| ***Annie Chun*** | | | | | |
| Chow Mein Noodles w/ Garlic Black Bean Sauce | 1 serv | 230 | 42 | 8 | 2 |
| Japanese Soba Noodles w/ Soy Ginger Sauce | 1 serv | 210 | 41 | 8 | 3 |
| ***Hunt's*** | | | | | |
| Noodles & Chicken | 1 cup (8.7 oz) | 176 | 21 | 3 | 2 |
| Noodles & Beef | 1 cup (8.7 oz) | 151 | 22 | 2 | 5 |
| **TAKE-OUT** | | | | | |
| noodle pudding | ½ cup | 132 | 11 | – | – |
| **NOODLES** | | | | | |
| cellophane | 1 cup | 492 | 121 | – | – |
| chow mein | 1 cup (1.6 oz) | 237 | 25 | – | 2 |
| egg | 1 cup (38 g) | 145 | 27 | – | – |
| egg cooked | 1 cup (5.6 oz) | 213 | 40 | – | 2 |
| japanese soba cooked | 1 cup (4 oz) | 113 | 24 | – | – |
| japanese somen cooked | 1 cup (6.2 oz) | 231 | 48 | – | – |
| korean acorn noodles not prep | 2 oz | 195 | 41 | – | tr |
| rice cooked | 1 cup (6.2 oz) | 192 | 44 | – | 2 |
| spinach/egg cooked | 1 cup (5.6 oz) | 211 | 39 | – | 4 |
| ***Annie Chun*** | | | | | |
| Chow Mein | 2 oz | 200 | 39 | 1 | 3 |
| Rice | 2 oz | 210 | 50 | 0 | 0 |

| FOOD | PORTION | CALS | CARB | SUGAR | FIBER |
|---|---|---|---|---|---|
| Rice Hunan | 2 oz | 210 | 50 | 0 | 0 |
| Rice Pad Thai | 2 oz | 210 | 50 | 0 | 0 |
| Rice Pad Thai Basil | 2 oz | 210 | 50 | 0 | 0 |
| ***Azumaya*** | | | | | |
| Spinach | 1 cup | 210 | 42 | 1 | 2 |
| Thin Cut | 1 cup | 210 | 43 | 1 | 2 |
| Wide Cut | 1 cup | 210 | 43 | 1 | 2 |
| ***Chun King*** | | | | | |
| Chow Mein | ½ cup (1 oz) | 137 | 19 | 0 | 1 |
| ***Eden*** | | | | | |
| Kudzu | 2 oz | 200 | 48 | 0 | 2 |
| ***Hodgson Mill*** | | | | | |
| Four Color Veggie Egg | 2 oz | 200 | 37 | 0 | 2 |
| Whole Wheat Egg not prep | 2 oz | 190 | 34 | 0 | 4 |
| ***La Choy*** | | | | | |
| Chow Mein | ½ cup (1 oz) | 137 | 19 | 0 | 1 |
| Chow Mein Crispy Wide | ½ cup (1 oz) | 148 | 16 | 0 | 1 |
| Rice | ½ cup (1 oz) | 121 | 21 | 0 | tr |
| ***Manischewitz*** | | | | | |
| Fine Yolk Free | 1½ cups | 210 | 40 | 2 | 2 |
| Fine Egg | 1½ cups | 220 | 40 | 2 | 2 |
| Wide Yolk Free | 1¾ cups | 210 | 40 | 2 | 2 |
| ***Nasoya*** | | | | | |
| Chinese | 1 cup | 210 | 43 | 1 | 2 |
| Japanese | 1 cup | 210 | 43 | 1 | 2 |
| Spinach | 1 cup | 210 | 42 | 1 | 2 |
| **NOPALES** | | | | | |
| cooked | 1 cup (5.2 oz) | 23 | 5 | – | – |
| raw sliced | 1 cup (3 oz) | 14 | 3 | – | – |
| **NUTMEG** | | | | | |
| ground | 1 tsp | 12 | 1 | – | – |
| **NUTRITION SUPPLEMENTS** *(see* CEREAL BARS, ENERGY BARS, ENERGY DRINKS*)* | | | | | |
| ***Boost*** | | | | | |
| High Protein Powder Vanilla as prep w/ water | 1 serv (8 oz) | 200 | 36 | 35 | 0 |
| ***Enlive!*** | | | | | |
| Drink All Flavors | 1 box (8.1 oz) | 300 | 65 | 15 | 0 |

| FOOD | PORTION | CALS | CARB | SUGAR | FIBER |
|---|---|---|---|---|---|
| ***Ensure*** | | | | | |
| Supplement All Flavors | 1 can (8 fl oz) | 250 | 40 | 18 | 0 |
| ***GeniSoy*** | | | | | |
| Soy Natural Protein Powder | 1 scoop (1 oz) | 100 | 0 | 0 | 0 |
| ***Glucerna*** | | | | | |
| Shakes All Flavors | 1 can (8 oz) | 220 | 29 | 7 | 3 |
| ***Juven*** | | | | | |
| Grape "w/ Arginine," "Glutamine, HMB" | 1 pkg (0.8 oz) | 90 | 2 | 2 | – |
| ***Met-Rx*** | | | | | |
| Lite | 1 pkg (1.6 oz) | 170 | 16 | 3 | 1 |
| Mass Action | 1 scoop (0.9 oz) | 60 | 15 | 9 | – |
| Original | 1 pkg (2.5 oz) | 250 | 22 | 3 | tr |
| Protein Shake | 1 can | 200 | 20 | 1 | 2 |
| Ultra | 1 pkg (2.6 oz) | 250 | 19 | 5 | 2 |
| ***Nestle*** | | | | | |
| Additions | 2⅓ tsp (0.7 oz) | 100 | 9 | 1 | 0 |
| ***NutraBalance*** | | | | | |
| EggPro | 1 tbsp (7.5 g) | 30 | 1 | 0 | 0 |
| ***Nutribar*** | | | | | |
| Shake Chocolate Supreme as prep w/ 2% milk | 1 serv (10 oz) (4.6 oz) | 262 | 34 | – | 2 |
| Shake Vanilla as prep w/ 2% milk | 1 (10 oz) | 259 | 35 | – | 2 |
| ***PermaLean*** | | | | | |
| Protein Powder Bodacious Berry | 1 scoop (1 oz) | 104 | 1 | 3 | – |
| Protein Powder Chocoholic Chocolate | 1 scoop (1 oz) | 104 | 5 | 3 | – |
| ***Pounds Off*** | | | | | |
| All Flavors | 1 bar (2.1 oz) | 210 | 32 | 18 | 2 |
| **NUTS MIXED** *(see also individual names)* | | | | | |
| dry roasted w/ peanuts | 1 oz | 169 | 7 | – | – |
| dry roasted w/ peanuts salted | 1 oz | 169 | 7 | – | – |
| mixed nuts chocolate covered | ¼ cup (1.5 oz) | 240 | 20 | 17 | 2 |
| oil roasted w/ peanuts | 1 oz | 175 | 6 | – | – |

| FOOD | PORTION | CALS | CARB | SUGAR | FIBER |
|---|---|---|---|---|---|
| oil roasted w/ peanuts salted | 1 oz | 175 | 6 | – | – |
| oil roasted w/o peanuts | 1 oz | 175 | 6 | – | – |
| oil roasted w/o peanuts salted | 1 oz | 175 | 6 | – | – |
| ***Estee*** | | | | | |
| Fruit & Nut Mix | ¼ cup | 210 | 19 | 10 | 2 |
| ***Judy's*** | | | | | |
| Sugar Free Mixed Nut Brittle | ¼ piece (1 oz) | 120 | 3 | 0 | tr |
| ***Maranatha*** | | | | | |
| Cashew Macadamia Butter | 2 tbsp | 210 | 8 | 2 | 2 |
| Tamari Organic | ¼ cup | 160 | 7 | 1 | 2 |
| Tamari Roasted | ¼ cup | 160 | 7 | 1 | 2 |
| **OCTOPUS** | | | | | |
| fresh steamed | 3 oz | 140 | 4 | – | – |
| **OHELOBERRIES** | | | | | |
| fresh | 1 cup | 39 | 10 | – | – |
| **OIL** | | | | | |
| almond | 1 cup | 1927 | 0 | 0 | 0 |
| almond | 1 tbsp | 120 | 0 | 0 | 0 |
| apricot kernel | 1 tbsp | 120 | 0 | 0 | 0 |
| apricot kernel | 1 cup | 1927 | 0 | 0 | 0 |
| avocado | 1 tbsp | 124 | 0 | 0 | 0 |
| avocado | 1 cup | 1927 | 0 | 0 | 0 |
| babassu palm | 1 tbsp | 120 | 0 | 0 | 0 |
| butter oil | 1 tbsp | 112 | 0 | 0 | 0 |
| butter oil | 1 cup | 1795 | 0 | 0 | 0 |
| canola | 1 cup | 1927 | 0 | 0 | 0 |
| canola | 1 tbsp | 124 | 0 | 0 | 0 |
| coconut | 1 tbsp | 117 | 0 | 0 | 0 |
| corn | 1 tbsp | 120 | 0 | 0 | 0 |
| corn | 1 cup | 1927 | 0 | 0 | 0 |
| cottonseed | 1 cup | 1927 | 0 | 0 | 0 |
| cottonseed | 1 tbsp | 120 | 0 | 0 | 0 |
| cupu assu | 1 tbsp | 120 | 0 | 0 | 0 |
| grapeseed | 1 tbsp | 120 | 0 | 0 | 0 |
| hazelnut | 1 tbsp | 120 | 0 | 0 | 0 |
| hazelnut | 1 cup | 1927 | 0 | 0 | 0 |
| mustard | 1 cup | 1927 | 0 | 0 | 0 |
| mustard | 1 tbsp | 124 | 0 | 0 | 0 |

| FOOD | PORTION | CALS | CARB | SUGAR | FIBER |
|---|---|---|---|---|---|
| oat | 1 tbsp | 120 | 0 | 0 | 0 |
| olive | 1 cup | 1909 | 0 | 0 | 0 |
| olive | 1 tbsp | 119 | 0 | 0 | 0 |
| palm | 1 tbsp | 120 | 0 | 0 | 0 |
| palm | 1 cup | 1927 | 0 | 0 | 0 |
| palm kernel | 1 tbsp | 117 | 0 | 0 | 0 |
| palm kernel | 1 cup | 1879 | 0 | 0 | 0 |
| peanut | 1 cup | 1909 | 0 | 0 | 0 |
| peanut | 1 tbsp | 119 | 0 | 0 | 0 |
| poppyseed | 1 tbsp | 120 | 0 | 0 | 0 |
| pumpkin seed | 1 oz | 217 | 0 | 0 | 0 |
| rice bran | 1 tbsp | 120 | 0 | 0 | 0 |
| safflower | 1 tbsp | 120 | 0 | 0 | 0 |
| safflower | 1 cup | 1927 | 0 | 0 | 0 |
| sesame | 1 tbsp | 120 | 0 | 0 | 0 |
| sheanut | 1 tbsp | 120 | 0 | 0 | 0 |
| soybean | 1 cup | 1927 | 0 | 0 | 0 |
| soybean | 1 tbsp | 120 | 0 | 0 | 0 |
| soybean organic | 1 tbsp | 120 | 0 | 0 | 0 |
| sunflower | 1 tbsp | 120 | 0 | 0 | 0 |
| sunflower | 1 cup | 1927 | 0 | 0 | 0 |
| teaseed | 1 tbsp | 120 | 0 | 0 | 0 |
| tomatoseed | 1 tbsp | 120 | 0 | 0 | 0 |
| vegetable | 1 cup | 1927 | 0 | 0 | 0 |
| vegetable | 1 tbsp | 120 | 0 | 0 | 0 |
| walnut | 1 cup | 1927 | 0 | 0 | 0 |
| walnut | 1 tbsp | 120 | 0 | 0 | 0 |
| wheat germ | 1 tbsp | 120 | 0 | 0 | 0 |
| ***Eden*** | | | | | |
| Olive Spanish Extra Virgin | 1 tbsp | 120 | 0 | 0 | 0 |
| ***Enova*** | | | | | |
| Oil | 1 tbsp | 120 | 0 | 0 | 0 |
| ***Mazola*** | | | | | |
| Oil | 1 tbsp (14 g) | 120 | 0 | – | – |
| ***Monini*** | | | | | |
| Olive Extra Virgin | 1 tbsp | 118 | 0 | 0 | 0 |
| ***Orville Redenbacher's*** | | | | | |
| Popping | 1 tbsp (0.5 oz) | 120 | 0 | 0 | 0 |
| ***Progresso*** | | | | | |
| Olive Extra Mild | 1 tbsp (0.5 oz) | 120 | 0 | 0 | 0 |

| FOOD | PORTION | CALS | CARB | SUGAR | FIBER |
|---|---|---|---|---|---|
| Olive Extra Virgin | 1 tbsp (0.5 oz) | 120 | 0 | 0 | 0 |
| Olive Riviera Blend | 1 tbsp (0.5 oz) | 120 | 0 | 0 | 0 |
| ***Tree Of Life*** | | | | | |
| Olive Extra Virgin Organic | 1 tbsp (0.5 g) | 130 | 0 | – | – |
| ***Weight Watchers*** | | | | | |
| Butter Spray | ⅓ sec spray | 0 | 0 | 0 | 0 |
| Cooking Spray | ⅓ sec spray | 0 | 0 | 0 | 0 |
| ***Wesson*** | | | | | |
| Canola | 1 tbsp | 120 | 0 | 0 | 0 |

## OKRA

| FOOD | PORTION | CALS | CARB | SUGAR | FIBER |
|---|---|---|---|---|---|
| **FRESH** | | | | | |
| sliced cooked | ½ cup | 25 | 6 | – | – |
| sliced cooked | 8 pods | 27 | 6 | – | – |
| **FROZEN** | | | | | |
| sliced cooked | 1 pkg (10 oz) | 94 | 21 | – | – |
| sliced cooked | ½ cup | 34 | 8 | – | – |
| ***Birds Eye*** | | | | | |
| Cut | ¾ cup | 25 | 5 | 1 | 3 |
| Whole | 9 pods | 25 | 5 | 1 | 3 |

## OLIVES

| FOOD | PORTION | CALS | CARB | SUGAR | FIBER |
|---|---|---|---|---|---|
| green | 3 extra lg | 15 | tr | – | tr |
| green | 4 med | 15 | tr | – | tr |
| green olive tapenade | 1 tbsp | 25 | 1 | 1 | 0 |
| ripe | 1 sm | 4 | tr | – | tr |
| ripe | 1 lg | 5 | tr | – | tr |
| ripe | 1 jumbo | 7 | tr | – | – |
| ripe | 1 colossal | 12 | 1 | – | – |
| spanish stuffed | 5 (0.5 oz) | 15 | 1 | 0 | 0 |
| ***Progresso*** | | | | | |
| Olive Salad (drained) | 2 tbsp (0.8 oz) | 25 | 1 | tr | tr |
| ***Vlasic*** | | | | | |
| Ripe Colossal Pitted | 2 (0.6 oz) | 20 | 1 | 0 | 0 |
| Ripe Jumbo Pitted | 3 (0.6 oz) | 25 | 1 | 0 | 0 |
| Ripe Large Pitted | 4 (0.5 oz) | 25 | 1 | 0 | 0 |
| Ripe Medium Pitted | 5 (0.5 oz) | 25 | 1 | 0 | 0 |
| Ripe Sliced | ¼ cup (0.5 oz) | 25 | 1 | 0 | 0 |
| Ripe Small Pitted | 6 (0.5 oz) | 25 | 1 | 0 | 0 |

| FOOD | PORTION | CALS | CARB | SUGAR | FIBER |
|---|---|---|---|---|---|
| **ONION** | | | | | |
| **CANNED** | | | | | |
| chopped | ½ cup | 21 | 5 | – | – |
| whole | 1 (2.2 oz) | 12 | 3 | – | – |
| ***Boar's Head*** | | | | | |
| Sweet Vidalia In Sauce | 1 tbsp | 10 | 2 | 2 | 0 |
| **DRIED** | | | | | |
| flakes | 1 tbsp | 16 | 4 | – | – |
| powder | 1 tsp | 7 | 2 | – | – |
| shallots | 1 tbsp | 3 | 1 | – | – |
| **FRESH** | | | | | |
| chopped cooked | ½ cup | 47 | 11 | – | – |
| raw chopped | 1 tbsp | 4 | 1 | – | tr |
| raw chopped | ½ cup | 30 | 7 | – | – |
| scallions raw chopped | 1 tbsp | 2 | tr | – | tr |
| scallions raw sliced | ½ cup | 16 | 4 | – | 1 |
| shallots raw chopped | 1 tbsp | 7 | 2 | – | – |
| welsh raw | 3½ oz | 34 | 7 | – | – |
| ***Antioch Farms*** | | | | | |
| Vidalia | 1 med | 60 | 14 | – | 3 |
| **FROZEN** | | | | | |
| chopped cooked | 1 tbsp | 4 | 1 | – | – |
| chopped cooked | ½ cup | 30 | 7 | – | – |
| rings | 7 (2.5 oz) | 285 | 27 | – | – |
| rings cooked | 2 (0.7 oz) | 81 | 8 | – | – |
| whole cooked | 3½ oz | 28 | 7 | – | – |
| ***Birds Eye*** | | | | | |
| Diced | ⅔ cup | 30 | 6 | 5 | 1 |
| Pearl Onions In Real Cream Sauce | ½ cup | 60 | 8 | 6 | 1 |
| ***McKenzie's*** | | | | | |
| Onion Rounds | 1 serv (3.2 oz) | 220 | 28 | 3 | 6 |
| **TAKE-OUT** | | | | | |
| fried | ½ cup (7.5 oz) | 176 | 17 | – | – |
| rings breaded & fried | 8 to 9 | 275 | 31 | – | – |
| **OPOSSUM** | | | | | |
| roasted | 3 oz | 188 | 0 | 0 | 0 |

| FOOD | PORTION | CALS | CARB | SUGAR | FIBER |
|---|---|---|---|---|---|
| **ORANGE** | | | | | |
| **CANNED** | | | | | |
| ***Del Monte*** | | | | | |
| Mandarin In Light Syrup | ½ cup (4.5 oz) | 80 | 19 | 19 | 1 |
| ***Dole*** | | | | | |
| FruitBowls Mandarin Oranges | 1 pkg (4 oz) | 70 | 18 | 17 | 0 |
| **FRESH** | | | | | |
| california navel | 1 | 65 | 16 | – | 3 |
| california valencia | 1 | 59 | 14 | – | 3 |
| florida | 1 | 69 | 17 | – | 4 |
| peel | 1 tbsp | 6 | 2 | – | – |
| sections | 1 cup | 85 | 21 | – | 4 |
| **ORANGE JUICE** | | | | | |
| canned | 1 cup | 104 | 25 | – | – |
| chilled | 1 cup | 110 | 25 | – | – |
| fresh | 1 cup | 111 | 26 | – | – |
| frzn as prep | 1 cup | 112 | 27 | – | 1 |
| frzn not prep | 6 oz | 339 | 81 | – | 2 |
| mandarin orange | 7 oz | 94 | 20 | – | – |
| orange drink | 6 oz | 94 | 24 | – | – |
| ***Big Juicy*** | | | | | |
| Drink | 8 oz | 110 | 28 | 28 | – |
| ***Fresh Samantha*** | | | | | |
| Juice | 1 cup (8 oz) | 100 | 8 | – | 0 |
| ***Horizon Organic*** | | | | | |
| Juice Pulp Free | 8 fl oz | 110 | 26 | 22 | – |
| ***Juicy Juice*** | | | | | |
| Punch | 1 box (4.23 oz) | 60 | 15 | 14 | 0 |
| Punch | 1 box (8.45 oz) | 130 | 33 | 28 | 0 |
| ***Minute Maid*** | | | | | |
| Original | 8 fl oz | 110 | 27 | 24 | – |
| Original Calcium + Vitamin D | 8 oz | 110 | 27 | 24 | – |
| Plus Calcium | 8 fl oz | 110 | 27 | 24 | – |
| Simply Orange 100% | 8 fl oz | 110 | 26 | 22 | – |
| Simply Orange Calcium Fortified | 8 fl oz | 110 | 26 | 22 | – |
| Simply Orange Grove Made | 8 fl oz | 110 | 26 | 22 | – |

| FOOD | PORTION | CALS | CARB | SUGAR | FIBER |
|---|---|---|---|---|---|
| ***Mott's*** | | | | | |
| 100% Juice | 1 box (8 oz) | 130 | 31 | – | – |
| 100% Juice | 8 fl oz | 130 | 31 | – | – |
| ***Nantucket Nectars*** | | | | | |
| 100% Juice | 8 oz | 120 | 28 | 22 | – |
| ***NutraShake*** | | | | | |
| Fortified | 1 pkg (4 oz) | 50 | 12 | – | 4 |
| ***Ocean Spray*** | | | | | |
| 100% Juice | 8 oz | 120 | 31 | 31 | 0 |
| ***Odwalla*** | | | | | |
| Organic | 8 fl oz | 110 | 25 | 24 | – |
| ***Simply Orange*** | | | | | |
| Pulp Free w/ Calcium | 8 oz | 110 | 26 | 22 | – |
| ***Snapple*** | | | | | |
| Orangeade | 8 fl oz | 120 | 29 | 29 | – |
| ***Squeezit*** | | | | | |
| Smarty Arty Orange | 1 bottle (7 oz) | 110 | 27 | 26 | 0 |
| ***Tropicana*** | | | | | |
| Double Vitamin C | 8 fl oz | 110 | 26 | – | – |
| Light'N Healthy | 8 oz | 70 | 17 | 14 | – |
| Original No Pulp | 8 oz | 110 | 26 | 22 | – |
| Ruby Red | 8 oz | 110 | 26 | – | – |
| Season's Best | 8 oz | 110 | 27 | – | – |
| Season's Best Homestyle | 8 fl oz | 110 | 27 | – | – |
| With Calcium + Vitamin D | 8 oz | 110 | 26 | 22 | – |
| ***Turkey Hill*** | | | | | |
| Orangeade | 1 cup | 120 | 30 | 30 | – |
| **TAKE-OUT** | | | | | |
| orange julius | 1 serv (24 oz) | 443 | 118 | – | 1 |

## OREGANO

| | | | | | |
|---|---|---|---|---|---|
| ground | 1 tsp | 5 | 1 | – | – |

**ORGAN MEATS** *(see* BRAINS, GIBLETS, GIZZARD, HEART, KIDNEY, LIVER, SWEETBREADS*)*

## OYSTERS

| | | | | | |
|---|---|---|---|---|---|
| canned eastern | 3 oz | 58 | 3 | – | – |
| canned eastern | 1 cup | 170 | 10 | – | – |
| eastern cooked | 6 med | 58 | 3 | – | – |
| eastern cooked | 3 oz | 117 | 7 | – | – |

| FOOD | PORTION | CALS | CARB | SUGAR | FIBER |
|---|---|---|---|---|---|
| eastern raw | 6 med | 58 | 3 | – | – |
| eastern raw | 1 cup | 170 | 10 | – | – |
| pacific raw | 1 med | 41 | 2 | – | – |
| pacific raw | 3 oz | 69 | 4 | – | – |
| steamed | 3 oz | 138 | 8 | – | – |
| steamed | 1 med | 41 | 2 | – | – |
| ***Bumble Bee*** | | | | | |
| Fancy Whole | 2 oz | 70 | 3 | 0 | 0 |
| Smoked | ½ can (1.9 oz) | 120 | 6 | 0 | 0 |
| **TAKE-OUT** | | | | | |
| breaded & fried | 6 (4.9 oz) | 368 | 40 | – | – |
| oysters rockefeller | 3 oysters | 66 | 5 | – | – |
| stew | 1 cup | 278 | 15 | – | tr |
| **PANCAKE/WAFFLE SYRUP** | | | | | |
| low calorie | 1 tbsp | 12 | 3 | – | 0 |
| maple | 1 tbsp (0.8 oz) | 52 | 13 | 12 | – |
| maple | 1 cup (11.1 oz) | 824 | 212 | 191 | – |
| pancake syrup | 1 tbsp (0.7 oz) | 57 | 15 | – | – |
| pancake syrup | 1 cup (11 oz) | 903 | 238 | – | – |
| pancake syrup light | 1 oz | 46 | 13 | – | – |
| pancake syrup w/ butter | 1 cup (11 oz) | 933 | 234 | – | – |
| pancake syrup w/ butter | 1 tbsp (0.7 oz) | 59 | 15 | – | – |
| ***Atkins*** | | | | | |
| Sugar Free | ¼ cup | 0 | 0 | 0 | 0 |
| ***Aunt Jemima*** | | | | | |
| Original | ¼ cup | 210 | 52 | 32 | – |
| ***Country Cupboard*** | | | | | |
| Boysenberry | ¼ cup | 0 | 0 | 0 | 0 |
| Maple Butter | ¼ cup | 0 | 2 | 0 | 0 |
| Strawberry | ¼ cup | 0 | 1 | 0 | 0 |
| ***Estee*** | | | | | |
| Maple | ¼ cup | 80 | 20 | 20 | 0 |
| ***Keto*** | | | | | |
| Maple Butter | ¼ cup | 0 | 1 | 1 | 0 |
| ***Ketogenics*** | | | | | |
| Zero Carb | ¼ cup | 0 | 0 | 0 | 0 |
| ***Log Cabin*** | | | | | |
| Original | ¼ cup | 210 | 53 | 39 | 0 |

| FOOD | PORTION | CALS | CARB | SUGAR | FIBER |
|---|---|---|---|---|---|
| ***Mrs. Butterworth's*** | | | | | |
| Lite | ¼ cup | 100 | 25 | 24 | – |
| Original | ¼ cup (2 oz) | 230 | 56 | 35 | – |
| ***Smucker's*** | | | | | |
| Breakfast Syrup Sugar Free | ¼ cup (2 oz) | 30 | 8 | 0 | – |
| ***Stonewall Kitchen*** | | | | | |
| Maine Maple | ¼ cup | 210 | 54 | 51 | 0 |

## PANCAKES

| FOOD | PORTION | CALS | CARB | SUGAR | FIBER |
|---|---|---|---|---|---|
| **FROZEN** | | | | | |
| buttermilk | 1 4 in diam | 83 | 16 | – | – |
| plain | 1 4 in diam | 83 | 16 | – | – |
| **MIX** | | | | | |
| buckwheat | 1 (4 in diam) | 62 | 9 | – | – |
| buttermilk | 1 (4 in diam) | 74 | 14 | – | tr |
| plain | 1 (4 in diam) | 74 | 14 | – | tr |
| sugar free low sodium | 1 (3 in diam) | 44 | 9 | – | – |
| whole wheat | 1 (4 in diam) | 92 | 13 | – | – |
| ***Atkins*** | | | | | |
| Quick Quisine Buttermilk not prep | ⅓ cup | 100 | 13 | 1 | 5 |
| Quick Quisine Original not prep | ¼ cup | 80 | 6 | 0 | 3 |
| ***Aunt Paula's*** | | | | | |
| Pancake & Waffle Mix as prep | 2 | 132 | 6 | 0 | 4 |
| ***Betty Crocker*** | | | | | |
| Buttermilk as prep | 3 | 200 | 20 | 3 | 1 |
| Original as prep | 3 | 200 | 39 | 9 | 2 |
| ***Bisquick*** | | | | | |
| Shake 'N Pour Blueberry as prep | 3 | 210 | 40 | 8 | 1 |
| ***Bruce*** | | | | | |
| Sweet Potato Pancakes | 2 | 210 | 39 | 5 | 2 |
| ***Carbolite*** | | | | | |
| Low Carb Mix not prep | ⅓ cup | 100 | 10 | 0 | tr |
| ***Carbsense*** | | | | | |
| Buckwheat not prep | ½ cup | 140 | 10 | 0 | 7 |
| Buttermilk not prep | ½ cup | 140 | 10 | 0 | 7 |
| ***Estee*** | | | | | |
| Pancake Mix as prep | 4 (4 in diam) | 180 | 40 | tr | 1 |

| FOOD | PORTION | CALS | CARB | SUGAR | FIBER |
|---|---|---|---|---|---|
| ***Hodgson Mill*** | | | | | |
| Buckwheat | ⅓ cup (1.8 oz) | 160 | 36 | 2 | 5 |
| ***Keto*** | | | | | |
| Banana not prep | ⅓ cup | 114 | 6 | 0 | 2 |
| Original not prep | ⅓ cup | 114 | 5 | 0 | 2 |
| ***Ketogenics*** | | | | | |
| Low Carb not prep | ⅔ cup | 185 | 15 | 1 | 6 |
| ***MiniCarb*** | | | | | |
| Apple Cinnamon as prep | 2 | 150 | 17 | 2 | 13 |
| ***Robin Hood*** | | | | | |
| Buttermilk as prep | 3 | 230 | 35 | 6 | 1 |
| **TAKE-OUT** | | | | | |
| blueberry | 1 (4 in diam) | 84 | 11 | – | – |
| plain | 1 (4 in diam) | 86 | 11 | – | – |
| potato | 1 (4 in diam) | 78 | 4 | – | tr |
| w/ butter & syrup | 2 (8.1 oz) | 520 | 91 | – | – |
| **PAPAYA** | | | | | |
| fresh | 1 | 117 | 30 | – | – |
| fresh cubed | 1 cup | 54 | 14 | – | – |
| ***SunFresh*** | | | | | |
| In Extra Light Syrup | ½ cup (4.5 oz) | 70 | 17 | 16 | 1 |
| **PAPAYA JUICE** | | | | | |
| nectar | 1 cup | 142 | 36 | – | – |
| ***Nantucket Nectars*** | | | | | |
| Cocktail | 8 oz | 120 | 30 | 27 | – |
| **PAPRIKA** | | | | | |
| paprika | 1 tsp | 6 | 1 | – | – |
| **PARSLEY** | | | | | |
| dry | 1 tsp | 1 | tr | – | – |
| dry | 1 tbsp | 1 | tr | – | – |
| fresh chopped | ½ cup | 11 | 2 | – | – |
| **PARSNIPS** | | | | | |
| fresh cooked | 1 (5.6 oz) | 130 | 31 | – | – |
| fresh sliced cooked | ½ cup | 63 | 15 | – | – |
| **PASSION FRUIT** | | | | | |
| purple fresh | 1 | 18 | 4 | – | – |

| FOOD | PORTION | CALS | CARB | SUGAR | FIBER |
|---|---|---|---|---|---|
| **PASSION FRUIT JUICE** | | | | | |
| purple | 1 cup | 126 | 34 | – | – |
| yellow | 1 cup | 149 | 36 | – | – |
| **PASTA** *(see also* NOODLES, PASTA DINNERS, PASTA SALAD*)* | | | | | |
| **DRY** | | | | | |
| corn cooked | 1 cup (4.9 oz) | 176 | 39 | – | 7 |
| corn spaghetti | 2 oz | 180 | 35 | 3 | 3 |
| elbows | 1 cup | 389 | 78 | – | – |
| elbows cooked | 1 cup (4.9 oz) | 197 | 40 | – | 2 |
| shells small cooked | 1 cup (4 oz) | 162 | 33 | – | 2 |
| shells small protein fortified cooked | 1 cup (4 oz) | 189 | 36 | – | – |
| spaghetti cooked | 1 cup (4.9 oz) | 197 | 40 | – | 2 |
| spaghetti protein fortified cooked | 1 cup (4.9 oz) | 230 | 44 | – | 2 |
| spinach spaghetti cooked | 1 cup (4.9 oz) | 182 | 37 | – | – |
| spirals cooked | 1 cup (4.7 oz) | 189 | 38 | – | 2 |
| vegetable cooked | 1 cup (4.7 oz) | 172 | 36 | – | 6 |
| whole wheat cooked | 1 cup (4.9 oz) | 174 | 37 | – | 4 |
| whole wheat spaghetti cooked | 1 cup (4.9 oz) | 174 | 37 | – | 6 |
| ***Annie Chun's*** | | | | | |
| Soba Noodles | 2 oz | 200 | 39 | 1 | 3 |
| ***Atkins*** | | | | | |
| All Shapes not prep | 2 oz | 230 | 15 | 2 | 9 |
| Quick Quisine All Shapes as prep | ¾ cup | 210 | 13 | 2 | 8 |
| ***Barilla*** | | | | | |
| Tortelloni Porcini Mushroom | ¾ cup | 240 | 32 | 3 | 5 |
| Tortelloni Ricotta & Asparagus | ¾ cup | 240 | 32 | 2 | 5 |
| Tortelloni Ricotta & Spinach | ¾ cup | 220 | 28 | 3 | 4 |
| ***Bella Vita*** | | | | | |
| Low Carb Penne Rigate | 2 oz | 190 | 18 | 3 | 8 |
| ***DaVinci*** | | | | | |
| Rotini | 1 cup | 210 | 43 | 3 | 2 |
| Spaghetti | 2 oz | 210 | 43 | 3 | 2 |
| ***Darielle*** | | | | | |
| All Shapes not prep | 2 oz | 160 | 18 | 3 | 8 |
| ***Duc Amici*** | | | | | |
| Pasta Lite Low Carb Fusilli | 2 oz | 160 | 10 | 3 | 7 |

| FOOD | PORTION | CALS | CARB | SUGAR | FIBER |
|---|---|---|---|---|---|
| ***Eden*** | | | | | |
| Organic Extra Fine | 2 oz | 210 | 40 | 1 | 3 |
| Organic Gemelli | 2 oz | 210 | 40 | 2 | 5 |
| Organic Pesto Gemelli | 2 oz | 210 | 41 | 2 | 4 |
| Organic Ribbons Saffron | 2 oz | 210 | 40 | 1 | 3 |
| Organic Spaghetti Semolina | 2 oz | 200 | 40 | 1 | 2 |
| Organic Spaghetti 50% Whole Grain | 2 oz | 210 | 41 | 2 | 4 |
| Organic Spirals Kamut Vegetable | 2 oz | 210 | 40 | 3 | 6 |
| Organic Spirals Sesame Rice | 2 oz | 200 | 37 | 1 | 4 |
| Organic Spirals Mixed Grain | 2 oz | 210 | 41 | 3 | 7 |
| Organic Spirals Spinach | 2 oz | 210 | 41 | 2 | 4 |
| Organic Vegetable Alphabets | 2 oz | 200 | 40 | 1 | 2 |
| Spirals Rye | 2 oz | 200 | 44 | 1 | 8 |
| ***Goya*** | | | | | |
| Coditos not prep | ½ cup | 230 | 47 | 2 | 3 |
| ***Hodgson Mill*** | | | | | |
| Four Color Veggie Bows | 2 oz | 200 | 41 | 0 | 1 |
| Four Color Veggie Rotini Spirals | 2 oz | 200 | 41 | 0 | 1 |
| Pastamania! Durum Wheat Fettuccine | 2 oz | 200 | 38 | 0 | 1 |
| Pastamania! Fettuccine Garlic & Parsley | 2 oz | 200 | 38 | 0 | 1 |
| Pastamania! Fettuccine w/ Jerusalem Artichoke | 2 oz | 210 | 41 | 0 | 2 |
| Pastamania! Fettucinne w/ Mushroom | 2 oz | 210 | 41 | 1 | 2 |
| Pastamania! Fusilli Tre Colore w/ Tomato & Spinach | 2 oz | 200 | 40 | 2 | 2 |
| Pastamania! Sea Shell Mix | 2 oz | 200 | 40 | 0 | 1 |
| Pastamania! Spinach Fettuccine | 2 oz | 200 | 37 | 0 | 2 |
| Pastamania! Thin Linguine | 2 oz | 200 | 38 | 0 | 1 |
| Pastamania! Tomato Spinach & Durum Wheat | 2 oz | 210 | 40 | 1 | 2 |
| Spaghetti Whole Wheat not prep | 2 oz | 190 | 34 | 0 | 6 |
| Whole Wheat Lasagne not prep | 2 oz | 190 | 34 | 0 | 6 |
| Whole Wheat Spinach Spaghetti not prep | 2 oz | 190 | 35 | 0 | 5 |

| FOOD | PORTION | CALS | CARB | SUGAR | FIBER |
|---|---|---|---|---|---|
| ***Keto*** | | | | | |
| Elbows not prep | 1.6 oz | 108 | 5 | 0 | 1 |
| Spaghetti not prep | 1.3 oz | 130 | 7 | 0 | 2 |
| ***Lundberg*** | | | | | |
| Spaghetti Organic Brown Rice | 2 oz | 210 | 44 | 3 | 3 |
| ***Pastalia*** | | | | | |
| Heart Health Low Carb not prep | 2 oz | 176 | 10 | tr | 3 |
| ***Real Torino*** | | | | | |
| Tirali not prep | 1 cup (2 oz) | 210 | 43 | 3 | 2 |
| ***Revival*** | | | | | |
| Soy Penne | ⅙ box | 200 | 34 | 2 | 1 |
| Soy Thin Spaghetti | ⅙ box | 200 | 34 | 2 | 1 |
| ***Ronzoni*** | | | | | |
| Elbows not prep | ½ cup (2 oz) | 210 | 42 | 2 | 2 |
| Lasagne | 2½ pieces (2 oz) | 210 | 42 | 2 | 2 |
| Tradizione D'Italia All Shapes | 2 oz | 210 | 42 | 2 | 2 |
| ***San Giorgio*** | | | | | |
| Healthy Harvest Whole Wheat Blend | 2 oz | 210 | 42 | 3 | 2 |
| ***Soy7*** | | | | | |
| Pasta All Shapes | 2 oz | 200 | 33 | 2 | 2 |
| ***Whey Cool*** | | | | | |
| High Protein Xtreme Rotini | 1 serv (2 oz) | 210 | 8 | 4 | 1 |
| **FRESH** | | | | | |
| cooked | 2 oz | 75 | 14 | – | – |
| spinach cooked | 2 oz | 74 | 14 | – | – |

**PASTA DINNERS** *(see also* PASTA SALAD*)*

| | | | | | |
|---|---|---|---|---|---|
| **CANNED** | | | | | |
| ***Chef Boyardee*** | | | | | |
| 99% Fat Free Beef Ravioli | 1 cup (8.6 oz) | 210 | 41 | 6 | 3 |
| 99% Fat Free Cheese Ravioli | 1 cup (8.8 oz) | 210 | 44 | 9 | 4 |
| Beef Ravioli | 1 cup (8.6 oz) | 230 | 37 | 5 | 4 |
| Beefaroni | 1 cup (8.7 oz) | 260 | 37 | 9 | 5 |
| Macaroni & Cheese | ½ can (7.5 oz) | 180 | 35 | 0 | 2 |
| Mini Ravioli | 1 cup (8.8 oz) | 252 | 37 | 5 | 3 |
| Spaghetti & Meat Balls | 1 cup (8.4 oz) | 240 | 32 | 7 | 3 |
| Tortellini Cheese | ½ can (7 oz) | 230 | 48 | 12 | 5 |
| Tortellini Meat | ½ can (7 oz) | 260 | 48 | 12 | 4 |

| FOOD | PORTION | CALS | CARB | SUGAR | FIBER |
|---|---|---|---|---|---|
| ***Franco-American*** | | | | | |
| Beef Raviolios | 1 can (7.7 oz) | 250 | 39 | 10 | 4 |
| Beefy Mac | 1 can (7.5 oz) | 228 | 30 | 10 | 3 |
| Elbow Macaroni & Cheese | 1 can (7.5 oz) | 187 | 25 | 2 | 2 |
| Spaghetti 'N Beef | 1 can (7.5 oz) | 226 | 30 | 9 | 3 |
| Spaghetti w/ Meatballs | 1 can (7.2 oz) | 249 | 33 | 12 | 4 |
| ***Progresso*** | | | | | |
| Beef Ravioli | 1 cup (9.1 oz) | 260 | 45 | 9 | 4 |
| Cheese Ravioli | 1 cup (9.1 oz) | 220 | 43 | 9 | 4 |
| **FROZEN** | | | | | |
| ***Amy's*** | | | | | |
| Bowl Stuffed Pasta Shells | 1 pkg (10 oz) | 300 | 30 | 7 | 5 |
| Cannelloni w/ Vegetables | 1 pkg (9 oz) | 330 | 34 | 10 | 6 |
| Lasagna Cheese | 1 pkg (10.25 oz) | 330 | 38 | 6 | 5 |
| Lasagna Garden Vegetable | 1 pkg (10.25 oz) | 290 | 41 | 7 | 5 |
| Macaroni & Cheese | 1 pkg (9 oz) | 410 | 47 | 6 | 3 |
| Macaroni & Soy Cheese | 1 pkg (9 oz) | 370 | 42 | 2 | 4 |
| Pasta & Vegetable Alfredo | 1 cup | 220 | 27 | 6 | 4 |
| Pasta Primavera | 1 pkg (9 oz) | 300 | 37 | 7 | 3 |
| Ravioli w/ Sauce | 1 pkg (8 oz) | 340 | 43 | 3 | 3 |
| Rice Mac & Cheese | 1 pkg (9 oz) | 140 | 47 | 6 | 3 |
| Skillet Meals | 1 cup | 250 | 27 | 3 | 3 |
| Tofu Vegetable Lasagna | 1 pkg (9.5 oz) | 300 | 41 | 6 | 6 |
| Vegetable Lasagna | 1 pkg (9.5 oz) | 280 | 29 | 5 | 3 |
| ***Banquet*** | | | | | |
| Chicken Pasta Primavera | 1 meal (9.5 oz) | 320 | 40 | 9 | 6 |
| Family Size Egg Noodles w/ Beef & Brown Gravy | 1 serv | 150 | 16 | 1 | 2 |
| Family Size Lasagna w/ Meat Sauce | 1 cup | 270 | 33 | 3 | 2 |
| Family Size Macaroni & Cheese | 1 cup | 230 | 32 | 7 | 3 |
| Fettuccine Alfredo | 1 meal (9.5 oz) | 350 | 40 | 5 | 4 |
| Homestyle Noodles & Chicken | 1 meal (12 oz) | 390 | 44 | 5 | 7 |
| Lasagna w/ Meat Sauce | 1 meal (9.5 oz) | 260 | 38 | 10 | 3 |

| FOOD | PORTION | CALS | CARB | SUGAR | FIBER |
|---|---|---|---|---|---|
| Macaroni & Cheese | 1 meal (12 oz) | 420 | 57 | 7 | 5 |
| ***Birds Eye*** | | | | | |
| Easy Recipe Creations Basil Herb Primavera | 2¼ cup | 260 | 31 | 5 | 3 |
| Easy Recipe Creations Tortellini Parmigiana | 2¼ cups | 240 | 25 | 5 | 4 |
| Pasta Secrets Italian Pesto | 2⅓ cups | 240 | 32 | 6 | 2 |
| Pasta Secrets Primavera | 2⅓ cups | 230 | 26 | 4 | 3 |
| Pasta Secrets Ranch | 2⅓ cups | 300 | 29 | 8 | 2 |
| Pasta Secrets Three Cheese | 2 cups | 230 | 31 | 8 | 2 |
| Pasta Secrets White Cheddar | 2 cups | 240 | 30 | 7 | 2 |
| Pasta Secrets Zesty Garlic | 2 cups | 240 | 31 | 6 | 2 |
| ***Healthy Choice*** | | | | | |
| Beef Macaroni | 1 meal (8.5 oz) | 220 | 34 | 9 | 5 |
| Bowls Cheese & Chicken Tortellini | 1 meal (8.7 oz) | 250 | 40 | 5 | 6 |
| Breaded Chicken Breast Stips w/ Macaroni & Cheese | 1 meal (8 oz) | 270 | 34 | 9 | 1 |
| Cheese Ravioli Parmigiana | 1 meal (9 oz) | 260 | 44 | 14 | 6 |
| Chicken Fettuccine Alfredo | 1 meal (8.5 oz) | 280 | 30 | 3 | 4 |
| Fettuccine Alfredo | 1 meal (8 oz) | 240 | 37 | 4 | 2 |
| Lasagna Roma | 1 meal (13.5 oz) | 420 | 59 | 14 | 6 |
| Macaroni & Cheese | 1 meal (9 oz) | 240 | 36 | 8 | 3 |
| Manicotti w/ Three Cheeses | 1 meal (11 oz) | 300 | 40 | 14 | 5 |
| Spaghetti & Sauce w/ Seasoned Beef | 1 meal (10 oz) | 260 | 43 | 7 | 5 |
| Stuffed Pasta Shells | 1 meal (10.35 oz) | 370 | 60 | 12 | 5 |
| ***Joseph's Pasta*** | | | | | |
| Grilled Chicken Ravioli w/ Roasted Red Pepper Sauce | 1 pkg (14 oz) | 540 | 66 | 3 | 6 |
| ***Kid Cuisine*** | | | | | |
| Magical Macaroni & Cheese | 1 meal (10.6 oz) | 440 | 72 | 25 | 4 |

| FOOD | PORTION | CALS | CARB | SUGAR | FIBER |
|---|---|---|---|---|---|
| ***Lean Cuisine*** | | | | | |
| Cafe Classics Bow Tie Pasta & Chicken | 1 pkg (9.5 oz) | 220 | 32 | 6 | 5 |
| Cafe Classics Cheese Lasagna w/ Chicken Scaloppini | 1 pkg (10 oz) | 270 | 27 | 7 | 4 |
| Cafe Classics Shrimp & Angel Hair Pasta | 1 pkg (10 oz) | 240 | 35 | 7 | 2 |
| Everyday Favorites Alfredo Pasta Primavera | 1 pkg (10 oz) | 290 | 46 | 6 | 3 |
| Everyday Favorites Angel Hair Pasta | 1 pkg (10 oz) | 240 | 43 | 11 | 4 |
| Everyday Favorites Cheese Cannelloni | 1 pkg (9.1 oz) | 230 | 28 | 8 | 4 |
| Everyday Favorites Cheese Lasagna Casserole | 1 pkg (10 oz) | 270 | 40 | 6 | 5 |
| Everyday Favorites Cheese Ravioli | 1 pkg (8.5 oz) | 260 | 38 | 8 | 4 |
| Everyday Favorites Chicken Lasagna | 1 pkg (10 oz) | 280 | 34 | 6 | 2 |
| Everyday Favorites Classic Cheese Lasagna | 1 pkg (11.5 oz) | 290 | 38 | 9 | 4 |
| Everyday Favorites Fettucini Alfredo | 1 pkg (9.25 oz) | 280 | 42 | 6 | 3 |
| Everyday Favorites Fettucini Primavera | 1 pkg (10 oz) | 270 | 38 | 8 | 4 |
| Everyday Favorites Lasagna w/ Meat Sauce | 1 pkg (10.5 oz) | 300 | 35 | 7 | 4 |
| Everyday Favorites Macaroni & Cheese | 1 pkg (10 oz) | 290 | 42 | 5 | 2 |
| Everyday Favorites Macaroni & Beef | 1 pkg (10 oz) | 270 | 43 | 9 | 4 |
| Everyday Favorites Penne Pasta | 1 pkg (10 oz) | 260 | 47 | 13 | 5 |
| Everyday Favorites Spaghetti w/ Meat Sauce | 1 pkg (11.5 oz) | 290 | 50 | 10 | 7 |
| Everyday Favorites Spaghetti w/ Meatballs | 1 pkg (9.5 oz) | 270 | 37 | 6 | 4 |
| Family Style Favorites Five Cheese Lasagna | 1 serv (8 oz) | 210 | 27 | 6 | 3 |

| FOOD | PORTION | CALS | CARB | SUGAR | FIBER |
|---|---|---|---|---|---|
| Skillet Sensations Chicken Alfredo | 1 serv | 280 | 36 | 6 | 3 |
| ***Marie Callender's*** | | | | | |
| Cheese Ravioli In Marinara Sauce w/ Spirals & Garlic Bread | 1 meal (16 oz) | 750 | 96 | 18 | 11 |
| Extra Cheese Lasagna | 1 meal (15 oz) | 590 | 61 | 19 | 7 |
| Fettuccine Alfredo & Garlic Bread | 1 meal (14 oz) | 920 | 62 | 5 | 3 |
| Fettuccine Alfredo Supreme | 1 meal (13 oz) | 450 | 35 | 1 | 4 |
| Fettuccine Primavera w/ Tortellini | 1 meal (14 oz) | 750 | 57 | 10 | 6 |
| Fettuccine w/ Broccoli & Chicken | 1 meal (13 oz) | 710 | 53 | 7 | 6 |
| Lasagna w/ Meat Sauce | 1 meal (15 oz) | 630 | 59 | 24 | 3 |
| Macaroni & Cheese | 1 meal (12 oz) | 540 | 55 | 12 | 5 |
| Skillet Meal Chicken Alfredo | ½ pkg | 490 | 32 | 5 | 7 |
| Skillet Meal Penne Pasta & Meatballs | ½ pkg | 600 | 53 | 4 | 4 |
| Skillet Meal Rigatoni Vegetables In Cheese Sauce | 1 cup | 290 | 32 | 16 | 4 |
| Spaghetti w/ Meat Sauce & Garlic Bread | 1 meal (17 oz) | 670 | 65 | 20 | 9 |
| Stuffed Pasta Trio | 1 meal (10.5 oz) | 380 | 40 | 26 | 5 |
| ***Morton*** | | | | | |
| Macaroni & Cheese | 1 serv (8 oz) | 240 | 34 | 10 | 3 |
| Spaghetti w/ Meat Sauce | 1 meal (8.5 oz) | 200 | 30 | 13 | 4 |
| ***Quorn*** | | | | | |
| Fettuccine Alfredo | 1 pkg (10.5 oz) | 360 | 40 | 5 | 4 |
| Lasagna | 1 pkg (10.5 oz) | 360 | 43 | 13 | 4 |
| ***Weight Watchers*** | | | | | |
| Garden Lasagna | 1 pkg (11 oz) | 270 | 36 | 6 | 5 |
| Homestyle Macaroni & Cheese | 1 pkg (9 oz) | 290 | 45 | 2 | 2 |
| Smart Ones Angel Hair Pasta | 1 pkg (9 oz) | 180 | 32 | 4 | 4 |
| Smart Ones Bowtie Pasta & Mushrooms Marsala | 1 pkg (9.65 oz) | 270 | 40 | 3 | 4 |

| FOOD | PORTION | CALS | CARB | SUGAR | FIBER |
|---|---|---|---|---|---|
| Smart Ones Chicken Fettucini | 1 pkg (10 oz) | 300 | 39 | 4 | 4 |
| Smart Ones Creamy Rigatoni w/ Broccoli & Chicken | 1 pkg (9 oz) | 230 | 40 | 5 | 4 |
| Smart Ones Fettucini Alfredo w/ Broccoli | 1 pkg (8.5 oz) | 230 | 32 | 8 | 3 |
| Smart Ones Lasagna Florentine | 1 pkg (10 oz) | 200 | 33 | 5 | 5 |
| Smart Ones Lasagna Alfredo | 1 pkg (9 oz) | 300 | 46 | 6 | 3 |
| Smart Ones Lasagna w/ Meat Sauce | 1 pkg (9 oz) | 240 | 43 | 5 | 4 |
| Smart Ones Lasagna w/ Meat Sauce | 1 pkg (10.25 oz) | 270 | 36 | 8 | 6 |
| Smart Ones Macaroni & Cheese | 1 pkg (9 oz) | 220 | 42 | 5 | 4 |
| Smart Ones Pasta & Spinach Romano | 1 pkg (10.4 oz) | 260 | 35 | 7 | 4 |
| Smart Ones Pasta w/ Tomato Basil Sauce | 1 pkg (9.6 oz) | 260 | 40 | 4 | 3 |
| Smart Ones Penne Pasta w/ Sun-Dried Tomatoes | 1 pkg (10 oz) | 280 | 40 | 5 | 3 |
| Smart Ones Penne Pollo | 1 pkg (10 oz) | 290 | 38 | 5 | 3 |
| Smart Ones Ravioli Florentine | 1 pkg (8.5 oz) | 220 | 43 | 5 | 4 |
| Smart Ones Spaghetti Marinara | 1 pkg (9 oz) | 280 | 46 | 7 | 4 |
| Smart Ones Spaghetti w/ Meat Sauce | 1 pkg (10 oz) | 280 | 41 | 8 | 4 |
| Smart Ones Spicy Penne & Ricotta | 1 pkg (10.2 oz) | 280 | 45 | 5 | 4 |
| Smart Ones Tuna Noodle Casserole | 1 pkg (9.5 oz) | 270 | 38 | 6 | 4 |
| Smart Ones Zita Mozzarella | 1 pkg (9 oz) | 290 | 47 | 5 | 5 |
| ***Yves*** | | | | | |
| Veggie Lasagna | 1 pkg (10.5 oz) | 300 | 51 | 9 | 4 |
| Veggie Macaroni | 1 pkg (10.5 oz) | 230 | 38 | 6 | 3 |
| Veggie Penne | 1 pkg (10.5 oz) | 220 | 36 | 7 | 4 |
| **MIX** | | | | | |
| ***Annie's Homegrown*** | | | | | |
| Mac & Cheese Meals | 1 pkg | 230 | 40 | 0 | tr |
| ***Aramana*** | | | | | |
| Cheddar Cheeseburger as prep | 1 cup | 260 | 11 | 2 | 4 |

| FOOD | PORTION | CALS | CARB | SUGAR | FIBER |
|---|---|---|---|---|---|
| Creamy Chicken Alfredo as prep | 1 cup | 260 | 12 | 2 | 5 |
| Mild Mexican as prep | 1 cup | 260 | 12 | 2 | 5 |
| ***Atkins*** | | | | | |
| Quick Quisine Elbows & Cheese as prep | 1 cup | 250 | 17 | 0 | 9 |
| Quick Quisine Fettuccine Alfredo as prep | 1 cup | 210 | 16 | 1 | 9 |
| Quick Quisine Pesto Cream as prep | 1 cup | 240 | 17 | 1 | 10 |
| ***Hamburger Helper*** | | | | | |
| Ravioli as prep | 1 cup | 280 | 30 | 5 | 1 |
| Ravioli w/ White Cheese Topping as prep | 1 cup | 310 | 34 | 7 | 1 |
| ***Hodgson Mill*** | | | | | |
| Macaroni & Cheese Whole Wheat | 1 serv | 250 | 45 | 8 | 6 |
| ***Keto*** | | | | | |
| Macaroni & Cheese not prep | 1 serv | 112 | 5 | 0 | 1 |
| ***Whey Cool*** | | | | | |
| High Protein Macaroni & Cheese as prep | 1 serv | 260 | 12 | 7 | 1 |
| **READY-TO-EAT** | | | | | |
| ***Tyson*** | | | | | |
| Rosemary Penne | 1 pkg (12.5 oz) | 330 | 45 | 2 | 5 |
| **SHELF-STABLE** | | | | | |
| ***It's Pasta Anytime*** | | | | | |
| Penne With Tomato Italian Sausage Sauce | 1 pkg (15.25 oz) | 540 | 100 | 17 | 12 |
| ***Lunch Bucket*** | | | | | |
| Beef Ravioli In Tomato Sauce | 1 pkg (7.5 oz) | 180 | 32 | 8 | 3 |
| Italian Pasta w/ Chicken | 1 pkg (7.5 oz) | 130 | 24 | 7 | 2 |
| Lasagna 'n Meatsauce | 1 pkg (7.5 oz) | 160 | 29 | 9 | 2 |
| Macaroni 'n Beef in Meatsauce | 1 pkg (7.5 oz) | 180 | 10 | 0 | 8 |
| Macaroni 'n Cheese | 1 pkg (7.5 oz) | 190 | 24 | 0 | 2 |
| Pasta'n Chicken | 1 pkg (7.5 oz) | 150 | 22 | 1 | 2 |
| Spaghetti'n Meatsauce | 1 pkg (7.5 oz) | 160 | 29 | 9 | 2 |

| FOOD | PORTION | CALS | CARB | SUGAR | FIBER |
|---|---|---|---|---|---|
| **TAKE-OUT** | | | | | |
| lasagna | 1 piece (2.5 in x 2.5 in) | 374 | 25 | – | 2 |
| macaroni & cheese | 1 cup | 230 | 26 | – | – |
| manicotti | ¾ cup (6.4 oz) | 273 | 28 | – | 2 |
| rigatoni w/ sausage sauce | ¾ cup | 260 | 28 | – | 3 |
| spaghetti w/ meatballs & cheese | 1 cup | 407 | 38 | – | – |

## PASTA SALAD

| FOOD | PORTION | CALS | CARB | SUGAR | FIBER |
|---|---|---|---|---|---|
| **MIX** | | | | | |
| ***Kraft*** | | | | | |
| Pasta Salad Italian 97% Fat Free as prep | ¾ cup (4.9 oz) | 190 | 35 | 5 | 2 |
| ***Suddenly Salad*** | | | | | |
| Classic Pasta | ¾ cup | 250 | 38 | 5 | 2 |
| Classic Pasta Reduced Fat Recipe | ¾ cup | 210 | 38 | 5 | 2 |
| Garden Italian 98% Fat Free | ¾ cup | 140 | 28 | 4 | 2 |
| **TAKE-OUT** | | | | | |
| elbow macaroni salad | 3.5 oz | 160 | 26 | – | – |
| italian style pasta salad | 3.5 oz | 140 | 15 | – | – |
| mustard macaroni salad | 3.5 oz | 190 | 23 | – | – |
| pasta salad w/ vegetables | 3.5 oz | 140 | 21 | – | – |

## PÂTÉ

| FOOD | PORTION | CALS | CARB | SUGAR | FIBER |
|---|---|---|---|---|---|
| chicken liver canned | 1 tbsp (13 g) | 109 | 1 | – | – |
| duck pâté | 1 oz | 96 | 1 | tr | – |
| fish pâté | 1 oz | 76 | 1 | – | – |
| goose liver smoked canned | 1 tbsp (13 g) | 60 | 1 | – | – |
| liver canned | 1 tbsp (13 g) | 41 | tr | – | – |
| mushroom anchovy pâté | 1 can (2.25 oz) | 130 | 7 | 1 | 1 |
| pâté foie gras | 1 oz | 127 | 1 | – | – |
| pork pâté | 1 oz | 107 | 1 | 1 | 0 |
| pork pâté en croute | 1 oz | 91 | 3 | tr | tr |
| rabbit pâté | 1 oz | 66 | 1 | – | – |
| shrimp | 1 can (2.25 oz) | 140 | 7 | 1 | 0 |

| FOOD | PORTION | CALS | CARB | SUGAR | FIBER |
|---|---|---|---|---|---|
| **PEACH** | | | | | |
| **CANNED** | | | | | |
| halves in heavy syrup | 1 half | 60 | 16 | – | – |
| halves in light syrup | 1 half | 44 | 12 | – | – |
| halves juice pack | 1 half | 34 | 9 | – | – |
| halves water pack | 1 half | 18 | 5 | – | – |
| peachsauce | ½ cup | 120 | 32 | 31 | 1 |
| spiced in heavy syrup | 1 fruit | 66 | 18 | – | – |
| spiced in heavy syrup | 1 cup | 180 | 49 | – | – |
| ***Del Monte*** | | | | | |
| Fruit Cup Diced Extra Light Syrup | 1 pkg (4 oz) | 50 | 13 | 12 | 1 |
| Fruit Cup Diced In Heavy Syrup | 1 serv (4 oz) | 80 | 20 | 19 | 1 |
| Fruit Cup Fruit Naturals Diced | 1 pkg (4 oz) | 50 | 13 | 12 | 1 |
| Fruit Pleasures Raspberry Flavor | ½ cup (4.5 oz) | 80 | 20 | 19 | 1 |
| Fruit To Go Banana Berry Peaches | 1 pkg (4 oz) | 70 | 17 | 16 | 1 |
| Fruitrageous Peachy Pie | 1 pkg (4 oz) | 80 | 21 | 20 | 1 |
| Fruitrageous Wild Raspberry Flavor | 1 pkg (4 oz) | 80 | 20 | 19 | 1 |
| Halves Ginger Flavor | ½ cup (4.5 oz) | 90 | 22 | 19 | 1 |
| Halves In Extra Light Syrup | ½ cup (4.5 oz) | 60 | 15 | 14 | 1 |
| Halves In Heavy Syrup | ½ cup (4.5 oz) | 100 | 24 | 23 | 1 |
| Halves Melba In Heavy Syrup | ½ cup (4.5 oz) | 100 | 24 | 23 | 1 |
| Orchard Select Sliced Cling | ½ cup | 80 | 22 | 19 | tr |
| Slice Fruit Natural | ½ cup (4.4 oz) | 60 | 15 | 14 | 1 |
| Sliced In Extra Light Syrup | ½ cup (4.4 oz) | 60 | 14 | 13 | 1 |
| Sliced Natural Raspberry Flavor | ½ cup (4.4 oz) | 80 | 20 | 19 | 1 |
| Sliced Natural Harvest Spice Flavor | ½ cup (4.5 oz) | 80 | 21 | 20 | 1 |
| Whole Spiced In Heavy Syrup | ½ cup (4.2 oz) | 100 | 24 | 23 | 1 |
| ***Dole*** | | | | | |
| All Natural Yellow Cling Sliced | ½ cup | 80 | 17 | 16 | tr |
| **DRIED** | | | | | |
| halves | 1 cup | 383 | 98 | – | 13 |
| halves | 10 | 311 | 80 | – | 11 |
| halves cooked w/ sugar | ½ cup | 139 | 36 | – | – |
| halves cooked w/o sugar | ½ cup | 99 | 25 | – | – |

| FOOD | PORTION | CALS | CARB | SUGAR | FIBER |
|---|---|---|---|---|---|
| **FRESH** | | | | | |
| peach | 1 | 37 | 10 | – | 1 |
| sliced | 1 cup | 73 | 19 | – | – |
| ***Chiquita*** | | | | | |
| Peach | 1 med (3.4 oz) | 40 | 10 | 9 | 2 |
| **FROZEN** | | | | | |
| slices sweetened | 1 cup | 235 | 60 | – | – |
| **PEACH JUICE** | | | | | |
| nectar | 1 cup | 134 | 35 | – | – |
| ***Nantucket Nectars*** | | | | | |
| The Original | 8 oz | 120 | 30 | 26 | – |
| **PEANUT BUTTER** | | | | | |
| chunky | 1 cup | 1520 | 56 | – | 17 |
| chunky | 2 tbsp | 188 | 7 | – | 2 |
| chunky w/o salt | 2 tbsp | 188 | 7 | – | 2 |
| chunky w/o salt | 1 cup | 1520 | 56 | – | 17 |
| smooth | 1 cup | 1517 | 53 | – | 15 |
| smooth | 2 tbsp | 188 | 7 | – | 2 |
| smooth w/o salt | 1 cup | 1517 | 53 | – | 15 |
| smooth w/o salt | 2 tbsp | 188 | 7 | – | 2 |
| ***Carb Options*** | | | | | |
| Creamy | 2 tbsp | 190 | 5 | tr | 2 |
| ***Estee*** | | | | | |
| Creamy Low Sodium | 2 tbsp (1 oz) | 190 | 7 | 2 | 2 |
| ***Jif*** | | | | | |
| Apple Cinnamon | 2 tbsp (1.3 oz) | 200 | 11 | 8 | 2 |
| Berry Blend | 2 tbsp (1.2 oz) | 200 | 10 | 7 | 1 |
| Chocolate Silk | 2 tbsp (1.3 oz) | 190 | 14 | 12 | 1 |
| Creamy | 2 tbsp (1.1 oz) | 190 | 7 | 3 | 2 |
| Extra Crunchy | 2 tbsp (1.1 oz) | 190 | 7 | 3 | 2 |
| Reduced Fat Creamy | 2 tbsp (1.3 oz) | 190 | 15 | 4 | 2 |
| Reduced Fat Crunchy | 2 tbsp (1.3 oz) | 190 | 15 | 4 | 2 |
| Simply | 2 tbsp (1.1 oz) | 190 | 6 | 2 | 2 |
| ***Maranatha*** | | | | | |
| Crunchy | 2 tbsp | 190 | 7 | 2 | 2 |
| Salted | 2 tbsp | 190 | 7 | 2 | 2 |
| ***P.B.*** | | | | | |
| Slices | 1 slice (1 oz) | 170 | 5 | 3 | 1 |

| FOOD | PORTION | CALS | CARB | SUGAR | FIBER |
|---|---|---|---|---|---|
| ***Peanut Wonder*** | | | | | |
| Low Sodium | 2 tbsp | 100 | 13 | 5 | 0 |
| Regular | 2 tbsp | 100 | 13 | 5 | 0 |
| ***Reese's*** | | | | | |
| Peanut Butter Chips | 1 tbsp (0.5 oz) | 80 | 7 | – | – |
| ***Skippy*** | | | | | |
| Creamy | 2 tbsp | 190 | 7 | 3 | 2 |
| Creamy w/ 2 slices white bread | 1 sandwich | 340 | 33 | – | – |
| Reduced Fat Creamy | 2 tbsp | 190 | 15 | 5 | 2 |
| ***Tropical Source*** | | | | | |
| Chips Dairy Free | 13 pieces (1.5 oz) | 80 | 9 | 7 | 0 |
| **PEANUTS** | | | | | |
| chocolate coated | 10 (1.4 oz) | 208 | 20 | – | – |
| chocolate coated | 1 cup (5.2 oz) | 773 | 74 | – | – |
| cooked | ½ cup | 102 | 7 | – | – |
| dry roasted | 1 cup | 855 | 31 | – | 12 |
| dry roasted w/ salt | 30 nuts (1 oz) | 170 | 6 | 2 | 2 |
| ***At Last!*** | | | | | |
| Chocolate Covered | 1 pkg (0.9 oz) | 150 | 18 | 0 | 5 |
| ***Estee*** | | | | | |
| Candy Coated | ¼ cup | 200 | 23 | 6 | 1 |
| ***Frito Lay*** | | | | | |
| Honey Roasted | 1 serv (1.5 oz) | 270 | 10 | 5 | 3 |
| Hot | 1 serv (1.1 oz) | 190 | 6 | 2 | 2 |
| Salted | 1 oz | 200 | 5 | 1 | 2 |
| ***Judy's*** | | | | | |
| Sugar Free Coconut Peanut Brittle | ¼ piece (1 oz) | 90 | 2 | 0 | 1 |
| ***Lance*** | | | | | |
| Honey Toasted | 1 pkg (1⅜ oz) | 220 | 13 | 5 | 3 |
| Roasted | 1 pkg (1¾ oz) | 190 | 6 | 1 | 4 |
| Salted | 1 pkg (1⅛ oz) | 200 | 6 | 0 | 4 |
| Salted Long Tube | ¼ cup (1 oz) | 180 | 5 | 0 | 3 |
| ***Little Debbie*** | | | | | |
| Salted | ¼ cup (1 oz) | 160 | 5 | 1 | 2 |
| ***Low Carb Creations*** | | | | | |
| Soft Peanut Brittle | 2 pieces (1 oz) | 140 | 8 | 2 | 2 |

| FOOD | PORTION | CALS | CARB | SUGAR | FIBER |
|---|---|---|---|---|---|
| ***Sweet Delight*** | | | | | |
| Peanut Roasters | ⅓ pkg (1 oz) | 160 | 7 | tr | 3 |
| ***Tom's*** | | | | | |
| Double Coated | 1 pkg (1.35 oz) | 220 | 15 | 10 | 1 |
| Toasted | 1 pkg (1.4 oz) | 240 | 7 | 1 | 2 |
| ***Weight Watchers*** | | | | | |
| Honey Roasted | 1 pkg (0.7 oz) | 100 | 7 | 3 | 2 |
| **PEAR** | | | | | |
| **CANNED** | | | | | |
| halves in heavy sirup | 1 cup | 188 | 49 | – | – |
| halves in heavy syrup | 1 half | 68 | 15 | – | – |
| halves in light syrup | 1 half | 45 | 12 | – | – |
| halves juice pack | 1 cup | 123 | 32 | – | – |
| halves water pack | 1 half | 22 | 6 | – | – |
| ***Del Monte*** | | | | | |
| Fruit Cup Diced In Heavy Syrup | 1 pkg (4 oz) | 80 | 20 | 19 | 1 |
| Fruit Cup Diced Extra Light Syrup | 1 pkg (4 oz) | 50 | 13 | 12 | 1 |
| Fruit To Go Peachy Peaches | 1 pkg (4 oz) | 70 | 17 | 16 | 1 |
| Halves Fruit Naturals | ½ cup (4.4 oz) | 60 | 15 | 14 | 1 |
| Halves In Extra Light Syrup | ½ cup (4.4 oz) | 60 | 15 | 14 | 1 |
| Halves In Heavy Syrup | ½ cup (4.5 oz) | 100 | 24 | 33 | 1 |
| Orchard Select Sliced Bartlett | ½ cup | 80 | 20 | 19 | 2 |
| Sliced In Extra Light Syrup | ½ cup (4.5 oz) | 60 | 15 | 14 | 1 |
| **DRIED** | | | | | |
| halves | 10 | 459 | 122 | – | – |
| halves | 1 cup | 472 | 125 | – | – |
| halves cooked w/ sugar | ½ cup | 196 | 52 | – | – |
| halves cooked w/o sugar | ½ cup | 163 | 43 | – | – |
| **FRESH** | | | | | |
| asian | 1 (4.3 oz) | 51 | 13 | – | – |
| pear | 1 | 98 | 25 | – | 4 |
| sliced w/ skin | 1 cup | 97 | 25 | – | 4 |
| ***Chiquita*** | | | | | |
| Pear | 1 med (5.8 oz) | 100 | 25 | 17 | 4 |
| **PEAR JUICE** | | | | | |
| nectar | 1 cup | 149 | 39 | – | – |

| FOOD | PORTION | CALS | CARB | SUGAR | FIBER |
|---|---|---|---|---|---|
| **PEAS** | | | | | |
| **CANNED** | | | | | |
| green | ½ cup | 59 | 11 | – | – |
| green low sodium | ½ cup | 59 | 11 | – | – |
| ***Del Monte*** | | | | | |
| Sweet | ½ cup (4.4 oz) | 60 | 13 | 6 | 4 |
| Sweet No Salt Added | ½ cup (4.4 oz) | 60 | 11 | 6 | 4 |
| Sweet Very Young Small | ½ cup (4.4 oz) | 60 | 10 | 5 | 4 |
| ***S&W*** | | | | | |
| Petite | ½ cup (4.4 oz) | 70 | 12 | 4 | 4 |
| Small | ½ cup (4.4 oz) | 70 | 12 | 4 | 4 |
| ***Veg-All*** | | | | | |
| Tender Sweet | ½ cup | 60 | 10 | 4 | 3 |
| **DRIED** | | | | | |
| split cooked | 1 cup | 231 | 41 | – | – |
| **FRESH** | | | | | |
| green cooked | ½ cup | 67 | 13 | – | – |
| green raw | ½ cup | 58 | 11 | – | – |
| snap peas cooked | ½ cup | 34 | 6 | – | 2 |
| snap peas raw | ½ cup | 30 | 5 | – | 2 |
| **FROZEN** | | | | | |
| green cooked | ½ cup | 63 | 11 | – | – |
| snap peas cooked | 1 pkg (10 oz) | 132 | 23 | – | – |
| snap peas cooked | ½ cup | 42 | 7 | – | – |
| ***Birds Eye*** | | | | | |
| Butter Peas | ½ cup | 110 | 20 | 1 | 4 |
| Crowder | ½ cup | 120 | 22 | 1 | 4 |
| Field Peas w/ Snaps | ⅔ cup | 130 | 24 | 1 | 4 |
| Purple Hull Peas | ½ cup | 110 | 21 | 1 | 4 |
| ***Fresh Like*** | | | | | |
| Garden | 3.5 oz | 85 | 14 | – | 2 |
| ***La Choy*** | | | | | |
| Snow Pea Pods | ½ pkg (3 oz) | 35 | 4 | 2 | 2 |
| ***Tree Of Life*** | | | | | |
| Peas | ⅔ cup (3.1 oz) | 70 | 12 | 6 | 4 |
| **SHELF-STABLE** | | | | | |
| ***TastyBite*** | | | | | |
| Agra Peas & Greens | ½ pkg (5 oz) | 260 | 26 | 1 | 1 |
| **TAKE-OUT** | | | | | |
| pea & potato curry | 1 serv (7 oz) | 284 | 19 | – | 6 |

| FOOD | PORTION | CALS | CARB | SUGAR | FIBER |
|---|---|---|---|---|---|
| pea curry | 1 serv (4.4 oz) | 438 | 11 | – | 4 |
| **PECANS** | | | | | |
| dry roasted | 1 oz | 187 | 6 | – | – |
| dry roasted salted | 1 oz | 187 | 6 | – | – |
| halves dry roasted w/ salt | 20 (1 oz) | 200 | 4 | 1 | 3 |
| halves dried | 1 cup | 721 | 20 | – | 7 |
| oil roasted | 1 oz | 195 | 5 | – | – |
| oil roasted salted | 1 oz | 195 | 5 | – | – |
| ***Keto*** | | | | | |
| Chocolately Covered | 1 oz | 207 | 6 | 0 | 5 |
| ***Sweet Delights*** | | | | | |
| Pecan Roasters | ⅓ pkg (1 oz) | 210 | 4 | 1 | 2 |
| **PECTIN** | | | | | |
| powder | ¼ pkg (0.4 oz) | 39 | 11 | – | – |
| powder | 1 pkg (1.75 oz) | 163 | 45 | – | – |
| ***Slim Set*** | | | | | |
| Packet | 1 pkg | 208 | 44 | – | 14 |
| Powder | 1 tbsp | 3 | 1 | – | tr |
| ***Sure Jell*** | | | | | |
| For Lower Sugar Recipes | 1 tsp (2.8 g) | 20 | 4 | 4 | 0 |
| Fruit Pectin | 1 tsp (3.6 g) | 20 | 4 | 4 | 0 |
| **PEPEAO** | | | | | |
| dried | ½ cup | 36 | 10 | – | – |
| raw sliced | 1 cup | 25 | 7 | – | – |
| **PEPPER** | | | | | |
| black | 1 tsp | 5 | 1 | – | – |
| cayenne | 1 tsp | 6 | 1 | – | – |
| red | 1 tsp | 6 | 1 | – | – |
| white | 1 tsp | 7 | 2 | – | – |
| ***McCormick*** | | | | | |
| Lemon & Pepper Seasoning Salt | ¼ tsp | 0 | 0 | 0 | 0 |
| **PEPPERS** | | | | | |
| **CANNED** | | | | | |
| chili green | 1 cup (5.5 oz) | 29 | 6 | – | 2 |
| chili green hot chopped | ½ cup | 17 | 4 | – | – |
| chili red hot | 1 (2.6 oz) | 18 | 4 | – | – |

| FOOD | PORTION | CALS | CARB | SUGAR | FIBER |
|---|---|---|---|---|---|
| chili red hot chopped | ½ cup | 17 | 4 | – | – |
| green halves | ½ cup | 13 | 3 | – | – |
| jalapeno chopped | ½ cup | 17 | 3 | – | – |
| red halves | ½ cup | 13 | 3 | – | – |
| ***Old El Paso*** | | | | | |
| Green Chiles Chopped | 2 tbsp (1 oz) | 5 | 1 | 0 | 1 |
| ***Progresso*** | | | | | |
| Cherry Sliced & So Hot | 2 tbsp (1 oz) | 25 | 2 | 1 | 1 |
| Hot Cherry | 1 (1 oz) | 10 | 2 | 0 | tr |
| Pepper Salad (drained) | 2 tbsp (1 oz) | 15 | 1 | tr | tr |
| Roasted | 1 piece (1 oz) | 10 | 3 | tr | 0 |
| Sweet Fried w/ Onions | 2 tbsp (0.9 oz) | 20 | 2 | 1 | 1 |
| Tuscan | 3 (1 oz) | 10 | 2 | 0 | 1 |
| ***Rosarita*** | | | | | |
| Chilies Diced Green | 2 tbsp (1 oz) | 6 | 1 | tr | 1 |
| Chilies Green Strips | ¼ cup (1.2 oz) | 5 | 1 | 1 | 1 |
| Chilies Whole Green | 2 tbsp (1.2 oz) | 5 | 1 | 1 | 1 |
| Jalapeno Whole w/ Escabeche | ¼ cup (1.2 oz) | 8 | 1 | tr | 1 |
| Jalapenos Diced | 2 tbsp (1 oz) | 5 | 1 | tr | 1 |
| Jalapenos Nacho Sliced | 2 tbsp (1 oz) | 2 | 1 | tr | tr |
| ***Vlasic*** | | | | | |
| Hot Sliced Cherry | 1 oz | 5 | 1 | 1 | – |
| Jalapeno Sliced | 1 oz | 10 | 2 | 2 | – |
| Mild Cherry | 1 oz | 5 | 1 | 1 | – |
| Pepper Rings Hot | 1 oz | 5 | 1 | 1 | – |
| Pepper Rings Mild | 1 oz | 5 | 1 | 1 | – |
| **DRIED** | | | | | |
| ancho | 1 (0.6 oz) | 48 | 9 | – | 4 |
| green | 1 tbsp | 1 | tr | – | – |
| pasilla | 1 (7 g) | 24 | 4 | – | 2 |
| red | 1 tbsp | 1 | tr | – | – |
| **FRESH** | | | | | |
| banana | 1 cup (4.4 oz) | 33 | 7 | – | 4 |
| banana | 1 (4 in) (1.2 oz) | 9 | 2 | – | 1 |
| chili green hot | 1 | 18 | 4 | – | – |
| chili green hot chopped | ½ cup | 30 | 7 | – | – |
| chili red chopped | ½ cup | 30 | 7 | – | – |
| chili red hot | 1 (1.6 oz) | 18 | 4 | – | – |
| green | 1 (2.6 oz) | 20 | 5 | – | 1 |

| FOOD | PORTION | CALS | CARB | SUGAR | FIBER |
|---|---|---|---|---|---|
| green chopped | ½ cup | 13 | 3 | – | 1 |
| green chopped cooked | ½ cup | 19 | 5 | – | – |
| green cooked | 1 (2.6 oz) | 20 | 5 | – | – |
| habanero chile | 1 tsp | 9 | 2 | – | 1 |
| hungarian | 1 (0.9 oz) | 8 | 2 | – | 0 |
| jalapeno | 1 (0.5 oz) | 4 | 1 | – | tr |
| jalapeno sliced | 1 cup (3.2 oz) | 27 | 5 | – | 3 |
| red | 1 (2.6 oz) | 20 | 5 | – | 1 |
| red chopped | ½ cup | 13 | 3 | – | 1 |
| red chopped cooked | ½ cup | 19 | 5 | – | – |
| red cooked | 1 (2.6 oz) | 20 | 5 | – | – |
| serrano | 1 (6 g) | 2 | tr | – | tr |
| serrano chopped | 1 cup (3.7 oz) | 34 | 7 | 4 | 4 |
| yellow | 1 (6.5 oz) | 50 | 12 | – | – |
| yellow | 10 strips | 14 | 3 | – | – |
| ***Chiquita*** | | | | | |
| Pepper | 1 med (5.2 oz) | 30 | 7 | 4 | 2 |
| **FROZEN** | | | | | |
| green chopped | 1 oz | 6 | 1 | – | – |
| red chopped | 1 oz | 6 | 1 | – | – |
| ***Birds Eye*** | | | | | |
| Diced Green | ¾ cup | 20 | 4 | 3 | 2 |
| **PERCH** | | | | | |
| **FRESH** | | | | | |
| cooked | 1 fillet (1.6 oz) | 54 | 0 | 0 | 0 |
| cooked | 3 oz | 99 | 0 | 0 | 0 |
| ocean perch atlantic cooked | 3 oz | 103 | 0 | 0 | 0 |
| ocean perch atlantic cooked | 1 fillet (1.8 oz) | 60 | 0 | 0 | 0 |
| ocean perch atlantic raw | 3 oz | 80 | 0 | 0 | 0 |
| **PERSIMMONS** | | | | | |
| dried japanese | 1 | 93 | 25 | – | – |
| fresh | 1 | 32 | 8 | – | – |
| fresh japanese | 1 | 118 | 31 | – | – |
| **PHEASANT** | | | | | |
| breast w/o skin raw | ½ breast (6.4 oz) | 243 | 0 | 0 | 0 |
| leg w/o skin raw | 1 (3.6 oz) | 143 | 0 | 0 | 0 |

| FOOD | PORTION | CALS | CARB | SUGAR | FIBER |
|---|---|---|---|---|---|
| roasted | 3.5 oz | 215 | 0 | 0 | 0 |
| w/ skin raw | ½ pheasant (14 oz) | 723 | 0 | 0 | 0 |
| w/o skin raw | ½ pheasant (12.4 oz) | 470 | 0 | 0 | 0 |
| **PHYLLO** | | | | | |
| phyllo dough | 1 oz | 85 | 15 | – | – |
| sheet | 1 | 57 | 10 | – | – |
| ***Ekizian*** | | | | | |
| Sheets | ¼ lb | 433 | 76 | 2 | – |
| ***Fillo Factory*** | | | | | |
| Fillo Dough Spelt Vegan | 3 sheets (2 oz) | 180 | 31 | 0 | 4 |
| Fillo Dough Vegan | 3 sheets (2 oz) | 170 | 36 | 1 | 1 |
| Fillo Dough Whole Wheat Vegan | 3 sheets (2 oz) | 190 | 40 | 0 | 3 |
| Pastry Shells Vegan | 3 (0.4 oz) | 45 | 7 | 0 | 0 |
| **PICANTE** *(see* SALSA*)* | | | | | |
| **PICKLES** | | | | | |
| dill | 1 (2.3 oz) | 12 | 3 | – | – |
| dill low sodium | 1 (2.3 oz) | 12 | 3 | – | 1 |
| dill low sodium sliced | 1 slice | 1 | tr | – | tr |
| dill sliced | 1 slice | 1 | tr | – | tr |
| gerkins | 1 oz | 6 | 1 | – | – |
| kosher dill | 1 (2.3 oz) | 12 | 3 | – | 1 |
| polish dill | 1 (2.3 oz) | 12 | 3 | – | 1 |
| quick sour | 1 (1.2 oz) | 4 | 1 | – | – |
| quick sour low sodium | 1 (1.2 oz) | 4 | 1 | – | – |
| quick sour sliced | 1 slice | 1 | tr | – | – |
| sweet | 1 (1.2 oz) | 41 | 11 | – | tr |
| sweet gherkin | 1 sm (½ oz) | 20 | 5 | – | – |
| sweet low sodium | 1 (1.2 oz) | 41 | 11 | – | tr |
| sweet sliced | 1 slice | 7 | 2 | – | tr |
| ***Claussen*** | | | | | |
| Bread 'N Butter Chips | 4 slices (1 oz) | 20 | 4 | 3 | 0 |
| Deli Style Hearty Garlic Whole | ½ (1 oz) | 5 | 1 | tr | 0 |

| FOOD | PORTION | CALS | CARB | SUGAR | FIBER |
|---|---|---|---|---|---|
| Kosher Dill Spears | 1 spear (1.2 oz) | 5 | 1 | 0 | 0 |
| Kosher Dills Halves | 1 half (1 oz) | 5 | 1 | 0 | 0 |
| Kosher Dills Mini | 1 (0.8 oz) | 5 | 1 | 0 | 0 |
| Kosher Dills Whole | ½ (1 oz) | 5 | 1 | 0 | 0 |
| New York Deli Style Half Sours Whole | ½ (1 oz) | 5 | 1 | tr | 0 |
| Sandwich Slices Bread 'N Butter | 2 (1.2 oz) | 25 | 5 | 3 | 0 |
| Sandwich Slices Deli Style Hearty Garlic | 2 (1.2 oz) | 5 | 1 | tr | 0 |
| Sandwich Slices Kosher Dills | 2 (1.2 oz) | 5 | 1 | tr | 0 |
| Super Slices For Burgers | 1 (0.8 oz) | 5 | 1 | 0 | 0 |
| ***Mt Olive*** | | | | | |
| Bread & Butter No Sugar Added | 1 oz | 0 | tr | 0 | 0 |
| ***Vlasic*** | | | | | |
| Hamburger Dill Chips | 1 oz | 5 | 1 | 1 | – |
| Kosher Cross Cuts | 1 oz | 5 | 1 | 1 | – |
| Kosher Spears | 1 oz | 5 | 1 | 1 | – |
| Kosher Whole | 1 oz | 5 | 1 | 1 | – |
| Sweet Butter Chips | 1 oz | 30 | 7 | 7 | – |
| Sweet Gerkins | 1 oz | 35 | 9 | 9 | – |
| Whole Dills | 1 oz | 5 | 1 | 1 | – |

## PIE

### FROZEN

| FOOD | PORTION | CALS | CARB | SUGAR | FIBER |
|---|---|---|---|---|---|
| apple | ⅛ of 9 in pie (4.4 oz) | 297 | 43 | – | 2 |
| blueberry | ⅛ of 9 in pie (4.4 oz) | 289 | 44 | – | – |
| cherry | ⅛ of 9 in pie (4.4 oz) | 325 | 50 | – | 1 |
| chocolate creme | ⅙ of 8 in pie (4 oz) | 344 | 38 | – | – |
| coconut creme | ⅙ of 7 in pie (2.2 oz) | 191 | 24 | – | 1 |
| lemon meringue | ⅙ of 8 in pie (4.5 oz) | 303 | 53 | – | 1 |
| peach | ⅙ of 8 in pie (4.1 oz) | 261 | 39 | – | – |

| FOOD | PORTION | CALS | CARB | SUGAR | FIBER |
|---|---|---|---|---|---|
| ***Amy's*** | | | | | |
| Apple | 1 serv (4 oz) | 240 | 37 | 15 | 2 |
| ***Mrs. Smith's*** | | | | | |
| Apple | 1 slice (4.3 oz) | 350 | 41 | 8 | 3 |
| Blueberry | 1 slice (4.6 oz) | 330 | 43 | 16 | 3 |
| Cappuccino | 1 slice (4.2 oz) | 300 | 45 | 27 | 2 |
| Cherry | 1 slice (4.3 oz) | 320 | 41 | 7 | 2 |
| Cherry Crumb | 1 slice (4.2 oz) | 320 | 52 | 28 | 1 |
| Chocolate Cream | 1 slice (4.6 oz) | 340 | 43 | 25 | 2 |
| Chocolate Mint Cream | 1 slice (4.3 oz) | 360 | 53 | 32 | 2 |
| Coconut Custard | 1 slice (4.4 oz) | 260 | 28 | 16 | tr |
| Cookies 'N Cream | 1 slice (4.3 oz) | 360 | 52 | 32 | 2 |
| Dutch Apple | 1 slice (4.4 oz) | 330 | 50 | 25 | 2 |
| French Silk | 1 slice (4.4 oz) | 560 | 48 | 34 | 1 |
| Key West Lime | 1 slice (4.3 oz) | 430 | 62 | 49 | 1 |
| Lemon Cream | 1 slice (5 oz) | 440 | 49 | 32 | tr |
| Lemonade | 1 slice (4.3 oz) | 340 | 51 | 31 | 1 |
| Mince | 1 slice (4.6 oz) | 380 | 53 | 26 | 2 |
| Mixed Berry | 1 slice (4.2 oz) | 300 | 44 | 24 | 2 |
| Peach | 1 slice (4.6 oz) | 320 | 40 | 16 | 2 |
| Peach Lattice | 1 slice (4.2 oz) | 290 | 42 | 23 | 2 |
| Peanut Butter Silk | 1 slice (4.6 oz) | 600 | 51 | 36 | 2 |

| FOOD | PORTION | CALS | CARB | SUGAR | FIBER |
|---|---|---|---|---|---|
| Pecan | 1 slice (4.8 oz) | 560 | 75 | 33 | 2 |
| Pumpkin Custard | 1 slice (4.6 oz) | 270 | 35 | 18 | 2 |
| Raspberry | 1 slice (4.6 oz) | 330 | 44 | 18 | 1 |
| S'Mores Cream | 1 slice (4.3 oz) | 360 | 53 | 32 | 2 |
| Strawberry Banana | 1 slice (4.3 oz) | 330 | 48 | 27 | 1 |
| Sweet Potato Custard | 1 slice (4.6 oz) | 340 | 44 | 25 | 2 |
| ***Sara Lee*** | | | | | |
| Apple 45% Reduced Fat | ⅙ pie (4.5 oz) | 290 | 51 | 16 | 2 |
| Chocolate Silk | ⅕ pie (4.8 oz) | 500 | 49 | 35 | 2 |
| Coconut Cream | ⅕ pie (4.8 oz) | 480 | 47 | 35 | 2 |
| Homestyle Apple | ⅛ pie (4.6 oz) | 340 | 46 | 26 | 1 |
| Homestyle Blueberry | ⅛ pie (4.6 oz) | 360 | 54 | 26 | 2 |
| Homestyle Cherry | ⅛ pie (4.6 oz) | 320 | 42 | 27 | 2 |
| Homestyle Dutch Apple | ⅛ pie (4.6 oz) | 350 | 53 | 30 | 2 |
| Homestyle Mince | ⅛ pie (4.6 oz) | 390 | 56 | 30 | 3 |
| Homestyle Peach | ⅛ pie (4.6 oz) | 320 | 46 | 30 | 2 |
| Homestyle Pecan | ⅛ pie (4.2 oz) | 520 | 70 | 28 | 3 |
| Homestyle Pumpkin | ⅛ pie (4.6 oz) | 260 | 37 | 18 | 2 |
| Homestyle Raspberry | ⅛ pie (4.6 oz) | 380 | 48 | 20 | 2 |
| Lemon Meringue | ⅙ pie (5 oz) | 350 | 59 | 42 | 5 |
| ***Weight Watchers*** | | | | | |
| Mississippi Mud | 1 piece (2.45 oz) | 160 | 26 | 16 | 1 |
| **SNACK** | | | | | |
| apple | 1 (3 oz) | 266 | 33 | – | – |
| cherry | 1 (3 oz) | 266 | 33 | – | – |
| lemon | 1 (3 oz) | 266 | 33 | – | – |
| ***Dolly Madison*** | | | | | |
| Apple | 1 (4.5 oz) | 480 | 67 | 36 | 2 |
| Blueberry | 1 (4.5 oz) | 480 | 70 | 31 | 2 |
| Cherry | 1 (4.5 oz) | 470 | 65 | 35 | 1 |
| Chocolate Pudding | 1 (4.5 oz) | 530 | 71 | 31 | 1 |
| Lemon | 1 (4.5 oz) | 500 | 66 | 46 | 0 |
| Peach | 1 (4.5 oz) | 480 | 66 | 30 | 1 |

| FOOD | PORTION | CALS | CARB | SUGAR | FIBER |
|---|---|---|---|---|---|
| Pecan | 1 (3 oz) | 360 | 44 | 19 | 1 |
| Pecan Fried | 1 (4.5 oz) | 530 | 80 | 32 | 1 |
| Pineapple | 1 (4.5 oz) | 460 | 62 | 29 | 1 |
| ***Hostess*** | | | | | |
| Apple | 1 (4.5 oz) | 480 | 67 | 36 | 2 |
| Blackberry | 1 (4.5 oz) | 520 | 79 | 29 | 2 |
| Blueberry | 1 (4.5 oz) | 480 | 70 | 31 | 2 |
| Cherry | 1 (4.5 oz) | 470 | 65 | 35 | 1 |
| French Apple | 1 (4.5 oz) | 480 | 67 | 36 | 2 |
| Lemon | 1 (4.5 oz) | 500 | 66 | 46 | 0 |
| Peach | 1 (4.5 oz) | 480 | 68 | 30 | 1 |
| Pineapple | 1 (4.5 oz) | 460 | 62 | 29 | 1 |
| Strawberry | 1 (4.5 oz) | 510 | 71 | 35 | 2 |
| ***Lance*** | | | | | |
| Pecan | 1 (3 oz) | 350 | 46 | 35 | 3 |
| ***Tastykake*** | | | | | |
| Apple | 1 (4 oz) | 270 | 41 | 20 | 1 |
| Blueberry | 1 (4 oz) | 300 | 49 | 23 | 1 |
| Cherry | 1 (4 oz) | 290 | 46 | 16 | tr |
| Coconut Creme | 1 (4 oz) | 370 | 42 | 21 | 1 |
| French Apple | 1 (4.2 oz) | 310 | 52 | 30 | 1 |
| Lemon | 1 (4 oz) | 300 | 44 | 24 | tr |
| Peach | 1 (4 oz) | 280 | 43 | 21 | 1 |
| Pineapple | 1 (4 oz) | 290 | 45 | 24 | 1 |
| Pineapple Cheese | 1 (4 oz) | 320 | 50 | 26 | 1 |
| Pumpkin | 1 (4 oz) | 340 | 47 | 22 | 1 |
| Strawberry | 1 (3.5 oz) | 320 | 51 | 29 | 1 |
| Tastyklair | 1 (4 oz) | 400 | 50 | 26 | 0 |
| ***Tom's*** | | | | | |
| Apple | 1 pkg (3 oz) | 330 | 42 | 21 | 1 |
| Banana Marshmallow | 1 pkg (2.75 oz) | 320 | 54 | 33 | 0 |
| Cherry | 1 pkg (3 oz) | 320 | 37 | 24 | 1 |
| Chocolate Marshmallow | 1 pkg (2.75 oz) | 320 | 53 | 32 | tr |
| **TAKE-OUT** | | | | | |
| apple | ⅛ of 9 in pie (5.4 oz) | 411 | 58 | – | 3 |
| banana cream | ⅛ of 9 in pie (5.2 oz) | 398 | 49 | – | – |

| FOOD | PORTION | CALS | CARB | SUGAR | FIBER |
|---|---|---|---|---|---|
| blueberry | ⅛ of 9 in pie (5.2 oz) | 360 | 49 | – | – |
| butterscotch | ⅛ of 9 in pie (4.5 oz) | 355 | 42 | – | – |
| cherry | ⅛ of 9 in pie (6.3 oz) | 486 | 69 | – | – |
| coconut creme | ⅛ of 9 in pie (4.7 oz) | 396 | 46 | – | – |
| coconut custard | ⅙ of 8 in pie (3.6 oz) | 271 | 32 | – | – |
| custard | ⅛ of 9 in pie (4.5 oz) | 262 | 34 | – | 2 |
| lemon meringue | ⅛ of 9 in pie (4.5 oz) | 362 | 50 | – | 2 |
| mince | ⅛ of 9 in pie (5.8 oz) | 477 | 79 | – | – |
| pecan | ⅙ of 8 in pie (4 oz) | 452 | 65 | – | 4 |
| pumpkin | ⅙ of 8 in pie (3.8 oz) | 229 | 30 | – | 3 |
| vanilla cream | ⅛ of 9 in pie (4.4 oz) | 350 | 41 | – | – |
| **PIE CRUST** | | | | | |
| **FROZEN** | | | | | |
| baked | ⅛ of 9 in pie (0.6 oz) | 82 | 8 | – | – |
| baked | 9 in shell (4.4 oz) | 647 | 63 | – | – |
| puff pastry baked | 1 shell (1.4 oz) | 223 | 18 | – | – |
| ***Pepperidge Farm*** | | | | | |
| Puff Pastry Sheets | ⅙ sheet (1.4 oz) | 170 | 14 | 1 | 0 |
| Puff Pastry Shell | 1 (1.6 oz) | 190 | 16 | 2 | 0 |
| Puff Pastry Squares | 1 sq (2 oz) | 240 | 19 | 2 | 0 |
| ***Pet-Ritz*** | | | | | |
| Deep Dish | ⅛ pie (0.7 oz) | 90 | 10 | 0 | 0 |
| Regular | ⅛ pie (0.7 oz) | 80 | 9 | tr | 0 |
| Tart Shells | 1 (1 oz) | 130 | 13 | 0 | 0 |

| FOOD | PORTION | CALS | CARB | SUGAR | FIBER |
|---|---|---|---|---|---|
| **MIX** | | | | | |
| as prep | 9 in crust (5.6 oz) | 801 | 81 | – | – |
| as prep | ⅛ of 9 in pie (0.7 oz) | 100 | 10 | – | – |
| ***Betty Crocker*** | | | | | |
| Pie Crust as prep | ⅛ crust | 110 | 9 | – | – |
| ***MiniCarb*** | | | | | |
| Pie Crust Mix | 1 slice | 105 | 1 | 0 | 0 |
| **READY-TO-EAT** | | | | | |
| chocolate cookie crumb | ⅛ of 9 in pie (1 oz) | 139 | 15 | – | – |
| chocolate cookie crumb | 9 in crust (7.7 oz) | 1130 | 122 | – | – |
| graham cracker | 9 in crust (8.4 oz) | 1181 | 156 | – | – |
| graham cracker | ⅛ of 9 in pie (1 oz) | 148 | 20 | – | – |
| vanilla wafer cracker crumbs | 9 in crust (6.1 oz) | 937 | 89 | – | – |
| vanilla wafer cracker crumbs | ⅛ of 9 in pie (0.8 oz) | 119 | 11 | – | – |
| ***Keebler*** | | | | | |
| Graham Single Serve | 1 (0.8 oz) | 120 | 15 | 6 | tr |
| Reduced Fat Graham | ⅛ pie (0.7 oz) | 90 | 14 | 6 | 0 |
| **REFRIGERATED** | | | | | |
| ***All Ready*** | | | | | |
| Crust | ⅛ pie (0.9 oz) | 120 | 13 | tr | 0 |

## PIE FILLING

| FOOD | PORTION | CALS | CARB | SUGAR | FIBER |
|---|---|---|---|---|---|
| apple | 1 can (21 oz) | 599 | 156 | 143 | 6 |
| apple | ⅛ can (2.6 oz) | 74 | 19 | 18 | 1 |
| cherry | 1 can (21 oz) | 683 | 175 | – | – |
| cherry | ⅛ can (2.6 oz) | 85 | 22 | – | – |
| pumpkin pie mix | 1 cup | 282 | 71 | – | – |
| ***Colac*** | | | | | |
| All Flavors | 1 tbsp | 19 | 7 | 0 | 0 |
| ***Comstock*** | | | | | |
| MoreFruit Light Cherry | ⅓ cup (2.9 oz) | 60 | 13 | 11 | 0 |
| Red Ruby Cherry | ⅓ cup (3.1 oz) | 90 | 23 | 19 | 1 |

| FOOD | PORTION | CALS | CARB | SUGAR | FIBER |
|---|---|---|---|---|---|
| ***Libby*** | | | | | |
| Pumpkin Pie Mix | ⅓ cup | 90 | 20 | 17 | 2 |
| ***Smucker's*** | | | | | |
| Pie Glaze Strawberry | 2 oz | 80 | 21 | 20 | – |
| **PIEROGI** | | | | | |
| pierogi | ¾ cup (4.4 oz) | 307 | 24 | – | – |
| ***Health Is Wealth*** | | | | | |
| Potato & Cheddar | 2 (2.8 oz) | 140 | 27 | 1 | 3 |
| Potato & Onion | 2 (2.8 oz) | 140 | 27 | 1 | 3 |
| ***Mrs. T's*** | | | | | |
| Broccoli & Cheddar | 3 (4.2 oz) | 200 | 34 | 2 | 2 |
| Jalapeno & Cheddar | 3 (4.2 oz) | 190 | 34 | 2 | 2 |
| Potato & American Cheese | 3 (4.2 oz) | 220 | 39 | 1 | 2 |
| Potato & Roasted Garlic | 3 (4.2 oz) | 190 | 36 | 2 | 2 |
| Potato & Cheddar | 3 (4.2 oz) | 190 | 35 | 1 | 2 |
| Potato & Onion | 3 (4.2 oz) | 180 | 34 | 1 | 2 |
| Rogies Cheddar & Bacon | 7 (3 oz) | 140 | 24 | 1 | 1 |
| Rogies Jalapeno & Cheddar | 7 (3 oz) | 120 | 23 | 1 | 1 |
| Rogies Potato & Cheddar | 7 (3 oz) | 130 | 24 | 1 | 1 |
| **PIG'S EARS AND FEET** | | | | | |
| ear simmered | 1 | 184 | tr | – | 0 |
| feet pickled | 1 lb | 921 | tr | – | 0 |
| feet pickled | 1 oz | 58 | tr | – | 0 |
| feet simmered | 3 oz | 165 | 0 | 0 | 0 |
| **PIGEON** | | | | | |
| w/ skin & bone | 3.5 oz | 169 | 0 | 0 | 0 |
| **PIGEON PEAS** | | | | | |
| dried cooked | ½ cup | 102 | 20 | – | – |
| dried cooked | 1 cup | 204 | 39 | – | – |
| **PIGNOLIA** *(see* PINE NUTS*)* | | | | | |
| **PIKE** | | | | | |
| northern cooked | 3 oz | 96 | 0 | 0 | 0 |
| northern cooked | ½ fillet (5.4 oz) | 176 | 0 | 0 | 0 |
| northern raw | 3 oz | 75 | 0 | 0 | 0 |
| roe raw | 1 oz | 37 | tr | – | – |
| walleye baked | 3 oz | 101 | 0 | 0 | 0 |

| FOOD | PORTION | CALS | CARB | SUGAR | FIBER |
|---|---|---|---|---|---|
| walleye fillet baked | 4.4 oz | 147 | 0 | 0 | 0 |
| **PILLNUTS** | | | | | |
| canarytree dried | 1 oz | 204 | 1 | – | – |
| **PIMIENTOS** | | | | | |
| canned | 1 slice | 0 | tr | – | – |
| canned | 1 tbsp | 3 | 1 | – | – |
| ***Dromedary*** | | | | | |
| Peeled | ½ tsp (4 g) | 0 | 0 | 0 | 0 |
| Unpeeled | ½ tsp (4 g) | 0 | 0 | 0 | 0 |
| **PINE NUTS** | | | | | |
| pignolia dried | 1 oz | 146 | 4 | – | – |
| pignolia dried | 1 tbsp | 51 | 1 | – | – |
| pinyon dried | 1 oz | 161 | 5 | – | – |
| ***Progresso*** | | | | | |
| Pignoli | 1 jar (1 oz) | 170 | 2 | 0 | 0 |
| **PINEAPPLE** | | | | | |
| **CANNED** | | | | | |
| chunks in heavy syrup | 1 cup | 199 | 52 | – | – |
| chunks juice pack | 1 cup | 150 | 39 | – | – |
| crushed in heavy syrup | 1 cup | 199 | 52 | – | – |
| slices in heavy syrup | 1 slice | 45 | 12 | – | – |
| slices in light syrup | 1 slice | 30 | 8 | – | – |
| slices juice pack | 1 slice | 35 | 9 | – | – |
| slices water pack | 1 slice | 19 | 5 | – | – |
| tidbits in heavy syrup | 1 cup | 199 | 52 | – | – |
| tidbits in juice | 1 cup | 150 | 19 | – | – |
| tidbits in water | 1 cup | 79 | 20 | – | – |
| ***Del Monte*** | | | | | |
| Chunks In Heavy Syrup | ½ cup (4.3 oz) | 90 | 24 | 22 | 1 |
| Chunks In Its Own Juice | ½ cup (4.3 oz) | 70 | 17 | 15 | 1 |
| Crushed In Heavy Syrup | ½ cup (4.3 oz) | 90 | 24 | 22 | 1 |
| Crushed In Its Own Juice | ½ cup (4.3 oz) | 70 | 17 | 15 | 1 |
| Fruit Cup Tidbits | 1 pkg (4 oz) | 50 | 15 | 13 | 1 |
| Sliced In Heavy Syrup | 2 slices (4.1 oz) | 90 | 23 | 21 | 1 |
| Sliced In Its Own Juice | ½ cup (4 oz) | 60 | 16 | 14 | 1 |
| Spears In Its Own Juice | ½ cup (4.3 oz) | 70 | 17 | 15 | 1 |
| Tidbits In Its Own Juice | ½ cup (4.3 oz) | 70 | 17 | 15 | 1 |

| FOOD | PORTION | CALS | CARB | SUGAR | FIBER |
|---|---|---|---|---|---|
| Wedges In Its Own Juice | ½ cup (4.3 oz) | 70 | 17 | 15 | 1 |
| ***Dole*** | | | | | |
| All Natural Chunks | ½ cup | 60 | 16 | 13 | tr |
| Chunks Juice Pack | ½ cup | 60 | 15 | 13 | 1 |
| ***SunFresh*** | | | | | |
| In Lightly Sweetened Juice | ½ cup | 70 | 18 | 15 | tr |
| **FRESH** | | | | | |
| diced | 1 cup | 77 | 19 | – | 2 |
| slice | 1 slice | 42 | 10 | – | 1 |
| ***Bonita Hill*** | | | | | |
| Golden Extra Sweet | 2 slices (3.9 oz) | 60 | 16 | 13 | 1 |
| ***Frosty Fresh*** | | | | | |
| Peeled & Cored | ½ cup | 60 | 14 | 13 | 1 |
| **FROZEN** | | | | | |
| chunks sweetened | ½ cup | 104 | 27 | – | – |
| **PINEAPPLE JUICE** | | | | | |
| canned | 1 cup | 139 | 34 | – | – |
| frzn as prep | 1 cup | 129 | 32 | – | – |
| frzn not prep | 6 oz | 387 | 96 | – | – |
| ***Del Monte*** | | | | | |
| Juice | 6 fl oz | 80 | 20 | 17 | 0 |
| ***Dole*** | | | | | |
| Chilled | 8 oz | 130 | 30 | – | – |
| **PINK BEANS** | | | | | |
| dried cooked | 1 cup | 252 | 47 | – | – |
| **PINTO BEANS** | | | | | |
| **CANNED** | | | | | |
| pinto | 1 cup | 186 | 35 | – | – |
| ***Eden*** | | | | | |
| Organic Spicy | ½ cup (4.6 oz) | 125 | 24 | 7 | 2 |
| ***Progresso*** | | | | | |
| Pinto Beans | ½ cup (4.6 oz) | 110 | 18 | tr | 7 |
| **DRIED** | | | | | |
| cooked | 1 cup | 235 | 44 | – | – |
| **FROZEN** | | | | | |
| cooked | 3 oz | 152 | 29 | – | – |

| FOOD | PORTION | CALS | CARB | SUGAR | FIBER |
|---|---|---|---|---|---|
| **PISTACHIOS** | | | | | |
| dried | 1 cup | 739 | 32 | – | 14 |
| dry roasted | 1 oz | 172 | 8 | – | – |
| dry roasted salted | 1 oz | 172 | 8 | – | – |
| dry roasted salted | 1 cup | 776 | 35 | – | – |
| dry roasted w/ salt | 47 nuts (1 oz) | 160 | 8 | 2 | 3 |
| with shells dry roasted unsalted | ½ cup | 180 | 9 | 3 | 3 |
| ***Lance*** | | | | | |
| Pistachios | 1 pkg (1⅛ oz) | 90 | 4 | 0 | 2 |
| ***Sweet Delights*** | | | | | |
| Pistachio Roasters | ⅓ pkg (1 oz) | 190 | 9 | 3 | 3 |
| **PITANGA** | | | | | |
| fresh | 1 | 2 | 1 | – | – |
| fresh | 1 cup | 57 | 13 | – | – |
| **PIZZA** *(see also* PIZZA DOUGH, PIZZA SAUCE*)* | | | | | |
| ***Amy's*** | | | | | |
| Cheese | ⅓ pie | 300 | 38 | 4 | 2 |
| Mushroom & Olive | ⅓ pie | 250 | 33 | 3 | 2 |
| Pesto | ⅓ pie | 310 | 39 | 3 | 2 |
| Pocket Sandwich Cheese Pizza | 1 (4.5 oz) | 300 | 42 | 5 | 4 |
| Pocket Sandwich Vegetarian Pizza | 1 (4.5 oz) | 250 | 39 | 4 | 4 |
| Roasted Vegetable | ⅓ pie | 260 | 42 | 5 | 2 |
| Snacks Cheese | 5-6 pieces | 180 | 22 | 3 | 2 |
| Soy Cheese | ⅓ pie | 290 | 37 | 3 | 2 |
| Spinach | ⅓ pie | 300 | 38 | 4 | 2 |
| Veggie Combo | ⅓ pie | 280 | 36 | 4 | 2 |
| ***Appian Way*** | | | | | |
| Pizza Mix Thick Crust | ⅓ pie (4.2 oz) | 290 | 51 | 4 | 2 |
| Pizza Mix Thin Crust | ⅓ pie (4.1 oz) | 250 | 48 | 4 | 2 |
| ***Banquet*** | | | | | |
| Pepperoni | 1 pie (6.75 oz) | 490 | 56 | 30 | 5 |
| Pizza Snack Cheese | 6 pieces (7.5 oz) | 200 | 24 | 4 | 2 |
| Pizza Snack Pepperoni | 6 pieces (7.5 oz) | 230 | 23 | 4 | 2 |
| Pizza Snack Pepperoni & Sausage | 6 pieces (7.5 oz) | 210 | 24 | 4 | 2 |

| FOOD | PORTION | CALS | CARB | SUGAR | FIBER |
|---|---|---|---|---|---|
| ***Health Is Wealth*** | | | | | |
| Pizza Munchees | 6 (3 oz) | 190 | 9 | 0 | 1 |
| ***Healthy Choice*** | | | | | |
| French Bread Cheese | 1 piece (6 oz) | 340 | 51 | 9 | 5 |
| French Bread Pepperoni | 1 piece (6 oz) | 340 | 49 | 6 | 6 |
| French Bread Sausage | 1 piece (6 oz) | 320 | 48 | 9 | 5 |
| French Bread Supreme | 1 piece (6.35 oz) | 330 | 51 | 7 | 6 |
| French Bread Vegetable | 1 piece (6 oz) | 280 | 44 | 8 | 5 |
| ***Kid Cuisine*** | | | | | |
| Backpacking Pizza Snack | 6 pieces | 230 | 23 | 4 | 1 |
| Big League Hamburger | 1 meal (8.3 oz) | 400 | 61 | 32 | 5 |
| Fire Chief Cheese | 1 pie (5.2 oz) | 340 | 44 | 7 | 2 |
| Pirate Pizza w/ Cheese | 1 meal (8 oz) | 430 | 71 | 34 | 5 |
| Poolside Pepperoni | 1 (5.2 oz) | 380 | 44 | 7 | 2 |
| ***Lean Cuisine*** | | | | | |
| Everyday Favorites French Bread Cheese | 1 pkg (6 oz) | 320 | 48 | 6 | 4 |
| Everyday Favorites French Bread Deluxe | 1 pkg (6.1 oz) | 290 | 43 | 5 | 3 |
| Everyday Favorites French Bread Pepperoni | 1 pkg (5.25 oz) | 300 | 43 | 6 | 3 |
| Everyday Favorites French Bread Sun Dried Tomatoes | 1 serv (6 oz) | 340 | 48 | 8 | 3 |
| ***Marie Callender's*** | | | | | |
| French Bread Cheese | 1 (7.2 oz) | 530 | 50 | 5 | 4 |
| French Bread Pepperoni | 1 (7.5 oz) | 570 | 50 | 5 | 4 |
| French Bread Supreme | 1 (7.5 oz) | 510 | 50 | 5 | 4 |
| ***Pepperidge Farm*** | | | | | |
| Gourmet Crust Cheese | 1 (4.4 oz) | 390 | 39 | 11 | 6 |
| Gourmet Crust Pepperoni | 1 (4.5 oz) | 420 | 39 | 8 | 5 |
| ***Weight Watchers*** | | | | | |
| Smart Ones Deluxe Combo | 1 (6.75 oz) | 380 | 47 | 3 | 6 |
| Smart Ones Pepperoni | 1 (5.56 oz) | 390 | 46 | 3 | 4 |
| **TAKE-OUT** | | | | | |
| cheese | 12 in pie | 1121 | 164 | – | – |
| cheese | ⅛ of 12 in pie | 140 | 21 | – | – |
| cheese deep dish individual | 1 (5.5 oz) | 460 | 47 | 4 | 2 |
| cheese meat & vegetables | ⅛ of 12 in pie | 184 | 21 | – | – |

| FOOD | PORTION | CALS | CARB | SUGAR | FIBER |
|---|---|---|---|---|---|
| cheese meat & vegetables | 12 in pie | 1472 | 170 | – | – |
| pepperoni | 12 in pie | 1445 | 157 | – | – |
| pepperoni | ⅛ of 12 in pie | 181 | 20 | – | – |
| **PIZZA DOUGH** | | | | | |
| crust | 1 slice (1.7 oz) | 130 | 25 | 1 | 1 |
| ***Betty Crocker*** | | | | | |
| Italian Herb Crust Mix | ¼ crust (1.6 oz) | 180 | 32 | 1 | 1 |
| ***Boboli*** | | | | | |
| Thin Crust | ⅕ crust (2 oz) | 160 | 24 | 1 | 1 |
| ***Carbsense*** | | | | | |
| Garlic & Herb as prep | 1 slice | 100 | 7 | 0 | 4 |
| ***Keto*** | | | | | |
| Dough Mix as prep | 1 slice | 79 | 5 | tr | 3 |
| ***MiniCarb*** | | | | | |
| Parmesan Herb Mix as prep | 1 slice | 130 | 6 | 0 | 3 |
| ***Pillsbury*** | | | | | |
| Crust | ⅕ crust (2 oz) | 150 | 27 | 3 | tr |
| ***Robin Hood*** | | | | | |
| Crust | ¼ crust | 160 | 33 | 1 | 1 |
| **PIZZA SAUCE** | | | | | |
| ***Hunt's*** | | | | | |
| Fully Prepared | ¼ cup (2.2 oz) | 21 | 4 | 3 | 2 |
| Pizza Sauce | ¼ cup (2.2 oz) | 27 | 5 | 2 | 2 |
| Prima Choice Supper Heavy | ¼ cup (2.2 oz) | 28 | 6 | 3 | 3 |
| ***Muir Glen*** | | | | | |
| Organic | ¼ cup (2.2 oz) | 40 | 6 | 3 | 2 |
| ***Progresso*** | | | | | |
| Pizza Sauce | ¼ cup (2.1 oz) | 20 | 4 | 2 | 1 |
| **PLANTAINS** | | | | | |
| fresh uncooked | 1 (6.3 oz) | 218 | 57 | – | – |
| sliced cooked | ½ cup | 89 | 24 | – | – |
| **TAKE-OUT** | | | | | |
| ripe fried | 2.8 oz | 214 | 38 | – | 4 |
| **PLUMS** | | | | | |
| **CANNED** | | | | | |
| purple in heavy syrup | 3 | 119 | 31 | – | – |
| purple in heavy syrup | 1 cup | 320 | 60 | – | – |

| FOOD | PORTION | CALS | CARB | SUGAR | FIBER |
|---|---|---|---|---|---|
| purple in light syrup | 1 cup | 158 | 41 | – | – |
| purple in light syrup | 3 | 83 | 22 | – | – |
| purple juice pack | 3 | 55 | 14 | – | – |
| purple juice pack | 1 cup | 146 | 38 | – | – |
| purple water pack | 1 cup | 102 | 27 | – | – |
| purple water pack | 3 | 39 | 10 | – | – |
| ***Eden*** | | | | | |
| Umeboshi Paste | 1 tsp | 5 | 1 | 0 | 0 |
| Umeboshi Plums | 1 | 5 | 1 | 0 | 0 |
| **FRESH** | | | | | |
| plum | 1 | 36 | 9 | – | – |
| sliced | 1 cup | 91 | 21 | – | – |
| ***Chiquita*** | | | | | |
| Purple | 2 med (4.6 oz) | 80 | 19 | 10 | 2 |
| **POI** | | | | | |
| poi | ½ cup | 134 | 33 | – | – |
| **POKEBERRY SHOOTS** | | | | | |
| cooked | ½ cup | 16 | 3 | – | – |
| fresh | ½ cup | 18 | 3 | – | – |
| **POLENTA** | | | | | |
| ***Frieda's*** | | | | | |
| Dried Tomato | 4 oz | 80 | 17 | 1 | 2 |
| Italian Herb | 4 oz | 80 | 17 | 0 | 2 |
| Mexicana | 4 oz | 80 | 17 | 0 | 2 |
| Original | 4 oz | 80 | 16 | 0 | 2 |
| Wild Mushroom | 4 oz | 80 | 17 | 0 | 2 |
| ***Melissa's*** | | | | | |
| Original | 4 oz | 80 | 16 | 0 | 2 |
| **POLLACK** | | | | | |
| altantic fillet baked | 5.3 oz | 178 | 0 | 0 | 0 |
| atlantic baked | 3 oz | 100 | 0 | 0 | 0 |
| **POMEGRANATE** | | | | | |
| fresh | 1 | 104 | 26 | – | – |
| **POMEGRANATE JUICE** | | | | | |
| ***POM Wonderful*** | | | | | |
| Pomegranate Blueberry | 8 oz | 140 | 34 | 28 | 0 |

| FOOD | PORTION | CALS | CARB | SUGAR | FIBER |
|---|---|---|---|---|---|
| ***POM Wonderful*** | | | | | |
| Pomegranate Cherry | 8 oz | 140 | 33 | 28 | 0 |
| Pomegranate Tangerine | 8 oz | 150 | 37 | 31 | 0 |
| **POMPANO** | | | | | |
| florida cooked | 3 oz | 179 | 0 | 0 | 0 |
| florida raw | 3 oz | 140 | 0 | 0 | 0 |
| **POPCORN** *(see also* POPCORN CAKES*)* | | | | | |
| air-popped | 1 cup (0.3 oz) | 31 | 6 | – | 2 |
| caramel coated | 1 cup (1.2 oz) | 152 | 28 | 14 | 2 |
| carmel coated w/ peanuts | ⅔ cup (1 oz) | 114 | 23 | 11 | 1 |
| cheese | 1 cup (0.4 oz) | 58 | 6 | – | 1 |
| oil popped | 1 cup (0.4 oz) | 55 | 6 | tr | 1 |
| ***Chester's*** | | | | | |
| Butter | 3 cups | 160 | 15 | 0 | 2 |
| Caramel Craze | ¾ cup | 130 | 27 | 18 | 1 |
| Cheddar Cheese | 3 cups | 190 | 17 | 2 | 3 |
| Microwave Butter | 5 cups | 200 | 22 | tr | 4 |
| ***Cracker Jack*** | | | | | |
| Fat Free Butter Toffee | ¾ cup | 110 | 26 | 17 | 1 |
| Fat Free Caramel | ¾ cup | 110 | 26 | 17 | 1 |
| Original | ½ cup (1 oz) | 120 | 23 | 15 | 1 |
| ***Estee*** | | | | | |
| Caramel | 1 cup | 120 | 26 | 1 | 1 |
| ***Husman's*** | | | | | |
| Cheese Corn | 2¼ cups (1 oz) | 160 | 15 | 0 | 1 |
| ***Jolly Time*** | | | | | |
| America's Best 94% Fat Free | 1 cup | 20 | 5 | 0 | 1 |
| Blast O Butter | 1 cup | 45 | 5 | 0 | 1 |
| Blast O Butter Light | 1 cup | 30 | 4 | 0 | 1 |
| Butter Licious | 1 cup | 35 | 4 | 0 | 1 |
| Butter Licious Light | 1 cup | 30 | 4 | 0 | tr |
| Crispy & White | 1 cup | 40 | 4 | 0 | 1 |
| Crispy & White Light | 1 cup | 25 | 4 | 0 | 1 |
| Healthy Pop 94% Fat Free | 1 cup | 20 | 5 | 0 | 1 |
| White Air Popped | 5 cups | 100 | 24 | 0 | 6 |
| Yellow Air Popped | 5 cups | 100 | 24 | tr | 6 |

| FOOD | PORTION | CALS | CARB | SUGAR | FIBER |
|---|---|---|---|---|---|
| ***Judy's*** | | | | | |
| Sugar Free Popcorn Nut Brittle | ¼ piece (1 oz) | 100 | 3 | 0 | tr |
| ***Lance*** | | | | | |
| Cheese | 1 pkg (0.6 oz) | 90 | 9 | 0 | 2 |
| Plain | 1 pkg (0.5 oz) | 70 | 10 | 0 | 1 |
| White Cheddar | 1 pkg (0.6 oz) | 100 | 7 | 1 | 1 |
| White Cheddar | 1 pkg (0.9 oz) | 150 | 10 | 1 | 1 |
| ***Orville Redenbacher's*** | | | | | |
| Gourmet Original | 3 cups | 92 | 22 | 0 | 5 |
| Hot Air | 3 cups | 92 | 22 | 0 | 5 |
| Microwave Butter | 3 cups | 168 | 15 | 0 | 4 |
| Microwave Butter No Salt Added | 3 cups | 176 | 19 | 0 | 4 |
| Microwave Butter Light | 3 cups | 122 | 20 | 0 | 5 |
| Microwave Caramel | 1 serv | 179 | 23 | 12 | 3 |
| Microwave Golden Cheddar | 1 serv | 169 | 15 | 0 | 3 |
| Microwave Natural | 3 cups | 164 | 18 | 0 | 4 |
| Microwave Natural No Salt Added | 3 cups | 174 | 19 | 0 | 5 |
| Microwave Natural Light | 3 cups | 118 | 19 | 0 | 5 |
| Microwave Smartpop | 1 serv | 96 | 20 | 0 | 5 |
| Microwave Smartpop Butter Snack Size | 1 bag | 155 | 34 | 6 | 0 |
| Microwave Snack Size Butter | 1 bag | 287 | 25 | 0 | 6 |
| Microwave Snack Size Butter Light | 1 bag | 183 | 30 | 0 | 7 |
| Microwave White Cheddar | 1 serv | 169 | 15 | 0 | 3 |
| Redenbudders Microwave Herb & Garlic | 1 serv | 176 | 16 | 0 | 4 |
| Redenbudders Microwave Zesty Butter | 1 serv | 177 | 16 | 0 | 4 |
| Redenbudders Movie Theater Butter Light | 1 serv | 113 | 20 | 0 | 5 |
| Redenbudders Movie Theater Microwave Butter | 1 serv | 176 | 16 | 0 | 4 |
| Smart Pop Movie Theater Butter | 1 serv | 92 | 20 | 0 | 5 |
| White | 3 cups | 92 | 22 | 0 | 5 |
| ***Pop Secret*** | | | | | |
| 94% Fat Free Butter | 1 cup (5 g) | 20 | 4 | 0 | tr |

| FOOD | PORTION | CALS | CARB | SUGAR | FIBER |
|---|---|---|---|---|---|
| 94% Fat Free Natural | 1 cup (5 g) | 20 | 4 | 0 | tr |
| Butter | 1 cup (7 g) | 35 | 4 | 0 | tr |
| Cheddar Cheese | 1 cup (6 g) | 30 | 3 | 0 | tr |
| Jumbo Pop Butter | 1 cup (7 g) | 40 | 4 | 0 | tr |
| Jumbo Pop Movie Theater Butter | 1 cup (7 g) | 40 | 4 | 0 | tr |
| Light Butter | 1 cup (5 g) | 20 | 4 | 0 | tr |
| Light Movie Theater Butter | 1 cup (5 g) | 25 | 4 | 0 | tr |
| Light Natural | 1 cup (5 g) | 25 | 4 | 0 | tr |
| Movie Theater Butter | 1 cup (7 g) | 40 | 3 | 0 | tr |
| Nacho Cheese | 1 cup (6 g) | 30 | 3 | 0 | tr |
| Natural | 1 cup (7 g) | 35 | 4 | 0 | tr |
| Real Butter | 1 cup (7 g) | 35 | 4 | 0 | tr |
| ***Smartfood*** | | | | | |
| Butter | 3 cups | 150 | 15 | 2 | 1 |
| Low Fat Toffee Crunch | ¾ cup | 110 | 25 | 19 | 1 |
| Reduced Fat Golden Butter | 3⅓ cups | 130 | 21 | 0 | 4 |
| Reduced Fat White Cheddar | 3 cups | 140 | 19 | 1 | 3 |
| White Cheddar | 2 cups | 190 | 17 | 5 | 2 |
| ***Snyder's Of Hanover*** | | | | | |
| Butter | ⅝ oz | 110 | 6 | 0 | 0 |
| ***Tom's*** | | | | | |
| Caramel Corn | 1 pkg (1.6 oz) | 180 | 39 | 23 | 2 |
| ***Utz*** | | | | | |
| Au Natural | 3 cups (1 oz) | 120 | 25 | 0 | 5 |
| Butter | 2 cups (1 oz) | 170 | 13 | tr | 3 |
| Cheese | 2 cups (1 oz) | 150 | 14 | 1 | 3 |
| Hulless Puff'N Corn | 2 cups (1 oz) | 180 | 11 | 0 | 0 |
| Hulless Puff'N Corn Hot Cheese | 1 pkg (1.75 oz) | 290 | 21 | 3 | 0 |
| Hulless Pull'N Corn Cheese | 2 cups (1 oz) | 170 | 13 | 0 | 0 |
| White Cheddar | 2 cups (1 oz) | 150 | 15 | 3 | 3 |
| ***Weight Watchers*** | | | | | |
| Butter | 1 pkg (0.66 oz) | 90 | 14 | 0 | 3 |
| Butter Toffee | 1 pkg (0.9 oz) | 110 | 21 | 11 | 1 |
| Caramel | 1 pkg (0.9 oz) | 100 | 22 | 11 | 1 |
| Microwave | 1 pkg (1 oz) | 100 | 20 | 0 | 7 |
| White Cheddar Cheese | 1 pkg (0.66 oz) | 90 | 12 | 0 | 2 |

| FOOD | PORTION | CALS | CARB | SUGAR | FIBER |
|---|---|---|---|---|---|
| **POPCORN CAKES** | | | | | |
| ***Orville Redenbacher's*** | | | | | |
| BBQ Mini | 8 (0.5 oz) | 55 | 12 | 1 | 1 |
| Butter | 2 (0.6 oz) | 134 | 13 | 1 | 2 |
| Butter Mini | 8 (0.5 oz) | 56 | 11 | tr | 1 |
| Caramel | 1 (0.4 oz) | 34 | 8 | 2 | 1 |
| Caramel Mini | 7 (0.5 oz) | 50 | 12 | 3 | 1 |
| Nacho Cheese Mini | 8 (0.5 oz) | 56 | 11 | tr | 1 |
| Peanut Crunch Mini | 7 (0.5 oz) | 55 | 11 | 3 | 1 |
| White Cheddar | 2 (0.6 oz) | 63 | 13 | tr | 2 |
| White Cheddar Mini | 8 (0.5 oz) | 56 | 12 | tr | 1 |
| **POPOVER** | | | | | |
| home recipe as prep w/ 2% milk | 1 (1.4 oz) | 87 | 11 | – | – |
| home recipe as prep w/ whole milk | 1 (1.4 oz) | 90 | 11 | – | – |
| mix as prep | 1 (1.2 oz) | 67 | 10 | – | – |
| **POPPY SEEDS** | | | | | |
| poppy seeds | 1 tsp | 15 | 1 | – | – |
| **PORGY** | | | | | |
| fresh | 3 oz | 77 | 0 | 0 | 0 |
| **PORK** *(see also* HAM, PORK DISHES*)* | | | | | |
| **FRESH** | | | | | |
| boston blade roast lean & fat cooked | 3 oz | 229 | 0 | 0 | 0 |
| boston blade steak lean & fat cooked | 3 oz | 220 | 0 | 0 | 0 |
| center loin roast lean bone in cooked | 3 oz | 169 | 0 | 0 | 0 |
| center loin chop lean bone in cooked | 3 oz | 172 | 0 | 0 | 0 |
| center rib chop lean & fat bone in cooked | 3 oz | 213 | 0 | 0 | 0 |
| center rib roast lean & fat bone in cooked | 3 oz | 217 | 0 | 0 | 0 |
| fresh ham rump lean roasted | 3 oz | 175 | 0 | 0 | 0 |
| fresh ham rump lean & fat roasted | 3 oz | 214 | 0 | 0 | 0 |

| FOOD | PORTION | CALS | CARB | SUGAR | FIBER |
|---|---|---|---|---|---|
| fresh ham shank lean roasted | 3 oz | 183 | 0 | 0 | 0 |
| fresh ham shank lean & fat roasted | 3 oz | 246 | 0 | 0 | 0 |
| fresh ham whole lean roasted | 3 oz | 179 | 0 | 0 | 0 |
| fresh ham whole lean roasted diced | 1 cup | 285 | 0 | 0 | 0 |
| fresh ham whole lean & fat roasted | 3 oz | 232 | 0 | 0 | 0 |
| fresh ham whole lean & fat roasted diced | 1 cup | 369 | 0 | 0 | 0 |
| ground 97% fat free | 4 oz | 130 | 0 | 0 | 0 |
| ground cooked | 3 oz | 252 | 0 | 0 | 0 |
| loin chop lean bone in braised | 3 oz | 191 | 0 | 0 | 0 |
| loin roast lean bone in roasted | 3 oz | 210 | 0 | 0 | 0 |
| loin whole lean & fat braised | 3 oz | 203 | 0 | 0 | 0 |
| loin whole lean & fat broiled | 3 oz | 206 | 0 | 0 | 0 |
| loin whole lean & fat roasted | 3 oz | 211 | 0 | 0 | 0 |
| lungs braised | 3 oz | 84 | 0 | 0 | 0 |
| pancreas cooked | 3 oz | 186 | 0 | 0 | 0 |
| ribs country style lean & fat braised | 3 oz | 252 | 0 | 0 | 0 |
| shoulder arm picnic lean & fat roasted | 3 oz | 269 | 0 | 0 | 0 |
| shoulder whole lean & fat roasted | 3 oz | 248 | 0 | 0 | 0 |
| shoulder whole lean & fat roasted diced | 1 cup | 394 | 0 | 0 | 0 |
| shoulder whole lean roasted | 3 oz | 196 | 0 | 0 | 0 |
| shoulder whole lean roasted diced | 1 cup | 311 | 0 | 0 | 0 |
| sirloin chop lean & fat bone in braised | 3 oz | 208 | 0 | 0 | 0 |
| sirloin roast lean & fat bone in cooked | 3 oz | 222 | 0 | 0 | 0 |
| spareribs braised | 3 oz | 338 | 0 | 0 | 0 |
| spleen braised | 3 oz | 127 | 0 | 0 | 0 |
| tail simmered | 3 oz | 336 | 0 | 0 | 0 |
| tenderloin lean roasted | 3 oz | 139 | 0 | 0 | 0 |
| top loin chop boneless lean & fat cooked | 3 oz | 198 | 0 | 0 | 0 |

| FOOD | PORTION | CALS | CARB | SUGAR | FIBER |
|---|---|---|---|---|---|
| top loin roast bonless lean & fat cooked | 3 oz | 192 | 0 | 0 | 0 |
| ***Freirich*** | | | | | |
| Porkette | 4 oz | 220 | 1 | 1 | 0 |
| ***Hormel*** | | | | | |
| Extra Lean Teriyaki | 4 oz | 140 | 5 | 4 | 0 |
| Extra Lean Loin Lemon Garlic | 1 serv (4 oz) | 130 | 2 | 0 | 0 |
| ***Smithfield*** | | | | | |
| Tenderloin Garlic & Herb | 3 oz | 100 | 2 | 0 | tr |
| **READY-TO-EAT** | | | | | |
| ***Tyson*** | | | | | |
| Pork Pattie | 1 (3.8 oz) | 200 | 9 | 7 | 3 |
| **TAKE-OUT** | | | | | |
| chicharrones pork cracklings fried | 1 cup | 844 | 22 | – | tr |

## PORK DISHES

| FOOD | PORTION | CALS | CARB | SUGAR | FIBER |
|---|---|---|---|---|---|
| ***Hormel*** | | | | | |
| Pork Roast Au Jus | 1 serv (5 oz) | 180 | 0 | 0 | 0 |
| ***Smithfield*** | | | | | |
| Pulled Pork w/ Barbecue Sauce | 2 oz | 90 | 7 | 6 | – |
| ***Tyson*** | | | | | |
| Lemon Pepper Pork Roast | 1 serv (3 oz) | 110 | 2 | 2 | 0 |
| **TAKE-OUT** | | | | | |
| pork roast | 2 oz | 70 | 0 | 0 | 0 |
| tourtiere | 1 piece (4.9 oz) | 451 | 21 | – | – |

## PORK RINDS *(see* SNACKS)

## POT PIE

| FOOD | PORTION | CALS | CARB | SUGAR | FIBER |
|---|---|---|---|---|---|
| ***Amy's*** | | | | | |
| Broccoli | 1 (7.5 oz) | 430 | 46 | 3 | 4 |
| Country Vegetable | 1 (7.5 oz) | 370 | 47 | 5 | 4 |
| Shepherd's | 1 (8 oz) | 160 | 27 | 5 | 5 |
| Vegetable | 1 (7.5 oz) | 420 | 54 | 3 | 4 |
| Vegetable Non-Dairy | 1 (7.5 oz) | 320 | 50 | 3 | 4 |
| ***Banquet*** | | | | | |
| Beef | 1 (7 oz) | 400 | 38 | 8 | 1 |

| FOOD | PORTION | CALS | CARB | SUGAR | FIBER |
|---|---|---|---|---|---|
| Cheesy Potato & Broccoli w/ Ham | 1 (7 oz) | 410 | 40 | 8 | 2 |
| Chicken | 1 (7 oz) | 380 | 36 | 6 | 1 |
| Chicken & Broccoli | 1 (7 oz) | 350 | 32 | 9 | 2 |
| Family Size Hearty Chicken | 1 cup | 460 | 39 | 14 | 2 |
| Macaroni & Cheese | 1 pkg (6.5 oz) | 210 | 34 | 10 | 1 |
| Turkey | 1 (7 oz) | 370 | 38 | 6 | 3 |
| Vegetable Cheese | 1 (7 oz) | 340 | 39 | 19 | 1 |
| ***Healthy Choice*** | | | | | |
| Colonial Chicken | 1 (9.5 oz) | 310 | 40 | 15 | 5 |
| ***Lean Cuisine*** | | | | | |
| Everyday Favorites Chicken Pie | 1 pkg (9.5 oz) | 300 | 38 | 14 | – |
| Everyday Favorites Vegetable Eggroll | 1 pkg (9 oz) | 300 | 57 | 16 | 4 |
| ***Marie Callender's*** | | | | | |
| Beef | 1 (9.5 oz) | 680 | 53 | 7 | 1 |
| Chicken | 1 (9.5 oz) | 680 | 53 | 9 | 3 |
| Chicken & Broccoli | 1 (9.5 oz) | 670 | 54 | 11 | 4 |
| Chicken Au Gratin | 1 (9.5 oz) | 690 | 50 | 3 | 4 |
| Turkey | 1 (9.5 oz) | 680 | 56 | 10 | 5 |
| ***Morton*** | | | | | |
| Macaroni & Cheese | 1 (6.5 oz) | 210 | 34 | 10 | 1 |
| Vegetable w/ Beef | 1 (7 oz) | 340 | 33 | 8 | 2 |
| Vegetable w/ Chicken | 1 (7 oz) | 320 | 32 | 7 | 2 |
| Vegetable w/ Turkey | 1 (7 oz) | 310 | 29 | 8 | 2 |
| ***Swanson*** | | | | | |
| Beef | 1 (7 oz) | 376 | 39 | 4 | 5 |
| Chicken | 1 (7 oz) | 416 | 45 | 5 | 2 |
| Turkey | 1 (7 oz) | 440 | 44 | 5 | 2 |
| **TAKE-OUT** | | | | | |
| beef | ⅓ of 9 in pie (7.4 oz) | 515 | 39 | – | – |
| chicken | ⅓ of 9 in pie (8.1 oz) | 545 | 42 | – | – |

**POTATO** *(see also* CHIPS, KNISH, PANCAKES*)*

| | | | | | |
|---|---|---|---|---|---|
| **CANNED** | | | | | |
| potatoes | ½ cup | 54 | 12 | – | – |
| ***Del Monte*** | | | | | |
| New Sliced | ⅔ cup (5.4 oz) | 60 | 13 | 0 | 2 |

| FOOD | PORTION | CALS | CARB | SUGAR | FIBER |
|---|---|---|---|---|---|
| New Whole | 2 med (5.5 oz) | 60 | 13 | 0 | 2 |
| ***S&W*** | | | | | |
| Whole Small | 2 (5.5 oz) | 60 | 13 | 0 | 2 |
| **FRESH** | | | | | |
| baked skin only | 1 skin (2 oz) | 115 | 27 | – | 2 |
| baked w/ skin | 1 (6.5 oz) | 220 | 51 | – | – |
| baked w/o skin | 1 (5 oz) | 145 | 34 | – | 2 |
| baked w/o skin | ½ cup | 57 | 13 | – | 1 |
| boiled | ½ cup | 68 | 16 | – | 1 |
| microwaved | 1 (7 oz) | 212 | 49 | – | – |
| microwaved w/o skin | ½ cup | 78 | 18 | – | – |
| ***PurelyIdaho*** | | | | | |
| Oven Roasts | 1 serv (3 oz) | 70 | 17 | 1 | 2 |
| **FROZEN** | | | | | |
| french fries | 10 strips | 111 | 17 | – | 2 |
| french fries thick cut | 10 strips | 109 | 17 | – | – |
| hashed brown | ½ cup | 170 | 22 | – | – |
| potato puffs | ½ cup | 138 | 19 | – | – |
| potato puffs as prep | 1 | 16 | 2 | – | – |
| ***Birds Eye*** | | | | | |
| Baby Gourmet | 7 (4 oz) | 100 | 21 | 0 | 1 |
| Whole | 3 | 50 | 13 | 0 | 1 |
| ***Fillo Factory*** | | | | | |
| Petite Fillo Puffs Potato & Herb | 7 (4.6 oz) | 280 | 44 | 0 | 1 |
| ***Healthy Choice*** | | | | | |
| Cheddar Broccoli Potatoes | 1 meal (10.5 oz) | 330 | 53 | 8 | 6 |
| ***Lean Cuisine*** | | | | | |
| Everyday Favorites Deluxe Cheddar Potato | 1 pkg (10.4 oz) | 250 | 37 | 6 | 5 |
| Everyday Favorites Roasted Potatoes w/ Broccoli | 1 pkg (10.25 oz) | 260 | 39 | 7 | 7 |
| ***Oh Boy!*** | | | | | |
| Stuffed With Cheddar Cheese | 1 (5 oz) | 130 | 22 | 0 | 2 |
| ***Tree Of Life*** | | | | | |
| Organic French Fries | 20 pieces (3 oz) | 110 | 19 | tr | 1 |
| ***Weight Watchers*** | | | | | |
| Smart Ones Baked Broccoli & Cheese | 1 pkg (10 oz) | 250 | 39 | 9 | 6 |

| FOOD | PORTION | CALS | CARB | SUGAR | FIBER |
|---|---|---|---|---|---|
| **MIX** | | | | | |
| au gratin as prep | ½ cup | 160 | 14 | – | – |
| instant mashed flakes as prep w/ whole milk & butter | ½ cup | 118 | 16 | – | – |
| instant mashed flakes not prep | ½ cup | 78 | 18 | – | – |
| instant mashed granules as prep w/ whole milk & butter | ½ cup | 114 | 15 | – | – |
| instant mashed granules not prep | ½ cup | 372 | 86 | – | – |
| scalloped | ½ cup | 105 | 13 | – | – |
| ***Betty Crocker*** | | | | | |
| Au Gratin Low Fat Recipe | ½ cup | 110 | 22 | 3 | 1 |
| Au Gratin as prep | ½ cup | 150 | 22 | 3 | 1 |
| Cheddar & Bacon | ½ cup | 150 | 21 | 2 | 1 |
| Cheddar & Bacon Low Fat Recipe | ½ cup | 120 | 21 | 2 | 1 |
| Cheddar & Sour Cream | ½ cup | 130 | 25 | 3 | 1 |
| Chicken & Vegetable | ⅔ cup | 140 | 23 | 4 | 2 |
| Chicken & Vegetable Low Fat Recipe | ⅔ cup | 120 | 23 | 4 | 2 |
| Hash Browns | ½ cup | 190 | 30 | 0 | 3 |
| Homestyle Broccoli Au Gratin | ½ cup | 140 | 21 | 6 | 2 |
| Homestyle Broccoli Au Gratin Low Fat Recipe | ½ cup | 110 | 21 | 6 | 2 |
| Homestyle Cheddar Cheese | ½ cup | 120 | 21 | 2 | 1 |
| Homestyle Cheddar Cheese Stove Top Recipe | ½ cup | 140 | 21 | 2 | 1 |
| Homestyle Cheesy Scalloped | ½ cup | 140 | 21 | 5 | 2 |
| Homestyle Cheesy Scalloped Low Fat Recipe | ½ cup | 110 | 21 | 5 | 3 |
| Julienne | ½ cup | 150 | 21 | 5 | 1 |
| Mashed Butter & Herb | ½ cup | 160 | 20 | 2 | 1 |
| Mashed Butter & Herb Reduced Fat Recipe | ½ cup | 130 | 20 | 2 | 1 |
| Mashed Chicken & Herb | ½ cup | 150 | 21 | 2 | 1 |
| Mashed Chicken & Herb Reduced Fat Recipe | ½ cup | 120 | 21 | 2 | 1 |
| Mashed Four Cheese | ½ cup | 150 | 20 | 3 | 2 |
| Mashed Four Cheese Reduced Fat Recipe | ½ cup | 120 | 20 | 3 | 2 |

| FOOD | PORTION | CALS | CARB | SUGAR | FIBER |
|---|---|---|---|---|---|
| Mashed Potato Buds | ⅔ cup | 160 | 19 | 2 | 1 |
| Mashed Potato Buds Reduced Fat Recipe | ⅔ cup | 120 | 19 | 2 | 1 |
| Mashed Roasted Garlic | ½ cup | 150 | 19 | 2 | 2 |
| Mashed Roasted Garlic Reduced Fat Recipe | ½ cup | 130 | 19 | 2 | 2 |
| Mashed Sour Cream & Chives | ½ cup | 150 | 21 | 3 | 1 |
| Mashed Sour Cream & Chives Reduced Fat Recipe | ½ cup | 120 | 21 | 3 | 1 |
| Potato Shakers Original | ⅔ cup | 140 | 23 | 2 | 2 |
| Potato Shakers Original Low Fat Recipe | ⅔ cup | 120 | 23 | 2 | 2 |
| Ranch | ½ cup | 160 | 25 | 4 | 2 |
| Scalloped | ½ cup | 150 | 23 | 3 | 1 |
| Scalloped Low Fat Recipe | ⅔ cup | 110 | 23 | 3 | 1 |
| Sour Cream'n Chive | ½ cup | 160 | 22 | 5 | 2 |
| Three Cheese | ½ cup | 150 | 23 | 3 | 1 |
| Twice Baked Cheddar & Bacon Low Fat Recipe | ⅔ cup | 130 | 22 | 4 | 1 |
| Twice Baked Cheddar & Bacon as prep | ⅔ cup | 210 | 22 | 4 | 1 |
| ***Hungry Jack*** | | | | | |
| Mashed Potato Flakes as prep | ½ cup | 160 | 21 | 0 | 1 |
| **REFRIGERATED** | | | | | |
| ***Purely Idaho*** | | | | | |
| Cheddar Crusted | ¾ cup | 120 | 26 | tr | 2 |
| **SHELF-STABLE** | | | | | |
| ***Lunch Bucket*** | | | | | |
| Scalloped w/ Ham Chunks | 1 pkg (7.5 oz) | 170 | 24 | tr | 3 |
| ***TastyBite*** | | | | | |
| Bombay Potatoes | ½ pkg (5 oz) | 190 | 22 | 2 | 6 |
| Mumbai Pav Bhaji | ½ pkg (5 oz) | 229 | 23 | 7 | 7 |
| Simla Potatoes | ½ pkg (5 oz) | 180 | 23 | 2 | 1 |
| **TAKE-OUT** | | | | | |
| au gratin w/ cheese | ½ cup | 178 | 17 | – | – |
| baked topped w/ cheese sauce | 1 | 475 | 47 | – | – |
| baked topped w/ cheese sauce & bacon | 1 | 451 | 44 | – | – |
| baked topped w/ cheese sauce & broccoli | 1 | 402 | 47 | – | – |

| FOOD | PORTION | CALS | CARB | SUGAR | FIBER |
|---|---|---|---|---|---|
| baked topped w/ cheese sauce & chili | 1 | 481 | 56 | – | – |
| baked topped w/ sour cream & chives | 1 | 394 | 50 | – | – |
| curry | 1 serv (6 oz) | 292 | 36 | – | 4 |
| french fries | 1 reg | 235 | 29 | – | – |
| french fries | 1 lg | 355 | 44 | – | – |
| hash brown | ½ cup (2.5 oz) | 151 | 16 | – | – |
| indian yogurt potatoes | 1 serv | 315 | 52 | – | 0 |
| mashed | ½ cup | 111 | 18 | – | – |
| mustard potato salad | 3.5 oz | 120 | 16 | – | – |
| o'brien | 1 cup | 157 | 30 | – | – |
| potato dumpling | 3.5 oz | 334 | 74 | – | 3 |
| potato pancakes | 1 (1.3 oz) | 101 | 11 | – | – |
| potato salad | ½ cup | 179 | 14 | – | – |
| potato salad w/ vegetables | 3.5 oz | 120 | 20 | – | – |
| scalloped | ½ cup | 127 | 18 | – | – |
| twice backed w/ cheese | 1 half (10 oz) | 392 | 48 | – | 4 |
| **POTATO STARCH** | | | | | |
| potato starch | 1 oz | 96 | 24 | – | – |
| **POUT** | | | | | |
| ocean baked | 3 oz | 86 | 0 | 0 | 0 |
| ocean fillet baked | 4.8 oz | 139 | 0 | 0 | 0 |
| **PRETZELS** | | | | | |
| chocolate covered | 1 oz | 130 | 20 | – | – |
| dutch twist | 4 (2.1 oz) | 229 | 48 | – | 2 |
| milk chocolate covered twists | 4 (1 oz) | 140 | 19 | 11 | tr |
| pretzels | 1 oz | 108 | 23 | – | 1 |
| rods | 4 (2 oz) | 229 | 48 | – | 2 |
| sticks | 10 | 10 | 2 | – | – |
| sticks | 120 (2 oz) | 229 | 48 | – | 2 |
| twist | 1 (½ oz) | 65 | 13 | – | – |
| twists | 10 (2.1 oz) | 229 | 48 | – | 2 |
| whole wheat | 2 sm (1 oz) | 103 | 23 | – | – |
| whole wheat | 2 med (2 oz) | 205 | 46 | – | – |
| ***Aramana*** | | | | | |
| Soy Pretzels | 15 (1 oz) | 100 | 12 | 0 | 4 |

| FOOD | PORTION | CALS | CARB | SUGAR | FIBER |
|---|---|---|---|---|---|
| ***Bachman*** | | | | | |
| Thin'n Right | 12 (1 oz) | 120 | 23 | tr | 1 |
| ***Estee*** | | | | | |
| Chocolate Covered | 7 | 130 | 19 | 0 | tr |
| Dutch | 2 (1.1 oz) | 130 | 26 | tr | 1 |
| Unsalted | 23 (1 oz) | 120 | 25 | tr | 1 |
| ***Gardetto's*** | | | | | |
| Mustard | 1 pkg (0.5 oz) | 50 | 10 | 0 | tr |
| ***Lance*** | | | | | |
| Pretzels | 1 pkg (1.25 oz) | 140 | 28 | 1 | tr |
| ***Landies Candies*** | | | | | |
| Sugar Free Chocolate | 4 (1.5 oz) | 220 | 23 | 0 | tr |
| ***Little Debbie*** | | | | | |
| Mini Twists | 1 pkg (1.2 oz) | 140 | 28 | tr | 1 |
| ***Rold Gold*** | | | | | |
| Crispy's Thins | 4 (1 oz) | 110 | 22 | 1 | 1 |
| Fat Free Honey Mustard | 17 (1 oz) | 110 | 23 | 2 | 1 |
| Fat Free Sticks | 48 (1 oz) | 110 | 23 | 1 | 1 |
| Fat Free Thins | 12 pieces (1 oz) | 110 | 24 | tr | 1 |
| Fat Free Tiny Twists | 18 pieces (1 oz) | 110 | 23 | tr | 1 |
| Honey Mustard | 16 (1 oz) | 110 | 22 | 1 | 1 |
| Rods | 3 (1 oz) | 110 | 22 | 1 | 1 |
| Sharp Cheddar | 22 (1 oz) | 110 | 22 | tr | 1 |
| Sour Dough Nuggets | 11 (1 oz) | 110 | 24 | 1 | 1 |
| ***Snyder's Of Hanover*** | | | | | |
| Dips White Fudge | 1 oz | 130 | 19 | 12 | 0 |
| Hard Sourdough | 1 oz | 100 | 22 | 0 | 1 |
| Hard Sourdough Unsalted | 1 oz | 100 | 22 | 0 | 1 |
| Logs | 1 oz | 110 | 21 | 1 | tr |
| Mini | 1 oz | 120 | 25 | tr | tr |
| Mini Unsalted | 1 oz | 110 | 25 | tr | tr |
| Nibblers | 1 oz | 120 | 25 | tr | tr |
| Nibblers Honey Mustard & Onions | 1 oz | 130 | 23 | tr | tr |
| Nibblers Oat Bran | 1 oz | 130 | 23 | 1 | 3 |
| Nibblers Unsalted | 1 oz | 120 | 25 | tr | tr |
| Oat Bran | 1 oz | 100 | 22 | tr | 2 |

| FOOD | PORTION | CALS | CARB | SUGAR | FIBER |
|---|---|---|---|---|---|
| Old Fashioned Dipping Stix | 1 oz | 100 | 22 | tr | 1 |
| Old Tyme Unsalted | 1 oz | 120 | 24 | tr | 1 |
| Olde Tyme | 1 oz | 120 | 24 | tr | 1 |
| Olde Tyme Stix | 1 oz | 120 | 23 | tr | 1 |
| Pieces Buttermilk Ranch | 1 oz | 130 | 19 | tr | tr |
| Pieces Cheddar Cheese | 1 oz | 190 | 18 | tr | tr |
| Pieces Honey Mustard & Onions | 1 oz | 140 | 18 | 3 | tr |
| Pieces Peppered Pizza | 1 oz | 150 | 16 | 1 | tr |
| Rods | 1 oz | 120 | 24 | tr | tr |
| Snaps | 24 (1 oz) | 120 | 25 | tr | tr |
| Thin | 1 oz | 130 | 23 | 1 | tr |
| Whole Wheat Honey | 1 oz | 120 | 24 | 4 | 2 |
| ***Utz*** | | | | | |
| Country Store Stix | 5 (1 oz) | 110 | 22 | tr | 1 |
| Fat Free Hard | 1 (0.8 oz) | 90 | 18 | tr | tr |
| Fat Free Hard No Salt Added | 1 (0.8 oz) | 90 | 19 | tr | tr |
| Fat Free Sour Dough Nuggets | 10 (1 oz) | 100 | 22 | tr | 1 |
| Fat Free Stix | 14 (1 oz) | 100 | 23 | 1 | 1 |
| Fat Free Thin | 10 (1 oz) | 100 | 22 | 1 | 1 |
| Honey Mustard & Onion | ⅓ cup (1 oz) | 130 | 18 | 1 | tr |
| Rods | 3 (1 oz) | 120 | 24 | 1 | 1 |
| Specials | 5 (1 oz) | 110 | 21 | tr | 1 |
| Specials Extra Dark | 5 (1 oz) | 110 | 21 | tr | 1 |
| Specials Unsalted | 5 (1 oz) | 110 | 21 | tr | 1 |
| Wheels | 20 (1 oz) | 100 | 22 | 1 | 1 |
| ***Wege*** | | | | | |
| Honey Wheat | 1 (0.8 oz) | 120 | 24 | 4 | 1 |
| ***Weight Watchers*** | | | | | |
| Oat Bran Nuggets | 1 pkg (1.5 oz) | 170 | 33 | 0 | 3 |
| **PRUNE JUICE** | | | | | |
| canned | 1 cup | 181 | 45 | – | 3 |
| **PRUNES** | | | | | |
| canned in heavy syrup | 5 | 90 | 24 | – | – |
| canned in heavy syrup | 1 cup | 245 | 65 | – | – |
| dried | 10 | 201 | 53 | – | 6 |
| dried | 1 cup | 385 | 101 | – | 12 |
| dried cooked w/ sugar | ½ cup | 147 | 39 | – | 7 |
| dried cooked w/o sugar | ½ cup | 113 | 30 | – | 6 |

| FOOD | PORTION | CALS | CARB | SUGAR | FIBER |
|---|---|---|---|---|---|
| **PUDDING** | | | | | |
| **MIX** | | | | | |
| ***Betty Crocker*** | | | | | |
| Rice as prep | 1 serv | 200 | 33 | 21 | – |
| ***Jell-O*** | | | | | |
| Vanilla as prep w/ 2% milk | ½ cup (5.1 oz) | 150 | 30 | 19 | 0 |
| ***Keto*** | | | | | |
| Banana not prep | ½ scoop | 62 | 3 | 0 | 2 |
| Chocolate not prep | ½ scoop | 66 | 4 | 0 | 3 |
| French Vanilla not prep | ½ scoop | 62 | 3 | 0 | 2 |
| ***Louisiana Purchase*** | | | | | |
| Bread | 1 serv (1.3 oz) | 150 | 28 | 16 | 2 |
| ***Lundberg*** | | | | | |
| Elegant Rice Cinnamon Raisin | ½ cup (3.9 oz) | 70 | 16 | 7 | 1 |
| Elegant Rice Coconut | ½ cup (3.9 oz) | 70 | 13 | 5 | 1 |
| Elegant Rice Honey Almond | ½ cup (3.9 oz) | 70 | 15 | 5 | 1 |
| ***Uncle Ben's*** | | | | | |
| Rice Pudding Cinnamon & Raisins as prep | ½ cup (1.5 oz) | 160 | 37 | 16 | 1 |
| **READY-TO-EAT** | | | | | |
| ***Boost*** | | | | | |
| Vanilla | 1 pkg (5 oz) | 240 | 33 | 20 | 0 |
| ***Healthy Choice*** | | | | | |
| Low Fat Chocolate Raspberry | ½ cup (3.5 oz) | 102 | 19 | 15 | 0 |
| Low Fat Chocolate Almond | ½ cup (3.5 oz) | 109 | 21 | 15 | 0 |
| Low Fat Double Chocolate Fudge | ½ cup (3.5 oz) | 101 | 20 | 14 | 0 |
| Low Fat French Vanilla | ½ cup (3.5 oz) | 98 | 20 | 16 | 0 |
| Low Fat Tapioca | ½ cup (3.5 oz) | 101 | 21 | 14 | 0 |
| ***Hunt's*** | | | | | |
| Snack Pack Banana | 1 serv (3.5 oz) | 119 | 18 | 14 | 0 |
| Snack Pack Butterscotch | 1 serv (3.5 oz) | 130 | 21 | 14 | 0 |
| Snack Pack Chocolate | 1 serv (3.5 oz) | 143 | 22 | 17 | 0 |
| Snack Pack Chocolate Fudge | 1 serv (3.5 oz) | 147 | 23 | 17 | 0 |
| Snack Pack Chocolate Marshmallow | 1 serv (3.5 oz) | 134 | 21 | 16 | 0 |
| Snack Pack Fat Free Chocolate | 1 serv (3.5 oz) | 86 | 19 | 14 | 0 |
| Snack Pack Fat Free Tapioca | 1 serv (3.5 oz) | 82 | 18 | 14 | 0 |
| Snack Pack Fat Free Vanilla | 1 serv (3.5 oz) | 81 | 18 | 13 | 0 |
| Snack Pack Lemon | 1 serv (3.5 oz) | 124 | 24 | 21 | 0 |

| FOOD | PORTION | CALS | CARB | SUGAR | FIBER |
|---|---|---|---|---|---|
| Snack Pack Milk Chocolate Variety | 1 serv (3.5 oz) | 143 | 22 | 18 | 0 |
| Snack Pack Swirl Chocolate Caramel | 1 serv (3.5 oz) | 143 | 23 | 17 | 0 |
| Snack Pack Swirl Chocolate Peanut Butter | 1 serv (3.5 oz) | 146 | 21 | 15 | 0 |
| Snack Pack Swirl Smores | 1 serv (3.5 oz) | 136 | 21 | 18 | 0 |
| Snack Pack Tapioca | 1 serv (3.5 oz) | 125 | 21 | 15 | 0 |
| Snack Pack Toppers Chocolate Fudge w/ Rainbow Sprinkles | 1 serv (4 oz) | 164 | 25 | 16 | tr |
| Snack Pack Toppers Chocolate w/ Dinosaurs | 1 serv (4 oz) | 161 | 25 | 18 | tr |
| Snack Pack Toppers Chocolate w/ Fun Chips | 1 serv (4 oz) | 176 | 28 | 21 | tr |
| Snack Pack Toppers Vanilla w/ Chocolate Sprinkles | 1 serv (4 oz) | 164 | 26 | 16 | tr |
| Snack Pack Vanilla | 1 serv (3.5 oz) | 135 | 21 | 17 | 0 |
| ***Imagine*** | | | | | |
| Banana | 1 pkg (4 oz) | 150 | 30 | 19 | 0 |
| Butterscotch | 1 pkg (4 oz) | 150 | 31 | 17 | 0 |
| Chocolate | 1 pkg (4 oz) | 170 | 38 | 22 | 1 |
| Lemon | 1 pkg (4 oz) | 150 | 33 | 19 | 1 |
| ***Jell-O*** | | | | | |
| Fat Free Chocolate Fudge & Caramel | 1 serv (4 oz) | 100 | 24 | 17 | 0 |
| Fat Free Tapioca | 1 serv (4 oz) | 100 | 23 | 17 | 0 |
| ***NutraBalance*** | | | | | |
| Low Lactose All Flavors | 1 serv (4 oz) | 225 | 31 | – | – |
| ***Swiss Miss*** | | | | | |
| Butterscotch | 1 pkg (4 oz) | 156 | 24 | 19 | 0 |
| Chocolate | 1 pkg (4 oz) | 166 | 26 | 23 | 0 |
| Chocolate Fudge | 1 pkg (4 oz) | 175 | 28 | 22 | 0 |
| Fat Free Chocolate | 1 pkg (4 oz) | 98 | 22 | 16 | 0 |
| Fat Free Chocolate Fudge | 1 pkg (4 oz) | 101 | 23 | 17 | 0 |
| Fat Free Tapioca | 1 pkg (4 oz) | 98 | 22 | 14 | 0 |
| Fat Free Vanilla | 1 pkg (4 oz) | 93 | 21 | 14 | 0 |
| Fat Free Parfait Vanilla Chocolate | 1 pkg (4 oz) | 96 | 21 | 16 | 0 |
| Lemon Meringue Pie | 1 pkg (4 oz) | 150 | 30 | 24 | – |
| Low Fat Vanilla | 1 serv (4 oz) | 120 | 24 | 18 | – |

| FOOD | PORTION | CALS | CARB | SUGAR | FIBER |
|---|---|---|---|---|---|
| Milk Chocolate | 1 pkg (4 oz) | 166 | 26 | 20 | 0 |
| Parfait Vanilla Chocolate | 1 pkg (4 oz) | 164 | 25 | 22 | 0 |
| Swirl Chocolate Caramel | 1 pkg (4 oz) | 169 | 26 | 20 | 1 |
| Swirl Chocolate Vanilla | 1 pkg (4 oz) | 169 | 26 | 21 | 0 |
| Swirl Chocolate Vanilla Chocolate | 1 pkg (4 oz) | 169 | 26 | 22 | 0 |
| Tapioca | 1 pkg (4 oz) | 138 | 24 | 20 | 0 |
| Vanilla | 1 pkg (4 oz) | 156 | 24 | 19 | 0 |
| **TAKE-OUT** | | | | | |
| blancmange | 1 serv (4.7 oz) | 154 | 25 | – | tr |
| bread pudding | ½ cup (4.4 oz) | 212 | 31 | – | – |
| bread w/ raisins | ½ cup | 180 | 31 | – | – |
| chocolate | ½ cup (5.5 oz) | 221 | 40 | – | – |
| corn | ⅔ cup | 181 | 21 | – | – |
| queen of puddings | 1 serv (4.4 oz) | 266 | 41 | – | tr |
| rice pudding | 1 serv (6 oz) | 220 | 34 | – | tr |
| rice w/ raisins | ½ cup | 246 | 42 | – | 4 |
| tapioca | ½ cup (5.3 oz) | 189 | 26 | – | – |
| vanilla | ½ cup (4.3 oz) | 130 | 20 | – | – |
| yorkshire | 1 serv (3 oz) | 177 | 22 | – | tr |

## PUDDING POPS

| FOOD | PORTION | CALS | CARB | SUGAR | FIBER |
|---|---|---|---|---|---|
| chocolate | 1 (1.6 oz) | 72 | 12 | 10 | – |
| vanilla | 1 (1.6 oz) | 75 | 13 | 11 | – |

## PUFFERFISH

| FOOD | PORTION | CALS | CARB | SUGAR | FIBER |
|---|---|---|---|---|---|
| raw | 3 oz | 72 | 0 | 0 | 0 |

## PUMMELO

| FOOD | PORTION | CALS | CARB | SUGAR | FIBER |
|---|---|---|---|---|---|
| fresh | 1 | 228 | 59 | – | – |
| sections | 1 cup | 71 | 18 | – | – |

## PUMPKIN

| FOOD | PORTION | CALS | CARB | SUGAR | FIBER |
|---|---|---|---|---|---|
| butter | 1 tbsp | 32 | 8 | 8 | – |
| canned | ½ cup | 41 | 10 | – | – |
| cooked mashed | ½ cup | 24 | 6 | – | – |
| flowers cooked | ½ cup | 10 | 2 | – | – |
| flowers raw | 1 | 0 | tr | – | – |
| leaves cooked | ½ cup | 7 | 1 | – | – |
| leaves raw | ½ cup | 4 | tr | – | – |

| FOOD | PORTION | CALS | CARB | SUGAR | FIBER |
|---|---|---|---|---|---|
| ***Libby*** | | | | | |
| Solid Pack | ½ cup | 40 | 9 | 4 | 5 |
| **PUMPKIN SEEDS** | | | | | |
| dried | 1 oz | 154 | 5 | – | – |
| roasted | ¼ cup | 296 | 8 | – | – |
| salted & roasted | ¼ cup | 296 | 8 | – | – |
| whole roasted | 1 oz | 127 | 15 | – | – |
| whole roasted | ¼ cup | 71 | 9 | – | – |
| whole salted roasted | ¼ cup | 71 | 9 | – | – |
| **PURSLANE** | | | | | |
| cooked | 1 cup | 21 | 4 | – | – |
| fresh | 1 cup | 7 | 1 | – | – |
| **QUAIL** | | | | | |
| breast w/o skin raw | 1 (2 oz) | 69 | 0 | 0 | 0 |
| w/ skin raw | 1 quail (3.8 oz) | 210 | 0 | 0 | 0 |
| w/o skin raw | 1 quail (3.2 oz) | 123 | 0 | 0 | 0 |
| **QUICHE** | | | | | |
| ***Atkins*** | | | | | |
| Crustless Bacon & Onion | 1 serv | 320 | 2 | 2 | 0 |
| Crustless Four Cheese | 1 serv | 290 | 2 | 1 | 0 |
| Crustless Smoked Ham & Cheese | 1 serv | 290 | 2 | 2 | 0 |
| **TAKE-OUT** | | | | | |
| cheese | 1 slice (3 oz) | 283 | 16 | – | 1 |
| lorraine | ⅛ of 8 in pie | 600 | 29 | – | – |
| mushroom | 1 slice (3 oz) | 256 | 17 | – | 1 |
| **QUINCE** | | | | | |
| fresh | 1 | 53 | 14 | – | – |
| **QUINOA** | | | | | |
| quinoa not prep | 1 cup (6 oz) | 636 | 117 | – | 10 |
| **RABBIT** | | | | | |
| domestic w/o bone roasted | 3 oz | 167 | 0 | 0 | 0 |
| wild w/o bone stewed | 3 oz | 147 | 0 | 0 | 0 |

| FOOD | PORTION | CALS | CARB | SUGAR | FIBER |
|---|---|---|---|---|---|
| **RACCOON** | | | | | |
| roasted | 3 oz | 217 | 0 | 0 | 0 |
| **RADICCHIO** | | | | | |
| raw shredded | ½ cup | 5 | 1 | – | – |
| **RADISHES** | | | | | |
| chinese dried | ½ cup | 157 | 37 | – | – |
| chinese raw | 1 (12 oz) | 62 | 14 | – | – |
| chinese raw sliced | ½ cup | 8 | 2 | – | – |
| chinese sliced cooked | ½ cup | 13 | 3 | – | – |
| daikon dried | ½ cup | 157 | 37 | – | – |
| daikon raw | 1 (12 oz) | 62 | 14 | – | – |
| daikon raw sliced | ½ cup | 8 | 2 | – | – |
| daikon sliced cooked | ½ cup | 13 | 3 | – | – |
| red raw | 10 | 7 | 2 | – | – |
| red sliced | ½ cup | 10 | 2 | – | – |
| white icicle raw | 1 (½ oz) | 2 | tr | – | – |
| white icicle raw sliced | ½ cup | 7 | 1 | – | – |
| ***Eden*** | | | | | |
| Daikon Dried Shredded | 2 tbsp | 45 | 9 | 6 | 3 |
| Daikon Pickled | 2 slices | 5 | 1 | 0 | 0 |
| **TAKE-OUT** | | | | | |
| korean kimchee | ½ cup | 31 | 6 | – | – |
| moo namul saengche korean salad | 1 serv (3.7 oz) | 34 | 8 | 6 | 2 |
| **RAISINS** | | | | | |
| chocolate coated | 1 cup (6.7 oz) | 741 | 130 | – | – |
| chocolate coated | 10 (0.4 oz) | 39 | 7 | – | – |
| golden seedless | 1 cup | 437 | 115 | – | 8 |
| jumbo golden | ¼ cup | 130 | 31 | 29 | 2 |
| seedless | 1 cup | 434 | 115 | – | 8 |
| seedless | 1 tbsp | 27 | 7 | – | – |
| sultanas | 1 oz | 88 | 23 | – | 2 |
| ***Dole*** | | | | | |
| CinnaRaisins | 1 pkg (1 oz) | 95 | 22 | 20 | 2 |
| ***Estee*** | | | | | |
| Chocolate Covered | ¼ cup | 180 | 27 | 16 | 1 |

| FOOD | PORTION | CALS | CARB | SUGAR | FIBER |
|---|---|---|---|---|---|
| ***Mariana*** | | | | | |
| Fruit n Yogurt Milk Chocolate Covered Raisins | 32 pieces (1 oz) | 130 | 20 | 17 | 2 |
| ***Nestle*** | | | | | |
| Chocolate Covered | 1⅓ tbsp | 70 | 11 | 9 | tr |
| ***Tree Of Life*** | | | | | |
| Organic | ¼ cup (1.4 oz) | 130 | 31 | 29 | 2 |
| **RASPBERRIES** | | | | | |
| canned in heavy syrup | ½ cup | 117 | 30 | – | – |
| fresh | 1 cup | 61 | 14 | – | – |
| fresh | 1 pint | 154 | 36 | – | – |
| frozen sweetened | 1 cup | 256 | 65 | – | – |
| frozen sweetened | 1 pkg (10 oz) | 291 | 74 | – | – |
| ***Birds Eye*** | | | | | |
| Red | 5 oz | 90 | 22 | 22 | 5 |
| ***Tree Of Life*** | | | | | |
| Organic | ⅔ cup (5 oz) | 50 | 12 | 7 | 2 |
| **RASPBERRY JUICE** | | | | | |
| ***Dole*** | | | | | |
| Country Raspberry | 8 fl oz | 140 | 35 | – | – |
| ***Fresh Samantha*** | | | | | |
| Raspberry Dream | 1 cup (8 oz) | 120 | 10 | – | 8 |
| ***Squeezit*** | | | | | |
| Blue Raspberry | 1 bottle (7 oz) | 110 | 28 | 27 | 0 |
| **RED BEANS** | | | | | |
| **CANNED** | | | | | |
| ***Hunt's*** | | | | | |
| Small | ½ cup (4.5 oz) | 89 | 19 | 4 | 6 |
| ***Van Camp*** | | | | | |
| Red Beans | ½ cup (4.6 oz) | 90 | 20 | 3 | 5 |
| **MIX** | | | | | |
| ***Bean Cuisine*** | | | | | |
| Pasta & Beans Barcelona Red With Radiatore | 1 serv | 210 | 29 | 2 | 4 |
| **RELISH** | | | | | |
| cranberry orange | ½ cup | 246 | 64 | – | – |
| hamburger | 1 tbsp | 19 | 5 | – | – |

| FOOD | PORTION | CALS | CARB | SUGAR | FIBER |
|---|---|---|---|---|---|
| hamburger | ½ cup | 158 | 42 | – | – |
| hot dog | ½ cup | 111 | 28 | – | – |
| hot dog | 1 tbsp | 14 | 4 | – | – |
| piccalilli | 1.4 oz | 13 | 2 | – | 1 |
| sweet | 1 tbsp | 19 | 5 | – | – |
| sweet | ½ cup | 159 | 43 | – | – |
| ***Claussen*** | | | | | |
| Sweet Pickle | 1 tbsp (0.5 oz) | 15 | 3 | 2 | 0 |
| ***Matouk's*** | | | | | |
| Hot Chow | 2 tbsp | 20 | 5 | 2 | 0 |
| Kuchela | 1 tsp | 9 | tr | 0 | 0 |
| ***Vlasic*** | | | | | |
| Fancy Sweet | 1 tbsp | 15 | 4 | 4 | – |
| **RENNIN** | | | | | |
| tablet | 1 (0.9 g) | 1 | tr | – | – |
| **RHUBARB** | | | | | |
| fresh | ½ cup | 13 | 3 | – | – |
| frozen | ½ cup | 60 | 3 | – | – |
| frzn as prep w/ sugar | ½ cup | 139 | 37 | – | – |
| **RICE** *(see also* RICE CAKES, WILD RICE*)* | | | | | |
| arborio | ½ cup | 100 | 22 | – | – |
| brown long grain cooked | 1 cup (6.8 oz) | 216 | 45 | – | 4 |
| brown medium grain cooked | 1 cup (6.8 oz) | 218 | 46 | – | 4 |
| glutinous cooked | 1 cup (6.1 oz) | 169 | 37 | – | 2 |
| starch | 1 oz | 98 | 24 | – | – |
| white long grain cooked | 1 cup (5.5 oz) | 205 | 45 | – | 1 |
| white long grain instant cooked | 1 cup (5.8 oz) | 162 | 35 | – | 1 |
| white medium grain cooked | 1 cup (6.5 oz) | 242 | 53 | – | 1 |
| white short grain cooked | 1 cup (6.5 oz) | 242 | 53 | – | – |
| ***Amy's*** | | | | | |
| Bowls Brown Rice & Vegetables | 1 pkg (10 oz) | 240 | 36 | 7 | 5 |
| ***Birds Eye*** | | | | | |
| Rice & Broccoli In Cheese Sauce | 1 pkg | 290 | 15 | 4 | 2 |
| White & Wild w/ Green Beans | 1 cup (6.6 oz) | 180 | 31 | 2 | 2 |
| ***Carolina*** | | | | | |
| Black Beans & Rice Mix as prep | 1 serv | 200 | 39 | 0 | 5 |
| Gold as prep | 1 cup | 160 | 37 | 0 | tr |
| Spanish Rice Mix as prep | 1 serv | 180 | 42 | 1 | 2 |

| FOOD | PORTION | CALS | CARB | SUGAR | FIBER |
|---|---|---|---|---|---|
| ***Chun King*** | | | | | |
| Fried Rice Mix | ½ cup (1.4 oz) | 126 | 29 | 5 | 1 |
| ***Gourmet House*** | | | | | |
| Brown & White not prep | ¼ cup | 160 | 34 | 1 | 1 |
| ***La Choy*** | | | | | |
| Fried Rice | 1 cup (4.9 oz) | 236 | 53 | 6 | 2 |
| ***Lundberg*** | | | | | |
| One-Step Curry | 1 cup (7.4 oz) | 160 | 38 | 0 | 5 |
| Quick Brown Rice Savory Vegetarian Chicken | 1 cup (2.5 oz) | 260 | 53 | 1 | 5 |
| Risotto Tomato Basil | 1 serv | 140 | 30 | 2 | 1 |
| ***Mahatma*** | | | | | |
| Jambalaya as prep | 1 cup | 190 | 42 | 1 | 1 |
| Nacho Cheese Mix as prep | 1 serv | 250 | 49 | 5 | tr |
| Thai Jasmine as prep | ¾ cup | 160 | 36 | 0 | 2 |
| ***Minute*** | | | | | |
| Instant Brown as prep | ⅔ cup | 170 | 34 | – | 2 |
| ***River Rice*** | | | | | |
| Brown Long Grain not prep | ¼ cup | 150 | 32 | 0 | tr |
| ***S&W*** | | | | | |
| Arborio as prep | ¾ cup | 150 | 35 | 0 | tr |
| Basmati Mix as prep | ¾ cup | 160 | 36 | 0 | 0 |
| Brown Long Grain not prep | ¼ cup | 150 | 32 | 0 | 1 |
| Long Grain Organic not prep | ¼ cup | 150 | 35 | 0 | 0 |
| ***Success*** | | | | | |
| Beef Mix as prep | 1 cup | 240 | 42 | 2 | 2 |
| Broccoli & Cheese | ½ cup | 130 | 21 | 4 | tr |
| Brown | 1 cup | 150 | 33 | 0 | 2 |
| Brown & Wild Mix | ½ cup | 120 | 21 | 1 | 2 |
| Classic Chicken | ½ cup | 90 | 15 | 0 | 1 |
| Grilled Chicken & Broccoli Mix as prep | 1 cup | 240 | 42 | 1 | 1 |
| Long Grain & Wild | ½ cup | 120 | 21 | 2 | tr |
| Pilaf | ½ cup | 120 | 21 | 3 | 1 |
| Red Beans & Rice Mix as prep | 1 cup | 300 | 51 | 1 | 8 |
| Spanish | ½ cup | 120 | 21 | 2 | 1 |
| White as prep | 1 cup | 190 | 44 | 0 | 1 |
| Yellow Mix as pre | 1 cup | 170 | 33 | 0 | 1 |
| ***TastyBite*** | | | | | |
| Pilaf Curried Vegetable | ½ pkg (4.5 oz) | 180 | 26 | 3 | 9 |

| FOOD | PORTION | CALS | CARB | SUGAR | FIBER |
|---|---|---|---|---|---|
| Pilaf Green Peas | ½ pkg (4.5 oz) | 208 | 36 | 0 | 4 |
| Pilaf Vegetable Kofta | ½ pkg (4.5 oz) | 229 | 39 | 0 | 7 |
| ***Uncle Ben*** | | | | | |
| White Converted | 1 cup | 170 | 38 | – | – |
| ***Van Camp*** | | | | | |
| Spanish | ½ cup (4.5 oz) | 90 | 19 | 5 | 2 |
| ***Water Maid*** | | | | | |
| White Medium Grain not prep | ¼ cup | 160 | 37 | 0 | tr |
| ***Zatarain's*** | | | | | |
| Dirty Rice Mix as prep w/o meat and oil | ½ cup | 130 | 29 | 0 | 0 |
| Red Beans & Rice as prep w/o oil | ½ cup | 100 | 21 | 1 | 4 |
| **TAKE-OUT** | | | | | |
| coconut rice | 1 serv | 500 | 30 | – | 2 |
| congee | ½ cup (4.1 oz) | 44 | 10 | – | – |
| nasi goreng (fried rice) | 1 serv | 206 | 35 | – | 5 |
| nasi goreng indonesian rice & vegetables | 1 cup (4.9 oz) | 130 | 28 | 1 | 1 |
| paella | 1 serv (7 oz) | 308 | 17 | – | 3 |
| pilaf | ½ cup | 84 | 11 | – | 3 |
| risotto | 6.6 oz | 426 | 65 | – | 3 |
| spanish | ¾ cup | 363 | 19 | – | – |

## RICE CAKES *(see also* POPCORN CAKES*)*

| FOOD | PORTION | CALS | CARB | SUGAR | FIBER |
|---|---|---|---|---|---|
| ***Estee*** | | | | | |
| Banana Nut | 5 | 60 | 14 | 0 | 0 |
| Cinnamon Spice | 5 | 60 | 14 | 0 | 0 |
| Granny Smith Apple | 5 | 60 | 13 | 0 | 0 |
| Mixed Berry | 5 | 60 | 14 | 0 | 0 |
| Peanut Butter Crunch | 5 | 60 | 13 | 0 | tr |
| ***Lundberg*** | | | | | |
| Nutra Farmed Brown Rice | 1 (0.7 oz) | 70 | 15 | – | – |
| Nutra Farmed Sesame Tamari | 1 (0.7 oz) | 70 | 16 | – | 2 |
| Organic Koku Sesame | 1 (0.7 oz) | 80 | 17 | tr | 2 |
| ***Weight Watchers*** | | | | | |
| Apple Cinnamon | 1 oz | 110 | 25 | 8 | 1 |
| Butter | 1 oz | 110 | 21 | 0 | 1 |
| Caramel | 1 oz | 110 | 24 | 8 | 1 |
| White Cheddar | 1 oz | 100 | 22 | 0 | 1 |

| FOOD | PORTION | CALS | CARB | SUGAR | FIBER |
|---|---|---|---|---|---|
| **ROCKFISH** | | | | | |
| pacific cooked | 3 oz | 103 | 0 | 0 | 0 |
| pacific cooked | 1 fillet (5.2 oz) | 180 | 0 | 0 | 0 |
| pacific raw | 3 oz | 80 | 0 | 0 | 0 |
| **ROE** *(see also individual fish names)* | | | | | |
| fish | 1 oz | 11 | tr | – | – |
| fresh baked | 1 oz | 58 | 1 | – | – |
| fresh baked | 3 oz | 173 | 2 | – | – |
| **ROLL** | | | | | |
| **FROZEN** | | | | | |
| ***Pillsbury*** | | | | | |
| Dinner Rolls Crusty French | 1 | 110 | 19 | 2 | 0 |
| ***Sara Lee*** | | | | | |
| Deluxe Cinnamon Rolls w/o Icing | 1 (2.7 oz) | 370 | 41 | 21 | 1 |
| **READY-TO-EAT** | | | | | |
| bialy | 1 (2.2 oz) | 138 | 32 | – | 1 |
| brioche sweet roll | 1 (3.5 oz) | 410 | 41 | 5 | 3 |
| brown & serve | 1 (1 oz) | 85 | 14 | – | – |
| cheese | 1 (2.3 oz) | 238 | 29 | – | – |
| cinnamon raisin | 1 (2¾ in) | 223 | 31 | – | 1 |
| dinner | 1 (1 oz) | 85 | 14 | – | – |
| egg | 1 (2½ in) | 107 | 18 | – | 1 |
| french | 1 (1.3 oz) | 105 | 19 | – | – |
| hamburger | 1 (1½ oz) | 123 | 22 | – | – |
| hamburger multi-grain | 1 (1½ oz) | 113 | 19 | – | 2 |
| hamburger reduced calorie | 1 (1½ oz) | 84 | 18 | – | 3 |
| hard | 1 (3½ in) | 167 | 30 | – | – |
| hot cross bun | 1 | 202 | 38 | – | 1 |
| hotdog | 1 (1½ oz) | 123 | 22 | – | – |
| hotdog reduced calorie | 1 (1½ oz) | 84 | 18 | – | 3 |
| hotdog whole wheat | 1 (1.5 oz) | 110 | 19 | 2 | 2 |
| kaiser | 1 (3½ in) | 167 | 30 | – | – |
| oat bran | 1 (1.2 oz) | 78 | 13 | – | 1 |
| rye | 1 (1 oz) | 81 | 15 | – | – |
| submarine | 1 (4.7 oz) | 155 | 30 | – | – |
| wheat | 1 (1 oz) | 77 | 13 | – | – |
| whole wheat | 1 (1 oz) | 75 | 15 | – | – |

| FOOD | PORTION | CALS | CARB | SUGAR | FIBER |
|---|---|---|---|---|---|
| ***Bread Du Jour*** | | | | | |
| Cracked Wheat | 1 (1.2 oz) | 100 | 17 | 2 | 1 |
| Italian | 1 (1.2 oz) | 90 | 16 | 2 | 0 |
| Sourdough | 1 (1.2 oz) | 90 | 17 | 1 | 0 |
| ***Country Kitchen*** | | | | | |
| Wheat Light | 1 | 80 | 17 | 1 | 4 |
| ***Pepperidge Farm*** | | | | | |
| Brown & Serve Club | 1 (1.6 oz) | 120 | 22 | 1 | 2 |
| Dinner Rolls Finger Poppy | 1 (0.9 oz) | 80 | 12 | 2 | tr |
| Parker House | 1 (0.9 oz) | 80 | 13 | 2 | tr |
| ***Stroehmann*** | | | | | |
| Hamburger | 1 (1.4 oz) | 100 | 21 | 3 | tr |
| Hamburger Potato | 1 (1.9 oz) | 140 | 28 | 5 | tr |
| Hot Dog | 1 (1.4 oz) | 100 | 21 | 3 | tr |
| Hot Dog Potato | 1 (1.9 oz) | 140 | 28 | 5 | tr |
| ***Wonder*** | | | | | |
| Brown & Serve | 1 (1 oz) | 80 | 13 | 1 | 0 |
| Brown & Serve Sourdough | 1 (1 oz) | 70 | 13 | 1 | 0 |
| Brown & Serve Wheat | 1 (1 oz) | 80 | 13 | 1 | 0 |
| Bun | 1 (3 oz) | 220 | 42 | 6 | 1 |
| Club French | 1 (1.6 oz) | 120 | 23 | 2 | 0 |
| Club Grain | 1 (1.6 oz) | 120 | 23 | 2 | 1 |
| Club Sourdough | 1 (1.6 oz) | 120 | 23 | 1 | 0 |
| Dinner | 2 (1.6 oz) | 130 | 25 | 3 | 1 |
| Dinner Honey Rich | 1 (1.3 oz) | 100 | 17 | 3 | 0 |
| Dinner Wheat | 2 (1.6 oz) | 140 | 24 | 4 | 1 |
| Hamburger | 1 (2.5 oz) | 190 | 36 | 8 | 1 |
| Hamburger | 1 (2 oz) | 150 | 28 | 4 | 1 |
| Hamburger | 1 (1.5 oz) | 110 | 21 | 3 | 0 |
| Hamburger Wheat | 1 (1.9 oz) | 140 | 24 | 1 | 2 |
| Hamburger Wheat | 1 (1.5 oz) | 120 | 21 | 1 | 1 |
| Hoagie French | 1 (3 oz) | 220 | 41 | 3 | 1 |
| Hoagie Grain | 1 (3 oz) | 220 | 41 | 4 | 2 |
| Hoagie Sourdough | 1 (3 oz) | 220 | 41 | 2 | 1 |
| Hot Dog | 1 (2 oz) | 160 | 29 | 6 | 0 |
| Kaiser | 1 (2.2 oz) | 180 | 33 | 2 | 1 |
| Kaiser Hoagie | 1 (3 oz) | 220 | 41 | 3 | 1 |
| Multigrain | 1 (1.8 oz) | 140 | 25 | 4 | 1 |
| Potato Bun | 1 (1.5 oz) | 110 | 22 | 3 | 1 |
| Steak | 1 (2.5 oz) | 190 | 36 | 1 | 1 |

| FOOD | PORTION | CALS | CARB | SUGAR | FIBER |
|---|---|---|---|---|---|
| **REFRIGERATED** | | | | | |
| cinnamon w/ frosting | 1 | 109 | 17 | – | – |
| crescent | 1 (1 oz) | 98 | 14 | – | – |
| ***Pillsbury*** | | | | | |
| Apple Cinnamon | 1 (1.5 oz) | 150 | 23 | 11 | tr |
| Caramel | 1 (1.7 oz) | 170 | 24 | 10 | tr |
| Cinnamon w/ Icing | 1 (1.5 oz) | 150 | 23 | 10 | tr |
| Cinnamon w/ Icing Reduced Fat | 1 (1.5 oz) | 140 | 24 | 10 | tr |
| Cinnamon Raisin w/ Icing | 1 (1.7 oz) | 170 | 26 | 11 | tr |
| Cornbread Twists | 1 (1.4 oz) | 140 | 18 | 4 | 0 |
| Crescents Reduced Fat | 1 (1 oz) | 100 | 12 | 2 | 0 |
| Crescent | 1 (1 oz) | 110 | 11 | 2 | 0 |
| Dinner | 1 (1.4 oz) | 110 | 18 | 3 | 1 |
| Dinner Wheat | 1 (1.4 oz) | 110 | 18 | 3 | 1 |
| Orange Sweet Roll w/ Icing | 1 (1.7 oz) | 150 | 25 | 10 | tr |
| **ROSE APPLE** | | | | | |
| fresh | 3.5 oz | 32 | 7 | – | – |
| **ROSE HIP** | | | | | |
| fresh | 1 oz | 26 | 5 | – | – |
| **ROSELLE** | | | | | |
| fresh | 1 cup | 28 | 6 | – | – |
| **ROSEMARY** | | | | | |
| dried | 1 tsp | 4 | 1 | – | – |
| **ROUGHY** | | | | | |
| orange baked | 3 oz | 75 | 0 | 0 | 0 |
| **RUTABAGA** | | | | | |
| cooked mashed | ½ cup | 41 | 9 | – | – |
| **SABLEFISH** | | | | | |
| baked | 3 oz | 213 | 0 | 0 | 0 |
| fillet baked | 5.3 oz | 378 | 0 | 0 | 0 |
| smoked | 1 oz | 72 | 0 | 0 | 0 |
| smoked | 3 oz | 218 | 0 | 0 | 0 |
| **SAFFLOWER** | | | | | |
| seeds dried | 1 oz | 147 | 10 | – | – |

| FOOD | PORTION | CALS | CARB | SUGAR | FIBER |
|---|---|---|---|---|---|
| **SAFFRON** | | | | | |
| saffron | 1 tsp | 2 | tr | – | – |
| **SAGE** | | | | | |
| ground | 1 tsp | 2 | tr | – | – |
| **SALAD** | | | | | |
| **MIX** | | | | | |
| ***Dole*** | | | | | |
| All American Toss | 2 cups (3.5 oz) | 50 | 7 | 4 | 2 |
| American Blend | 1½ cups (3 oz) | 15 | 3 | 2 | 1 |
| Classic | 1½ cups (3 oz) | 15 | 4 | 2 | 1 |
| Classic Romaine Blend | 1½ cups (3 oz) | 15 | 3 | 2 | 1 |
| Coleslaw | 1½ cups (3 oz) | 25 | 5 | 3 | 2 |
| European Special Blend | 2 cups (3 oz) | 15 | 3 | 2 | 1 |
| Garlic Caesar Complete w/ Dressing | 1½ cups (3.5 oz) | 180 | 8 | 7 | 1 |
| Greek Marinade | 1½ cups (3.5 oz) | 100 | 5 | 3 | 1 |
| Greener Selection | 1½ cups (3 oz) | 15 | 3 | 2 | 1 |
| Light Caesar Complete w/ Dressing | 1½ cups (3.5 oz) | 60 | 10 | 5 | 2 |
| Light Herb Ranch Complete w/ Dressing | 1½ cups (3.5 oz) | 50 | 10 | 5 | 2 |
| Light Roasted Garlic Caesar Complete w/ Dressing | 1½ cups (3.5 oz) | 60 | 11 | 4 | 1 |
| Light Zesty Italian Complete w/ Dressing | 1½ cups (3.5 oz) | 50 | 11 | 5 | 1 |
| Mediterranean Marinade | 2 cups (3.5 oz) | 90 | 5 | 3 | 1 |
| Oriental Complete w/ Dressing | 1½ cups (3.5 oz) | 120 | 13 | 5 | 2 |
| Romano Complete w/ Dressing | 1½ cups (3.5 oz) | 150 | 9 | 2 | 2 |

| FOOD | PORTION | CALS | CARB | SUGAR | FIBER |
|---|---|---|---|---|---|
| Sunflower Ranch Complete w/ Dressing | 1½ cups (3.5 oz) | 160 | 5 | 3 | 2 |
| Tomato & Mozzarella Medley | 2 cups (3.5 oz) | 60 | 7 | 4 | 2 |
| Triple Cheese Toss | 2 cups (3.5 oz) | 80 | 4 | 2 | 1 |
| ***Earthbound Farm*** | | | | | |
| Baby Caesar Mix | 1 pkg (5 oz) | 25 | 3 | 3 | 2 |
| Baby Greens w/ Low Fat Honey Dijon Vinaigrette & Tomato Croutons | 1 serv (3.5 oz) | 90 | 15 | 6 | 2 |
| Caesar w/ Garlic Croutons | 1 serv (3.5 oz) | 170 | 7 | 1 | 1 |
| Italian Salad Organic | 1⅔ cups (2.9 oz) | 15 | 3 | 2 | 1 |
| Mixed Baby Greens Organic | 1 pkg (4 oz) | 30 | 4 | 0 | 2 |
| Organic Baby Greens w/ Vinaigrette & Garlic Croutons | 1 serv (3.5 oz) | 230 | 11 | 0 | 1 |
| Organic Baby Spinach w/ Sesame Soy Vinaigrette & Peanuts | 1 serv (3.5 oz) | 150 | 8 | 4 | 2 |
| Organic Italian Salad w/ Blue Cheese Dressing & Walnuts | 1 serv (3.5 oz) | 190 | 4 | 2 | 1 |
| Romaine Blend Organic | 1⅔ cups (2.9 oz) | 15 | 3 | 2 | 1 |
| ***Fresh Express*** | | | | | |
| Baby Spinach Trio | 4 cups (3 oz) | 20 | 4 | 1 | 1 |
| Fancy Field Greens | 1½ cups (3 oz) | 15 | 3 | 1 | 2 |
| Original Iceberg Garden w/ Zip | 1½ cups (3 oz) | 15 | 3 | 2 | 1 |
| Veggie Lover's | 1½ cups (3 oz) | 20 | 4 | 2 | 1 |
| ***Suddenly Salad*** | | | | | |
| Caesar | ¾ cup | 220 | 30 | 3 | 1 |
| Caesar Low Fat Recipe | ¾ cup | 170 | 30 | 3 | 1 |
| Italian Pepperoni | 1 cup | 190 | 35 | 7 | 2 |
| Italian Pepperoni Low Fat Recipe | 1 cup | 180 | 35 | 7 | 2 |
| Ranch & Bacon | ¾ cup | 330 | 30 | 3 | 1 |

| FOOD | PORTION | CALS | CARB | SUGAR | FIBER |
|---|---|---|---|---|---|
| Ranch & Bacon Low Fat Recipe | ¾ cup | 180 | 30 | 3 | 1 |
| ***Weight Watchers*** | | | | | |
| Caesar Salad | 1 serv (3.5 oz) | 60 | 11 | 1 | 1 |
| Caesar Salad w/ Cookies | 1 pkg (4.3 oz) | 160 | 29 | 12 | 3 |
| European Salad | 1 serv (3.5 oz) | 60 | 13 | 9 | 2 |
| European Salad w/ Cookies | 1 pkg (4.3 oz) | 160 | 31 | 11 | 2 |
| Garden Salad | 1 serv (3.5 oz) | 60 | 12 | 4 | 1 |
| Garden Salad w/ Cookies | 1 pkg (4 oz) | 120 | 24 | 10 | 2 |
| **TAKE-OUT** | | | | | |
| caesar | 2 cups (5 oz) | 235 | 11 | 3 | 1 |
| chef w/o dressing | 1½ cups | 386 | 9 | – | – |
| tossed w/o dressing | ¾ cup | 16 | 3 | – | – |
| tossed w/o dressing | 1½ cups | 32 | 7 | – | – |
| tossed w/o dressing w/ cheese & egg | 1½ cups | 102 | 5 | – | – |
| tossed w/o dressing w/ chicken | 1½ cups | 105 | 4 | – | – |
| tossed w/o dressing w/ pasta & seafood | 1½ cups (14.6 oz) | 380 | 32 | – | – |
| tossed w/o dressing w/ shrimp | 1½ cups | 107 | 7 | – | – |
| waldorf | ½ cup | 79 | 6 | – | 1 |
| **SALAD DRESSING** | | | | | |
| **MIX** | | | | | |
| ***Et Tu*** | | | | | |
| Caesar Salad Kit | 1 serv | 140 | 6 | 0 | 0 |
| ***McCormick*** | | | | | |
| Mediterrenean Potato Salad | 1 tbsp | 25 | 4 | 3 | 1 |
| Pasta Salad Vinagarette | 1 tsp (5 g) | 15 | 2 | 1 | – |
| **READY-TO-EAT** | | | | | |
| blue cheese | 1 tbsp | 77 | 1 | – | – |
| french | 1 tbsp | 67 | 3 | – | – |
| french reduced calorie | 1 tbsp | 22 | 4 | – | – |
| italian | 1 tbsp | 69 | 2 | – | – |
| italian reduced calorie | 1 tbsp | 16 | 1 | – | – |
| russian | 1 tbsp | 76 | 2 | – | – |
| russian reduced calorie | 1 tbsp | 23 | 5 | – | – |

| FOOD | PORTION | CALS | CARB | SUGAR | FIBER |
|---|---|---|---|---|---|
| sesame seed | 1 tbsp | 68 | 1 | – | – |
| thousand island | 1 tbsp | 59 | 2 | – | – |
| thousand island reduced calorie | 1 tbsp | 24 | 3 | – | – |
| ***Annie Chun*** | | | | | |
| Lemongrass | 2 tbsp | 60 | 6 | 5 | 0 |
| Sesame Cilantro | 1 tbsp | 4 | 4 | 4 | 0 |
| ***Carb Options*** | | | | | |
| Italian | 2 tbsp | 70 | 0 | 0 | 0 |
| Ranch | 2 tbsp | 150 | 0 | 0 | 0 |
| ***Drew's*** | | | | | |
| Low Carb Garlic Italian | 1 tbsp | 80 | 0 | 0 | 0 |
| Low Carb Lemon Tahini Goddess | 1 tbsp | 80 | 1 | 0 | 0 |
| Low Carb Sesame Orange | 1 tbsp | 80 | 2 | 0 | 0 |
| ***Estee*** | | | | | |
| Creamy French | 2 tbsp (1 oz) | 10 | 2 | 2 | – |
| Italian | 2 tbsp | 5 | 1 | 1 | 0 |
| ***Hellmann's*** | | | | | |
| Citrus Splash Ruby Red Ginger | 2 tbsp (1 oz) | 90 | 8 | 7 | – |
| ***LaMartinique*** | | | | | |
| Blue Cheese Vinaigrette | 2 tbsp | 160 | 0 | 0 | 0 |
| Poppy Seed | 2 tbsp | 170 | 8 | 7 | 0 |
| ***Nasoya*** | | | | | |
| Creamy Dill | 2 tbsp | 70 | 2 | 1 | 0 |
| Creamy Italian | 2 tbsp | 60 | 2 | 1 | 0 |
| Garden Herb | 2 tbsp | 70 | 2 | 1 | 0 |
| Sesame Garlic | 2 tbsp | 60 | 2 | 1 | 0 |
| Thousand Island | 2 tbsp | 70 | 3 | 2 | 0 |
| ***Old Dutch*** | | | | | |
| Sweet & Sour | 2 tbsp | 50 | 13 | 13 | 0 |
| ***Paul's*** | | | | | |
| No-Fat Raspberry & Balsamic | 2 tbsp | 20 | 5 | 5 | – |
| No-Oil Orange & Basil | 2 tbsp | 15 | 4 | 4 | 0 |
| ***Steel's*** | | | | | |
| Honey Mustard | 1 tbsp | 90 | 0 | 0 | 0 |
| Sweet Ginger Lime | 1 tbsp | 68 | 1 | 0 | 1 |
| ***Weight Watchers*** | | | | | |
| Fat Free Caesar | 2 tbsp | 10 | 1 | 1 | 0 |
| Fat Free Caesar | 1 pkg (0.75 oz) | 5 | 1 | 1 | 0 |

| FOOD | PORTION | CALS | CARB | SUGAR | FIBER |
| --- | --- | --- | --- | --- | --- |
| Fat Free Creamy Italian | 2 tbsp | 30 | 7 | 2 | 0 |
| Fat Free French Style | 2 tbsp | 40 | 9 | 6 | 0 |
| Fat Free Honey Dijon | 2 tbsp | 45 | 11 | 5 | 0 |
| Fat Free Italian | 2 tbsp | 10 | 2 | 1 | 0 |
| Fat Free Ranch | 2 tbsp | 35 | 7 | 3 | 0 |
| Fat Free Ranch | 1 pkg (0.75 oz) | 25 | 6 | 2 | 0 |
| **TAKE-OUT** | | | | | |
| vinegar & oil | 1 tbsp | 72 | tr | – | – |

## SALMON

| FOOD | PORTION | CALS | CARB | SUGAR | FIBER |
| --- | --- | --- | --- | --- | --- |
| **CANNED** | | | | | |
| chum w/ bone | 1 can (13.9 oz) | 521 | 0 | 0 | 0 |
| chum w/ bone | 3 oz | 120 | 0 | 0 | 0 |
| pink w/ bone | 1 can (15.9 oz) | 631 | 0 | 0 | 0 |
| pink w/ bone | 3 oz | 118 | 0 | 0 | 0 |
| sockeye w/ bone | 3 oz | 130 | 0 | 0 | 0 |
| sockeye w/ bone | 1 can (12.9 oz) | 566 | 0 | 0 | 0 |
| ***Bumble Bee*** | | | | | |
| Keta | ½ cup (3.5 oz) | 160 | 0 | 0 | 0 |
| Red | ½ cup (3.5 oz) | 180 | 0 | 0 | 0 |
| **FRESH** | | | | | |
| atlantic baked | 3 oz | 155 | 0 | 0 | 0 |
| chinook baked | 3 oz | 196 | 0 | 0 | 0 |
| chum baked | 3 oz | 131 | 0 | 0 | 0 |
| coho cooked | ½ fillet (5.4 oz) | 286 | 0 | 0 | 0 |
| coho cooked | 3 oz | 157 | 0 | 0 | 0 |
| coho raw | 3 oz | 124 | 0 | 0 | 0 |
| pink baked | 3 oz | 127 | 0 | 0 | 0 |
| roe raw | 1 oz | 59 | tr | – | – |
| sockeye cooked | ½ fillet (5.4 oz) | 334 | 0 | 0 | 0 |
| sockeye cooked | 3 oz | 183 | 0 | 0 | 0 |
| sockeye raw | 3 oz | 143 | 0 | 0 | 0 |
| **SMOKED** | | | | | |
| chinook | 1 oz | 33 | 0 | 0 | 0 |

| FOOD | PORTION | CALS | CARB | SUGAR | FIBER |
|---|---|---|---|---|---|
| chinook | 3 oz | 99 | 0 | 0 | 0 |
| ***Lascco*** | | | | | |
| Nova Sliced | 2 oz | 60 | 3 | 0 | 0 |
| **TAKE-OUT** | | | | | |
| roulette w/ spinach stuffing | 1 serv (4 oz) | 160 | 10 | 0 | tr |
| salmon cake | 1 (3 oz) | 241 | 6 | – | – |

## SALSA

| FOOD | PORTION | CALS | CARB | SUGAR | FIBER |
|---|---|---|---|---|---|
| black bean & corn | 2 tbsp (1 oz) | 15 | 3 | 1 | tr |
| cirtus | 2 tbsp (1 oz) | 10 | 2 | 2 | 0 |
| ***Del Salsa*** | | | | | |
| Fire Roasted All Flavors | 2 tbsp | 8 | 2 | 0 | 0 |
| ***Gringo Billy's*** | | | | | |
| Salsa Mix | 1 tsp | 5 | 1 | 0 | 1 |
| ***Guiltless Gourmet*** | | | | | |
| Roasted Red Pepper | 2 tbsp (1 oz) | 10 | 2 | 1 | 0 |
| Southwestern Grill | 2 tbsp (1 oz) | 10 | 2 | 1 | 0 |
| ***Hunt's*** | | | | | |
| Alfresco All Varieties | 2 tbsp (1.1 oz) | 10 | 2 | 2 | tr |
| Hot | 2 tbsp (1.1 oz) | 27 | 6 | 1 | 1 |
| Medium | 2 tbsp (1.1 oz) | 27 | 6 | 1 | 1 |
| Mild | 2 tbsp (1.1 oz) | 27 | 6 | 1 | 1 |
| Picante All Varieties | 2 tbsp (1.1 oz) | 11 | 2 | 1 | tr |
| Squeeze Mild & Medium | 2 tbsp (1.1 oz) | 27 | 6 | 2 | 1 |
| ***Muir Glen*** | | | | | |
| Black Bean & Corn Medium | 2 tbsp (1.1 oz) | 15 | 3 | 1 | tr |
| Chipotle Medium | 2 tbsp (1.1 oz) | 10 | 2 | 1 | 0 |
| Fire Roasted Tomato Medium | 2 tbsp (1.1 oz) | 10 | 2 | 1 | 0 |
| Garlic Cilantro Medium | 2 tbsp (1.1 oz) | 10 | 2 | 1 | 0 |
| Habanero Hot | 2 tbsp (1.1 oz) | 10 | 2 | 1 | 0 |
| Organic Medium | 2 tbsp (1.1 oz) | 10 | 2 | 1 | 0 |
| Organic Mild | 2 tbsp (1.1 oz) | 10 | 2 | 1 | 0 |
| Roasted Garlic Medium | 2 tbsp (1.1 oz) | 10 | 2 | 1 | 0 |
| ***Pace*** | | | | | |
| Picante Mild or Medium | 2 tbsp | 10 | 2 | 1 | 0 |
| Thick & Chunky Mild or Medium | 2 tbsp | 10 | 2 | 1 | 0 |
| ***Rosarita*** | | | | | |
| Extra Chunky Medium | 2 tbsp (1 oz) | 7 | 1 | 1 | tr |
| Green Tomatillo Medium | 2 tbsp (1 oz) | 8 | 2 | 2 | 1 |

| FOOD | PORTION | CALS | CARB | SUGAR | FIBER |
|---|---|---|---|---|---|
| Picante Zesty Jalapeno Hot | 2 tbsp (1 oz) | 8 | 2 | 1 | 1 |
| Picante Zesty Jalapeno Medium | 2 tbsp (1 oz) | 9 | 2 | 1 | 1 |
| Picante Zesty Jalapeno Mild | 2 tbsp (1 oz) | 8 | 2 | 1 | tr |
| Roasted Mild | 2 tbsp (1 oz) | 10 | 2 | 1 | 1 |
| Traditional Medium | 2 tbsp (1 oz) | 7 | 2 | 1 | 1 |
| Traditional Mild | 2 tbsp (1 oz) | 7 | 1 | 1 | 1 |
| ***Snyder's Of Hanover*** | | | | | |
| Mild | 2 tbsp | 10 | 2 | 2 | 0 |
| ***Tostitos*** | | | | | |
| Con Queso | 2.3 oz | 80 | 10 | tr | 2 |
| Hot | 2.3 oz | 30 | 6 | 2 | 2 |
| Low Fat Con Queso | 2.5 oz | 80 | 8 | tr | tr |
| Medium | 2.3 oz | 30 | 6 | 2 | 2 |
| Mild | 2.3 oz | 30 | 6 | 2 | 2 |
| Restaurant Style | 2.2 oz | 30 | 6 | 2 | 2 |
| Ultimate Garden | 2.4 oz | 30 | 6 | 2 | 2 |
| ***Tree Of Life*** | | | | | |
| Medium | 2 tbsp (1 oz) | 10 | 2 | 1 | – |
| Mild | 2 tbsp (1 oz) | 10 | 2 | 1 | – |
| ***Utz*** | | | | | |
| Chunky | 2 tbsp (1 oz) | 60 | 14 | 4 | 4 |
| **SALSIFY** | | | | | |
| fresh sliced cooked | ½ cup | 46 | 10 | – | – |
| raw sliced | ½ cup | 55 | 12 | – | – |
| **SALT SUBSTITUTES** | | | | | |
| ***Eden*** | | | | | |
| Shiso Leaf Powder | 1 tsp | 0 | 0 | 0 | 2 |
| ***Estee*** | | | | | |
| Salt-It | ¼ tsp | 0 | 0 | 0 | 0 |
| ***Halsosalt*** | | | | | |
| All Flavors | ¼ tsp (7 g) | 1 | 0 | – | – |
| ***Molly McButter*** | | | | | |
| Lite Sodium | 1 tsp | 5 | 2 | – | – |
| ***Morton*** | | | | | |
| Salt Substitute | ¼ tsp (1.2 g) | tr | tr | – | – |
| ***Mrs. Dash*** | | | | | |
| Onion & Herb | ¼ tsp | 0 | 0 | 0 | 0 |

| FOOD | PORTION | CALS | CARB | SUGAR | FIBER |
|---|---|---|---|---|---|
| **SALT/SEASONED SALT** | | | | | |
| salt | 1 tbsp (18 g) | 0 | 0 | 0 | 0 |
| salt | 1 tsp (6 g) | 0 | 0 | 0 | 0 |
| ***Eden*** | | | | | |
| Atlantic Sea Salt | ¼ tsp | 0 | 0 | 0 | 0 |
| Brittany Sea Salt | ¼ tsp | 0 | 0 | 0 | 0 |
| ***Morton*** | | | | | |
| Lite | ¼ tsp (1.4 g) | tr | tr | – | – |
| **SANDWICHES** | | | | | |
| ***Amy's*** | | | | | |
| Pocket Sandwich Broccoli & Cheese | 1 (4.5 oz) | 270 | 37 | 4 | 3 |
| Pocket Sandwich Roasted Vegetables | 1 (4.5 oz) | 220 | 35 | 5 | 4 |
| Pocket Sandwich Spinach Feta | 1 (4.5 oz) | 250 | 34 | 4 | 3 |
| Pocket Sandwich Tofu Scramble | 1 (4 oz) | 160 | 23 | 2 | tr |
| Pocket Sandwich Vegetable Pie | 1 (5 oz) | 300 | 45 | 5 | 3 |
| Toaster Pops Grilled Cheese | 1 | 180 | 19 | 3 | 0 |
| ***Healthy Choice*** | | | | | |
| Bread Stuffs Chicken & Broccoli | 1 (6.1 oz) | 310 | 50 | 11 | 2 |
| Bread Stuffs Ham & Cheese w/ Broccoli | 1 (6.1 oz) | 320 | 46 | 10 | 1 |
| Bread Stuffs Italian Style Meatball | 1 (6.1 oz) | 330 | 52 | 12 | 4 |
| Bread Stuffs Philly Beef Steal | 1 (6.1 oz) | 310 | 50 | 10 | 3 |
| ***Smucker's*** | | | | | |
| Uncrustables Grape | 1 (2 oz) | 200 | 27 | 12 | 2 |
| **TAKE-OUT** | | | | | |
| chicken fillet plain | 1 | 515 | 39 | – | – |
| chicken fillet w/ cheese lettuce mayonnaise & tomato | 1 | 632 | 42 | – | – |
| croque monsieur | 1 (12.4 oz) | 765 | 43 | 9 | 2 |
| fish fillet w/ tartar sauce | 1 | 431 | 41 | – | – |
| fish fillet w/ tartar sauce & cheese | 1 | 524 | 48 | – | – |
| fried egg w/ cheese | 1 | 340 | 26 | – | – |
| fried egg w/ cheese & ham | 1 | 348 | 31 | – | – |
| ham w/ cheese | 1 | 353 | 33 | – | – |

| FOOD | PORTION | CALS | CARB | SUGAR | FIBER |
|---|---|---|---|---|---|
| roast beef submarine sandwich w/ tomato lettuce & mayonnaise | 1 | 411 | 44 | – | – |
| roast beef w/ cheese | 1 | 402 | 27 | – | – |
| roast beef plain | 1 | 346 | 33 | – | – |
| steak w/ tomato lettuce salt & mayonnaise | 1 | 459 | 52 | – | – |
| submarine w/ salami ham cheese lettuce tomato onion & oil | 1 | 456 | 51 | – | – |
| tuna salad submarine sandwich w/ lettuce & oil | 1 | 584 | 55 | – | – |
| **SAPODILLA** | | | | | |
| fresh | 1 | 140 | 34 | – | – |
| fresh cut up | 1 cup | 199 | 48 | – | – |
| **SAPOTES** | | | | | |
| fresh | 1 | 301 | 76 | – | – |
| **SARDINES** | | | | | |
| **CANNED** | | | | | |
| atlantic in oil w/ bone | 2 | 50 | 0 | 0 | 0 |
| atlantic in oil w/ bone | 1 can (3.2 oz) | 192 | 0 | 0 | 0 |
| pacific in tomato sauce w/ bone | 1 can (13 oz) | 658 | 0 | 0 | 0 |
| pacific in tomato sauce w/ bone | 1 | 68 | 0 | 0 | 0 |
| ***Bumble Bee*** | | | | | |
| In Hot Sauce | ½ can (2 oz) | 109 | tr | tr | 0 |
| In Mustard | ½ can (2 oz) | 88 | 1 | tr | 0 |
| In Oil | ½ can (2 oz) | 125 | 0 | 0 | 0 |
| In Water | ½ can (2 oz) | 83 | 0 | 0 | 0 |
| ***King Oscar*** | | | | | |
| Skinless Boneless In Soya Oil | 3 pieces (1.9 oz) | 120 | 0 | 0 | 0 |
| **SAUCE** (*see also* BARBECUE SAUCE, GRAVY, PIZZA SAUCE, SPAGHETTI SAUCE) | | | | | |
| **JARRED** | | | | | |
| fish sauce chinese | 1 tbsp | 9 | tr | – | 0 |
| fish sauce vietnamese nuoc mam | 1 tbsp | 6 | 1 | – | 0 |
| hoisin | 1 tbsp | 35 | 7 | – | tr |
| morroccan tangerine | ½ cup (4 oz) | 70 | 10 | 10 | 1 |

| FOOD | PORTION | CALS | CARB | SUGAR | FIBER |
|---|---|---|---|---|---|
| oyster | 1 tbsp | 8 | 2 | – | 0 |
| teriyaki | 1 oz | 30 | 6 | – | – |
| teriyaki | 1 tbsp | 15 | 3 | – | – |
| ***A1*** | | | | | |
| Bold Steak Sauce | 1 tbsp | 20 | 5 | 4 | – |
| ***Annie Chun*** | | | | | |
| Shiitake Mushroom | 1 tbsp | 15 | 3 | 2 | 0 |
| Thai Peanut | 2 tbsp | 120 | 10 | 8 | 1 |
| ***Armour*** | | | | | |
| Chili Hot Dog | ¼ cup (2.2 oz) | 120 | 5 | 2 | 0 |
| Meatless Sloppy Joe Sauce | ¼ cup (2.2 oz) | 30 | 7 | 6 | 0 |
| ***Atkins*** | | | | | |
| Steak Sauce | 1 tbsp | 5 | 1 | 0 | 0 |
| Teriyaki | 1 tbsp | 10 | 1 | 0 | 0 |
| ***Boar's Head*** | | | | | |
| Ham Glaze Brown Sugar & Spice | 2 tbsp (1.4 oz) | 120 | 30 | 29 | 0 |
| ***Carb Options*** | | | | | |
| Alfredo | ¼ cup | 110 | 2 | 0 | 0 |
| Asian Teriyaki Marinade | 1 tbsp | 5 | 1 | 0 | 0 |
| Cheese | ¼ cup | 90 | 2 | 0 | 0 |
| Garden Style | ½ cup | 80 | 7 | 4 | 2 |
| Steak Sauce | 1 tbsp | 5 | 1 | 0 | 0 |
| ***Chun King*** | | | | | |
| Sweet And Sour | 2 tbsp (1.2 oz) | 58 | 14 | 14 | 0 |
| Teriyaki | 1 tbsp (0.6 oz) | 17 | 3 | 2 | 0 |
| Teriyaki Hot | 1 tbsp (0.6 oz) | 17 | 3 | 2 | 0 |
| ***Del Monte*** | | | | | |
| Seafood Cocktail | ¼ cup (2.7 oz) | 100 | 24 | 22 | 0 |
| Sloppy Joe Hickory Flavor | ¼ cup (2.4 oz) | 70 | 18 | 15 | 0 |
| Sloppy Joe Original | ¼ cup (2.4 oz) | 70 | 16 | 13 | 0 |
| ***Fritos*** | | | | | |
| Texas-Style Chili Hearty Topping | 2.3 oz | 50 | 8 | 2 | 1 |
| Utimate Taco Hearty Topping | 2.3 oz | 50 | 8 | 2 | 1 |
| ***Gebhardt*** | | | | | |
| Enchilada Sauce | ¼ cup (2.2 oz) | 35 | 4 | 0 | 1 |
| Hot Dog Chili Sauce | ¼ cup (2.2 oz) | 60 | 6 | 0 | 2 |
| Hot Sauce | 1 tsp (5 g) | 1 | tr | 0 | 0 |

| FOOD | PORTION | CALS | CARB | SUGAR | FIBER |
|---|---|---|---|---|---|
| ***Gringo Billy's*** | | | | | |
| Chipotle Dipping & Grilling Sauce | 1 tsp | 5 | 1 | 0 | 0 |
| ***Hunt's*** | | | | | |
| Light w/ Mushrooms | ½ cup (4.4 oz) | 42 | 8 | 5 | 2 |
| Steak | 1 tbsp (0.6 oz) | 10 | 2 | 2 | tr |
| ***Jok'n'Al*** | | | | | |
| Cocktail | ¼ cup | 29 | 6 | 2 | – |
| Plum | 1 tbsp | 10 | 2 | 1 | – |
| ***Just Rite*** | | | | | |
| Hot Dog | ¼ cup (2.2 oz) | 50 | 5 | 0 | 2 |
| ***Kikkoman*** | | | | | |
| Teriyaki | 1 tbsp | 15 | 3 | 2 | 0 |
| ***La Choy*** | | | | | |
| Duck Sauce Sweet & Sour | 2 tbsp (1.3 oz) | 61 | 15 | 15 | 0 |
| Sweet & Sour | 2 tbsp (1.2 oz) | 58 | 14 | 14 | 0 |
| Teriyaki | 1 tbsp (0.6 oz) | 17 | 3 | 2 | 0 |
| ***Lea & Perrins*** | | | | | |
| Worcestershire | 1 tsp | 5 | 1 | 1 | – |
| ***Manwich*** | | | | | |
| BBQ Sloppy Joe | ¼ cup (2.2 oz) | 57 | 14 | 10 | 1 |
| Bold | ¼ cup (2.2 oz) | 62 | 13 | 11 | 1 |
| Mexican | ¼ cup (2.2 oz) | 27 | 5 | 5 | 1 |
| Original | ¼ cup (2.2 oz) | 32 | 6 | 5 | 1 |
| Taco Season | ¼ cup (2.2 oz) | 27 | 6 | 4 | 1 |
| Thick & Chunky | ¼ cup (2.3 oz) | 44 | 9 | 7 | 1 |
| ***Matouk's*** | | | | | |
| Flambeau Sauce | 1 tsp | 0 | 0 | 0 | 0 |
| ***McCormick*** | | | | | |
| Flavor Medleys Garlic & Herb | 2 tbsp | 50 | 5 | 4 | – |
| Flavor Medleys Italian Herb | 2 tbsp | 50 | 4 | 3 | – |
| Flavor Medleys Lemon Pepper | 2 tbsp | 50 | 4 | 3 | – |
| Flavor Medleys Tomato & Basil | 2 tbsp | 50 | 4 | 3 | – |
| ***Old El Paso*** | | | | | |
| Enchilada Mild | ¼ cup (2 oz) | 20 | 3 | tr | 0 |
| ***Open Range*** | | | | | |
| Hot Dog Chili | ¼ cup (2.2 oz) | 61 | 6 | 1 | 2 |
| ***Pace*** | | | | | |
| Enchilada Sauce | ¼ cup | 36 | 6 | 4 | 0 |
| Taco Sauce | ¼ cup | 32 | 4 | 2 | 0 |

| FOOD | PORTION | CALS | CARB | SUGAR | FIBER |
|---|---|---|---|---|---|
| ***Progresso*** | | | | | |
| Alfredo | ½ cup (4.4 oz) | 200 | 7 | 2 | 1 |
| ***Sauce Arturo*** | | | | | |
| Original | ¼ cup (2.2 fl oz) | 50 | 8 | 4 | 0 |
| ***Steel's*** | | | | | |
| Sugar Free Cocktail w/ Dill & Lemon | ¼ cup | 36 | 1 | 1 | 1 |
| Sugar Free Hoisin | 2 tbsp | 15 | 2 | 1 | 1 |
| Sugar Free Peanut Sauce | 1 tbsp | 34 | 7 | 0 | 5 |
| Sugar Free Sweet & Sour | 2 tbsp | 10 | 2 | 0 | 0 |
| ***Tostitos*** | | | | | |
| Beef Fiesta Nacho | 2.4 oz | 120 | 6 | 2 | tr |
| Chicken Quesadilla Topping | 2.5 oz | 90 | 6 | 2 | tr |
| ***Walden Farms*** | | | | | |
| Calorie Free Seafood Sauce | 1 tbsp | 0 | 0 | 0 | 0 |
| Scampi Sauce Calorie Free | 2 tbsp | 0 | 0 | 0 | 0 |
| ***Wild Thyme Farms*** | | | | | |
| Chili Ginger Honey | 1 tbsp | 30 | 8 | 8 | – |
| **MIX** | | | | | |
| cheese as prep w/ milk | 1 cup | 307 | 23 | – | – |
| curry as prep w/ milk | 1 cup | 270 | 26 | – | – |
| mushroom as prep w/ milk | 1 cup | 228 | 24 | – | – |
| sour cream as prep w/ milk | 1 cup | 509 | 45 | – | – |
| stroganoff as prep | 1 cup | 271 | 34 | – | – |
| sweet & sour as prep | 1 cup | 294 | 73 | – | – |
| teriyaki as prep | 1 cup | 131 | 28 | – | – |
| white as prep w/ milk | 1 cup | 241 | 21 | – | – |
| ***Durkee*** | | | | | |
| A La King as prep | 1 cup | 60 | 8 | 2 | 0 |
| Cheese as prep | ¼ cup | 25 | 4 | 0 | 0 |
| Hollandaise as prep | 2 tbsp | 10 | 2 | 0 | 0 |
| White as prep | ¼ cup | 20 | 5 | 0 | 0 |
| ***French's*** | | | | | |
| Cheese as prep | ¼ cup | 25 | 4 | 0 | 0 |
| Hollandaise as prep | 2 tbsp | 10 | 2 | 0 | 0 |
| ***Manwich*** | | | | | |
| Mix | ¼ oz | 22 | 5 | 0 | tr |
| ***McCormick*** | | | | | |
| Bernaise Blend | 1 tsp (3 g) | 10 | 1 | – | – |

| FOOD | PORTION | CALS | CARB | SUGAR | FIBER |
|---|---|---|---|---|---|
| Chicken Dijon Blend | 1⅓ tbsp (10 g) | 40 | 5 | 1 | – |
| Green Peppercorn Blend as prep | ¼ cup | 20 | 3 | 1 | – |
| Grill Mates Mesquite Marinade as prep | 1 tbsp | 15 | 2 | 2 | – |
| Grill Mates Southwest Marinade | 2 tsp (5 g) | 15 | 2 | – | tr |
| Hollandaise Blend | 2 tsp (4 g) | 15 | 1 | – | – |
| Hunter Blend as prep | ¼ cup | 25 | 4 | 1 | – |
| Meat Marinade | 1 tsp (4 g) | 15 | 2 | tr | – |
| Pepper Medley Blend as prep | ¼ cup | 30 | 3 | tr | – |
| White Blend | 2 tsp (6 g) | 20 | 3 | – | – |
| **TAKE-OUT** | | | | | |
| bearnaise | 1 oz | 177 | 1 | – | tr |
| **SAUERKRAUT** | | | | | |
| canned | ½ cup | 22 | 5 | – | – |
| ***B&G*** | | | | | |
| Sauerkraut | 2 tbsp (1 oz) | 6 | 1 | 0 | 1 |
| ***Boar's Head*** | | | | | |
| Sauerkraut | 2 tbsp (1 oz) | 5 | 1 | 0 | tr |
| ***Claussen*** | | | | | |
| Sauerkraut | ¼ cup (1.1 oz) | 5 | 1 | 0 | 1 |
| ***Del Monte*** | | | | | |
| Bavarian Style | 2 tbsp (1 oz) | 15 | 4 | 3 | 0 |
| Sauerkraut | 2 tbsp (1 oz) | 0 | 1 | 0 | 1 |
| ***Eden*** | | | | | |
| Organic | ½ cup | 25 | 4 | 1 | 3 |
| ***S&W*** | | | | | |
| Canned | 2 tbsp (1 oz) | 5 | 1 | 0 | 0 |
| Red Cabbage | 2 tbsp (1 oz) | 15 | 3 | 2 | 0 |
| **SAUSAGE** | | | | | |
| bierschinken | 3.5 oz | 174 | tr | – | – |
| bierwurst | 3.5 oz | 258 | 0 | 0 | 0 |
| blutwurst uncooked | 3.5 oz | 424 | 0 | 0 | 0 |
| bockwurst | 3.5 oz | 276 | 0 | 0 | 0 |
| bratwurst pork cooked | 1 link (3 oz) | 256 | 2 | – | – |
| bratwurst pork & beef | 1 link (2.5 oz) | 226 | 2 | – | – |
| chipolata | 3.5 oz | 342 | 1 | 1 | 0 |

| FOOD | PORTION | CALS | CARB | SUGAR | FIBER |
|---|---|---|---|---|---|
| chorizo | 3.5 oz | 499 | 4 | 4 | tr |
| fleischwurst | 3.5 oz | 305 | 0 | 0 | 0 |
| gelbwurst uncooked | 3.5 oz | 363 | 0 | 0 | 0 |
| italian pork cooked | 1 (3 oz) | 268 | 1 | – | – |
| jagdwurst | 3.5 oz | 211 | 0 | 0 | 0 |
| kielbasa pork | 1 oz | 88 | 1 | – | – |
| knockwurst pork & beef | 1 (2.4 oz) | 209 | 1 | – | – |
| mettwurst uncooked | 3.5 oz | 483 | 0 | 0 | 0 |
| plockwurst uncooked | 3.5 oz | 312 | 0 | 0 | 0 |
| polish pork | 1 (8 oz) | 739 | 4 | – | – |
| pork cooked | 1 link (½ oz) | 48 | tr | – | – |
| regensburger uncooked | 3.5 oz | 354 | 0 | 0 | 0 |
| vienna canned | 7 (4 oz) | 315 | 2 | – | – |
| vienna canned | 1 (½ oz) | 45 | tr | – | – |
| weisswurst uncooked | 3.5 oz | 305 | 0 | 0 | 0 |
| zungenwurst (tongue) | 3.5 oz | 285 | 0 | 0 | 0 |
| ***Armour*** | | | | | |
| Vienna Sausage 25% Less Fat | 3 (1.9 oz) | 130 | 1 | 0 | 0 |
| Vienna Sausage 50% Less Fat | 3 (1.9 oz) | 90 | 1 | 1 | 0 |
| Vienna Sausage Chicken & Beef | 3 (1.9 oz) | 120 | 1 | 1 | 0 |
| Vienna Sausage Hot'n Spicy | 3 (2.1 oz) | 150 | 2 | 0 | 0 |
| Vienna Sausage In BBQ Sauce | 3 (2.1 oz) | 150 | 3 | 3 | 0 |
| Vienna Sausage In Beef Stock | 3 (1.9 oz) | 150 | 0 | 0 | 0 |
| Vienna Sausage Jalapeno In Beef Stock | 3 (1.9 oz) | 170 | 1 | 0 | 0 |
| ***Banner*** | | | | | |
| Sausage Stomachs | 2 oz | 90 | 0 | 0 | 0 |
| Sausage Tripe | 2 oz | 90 | 2 | 0 | 0 |
| ***Boar's Head*** | | | | | |
| Bratwurst | 1 (4 oz) | 300 | 0 | 0 | 0 |
| Hot Smoked | 1 (3.2 oz) | 280 | 1 | 0 | 0 |
| Kielbasa | 2 oz | 120 | 0 | 0 | 0 |
| Knockwurst | 1 (4 oz) | 310 | 1 | 0 | 0 |
| ***Brown'N Serve*** | | | | | |
| Turkey | 3 (2.1 oz) | 120 | 2 | 1 | 0 |
| ***Jones*** | | | | | |
| Light 50% Less Fat | 2 (1.6 oz) | 100 | 1 | – | – |
| ***Perdue*** | | | | | |
| Hot Italian Turkey Cooked | 1 link (2.4 oz) | 150 | 1 | – | – |
| Sweet Italian Turkey Cooked | 1 link (2.4 oz) | 150 | 1 | – | – |

| FOOD | PORTION | CALS | CARB | SUGAR | FIBER |
|---|---|---|---|---|---|
| ***Turkey Store*** | | | | | |
| Breakfast | 2 links (2 oz) | 140 | 1 | – | – |
| ***Wampler*** | | | | | |
| Breakfast Turkey | 2 (2.4 oz) | 110 | 1 | 1 | – |
| Italian Turkey | 1 (2.7 oz) | 120 | 1 | 1 | – |
| **TAKE-OUT** | | | | | |
| pork | 1 patty (1 oz) | 100 | tr | – | – |
| pork | 1 link (0.5 oz) | 48 | tr | – | – |

## SAUSAGE DISHES

| FOOD | PORTION | CALS | CARB | SUGAR | FIBER |
|---|---|---|---|---|---|
| **TAKE-OUT** | | | | | |
| italian sausage w/ peppers & onions | 1 cup | 210 | 14 | – | – |
| sausage roll | 1 (2.3 oz) | 311 | 22 | – | 1 |

## SAUSAGE SUBSTITUTES

| FOOD | PORTION | CALS | CARB | SUGAR | FIBER |
|---|---|---|---|---|---|
| nonmeat sausage | 1 link (25 g) | 64 | 2 | – | – |
| nonmeat sausage | 1 patty (38 g) | 97 | 4 | – | – |
| ***Boca Burgers*** | | | | | |
| Breakfast Patties | 1 (1.3 oz) | 70 | 4 | 1 | 2 |
| ***Lightlife*** | | | | | |
| Gimme Lean | 2 oz | 70 | 8 | 1 | 1 |
| Lean Links Breakfast | 1 (1.2 oz) | 60 | 4 | 1 | 0 |
| Lean Links Italian | 1 (1.4 oz) | 60 | 5 | 1 | 0 |
| Light | 2 patties (2.3 oz) | 80 | 10 | 1 | 1 |
| ***Loma Linda*** | | | | | |
| Linketts | 1 (1.2 oz) | 70 | 1 | 0 | 1 |
| Little Links | 2 (1.6 oz) | 90 | 2 | 0 | 2 |
| ***Morningstar Farms*** | | | | | |
| Breakfast Links | 2 (1.6 oz) | 60 | 2 | 0 | 2 |
| Breakfast Patties | 1 (1.3 oz) | 80 | 3 | tr | 2 |
| Grillers | 1 patty (2.2 oz) | 140 | 5 | tr | 3 |
| Sausage Style Recipe Crumbles | ⅔ cup (1.9 oz) | 90 | 5 | tr | 2 |
| ***Natural Touch*** | | | | | |
| Vegan Sausage Crumbles | ½ cup (1.9 oz) | 60 | 4 | 0 | 2 |
| ***Quron*** | | | | | |
| Meat-Free Links | 2 (1.6 oz) | 70 | 2 | 0 | 1 |

| FOOD | PORTION | CALS | CARB | SUGAR | FIBER |
|---|---|---|---|---|---|
| ***Worthington*** | | | | | |
| Leanies | 1 link (1.4 oz) | 100 | 2 | tr | 1 |
| Prosage Links | 2 (1.6 oz) | 60 | 2 | 0 | 2 |
| ***Yves*** | | | | | |
| Veggie Breakfast Links | 1 (1.6 oz) | 60 | 3 | 1 | 2 |
| Veggie Breakfast Patties | 1 (2 oz) | 70 | 4 | 1 | 2 |
| **SAVORY** | | | | | |
| ground | 1 tsp | 4 | 1 | – | – |
| **SCALLOP** | | | | | |
| **TAKE-OUT** | | | | | |
| breaded & fried | 2 lg | 67 | 3 | – | – |
| **SCONE** | | | | | |
| ***Health Valley*** | | | | | |
| Apple Kiwi | 1 | 180 | 43 | 18 | 5 |
| Cinnamon Raisin | 1 | 180 | 43 | 18 | 5 |
| Cranberry Orange | 1 | 180 | 43 | 18 | 5 |
| Mountain Blueberry | 1 | 180 | 43 | 18 | 5 |
| Pineapple Banana | 1 | 180 | 43 | 18 | 5 |
| **TAKE-OUT** | | | | | |
| apricot | 1 | 232 | 39 | – | – |
| blueberry | 1 (3 oz) | 270 | 41 | 7 | 2 |
| cheese | 1 (3.5 oz) | 364 | 44 | – | 2 |
| orange poppy | 1 (3 oz) | 260 | 47 | 12 | 2 |
| plain | 1 (3.5 oz) | 362 | 54 | – | 2 |
| raisin | 1 (3 oz) | 270 | 43 | 12 | 2 |
| **SCUP** | | | | | |
| fresh baked | 3 oz | 115 | 0 | 0 | 0 |
| **SEA BASS** *(see BASS)* | | | | | |
| **SEA CUCUMBER** | | | | | |
| dried | 1 oz | 74 | 1 | – | 0 |
| fresh | 1 oz | 20 | tr | – | 0 |
| **SEATROUT** *(see TROUT)* | | | | | |
| **SEA URCHIN** | | | | | |
| canned | 1 oz | 39 | 3 | – | 0 |
| fresh | 1 oz | 36 | 3 | – | tr |
| roe paste | 1 tbsp | 19 | 3 | – | 0 |

| FOOD | PORTION | CALS | CARB | SUGAR | FIBER |
|---|---|---|---|---|---|
| **SEAWEED** | | | | | |
| agar dried | 1 oz | 87 | 23 | – | – |
| agar fresh | 1 oz | tr | 2 | – | – |
| hijiki dried | 1 tbsp | 9 | 2 | – | 1 |
| irishmoss fresh | 1 oz | 14 | 4 | – | – |
| kelp fresh | 1 oz | 12 | 3 | – | – |
| kombu fresh | 1 oz | 12 | 3 | – | – |
| laver fresh | 1 oz | 10 | 1 | – | – |
| nori fresh | 1 oz | 10 | 1 | – | – |
| nori sheet dried | 1 (8 x 8 in) | 5 | 1 | – | 1 |
| seahair dried | 1 tbsp | 13 | 3 | – | tr |
| spirulina dried | 1 oz | 83 | 7 | – | – |
| spirulina fresh | 1 oz | 7 | 1 | – | – |
| tangle fresh | 1 oz | 12 | 3 | – | – |
| wakame fresh | 1 oz | 13 | 3 | – | – |
| **SEITAN** *(see* WHEAT*)* | | | | | |
| **SEMOLINA** | | | | | |
| dry | 1 cup (5.9 oz) | 601 | 122 | – | 7 |
| **SESAME** | | | | | |
| seeds | 1 tsp | 16 | tr | – | – |
| sesame butter | 1 tbsp | 95 | 4 | – | 1 |
| sesame crunch candy | 20 pieces (1.2 oz) | 181 | 18 | – | – |
| sesame crunch candy | 1 oz | 146 | 14 | – | – |
| tahini from roasted & toasted kernels | 1 tbsp | 89 | 3 | – | – |
| tahini from stone ground kernels | 1 tbsp | 86 | 4 | – | – |
| tahini from unroasted kernels | 1 tbsp | 85 | 3 | – | – |
| ***Eden*** | | | | | |
| Organic Seaweed Gomasio | 1 serv (1.5 oz) | 10 | 0 | 0 | 0 |
| Organic Gomasio | ½ tsp | 10 | 0 | 0 | tr |
| Organic Gomasio Garlic | ½ tsp | 10 | 0 | 0 | tr |
| ***Maranatha*** | | | | | |
| Raw Tahini | 2 tbsp | 190 | 9 | 0 | 3 |
| Roasted Tahini | 2 tbsp | 210 | 10 | 0 | 2 |
| **SESBANIA** | | | | | |
| flower | 1 | 1 | tr | – | – |

| FOOD | PORTION | CALS | CARB | SUGAR | FIBER |
|---|---|---|---|---|---|
| flowers | 1 cup | 5 | 1 | – | – |
| flowers cooked | 1 cup | 23 | 5 | – | – |
| **SHAD** | | | | | |
| american baked | 3 oz | 214 | 0 | 0 | 0 |
| roe baked w/ butter & lemon | 1 oz | 36 | tr | – | – |
| roe raw | 1 oz | 37 | tr | – | – |
| **SHARK** | | | | | |
| batter-dipped & fried | 3 oz | 194 | 5 | – | – |
| raw | 3 oz | 111 | 0 | 0 | 0 |
| **SHEEPSHEAD FISH** | | | | | |
| cooked | 3 oz | 107 | 0 | 0 | 0 |
| cooked | 1 fillet (6.5 oz) | 234 | 0 | 0 | 0 |
| **SHELLFISH** *(see individual names,* SHELLFISH SUBSTITUTES*)* | | | | | |
| **SHELLFISH SUBSTITUTES** | | | | | |
| crab imitation | 3 oz | 87 | 1 | – | – |
| scallop imitation | 3 oz | 84 | 9 | – | – |
| shrimp imitation | 3 oz | 86 | 8 | – | – |
| surimi | 3 oz | 84 | 6 | – | – |
| surimi | 1 oz | 28 | 2 | – | – |
| ***Louis Kemp*** | | | | | |
| Crab Delights | ½ cup (3 oz) | 90 | 12 | 8 | 2 |
| Lobster Delights | ½ cup (3 oz) | 80 | 12 | 4 | 0 |
| Scallop Delights | 13 pieces (3 oz) | 80 | 12 | 3 | 0 |
| **SHELLIE BEANS** | | | | | |
| canned | ½ cup | 37 | 8 | – | – |
| **SHERBET** | | | | | |
| orange | ½ cup (4 fl oz) | 132 | 29 | – | – |
| orange | ½ gal | 2158 | 469 | – | – |
| orange | 1 bar (2.75 fl oz) | 91 | 20 | – | – |
| orange home recipe | ½ cup | 120 | 24 | – | – |
| ***Breyers*** | | | | | |
| Orange | ½ cup | 120 | 26 | 19 | 0 |
| Rainbow | ½ cup | 120 | 26 | 20 | 0 |

| FOOD | PORTION | CALS | CARB | SUGAR | FIBER |
|---|---|---|---|---|---|
| ***Turkey Hill*** | | | | | |
| Fruit Rainbow | ½ cup | 120 | 26 | – | – |
| Orange Grove | ½ cup | 120 | 26 | – | – |
| **SHRIMP** | | | | | |
| canned | 3 oz | 102 | 1 | – | – |
| canned | 1 cup | 154 | 1 | – | – |
| chinese shrimp paste | 1 tbsp | 15 | 1 | – | – |
| cooked | 3 oz | 84 | 0 | 0 | 0 |
| cooked | 4 large | 22 | 0 | 0 | 0 |
| ***Bumble Bee*** | | | | | |
| Medium | ⅓ can (2 oz) | 45 | 0 | 1 | 0 |
| Orleans Tiny Cocktail | ½ can (3 oz) | 44 | 0 | 1 | 0 |
| ***Gorton's*** | | | | | |
| Popcorn Garlic & Herb | 22 pieces (3.6 oz) | 270 | 24 | 3 | – |
| Popcorn Original | 20 pieces (3.2 oz) | 240 | 22 | 1 | – |
| **TAKE-OUT** | | | | | |
| breaded & fried | 3 oz | 206 | 10 | – | – |
| jambalaya | ¾ cup | 188 | 26 | – | 8 |
| **SMELT** | | | | | |
| rainbow cooked | 3 oz | 106 | 0 | 0 | 0 |
| rainbow raw | 3 oz | 83 | 0 | 0 | 0 |
| **SMOOTHIE** *(see* FRUIT DRINKS*)* | | | | | |
| **SNACKS** | | | | | |
| cheese puffs | 1 oz | 157 | 15 | – | tr |
| corn puffs cheese | 1 bag (8 oz) | 1256 | 122 | – | 2 |
| corn twists cheese | 1 oz | 157 | 15 | – | tr |
| corn twists cheese | 1 bag (8 oz) | 1256 | 122 | – | 2 |
| oriental mix | 1 oz | 155 | 9 | – | – |
| pork skins | 1 oz | 154 | 0 | 0 | 0 |
| pork skins barbecue | 1 oz | 152 | 1 | – | – |
| trail mix | 1 oz | 131 | 13 | – | – |
| trail mix | 1 cup (5.3 oz) | 693 | 67 | – | – |
| trail mix tropical | 1 oz | 115 | 19 | – | – |
| trail mix w/ chocolate chips | 1 cup (5.1 oz) | 707 | 66 | – | – |
| trail mix w/ chocolate chips | 1 oz | 137 | 13 | – | – |

| FOOD | PORTION | CALS | CARB | SUGAR | FIBER |
|---|---|---|---|---|---|
| ***Baken-ets*** | | | | | |
| BBQ | 9 (0.5 oz) | 70 | tr | 0 | tr |
| Hot N'Spicy | 7 (0.5 oz) | 70 | tr | 0 | tr |
| Hot N'Spicy Cracklins | 8 (0.5 oz) | 80 | tr | 0 | tr |
| Regular | 9 (0.5 oz) | 80 | tr | 0 | tr |
| Regular Cracklins | 8 (0.5 oz) | 40 | tr | 0 | tr |
| ***Barbara's Bakery*** | | | | | |
| Cheese Puffs Bakes | 1½ cups (1 oz) | 160 | 13 | 1 | 0 |
| Cheese Puffs Jalapeno | ¾ cup (1 oz) | 150 | 16 | 0 | 0 |
| Cheese Puffs Original | ¾ cup (1 oz) | 150 | 16 | 0 | 0 |
| ***Bowlby's*** | | | | | |
| Bits Almond | ½ cup | 100 | 5 | 1 | 1 |
| Bits Pecan | ½ cup | 200 | 5 | 1 | 1 |
| Bits Ranch | ½ cup | 170 | 7 | 2 | 0 |
| Bits Salsa | ½ cup | 170 | 7 | 2 | 0 |
| Bits Sour Cream Onion & Dill | ½ cup | 170 | 7 | 2 | 0 |
| Bits'N'Pops | ¾ cup | 130 | 16 | 13 | 1 |
| Mix-Ups Country Mix | ½ cup | 170 | 8 | 1 | 1 |
| Mix-Ups Nuttyest-Of-All | ½ cup | 160 | 8 | 2 | 1 |
| Mix-Ups Trail Mix | ½ cup | 165 | 11 | 6 | 1 |
| ***Bugles*** | | | | | |
| Baked Original | 1⅓ cup | 130 | 23 | 2 | – |
| Chile Con Queso | 1⅓ cups | 160 | 18 | 1 | – |
| Nacho | 1½ cups | 160 | 18 | 1 | – |
| Original | 1½ cups | 160 | 18 | 1 | tr |
| Smokin'BBQ | 1⅓ cups | 150 | 19 | 2 | – |
| ***Cheetos*** | | | | | |
| Crunchy | 21 pieces (1 oz) | 160 | 15 | 1 | tr |
| Curls | 15 pieces (1 oz) | 150 | 15 | 1 | 1 |
| Flamin' Hot | 21 pieces (1 oz) | 160 | 15 | 1 | tr |
| Nacho Cheese | 23 pieces (1 oz) | 160 | 15 | 0 | tr |
| Puffed Balls | 38 pieces (1 oz) | 150 | 15 | 1 | tr |
| Puffs | 29 pieces (1 oz) | 160 | 15 | tr | tr |

| FOOD | PORTION | CALS | CARB | SUGAR | FIBER |
|---|---|---|---|---|---|
| Zig Zags | 17 pieces (1 oz) | 170 | 17 | tr | tr |
| ***Chex Mix*** | | | | | |
| Cheddar | ⅔ cup | 140 | 21 | 2 | 2 |
| Hot'N Spicy | ⅔ cup | 130 | 21 | 2 | 2 |
| Nacho Fiesta | ⅔ cup | 120 | 22 | 2 | 1 |
| Party Blend Bold | ⅔ cup | 140 | 20 | 2 | 2 |
| Peanut Lovers | ⅔ cup | 140 | 19 | 2 | 1 |
| Traditional | ⅔ cup | 130 | 22 | 2 | 1 |
| ***Dakota Gourmet*** | | | | | |
| Amazing Corn Classic | 1 pkg (1 oz) | 360 | 78 | – | 5 |
| Amazing Corn Cool Ranch | 1 pkg (1 oz) | 367 | 74 | – | 5 |
| Amazing Corn Mesquite BBQ | 1 pkg (1 oz) | 369 | 76 | – | 5 |
| Heart Smart Toasted Corn | ⅓ cup (1 oz) | 110 | 22 | 0 | 3 |
| Toasted Corn Heart Smart | 1 pkg (1.75 oz) | 177 | 39 | 0 | 2 |
| Trail Mix Heart Smart | 1 pkg (1.75 oz) | 172 | 39 | 25 | 3 |
| ***Eden*** | | | | | |
| Rice Puffs Five Flavor Arare | 1 oz | 110 | 24 | 0 | 2 |
| ***Frito Lay*** | | | | | |
| Funyuns | 13 (1 oz) | 140 | 18 | tr | tr |
| Munchos | 16 (1 oz) | 160 | 16 | 0 | 1 |
| Munchos BBQ | 14 (1 oz) | 160 | 15 | 2 | 1 |
| ***Glenny's*** | | | | | |
| Soy Crisps All Flavors | 5 | 60 | 8 | 0 | 1 |
| ***Gram's Gourmet*** | | | | | |
| Crunchies Pork Rinds | ⅛ pkg (0.5 oz) | 70 | 0 | 0 | 0 |
| ***Health Valley*** | | | | | |
| Cheddar Lites Green Onion | 1¾ cups | 120 | 21 | 1 | 1 |
| Cheddar Lites Original | 1¾ cups | 120 | 21 | 1 | 1 |
| Corn Puffs Caramel | 2 cups | 120 | 25 | 7 | 1 |
| Low Fat Potato Puffs Cheddar Cheese | 1½ cups | 110 | 21 | 1 | 1 |
| Low Fat Potato Puffs Garlic w/ Cheese | 1½ cups | 260 | 21 | 1 | 1 |
| Low Fat Potato Puffs Zesty Ranch | 1½ cups | 110 | 21 | 1 | 1 |

| FOOD | PORTION | CALS | CARB | SUGAR | FIBER |
|---|---|---|---|---|---|
| ***J&J*** | | | | | |
| Microwave Pork Rinds All Flavors | 1 oz | 130 | tr | – | 0 |
| ***Lance*** | | | | | |
| Cheese Balls | 1 pkg (1 oz) | 150 | 16 | 1 | 0 |
| Crunchy Cheese Twists | 1 pkg (1.25 oz) | 190 | 15 | 0 | 0 |
| Gold-N-Chees | 1 pkg (1 oz) | 130 | 18 | 0 | 1 |
| Onion Rings | 1 pkg (0.9 oz) | 100 | 7 | 1 | 1 |
| Pork Skins | 1 pkg (0.4 oz) | 65 | 1 | 0 | 0 |
| Pork Skins BBQ | 1 pkg (0.4 oz) | 60 | 1 | 0 | 0 |
| ***Maranatha*** | | | | | |
| High Energy Mix | ¼ cup | 120 | 15 | 12 | 2 |
| Organic Harvest Mix | ¼ cup | 150 | 15 | 2 | 2 |
| Organic Nature Mix | ¼ cup | 150 | 15 | 2 | 2 |
| Snack Attack Mix | ¼ cup | 140 | 16 | 12 | 2 |
| Tail Mix Organic Raw | ¼ cup | 140 | 13 | 10 | 2 |
| Trail Mix Deluxe | ¼ cup | 150 | 11 | 8 | 2 |
| Trail Mix Navajo | ¼ cup | 140 | 13 | 8 | 4 |
| Trail Mix Olympic w/ Chocolate | ¼ cup | 140 | 16 | 13 | 2 |
| Trail Mix Organic Delight | ¼ cup | 150 | 12 | 8 | 2 |
| ***Old Dutch Foods*** | | | | | |
| Baked Cheese Curls | 2 cups (1.1 oz) | 180 | 15 | 1 | tr |
| Cheese Puffcorn Curls | 2 cups (1.1 oz) | 170 | 15 | 1 | 0 |
| ***Planters*** | | | | | |
| Cheez Mania Original | 42 pieces (1 oz) | 150 | 15 | tr | 1 |
| ***Pumpkorn*** | | | | | |
| Caramel | ⅓ cup | 150 | 4 | – | 2 |
| Chili | ⅓ cup | 150 | 4 | – | 2 |
| Curry | ⅓ cup | 150 | 4 | – | 2 |
| Maple Vanilla | ⅓ cup | 150 | 4 | – | 2 |
| Mesquite | ⅓ cup | 150 | 4 | – | 2 |
| Original | ⅓ cup | 150 | 4 | – | 2 |
| ***Robert's American Gourmet*** | | | | | |
| Pirate's Booty Puffed Rice & Corn w/ Cheddar | 1 oz | 120 | 22 | 0 | 4 |
| ***Rold Gold*** | | | | | |
| Snack Mix Colossal Cheddar | 1 pkg (1 oz) | 140 | 17 | 2 | 1 |

| FOOD | PORTION | CALS | CARB | SUGAR | FIBER |
|---|---|---|---|---|---|
| ***Snyder's Of Hanover*** | | | | | |
| Cheese Twists | 1 oz | 230 | 10 | 0 | 0 |
| Fried Pork Skins | 1 oz | 80 | 1 | 0 | 0 |
| Fried Pork Skins Barbecue | 1 oz | 80 | 1 | 0 | 0 |
| Kruncheez | 1.25 oz | 200 | 19 | tr | tr |
| Onion Toasters | 1 oz | 188 | 21 | tr | tr |
| ***Utz*** | | | | | |
| Caramel Corn Clusters | 1⅛ cups (1 oz) | 120 | 24 | 13 | tr |
| Cheese Balls | 50 (1 oz) | 150 | 16 | tr | tr |
| Cheese Curls | 18 (1 oz) | 150 | 16 | tr | tr |
| Cheese Curls Crunchy | 30 (1 oz) | 160 | 16 | tr | 0 |
| Cheese Curls Reduced Fat | 32 (1 oz) | 140 | 18 | tr | 2 |
| Onion Rings | 41 (1 oz) | 140 | 18 | 2 | 0 |
| Party Mix | ¾ cup (1 oz) | 140 | 19 | tr | 1 |
| Pork Cracklins | 0.5 oz | 90 | 0 | – | – |
| Pork Cracklins Hot & Spicy | 0.5 oz | 80 | 0 | – | – |
| Pork Rinds | 0.5 oz | 80 | 0 | – | – |
| Pork Rinds BBQ | 0.5 oz | 80 | 0 | – | – |
| ***Weight Watchers*** | | | | | |
| Cheese Curls | 1 pkg (0.5 oz) | 70 | 10 | 0 | 0 |
| **SNAIL** | | | | | |
| cooked | 3 oz | 233 | 13 | – | – |
| **TAKE-OUT** | | | | | |
| escargot cooked | 5 | 25 | 1 | – | 0 |
| **SNAKE** | | | | | |
| fresh | 3 oz | 78 | 3 | – | 0 |
| **SNAPPER** | | | | | |
| cooked | 1 fillet (6 oz) | 217 | 0 | 0 | 0 |
| cooked | 3 oz | 109 | 0 | 0 | 0 |
| **SODA** | | | | | |
| club | 12 oz | 0 | 0 | 0 | 0 |
| cola | 12 oz | 151 | 39 | – | – |
| cream | 12 oz | 191 | 49 | – | – |
| diet cola | 12 oz | 2 | tr | – | – |
| diet cola w/ equal | 12 oz | 2 | tr | – | – |
| diet cola w/ saccharin | 12 oz | 2 | tr | – | – |
| ginger ale | 12 oz can | 124 | 32 | – | – |

| FOOD | PORTION | CALS | CARB | SUGAR | FIBER |
|---|---|---|---|---|---|
| grape | 12 oz | 161 | 42 | – | – |
| lemon lime | 12 oz | 149 | 38 | – | – |
| orange | 12 oz | 177 | 46 | – | – |
| pepper type | 12 oz | 151 | 38 | – | – |
| quinine | 12 oz | 125 | 32 | – | – |
| root beer | 12 oz | 152 | 39 | – | – |
| shirley temple | 1 serv | 159 | 41 | – | 0 |
| tonic water | 12 oz | 125 | 32 | – | – |
| ***7 Up*** | | | | | |
| Diet | 8 oz | 0 | 0 | 0 | – |
| Original | 1 can | 140 | 39 | 39 | – |
| ***A & W*** | | | | | |
| Root Beer | 1 can (12 oz) | 170 | 46 | 46 | – |
| ***Barq's*** | | | | | |
| Root Beer | 1 can (12 oz) | 160 | 45 | 45 | – |
| ***Barritts*** | | | | | |
| Ginger Beer | 1 bottle (12 oz) | 200 | 49 | 49 | – |
| ***Best Health*** | | | | | |
| Root Beer | 1 bottle (12 oz) | 165 | 42 | 42 | – |
| Vanilla Cream | 1 bottle (12 oz) | 170 | 43 | 43 | – |
| ***Canada Dry*** | | | | | |
| Ginger Ale | 1 can (12 oz) | 140 | 35 | 35 | 0 |
| Tonic Water | 8 fl oz | 90 | 24 | 24 | 0 |
| ***Coca-Cola*** | | | | | |
| Classic | 1 can (12 oz) | 140 | 39 | 39 | – |
| Diet | 1 can (12 oz) | 0 | 0 | 0 | – |
| ***Dr Pepper*** | | | | | |
| Original | 1 can (12 oz) | 150 | 40 | 40 | – |
| ***Hansen's*** | | | | | |
| Black Cherry | 8 fl oz | 110 | 30 | 29 | – |
| Diet All Flavors | 1 can | 0 | 0 | 0 | – |
| Ginger Beer | 8 fl oz | 100 | 28 | 28 | – |
| Natural Black Cherry | 1 can | 160 | 44 | 43 | – |
| Natural Cherry Vanilla | 1 can | 140 | 39 | 39 | – |
| Natural Creamy Rootbeer | 1 can | 160 | 44 | 44 | – |
| Natural Ginger Ale | 1 can | 140 | 37 | 37 | – |
| Natural Grapefruit | 1 can | 130 | 38 | 36 | – |

| FOOD | PORTION | CALS | CARB | SUGAR | FIBER |
|---|---|---|---|---|---|
| Natural Key Lime | 1 can | 130 | 37 | 36 | – |
| Natural Kiwi Strawberry | 1 can | 130 | 38 | 36 | – |
| Natural Mandarin Lime | 1 can | 130 | 37 | 35 | – |
| Natural Orange Mango | 1 can | 170 | 46 | 46 | – |
| Natural Raspberry | 1 can | 130 | 36 | 37 | – |
| Natural Tangerine | 1 can | 160 | 43 | 35 | – |
| Natural Tropical Passion | 1 can | 160 | 43 | 42 | – |
| Natural Vanilla Cola | 1 can | 140 | 39 | 37 | – |
| Orange Creme | 8 fl oz | 110 | 31 | 31 | – |
| Sangria | 8 fl oz | 110 | 30 | 30 | – |
| Sarsaparilla | 8 fl oz | 110 | 30 | 30 | – |
| Sparkling Orangeade | 8 fl oz | 100 | 25 | 25 | – |
| Vanilla Creme | 8 fl oz | 110 | 30 | 30 | – |
| ***Health Valley*** | | | | | |
| Ginger Ale | 1 bottle | 160 | 40 | 40 | 0 |
| Rootbeer Old Fashioned | 1 bottle | 160 | 40 | 40 | 0 |
| Sarsaparilla Rootbeer | 1 bottle | 160 | 40 | 40 | 0 |
| ***IBC*** | | | | | |
| Root Beer | 1 can | 160 | 43 | 43 | – |
| ***Jones Soda*** | | | | | |
| Sugar Free All Flavors | 1 bottle (12 oz) | 0 | 0 | 0 | – |
| ***Lucozade*** | | | | | |
| Soda | 7 oz | 136 | 36 | – | 0 |
| ***Olde Brooklyn*** | | | | | |
| Flatbush Orange | 8 oz | 130 | 33 | 33 | – |
| Williamsburg Root Beer | 8 oz | 120 | 32 | 32 | – |
| ***Olde Philadelphia*** | | | | | |
| Black Cherry | 1 bottle (12 oz) | 180 | 45 | 45 | – |
| Cream | 1 bottle (12 oz) | 190 | 47 | 47 | – |
| Cream Diet | 1 bottle (12 oz) | 0 | 0 | 0 | – |
| Grape | 1 bottle (12 oz) | 180 | 45 | 45 | – |
| Orange Cream | 1 bottle (12 oz) | 190 | 49 | 49 | – |
| Pineapple | 1 bottle | 190 | 48 | 48 | – |

| FOOD | PORTION | CALS | CARB | SUGAR | FIBER |
|---|---|---|---|---|---|
| Root Beer | 1 bottle (12 oz) | 180 | 44 | 44 | – |
| ***Pennsylvania Dutch*** | | | | | |
| Birch Beer | 8 fl oz | 110 | 28 | 28 | – |
| ***Pepsi*** | | | | | |
| Blue Berry Cola Fusion | 8 fl oz | 100 | 28 | 27 | – |
| Diet | 1 can (12 oz) | 0 | 0 | 0 | – |
| Regular | 1 can (12 oz) | 150 | 41 | 41 | – |
| Vanilla | 1 can | 160 | 43 | 42 | – |
| Vanilla Diet | 1 can | 0 | 0 | 0 | 0 |
| ***Prism*** | | | | | |
| Green Tea Soda Cola | 8 oz | 105 | 26 | 26 | – |
| Lemon Lime | 8 oz | 117 | 29 | 29 | – |
| ***Qibla*** | | | | | |
| Cola | 1 bottle (18 oz) | 185 | 11 | – | – |
| Diet Cola | 1 bottle (18 oz) | 1 | 0 | 0 | 0 |
| ***Saranac*** | | | | | |
| Diet Root Beer | 1 bottle (12 oz) | 35 | 9 | 9 | – |
| Ginger Beer | 1 bottle (12 oz) | 160 | 42 | 42 | – |
| Root Beer | 1 bottle (12 oz) | 180 | 46 | 46 | – |
| ***Seagram's*** | | | | | |
| Ginger Ale | 1 can (12 oz) | 130 | 35 | 35 | – |
| ***Sex Cola*** | | | | | |
| All Flavors | 1 bottle (12 oz) | 0 | 0 | 0 | 0 |
| ***Ski*** | | | | | |
| Citrus | 1 bottle (10 oz) | 150 | 40 | 40 | – |
| ***Steap*** | | | | | |
| Green Tea Soda Root Beer | 8 oz | 90 | 23 | 23 | – |
| ***Stewart's*** | | | | | |
| Root Beer | 1 bottle (12 oz) | 160 | 41 | 41 | – |
| Strawberries N' Cream | 1 bottle | 200 | 50 | 50 | – |
| Wishniak Black Cherry | 1 bottle | 180 | 47 | 47 | – |

| FOOD | PORTION | CALS | CARB | SUGAR | FIBER |
|---|---|---|---|---|---|
| ***Sunkist*** | | | | | |
| Orange | 1 can | 190 | 52 | 52 | 0 |
| ***Vermont Sweetwater*** | | | | | |
| Coutry Apple Jack | 1 bottle | 180 | 42 | 42 | 0 |
| Kickin'Cow Cola | 1 bottle | 129 | 33 | 33 | 0 |
| Mango Moonshine | 1 bottle | 180 | 42 | 42 | 0 |
| Maple | 1 bottle | 101 | 27 | 27 | 0 |
| Raspberry Rhubarb Ramble | 1 bottle | 180 | 42 | 42 | 0 |
| Tangerine Cream Twister | 1 bottle | 180 | 42 | 42 | 0 |
| Vermont Maple Seltzer | 1 bottle | 53 | 12 | 12 | 0 |
| ***White T*** | | | | | |
| All Flavors | 1 bottle (12 oz) | 128 | 33 | 33 | 0 |
| Diet All Flavors | 1 bottle (12 oz) | 0 | 0 | 0 | 0 |
| ***Yoo-Hoo*** | | | | | |
| Original | 9 fl oz | 150 | 31 | – | tr |
| **SOLE** | | | | | |
| cooked | 3 oz | 99 | 0 | 0 | 0 |
| cooked | 1 fillet (4.5 oz) | 148 | 0 | 0 | 0 |
| lemon raw | 3.5 oz | 85 | 0 | 0 | 0 |
| **TAKE-OUT** | | | | | |
| battered & fried | 3.2 oz | 211 | 15 | – | – |
| breaded & fried | 3.2 oz | 211 | 15 | – | – |
| **SORGHUM** | | | | | |
| sorghum | 1 cup (6.7 oz) | 651 | 143 | – | – |
| **SOUFFLE** | | | | | |
| lemon chilled | 1 cup | 176 | 34 | – | – |
| raspberry chilled | 1 cup | 173 | 34 | – | – |
| spinach | 1 cup | 218 | 3 | – | – |
| **SOUP** | | | | | |
| **CANNED** | | | | | |
| ***Amy's*** | | | | | |
| Organic Barley | 1 cup | 50 | 10 | 4 | 2 |
| Organic Black Bean Vegetable | 1 cup | 110 | 22 | 6 | 5 |
| Organic Cream Of Mushroom | 1 cup | 120 | 10 | 2 | 2 |
| Organic Cream of Tomato | 1 cup | 100 | 17 | 11 | 4 |

| FOOD | PORTION | CALS | CARB | SUGAR | FIBER |
|---|---|---|---|---|---|
| Organic Lentil | 1 cup | 130 | 19 | 3 | 9 |
| Organic Minestrone | 1 cup | 90 | 17 | 5 | 3 |
| Organic No Chicken Noodle Soup | 1 cup | 90 | 12 | 4 | 2 |
| Organic Vegetable | 1 cup | 35 | 8 | 4 | 1 |
| ***Boston Market*** | | | | | |
| Chicken Broth Reduced Sodium | 1 cup | 15 | 1 | 0 | 0 |
| ***Butterball*** | | | | | |
| Chicken Broth Reduced Sodium 99% Fat Free | 1 cup | 10 | 2 | 0 | 0 |
| ***Campbell's*** | | | | | |
| 98% Fat Free Cream Of Chicken as prep | 1 cup | 80 | 10 | 0 | 0 |
| Bean With Bacon as prep | 1 cup | 168 | 26 | 3 | 8 |
| Beef Barley as prep | 1 cup | 81 | 11 | 1 | 2 |
| Cheddar Cheese | 1 cup | 110 | 12 | 2 | 1 |
| Cheddar Cheese as prep | 1 cup | 134 | 11 | 1 | 1 |
| Chicken Vegetable as prep | 1 cup | 74 | 9 | 1 | 1 |
| Chicken Gumbo as prep | 1 cup | 55 | 9 | 2 | 1 |
| Chunky Savory Chicken w/ White & Wild Rice | 1 cup | 140 | 18 | 2 | 2 |
| Chunky Classic Chicken Noodle | 1 cup (8.4 oz) | 130 | 15 | 4 | 1 |
| Clam Chowder New England as prep | 1 cup | 89 | 13 | tr | 1 |
| Classic Chicken Rice | 1 cup (8.4 oz) | 80 | 14 | 0 | 1 |
| Classics Beef Noodle | 1 cup | 70 | 8 | 1 | 1 |
| Consomme as prep | 1 cup | 24 | 1 | 1 | tr |
| Cream Of Asparagus as prep | 1 cup | 72 | 9 | 3 | 1 |
| Cream Of Mushroom as prep | 1 cup | 108 | 9 | 1 | 2 |
| Cream Of Celery as prep | 1 cup | 107 | 9 | 1 | 1 |
| Cream Of Chicken as prep | 1 cup | 120 | 10 | 1 | 1 |
| Cream Of Potato as prep | 1 cup | 102 | 15 | 1 | 1 |
| Cream of Chicken w/ Herbs | 1 cup | 90 | 10 | 2 | 1 |
| Fiesta Tomato as prep | 1 cup | 72 | 16 | 8 | 1 |
| Garden Vegetable as prep | 1 cup | 69 | 11 | 2 | 1 |
| Green Pea as prep | 1 cup | 173 | 29 | 4 | 4 |
| Healthy Request Chicken Noodle as prep | 1 cup | 70 | 9 | 1 | 0 |
| Healthy Request Chicken Rice as prep | 1 cup | 60 | 8 | 1 | tr |

| FOOD | PORTION | CALS | CARB | SUGAR | FIBER |
|---|---|---|---|---|---|
| Healthy Request Cream Of Mushroom as prep | 1 cup | 66 | 10 | 2 | 1 |
| Healthy Request Cream Of Chicken & Broccoli as prep | 1 cup | 78 | 10 | 2 | 1 |
| Healthy Request Cream Of Chicken as prep | 1 cup | 70 | 12 | 2 | tr |
| Healthy Request Hearty Pasta w/ Vegetables | 1 cup | 87 | 17 | 7 | 2 |
| Healthy Request Tomato as prep | 1 cup | 91 | 18 | 9 | 2 |
| Healthy Request Vegetable as prep | 1 cup | 84 | 17 | 5 | 2 |
| Home Cookin' Chicken Vegetable | 1 cup (8.4 oz) | 130 | 20 | 6 | 3 |
| Home Cookin' Chicken Rice | 1 cup | 110 | 20 | 3 | 2 |
| Home Cookin' Chicken With Egg Noodles | 1 cup (8.4 oz) | 90 | 13 | 2 | 1 |
| Home Cookin' Oriental Noodles w/ Vegetables | 1 cup (8.4 oz) | 100 | 18 | 5 | 3 |
| Italian Tomato as prep | 1 cup | 105 | 23 | 16 | 4 |
| Kitchen Classics Chicken Noodle | 1 cup | 980 | 13 | 1 | 1 |
| Low Sodium Chicken Broth | 1 can (10.75 oz) | 27 | 2 | 1 | tr |
| Low Sodium Chicken W/ Noodles | 1 can (10.75 oz) | 162 | 16 | 3 | 2 |
| Low Sodium Chunky Vegetable Beef | 1 can (10.75 oz) | 159 | 17 | 5 | 3 |
| Low Sodium Cream of Mushroom | 1 can (10.75 oz) | 200 | 18 | 5 | 2 |
| Low Sodium Green Pea | 1 can (10.75 oz) | 235 | 38 | 4 | 6 |
| Low Sodium Tomato w/ Pieces | 1 can (10.75 oz) | 170 | 28 | 17 | 3 |
| Minestrone as prep | 1 cup | 81 | 12 | 2 | 2 |
| Ready To Serve Bean w/ Bacon 'N Ham | 1 can (10.5 oz) | 274 | 41 | 8 | 11 |
| Ready To Serve Chicken Noodle | 1 cup | 80 | 11 | 1 | 1 |
| Ready To Serve Chicken w/ Rice | 1 can (10.5 oz) | 122 | 20 | 4 | 2 |

| FOOD | PORTION | CALS | CARB | SUGAR | FIBER |
|---|---|---|---|---|---|
| Ready-To-Serve Vegetable Beef | 1 can (10.5 oz) | 143 | 26 | 5 | 5 |
| Savory Tomato & Dill as prep | 1 cup | 99 | 20 | 11 | 2 |
| Select Chicken & Pasta With Roasted Garlic | 1 cup (8.4 oz) | 100 | 16 | 4 | 2 |
| Select Chicken Rice | 1 cup | 110 | 18 | 2 | 2 |
| Select Fiesta Vegetable | 1 cup (8.4 oz) | 120 | 24 | 7 | 3 |
| Select Herbed Chicken w/ Roasted Vegetables | 1 cup | 90 | 14 | 2 | 1 |
| Select Italian Style Wedding | 1 cup | 120 | 16 | 3 | 2 |
| Select Mushroom w/ White & Wild Rice | 1 cup | 90 | 16 | 2 | 2 |
| Select Roasted Chicken w/ Rotini & Penne Pasta | 1 cup | 90 | 16 | 4 | 2 |
| Select Rosemary Chicken w/ Roasted Potatoes | 1 cup | 110 | 18 | 2 | 2 |
| Select Split Pea w/ Ham | 1 cup (8.4 oz) | 170 | 30 | 6 | 6 |
| Select Tuscany Style Minestrone | 1 cup (8.4 oz) | 190 | 21 | 5 | 5 |
| Simply Home Chicken Noodle | 1 cup (8.4 oz) | 80 | 12 | 2 | 1 |
| Simply Home Chicken With Rice | 1 cup (8.4 oz) | 100 | 19 | 2 | 1 |
| Soup At Hand Blended Vegetable Medley | 1 pkg (10.75 oz) | 110 | 21 | 10 | 4 |
| Tomato as prep | 1 cup | 80 | 18 | 10 | 2 |
| Vegetable Beef as prep | 1 cup | 68 | 9 | 1 | 2 |
| Vegetarian Vegetable as prep | 1 cup | 79 | 14 | 3 | 2 |
| ***College Inn*** | | | | | |
| Beef Broth 99% Fat Free | 1 cup | 20 | 0 | 0 | 0 |
| Chicken Broth Fat Free 50% Less Sodium | 1 cup | 10 | 0 | 0 | 0 |
| ***Gold's*** | | | | | |
| Russian Borscht | 8 oz | 70 | 17 | 15 | 2 |
| ***Health Valley*** | | | | | |
| 5 Bean Vegetable | 1 cup | 250 | 32 | 9 | 10 |
| Beef Broth Fat Free | 1 cup | 20 | 0 | 2 | 0 |
| Beef Broth Fat Free No Salt | 1 cup | 20 | 0 | 2 | 0 |
| Black Bean & Vegetable | 1 cup | 110 | 24 | 8 | 9 |
| Chicken Broth | 1 cup | 45 | 0 | 0 | 0 |
| Chicken Broth Fat Free | 1 cup | 30 | 0 | 0 | 0 |
| Chicken Broth No Salt | 1 cup | 45 | 0 | 0 | 0 |
| Country Corn & Vegetable | 1 cup | 70 | 17 | 8 | 7 |

| FOOD | PORTION | CALS | CARB | SUGAR | FIBER |
|---|---|---|---|---|---|
| Garden Vegetable | 1 cup | 80 | 17 | 8 | 4 |
| Italian Plus Carotene | 1 cup | 80 | 19 | 5 | 6 |
| Lentil & Carrot | 1 cup | 100 | 25 | 7 | 10 |
| Organic Black Bean | 1 cup | 110 | 28 | 14 | 10 |
| Organic Lentil No Salt | 1 cup | 90 | 20 | 7 | 9 |
| Organic Minestrone | 1 cup | 100 | 23 | 6 | 8 |
| Organic Mushroom Barley No Salt | 1 cup | 60 | 15 | 5 | 5 |
| Organic Potato Leek | 1 cup | 70 | 15 | 5 | 3 |
| Organic Potato Leek No Salt | 1 cup | 70 | 15 | 5 | 3 |
| Organic Split Pea | 1 cup | 110 | 23 | 5 | 8 |
| Organic Split Pea No Salt | 1 cup | 110 | 23 | 5 | 8 |
| Organic Tomato | 1 cup | 90 | 22 | 20 | 4 |
| Organic Vegetable No Salt | 1 cup | 80 | 18 | 10 | 6 |
| Pasta Bolognese | 1 cup | 100 | 20 | 4 | 4 |
| Pasta Cacciatore | 1 cup | 100 | 20 | 6 | 4 |
| Pasta Romano | 1 cup | 100 | 20 | 6 | 4 |
| Real Italian Minestrone | 1 cup | 90 | 21 | 6 | 8 |
| Rotini & Vegetable | 1 cup | 100 | 20 | 4 | 4 |
| Split Pea & Carrots | 1 cup | 110 | 17 | 7 | 4 |
| Super Broccoli Carotene | 1 cup | 70 | 16 | 12 | 7 |
| Tomato Vegetable | 1 cup | 80 | 17 | 9 | 5 |
| Vegetable Barley | 1 cup | 90 | 19 | 4 | 4 |
| Vegetable Power Carotene | 1 cup | 70 | 17 | 7 | 6 |
| ***Healthy Choice*** | | | | | |
| Bean & Ham | 1 cup (8.7 oz) | 166 | 31 | 3 | 7 |
| Beef & Potato | 1 cup (8.5 oz) | 116 | 16 | 3 | tr |
| Broccoli Cheddar | 1 cup (8.4 oz) | 116 | 22 | 1 | 2 |
| Chicken Corn Chowder | 1 cup (8.8 oz) | 176 | 30 | 2 | 2 |
| Chicken Pasta | 1 cup (8.6 oz) | 119 | 18 | 0 | 1 |
| Chicken Rice | 1 cup (8.4 oz) | 119 | 19 | 3 | 3 |
| Chili Beef | 1 cup (9.1 oz) | 189 | 32 | 5 | 5 |
| Clam Chowder | 1 cup (8.8 oz) | 123 | 23 | 3 | 2 |
| Classic Italian Bean and Pasta | 1 cup (8 oz) | 100 | 17 | 0 | 3 |
| Country Vegetable | 1 cup (8.6 oz) | 112 | 24 | 5 | 3 |
| Cream Of Mushroom | 1 cup (8.8 oz) | 77 | 14 | 0 | 1 |
| Cream Of Celery as prep | 1 cup | 73 | 14 | 2 | 3 |
| Cream Of Chicken Vegetable | 1 cup (8.9 oz) | 127 | 21 | 0 | 1 |
| Cream Of Roasted Chicken as prep | 1 cup | 80 | 13 | 1 | 3 |

| FOOD | PORTION | CALS | CARB | SUGAR | FIBER |
|---|---|---|---|---|---|
| Cream Of Roasted Garlic as prep | 1 cup | 57 | 13 | 0 | 3 |
| Garden Tomato Herbs as prep | 1 cup | 80 | 18 | 11 | 3 |
| Garden Vegetable | 1 cup (8.6 oz) | 108 | 22 | 0 | 6 |
| Hearty Chicken | 1 cup (8.6 oz) | 136 | 20 | 1 | 3 |
| Lentil | 1 cup (8.7 oz) | 135 | 28 | 2 | 5 |
| Minestrone | 1 cup (8.6 oz) | 107 | 24 | 4 | 5 |
| Old Fashion Chicken Noodle | 1 cup (8.8 oz) | 137 | 19 | 0 | 1 |
| Split Pea & Ham | 1 cup (8.8 oz) | 164 | 26 | 6 | 5 |
| Tomato Garden | 1 cup (8.6 oz) | 101 | 19 | 8 | 5 |
| Turkey Wild Rice | 1 cup (8.4 oz) | 72 | 9 | 5 | 3 |
| Vegetable Beef | 1 cup (8.8 oz) | 96 | 14 | 3 | 2 |
| ***Imagine*** | | | | | |
| Creamy Broccoli | 1 serv (8 oz) | 70 | 10 | 4 | 2 |
| Creamy Butternut Squash | 1 serv (8 oz) | 120 | 23 | 14 | 2 |
| Creamy Mushroom | 1 serv (8 oz) | 80 | 10 | 1 | 2 |
| Creamy Potato Leek | 1 serv (8 oz) | 90 | 14 | tr | 2 |
| Creamy Sweet Corn | 1 serv (8 oz) | 100 | 15 | 6 | 1 |
| Creamy Tomato | 1 serv (8 oz) | 90 | 17 | 10 | 2 |
| Vegetable Broth | 1 serv (8 oz) | 45 | 7 | 5 | 1 |
| Zesty Gazpacho | 1 serv (8 oz) | 80 | 8 | 5 | tr |
| ***Manischewitz*** | | | | | |
| Clear Chicken Condensed | ½ cup | 15 | 2 | 0 | 2 |
| ***Natural Choice*** | | | | | |
| Orangic Vegan Classic Tomato | 1 cup | 100 | 22 | 8 | 2 |
| Organic Vegan Classic Mushroom | 1 cup | 50 | 9 | 3 | 2 |
| Organic Vegan Country Corn | 1 cup | 100 | 24 | 6 | 3 |
| Organic Vegan Kabocha Squash | 1 cup | 60 | 14 | 8 | 1 |
| Organic Vegan Southern Greens | 1 cup | 80 | 13 | 5 | 2 |
| Organic Vegan Split Pea | 1 cup | 120 | 21 | 4 | 7 |
| Organic Vegan Vegetable Curry | 1 cup | 110 | 17 | 4 | 2 |
| ***Pacific*** | | | | | |
| Free Range Organic Chicken Broth | 1 cup | 5 | 1 | – | – |
| ***Progresso*** | | | | | |
| 99% Fat Free Beef Barley | 1 cup (8.5 oz) | 140 | 20 | 4 | 3 |
| 99% Fat Free Beef Vegetable | 1 cup (8.5 oz) | 160 | 24 | 4 | 3 |
| 99% Fat Free Chicken Noodle | 1 cup | 90 | 13 | 2 | tr |

| FOOD | PORTION | CALS | CARB | SUGAR | FIBER |
|---|---|---|---|---|---|
| 99% Fat Free Chicken Rice w/ Vegetables | 1 cup (8.4 oz) | 110 | 16 | 2 | 1 |
| 99% Fat Free Creamy Mushroom Chicken | 1 cup (8.3 oz) | 90 | 12 | 2 | 1 |
| 99% Fat Free Lentil | 1 cup (8.5 oz) | 130 | 20 | 1 | 6 |
| 99% Fat Free Minestrone | 1 cup (8.5 oz) | 130 | 23 | 3 | 4 |
| 99% Fat Free Roasted Chicken w/ Italian Style Vegetable | 1 cup (8 oz) | 90 | 12 | 2 | 1 |
| 99% Fat Free Split Pea | 1 cup (8.9 oz) | 170 | 29 | 5 | 5 |
| 99% Fat Free Tomato Garden Vegetable | 1 cup (8.6 oz) | 100 | 19 | 7 | 2 |
| 99% Fat Free Vegetable | 1 cup (8.4 oz) | 70 | 13 | 3 | 2 |
| 99% Fat Free White Cheddar Potato | 1 cup (8.6 oz) | 140 | 26 | 2 | 2 |
| Basil Rotini Tomato | 1 cup (8.9 oz) | 120 | 22 | 6 | 2 |
| Bean & Ham | 1 cup (8.4 oz) | 160 | 25 | 3 | 8 |
| Beef & Vegetable | 1 cup | 130 | 16 | 4 | 2 |
| Beef Barley | 1 cup (8.5 oz) | 130 | 13 | 4 | 3 |
| Beef Minestrone | 1 cup (8.5 oz) | 140 | 18 | 3 | 3 |
| Beef Noodle | 1 cup (8.5 oz) | 140 | 15 | 2 | 1 |
| Cheese & Herb Tortellini Tomato | 1 cup (8.6 oz) | 140 | 23 | 9 | 2 |
| Chickarina | 1 cup (8.3 oz) | 130 | 12 | tr | tr |
| Chicken Minestrone | 1 cup (8.4 oz) | 110 | 15 | 2 | 2 |
| Chicken Vegetable | 1 cup (8.4 oz) | 90 | 13 | 2 | 2 |
| Chicken & Wild Rice | 1 cup (8.4 oz) | 100 | 15 | 1 | 1 |
| Chicken Barley | 1 cup (8.5 oz) | 110 | 16 | 2 | 3 |
| Chicken Broth | 1 cup (8.5 oz) | 20 | 1 | 0 | 0 |
| Chicken Noodle | 1 cup (8.4 oz) | 90 | 9 | 1 | tr |
| Chicken Rice w/ Vegetable | 1 cup (8.4 oz) | 90 | 13 | 1 | 1 |
| Clam & Rotini Chowder | 1 cup (8.8 oz) | 190 | 21 | 3 | 0 |
| Escarole In Chicken Broth | 1 cup (8.1 oz) | 25 | 3 | tr | 1 |
| Green Split Pea | 1 cup (8.6 oz) | 170 | 25 | 4 | 5 |
| Hearty Black Bean | 1 cup (8.5 oz) | 170 | 30 | 2 | 10 |
| Hearty Penne In Chicken Broth | 1 cup (8.4 oz) | 80 | 14 | 1 | tr |
| Hearty Tomato | 1 cup (8.7 oz) | 100 | 19 | 11 | 1 |
| Herb Rotini Vegetable | 1 cup (9.1 oz) | 120 | 21 | 5 | 4 |
| Homestyle Chicken w/ Vegetable | 1 cup (8.4 oz) | 90 | 11 | 1 | tr |
| Italian Herb Shells Minestrone | 1 cup (9.1 oz) | 120 | 22 | 4 | 4 |

| FOOD | PORTION | CALS | CARB | SUGAR | FIBER |
|---|---|---|---|---|---|
| Lentil | 1 cup (8.5 oz) | 140 | 22 | 2 | 7 |
| Macaroni & Bean | 1 cup (8.6 oz) | 160 | 23 | 1 | 6 |
| Manhattan Clam Chowder | 1 cup (8.4 oz) | 110 | 11 | 3 | 3 |
| Meatballs & Pasta Pearls | 1 cup (8.3 oz) | 140 | 13 | 0 | 0 |
| Minestrone | 1 cup (8.4 oz) | 120 | 21 | 4 | 5 |
| Minestrone Parmesan | 1 cup (8.3 oz) | 100 | 16 | 3 | 3 |
| New England Clam Chowder | 1 cup (8.4 oz) | 190 | 20 | 3 | 1 |
| Oregano Penne Italian Style Vegetable | 1 cup (8.7 oz) | 90 | 15 | 2 | 1 |
| Peppercorn Penne Vegetable | 1 cup (9.1 oz) | 100 | 20 | 3 | 2 |
| Potato Broccoli & Cheese | 1 cup (8.8 oz) | 160 | 21 | 4 | 1 |
| Potato Ham & Cheese | 1 cup (8.6 oz) | 170 | 21 | 3 | 1 |
| Rich & Hearty Beef Pot Roast | 1 cup | 130 | 17 | 4 | 2 |
| Roasted Garlic Pasta Lentil | 1 cup (9.3 oz) | 120 | 20 | 2 | 5 |
| Rotisserie Seasoned Chicken | 1 cup (8.5 oz) | 100 | 15 | 2 | 2 |
| Spicy Chicken & Penne | 1 cup (8.5 oz) | 110 | 14 | 2 | 1 |
| Split Pea w/ Ham | 1 cup (8.4 oz) | 150 | 20 | 3 | 5 |
| Tomato | 1 cup (8.5 oz) | 100 | 19 | 10 | 1 |
| Tomato Basil | 1 cup (8.8 oz) | 100 | 19 | 10 | 1 |
| Tomato Vegetable | 1 cup (8.5 oz) | 90 | 15 | 8 | 4 |
| Tortellini In Chicken Broth | 1 cup (8.3 oz) | 70 | 10 | 1 | 2 |
| Turkey Noodle | 1 cup (8.4 oz) | 90 | 11 | 2 | tr |
| Turkey Rice w/ Vegetables | 1 cup (8.5 oz) | 110 | 18 | 2 | 1 |
| Vegetable | 1 cup (8.4 oz) | 90 | 15 | 3 | 2 |
| White Meat Roasted Chicken Rotini | 1 cup (8.1 oz) | 80 | 11 | 1 | tr |
| ***Streit's*** | | | | | |
| Hearty Vegetarian Vegetable | 1 cup | 90 | 19 | 7 | 3 |
| Mushroom Barley | 1 cup | 100 | 17 | 4 | 3 |
| ***Swanson*** | | | | | |
| Beef Broth 100% Fat Free Lower Sodium | 1 cup | 15 | 1 | 1 | – |
| Beef Broth 99% Fat Free | 1 cup | 10 | 0 | 0 | 0 |
| Beef Broth Onion Seasoned | 1 cup (8.4 oz) | 20 | 2 | 1 | tr |
| Chicken Broth 100% Fat Free 33% Less Sodium | 1 cup | 15 | 1 | 1 | – |
| Chicken Broth Seasoned Italian Herbs | 1 cup (8.4 oz) | 20 | 3 | 0 | tr |
| Vegetable Broth | 1 cup | 19 | 3 | 3 | 0 |

| FOOD | PORTION | CALS | CARB | SUGAR | FIBER |
|---|---|---|---|---|---|
| ***Walnut Acres*** | | | | | |
| Organic Country Corn Chowder | 1 cup (8.8 oz) | 150 | 28 | 8 | 2 |
| ***Weight Watchers*** | | | | | |
| Chicken & Rice | 1 can (10.5 oz) | 110 | 17 | 11 | 4 |
| Chicken Noodle | 1 can (10.5 oz) | 150 | 25 | 15 | 4 |
| Minestrone | 1 can (10.5 oz) | 130 | 23 | 7 | 6 |
| Vegetable | 1 can (10.5 oz) | 130 | 27 | 11 | 6 |
| **FROZEN** | | | | | |
| ***Birds Eye*** | | | | | |
| Hearty Spoonfuls Pasta & Chicken | 1 bowl (11.2 oz) | 140 | 19 | 3 | 2 |
| ***Nature's Entree*** | | | | | |
| Chowder | 1 pkg (12 oz) | 230 | 26 | 5 | 5 |
| Tortellini Minestrone | 1 pkg (12 oz) | 360 | 48 | 6 | 5 |
| **MIX** | | | | | |
| ***Alpine Aire*** | | | | | |
| Low Carb Bay Shrimp Bisque | 1 pkg | 150 | 6 | 1 | 1 |
| Low Carb Beefy Vegetable | 1 pkg | 100 | 7 | 1 | 1 |
| Low Carb Broccoli Cheddar | 1 pkg | 140 | 6 | 1 | 2 |
| Low Carb Mushroom & Chicken w/ Roasted Garlic | 1 pkg | 130 | 7 | 2 | 1 |
| ***Armour*** | | | | | |
| Bouillon Cubes Beef | 1 (4 g) | 5 | 1 | 0 | 0 |
| Bouillon Cubes Chicken | 1 (4 g) | 5 | 1 | 0 | 0 |
| ***Azumaya*** | | | | | |
| Thin Cut Noodle | 1 cup | 120 | 24 | 2 | tr |
| Wide Cut Noodle | 1 cup | 120 | 24 | 2 | tr |
| ***Bean Cuisine*** | | | | | |
| 13 Bean Bouillabisse | 1 cup | 220 | 17 | 1 | 5 |
| Island Black Bean | 1 cup | 210 | 17 | 1 | 7 |
| Lots of Lentil | 1 cup | 230 | 17 | 1 | 5 |
| Mesa Maize | 1 cup | 160 | 18 | 2 | 6 |
| White Bean Provencal | 1 cup | 250 | 32 | 4 | 11 |
| ***Health Valley*** | | | | | |
| Chicken Noodles w/ Vegetables | 1 serv | 110 | 24 | 1 | 3 |
| Corn Chowder w/ Tomatoes | 1 serv | 100 | 21 | 1 | 3 |

| FOOD | PORTION | CALS | CARB | SUGAR | FIBER |
|---|---|---|---|---|---|
| Creamy Potato w/ Broccoli | 1 serv | 70 | 17 | 2 | 3 |
| Garden Split Pea w/ Carrots | 1 serv | 130 | 22 | 2 | 2 |
| Lentil w/ Couscous | 1 serv | 130 | 28 | 1 | 5 |
| Pasta Italiano | 1 serv | 140 | 31 | 1 | 3 |
| Pasta Marinara | 1 serv | 100 | 20 | 1 | 1 |
| Pasta Parmesan | 1 serv | 100 | 20 | 1 | 1 |
| Spicy Black Bean w/ Couscous | 1 serv | 130 | 29 | 3 | 5 |
| Zesty Black Bean w/ Rice | 1 serv | 100 | 22 | 2 | 4 |
| ***Hodgson Mill*** | | | | | |
| Choice Bean not prep | ¼ cup (1.5 oz) | 150 | 27 | 2 | 11 |
| ***MiniCarb*** | | | | | |
| Miso w/ Tofu & Shitake | 1 pkg | 33 | 5 | 2 | 1 |
| Szechuan Beef | 1 pkg | 24 | 4 | 0 | 0 |
| Thai Coconut Cream | 1 pkg | 100 | 9 | 0 | 1 |
| ***Miso-Cup*** | | | | | |
| Golden Vegetable as prep | 1 cup | 30 | 3 | 1 | tr |
| Miso Reduced Sodium as prep | 1 cup | 25 | 3 | tr | tr |
| Organic Miso as prep | 1 cup | 35 | 4 | tr | tr |
| Savory Seaweed as prep | 1 cup | 30 | 3 | 1 | tr |
| ***Ramen Noodle*** | | | | | |
| Beef Low Fat as prep | 1 pkg (2.2 oz) | 216 | 45 | 3 | 2 |
| Beef as prep | 1 pkg (2.2 oz) | 280 | 40 | 3 | 3 |
| Chicken Low Fat as prep | 1 pkg (2.2 oz) | 216 | 44 | 3 | 2 |
| Chicken as prep | 1 pkg (2.2 oz) | 279 | 40 | 3 | 6 |
| Oriental Low Fat as prep | 1 pkg (2.2 oz) | 217 | 45 | 3 | 2 |
| Shrimp Low Fat as prep | 1 pkg (2.2 oz) | 218 | 45 | 3 | 3 |
| Shrimp as prep | 1 pkg (2.2 oz) | 294 | 39 | 3 | 3 |
| Tomato as prep | 1 pkg (2.2 oz) | 295 | 39 | 4 | 2 |
| ***Rapunzel*** | | | | | |
| Cubes Vegetable Bouillon No Salt Added | ½ cube | 25 | 0 | 0 | 0 |
| Cubes Vegetable Bouillon w/ Sea Salt | ½ cube | 15 | 0 | 0 | 0 |
| Cubes Vegetable Bouillon w/ Sea Salt & Herbs | ½ cube | 15 | 0 | 0 | 0 |
| ***Slim-Fast*** | | | | | |
| Creamy Broccoli | 1 pkg | 210 | 30 | 13 | 5 |
| Creamy Chicken | 1 pkg | 220 | 33 | 15 | 5 |
| Creamy Potato Cheddar & Chive | 1 pkg | 220 | 35 | 15 | 5 |

| FOOD | PORTION | CALS | CARB | SUGAR | FIBER |
|---|---|---|---|---|---|
| ***Steero*** | | | | | |
| Beef Bouillon Cube | 1 (3.5 g) | 5 | 1 | – | – |
| Beef Bouillon Cube Reduced Sodium | 1 cube (3.5 oz) | 5 | 1 | – | – |
| Beef Bouillon Instant | 1 tsp (3.5 oz) | 5 | 1 | – | – |
| Beef Bouillon Instant Reduced Sodium | 1 tsp (3.5 oz) | 5 | 1 | – | – |
| Chicken Bouillon Cube | 1 (3.5 g) | 5 | 1 | – | – |
| Chicken Bouillon Cube Reduced Sodium | 1 (3.5 g) | 5 | 1 | – | – |
| Chicken Bouillon Cube Reduced Sodium | 1 (3.5 g) | 5 | 1 | – | – |
| Chicken Bouillon Instant | 1 tsp (3.5 g) | 5 | 1 | – | – |
| Chicken Bouillon Instant Reduced Sodium | 1 tsp (3.5 g) | 5 | 1 | – | – |
| ***Thai Kitchen*** | | | | | |
| Instant Rice Noodle Bangkok Curry | 1 pkg | 192 | 35 | 2 | 0 |
| Rice Noodle Bowl Roasted Garlic | 1 bowl | 170 | 35 | 2 | 0 |
| Rice Noodle Bowl Spring Onion | 1 bowl | 170 | 35 | 2 | 0 |
| ***Weight Watchers*** | | | | | |
| Instant Beef Broth | 1 pkg (0.16 oz) | 10 | 2 | 2 | 0 |
| Instant Chicken Broth | 1 pkg (0.16 oz) | 10 | 2 | 2 | 0 |
| ***Wyler's*** | | | | | |
| Beef Bouillon Cube | 1 (3.5 g) | 5 | 1 | – | – |
| Beef Bouillon Cube Reduced Sodium | 1 (3.5 g) | 5 | 1 | – | – |
| Beef Bouillon Instant | 1 tsp (3.5 g) | 5 | 1 | – | – |
| Beef Bouillon Instant Reduced Sodium | 1 tsp (3.5 g) | 5 | 1 | – | – |
| Chicken Bouillon Cube | 1 (3.5 g) | 5 | 1 | – | – |
| Chicken Bouillon Cube Reduced Sodium | 1 (3.5 g) | 5 | 1 | – | – |
| Chicken Bouillon Instant | 1 tsp (3.5) | 5 | 1 | – | – |
| Chicken Bouillon Instant Reduced Sodium | 1 tsp (3.5 g) | 5 | 1 | – | – |

| FOOD | PORTION | CALS | CARB | SUGAR | FIBER |
|---|---|---|---|---|---|
| **SHELF-STABLE** | | | | | |
| ***Annie Chun*** | | | | | |
| Ginger Chicken | 1 cup | 30 | 3 | 3 | 0 |
| Shiitake Mushroom | 1 cup | 25 | 3 | 2 | 0 |
| Traditional Miso | 1 cup | 35 | 5 | 2 | 1 |
| ***Campbell's*** | | | | | |
| Soup At Hand Blended Vegetable Medley | 1 pkg (10.75 oz) | 110 | 21 | 10 | 4 |
| ***Lunch Bucket*** | | | | | |
| Chicken Noodle | 1 pkg (7.25 oz) | 80 | 13 | 0 | 0 |
| Country Vegetable | 1 pkg (7.25 oz) | 60 | 14 | 1 | 3 |
| ***TastyBite*** | | | | | |
| Tom Yum | ½ pkg (5.3 oz) | 92 | 6 | 0 | 1 |
| **TAKE-OUT** | | | | | |
| beef stew soup | 1 cup (8.8 oz) | 221 | 20 | – | – |
| black bean turtle soup | 1 cup | 241 | 45 | – | 10 |
| brunswick stew soup | 1 cup (8.5 oz) | 232 | 17 | – | – |
| corn & cheese chowder | ¾ cup | 215 | 21 | – | 3 |
| gazpacho | 1 cup | 46 | 5 | – | – |
| greek lemon | ¾ cup | 63 | 7 | – | 2 |
| hot & sour | 1 serv (14 oz) | 173 | 8 | 1 | 1 |
| onion soup gratinee | 1 serv | 492 | 38 | 6 | 4 |
| oxtail | 5 oz | 64 | 7 | – | – |
| pasta e fagioli | 1 cup (8.8 oz) | 194 | 30 | – | – |
| ratatouille | 1 cup (7.5 oz) | 266 | 12 | – | – |
| thai lemon grass | 1 bowl | 100 | 5 | – | – |
| vietnamese pho beef noodle | 1 serv (7.8 oz) | 480 | 78 | 2 | 1 |
| wonton soup | 1 cup | 205 | 26 | – | 1 |
| zupa koprowa polish dill soup | 1 bowl | 54 | 6 | – | – |

## SOUR CREAM

| FOOD | PORTION | CALS | CARB | SUGAR | FIBER |
|---|---|---|---|---|---|
| sour cream | 1 cup (8 oz) | 493 | 10 | – | – |
| sour cream | 1 tbsp (0.4 oz) | 26 | 1 | – | – |
| ***Cabot*** | | | | | |
| Light | 2 tbsp | 35 | 2 | 0 | 0 |
| No Fat | 2 tbsp | 20 | 3 | 2 | 0 |
| Sour Cream | 2 tbsp | 50 | 1 | 0 | 0 |

| FOOD | PORTION | CALS | CARB | SUGAR | FIBER |
|---|---|---|---|---|---|
| ***Land O Lakes*** | | | | | |
| Fat Free | 2 tbsp (1.1 oz) | 25 | 4 | 2 | 0 |
| Light | 2 tbsp (1 oz) | 40 | 3 | 2 | 0 |
| Sour Cream | 2 tbsp (1 oz) | 60 | 1 | 1 | 0 |
| **SOUR CREAM SUBSTITUTES** | | | | | |
| nondairy | 1 cup | 479 | 15 | – | – |
| nondairy | 1 oz | 59 | 2 | – | – |
| **SOURSOP** | | | | | |
| fresh | 1 | 416 | 105 | – | – |
| fresh cut up | 1 cup | 150 | 38 | – | – |
| **SOY** *(see also* CHEESE SUBSTITUTES, ICE CREAM FROZEN DESSERTS, MILK SUBSTITUTES, MISO, SOY SAUCE, SOYBEANS, TEMPEH, TOFU, YOGURT FROZEN*)* | | | | | |
| lecithin | 1 tbsp | 104 | 0 | 0 | 0 |
| soy milk | 1 cup | 79 | 4 | – | – |
| soya cheese | 1.4 oz | 128 | tr | – | 0 |
| ***Bob's Red Mill*** | | | | | |
| Flour | ⅓ cup | 130 | 11 | 0 | 5 |
| ***Fearn*** | | | | | |
| Granules | ¼ cup | 110 | 13 | 5 | 8 |
| Powder | ¼ cup | 100 | 7 | 0 | 4 |
| ***GeniSoy*** | | | | | |
| Soy Nuts Deep Sea Salted | 1 oz | 120 | 9 | 3 | 5 |
| Soy Nuts Old Hickory Smoked | 1 oz | 120 | 9 | 5 | 5 |
| Soy Nuts Praline | 55 pieces (1 oz) | 120 | 18 | 16 | 2 |
| Soy Nuts Unsalted | 1 oz | 120 | 9 | 3 | 5 |
| Soy Nuts Zesty Barbeque | 1 oz | 120 | 9 | 5 | 5 |
| ***Health Trip*** | | | | | |
| Soynut Butter Honey Sweet | 2 tbsp | 170 | 9 | 3 | 1 |
| Soynut Butter Original | 2 tbsp | 180 | 8 | 1 | 1 |
| Soynut Butter Unsalted | 2 tbsp | 180 | 8 | 1 | 1 |
| ***I.M. Healthy*** | | | | | |
| SoyNut Butter Chocolate | 2 tbsp (1.1 oz) | 190 | 12 | 7 | 4 |
| SoyNut Butter Honey Creamy | 2 tbsp (1.1 oz) | 170 | 12 | 2 | 2 |
| SoyNut Butter Original Creamy | 2 tbsp (1.1 oz) | 170 | 10 | 3 | 1 |

| FOOD | PORTION | CALS | CARB | SUGAR | FIBER |
|---|---|---|---|---|---|
| SoyNut Butter Unsweetened Chunky | 2 tbsp (1.1 oz) | 160 | 5 | 1 | 5 |
| SoyNut Butter Unsweetened Creamy | 2 tbsp (1.1 oz) | 160 | 5 | 1 | 5 |
| ***Loma Linda*** | | | | | |
| Soyagen All Purpose | ¼ cup (1 oz) | 130 | 12 | 7 | 3 |
| Soyagen Carob | ¼ cup (1 oz) | 130 | 13 | 7 | 2 |
| Soyagen No Sucrose | ¼ cup (1 oz) | 130 | 12 | 7 | 3 |
| ***Natural Touch*** | | | | | |
| Roasted Soy Butter | 2 tbsp (1.1 oz) | 170 | 10 | 3 | 1 |
| ***Revival*** | | | | | |
| Shake Chocolate Daydream Fructose | 1 pkg | 240 | 36 | 32 | 2 |
| Shake Strawberry Smile Unsweetened | 1 pkg | 130 | 4 | 0 | 0 |
| Shake Strawberry Smile Fructose | 1 pkg | 225 | 33 | 29 | 0 |
| Shake Strawberry Smile Splenda | 1 pkg | 130 | 4 | 1 | 0 |
| Soy Shake Plain | 1 pkg | 110 | 2 | 1 | 0 |
| Soy Shake Vanilla Pleasure | 1 pkg | 220 | 31 | 28 | 0 |
| Soy Shake Vanilla Pleasure Splenda | 1 pkg | 120 | 6 | 1 | 0 |
| Soy Shake Vanilla Pleasure Unsweetened | 1 pkg | 120 | 6 | 1 | 0 |
| Soynuts Chocolate Covered | ⅙ cup | 70 | 7 | 6 | tr |
| Soynuts Hot Jalapeno & Cheddar | ⅙ cup | 78 | 5 | tr | 2 |
| Soynuts Unsalted | ⅙ cup | 78 | 5 | tr | 2 |
| Soynuts Yogurt Covered | ⅙ cup | 720 | 8 | 7 | tr |
| ***Soy Juicy*** | | | | | |
| All Flavors | 8 oz | 160 | 25 | 24 | 1 |
| ***Soy Wonder*** | | | | | |
| Creamy | 2 tbsp | 170 | 10 | 3 | 1 |
| Crunchy | 2 tbsp | 170 | 10 | 3 | 1 |
| **SOY SAUCE** | | | | | |
| shoyu | 1 tbsp | 9 | 2 | – | – |
| soy sauce | 1 tbsp | 7 | 1 | – | – |
| tamari | 1 tbsp | 11 | 1 | – | – |

| FOOD | PORTION | CALS | CARB | SUGAR | FIBER |
|---|---|---|---|---|---|
| ***Chun King*** | | | | | |
| Lite | 1 tbsp (0.5 oz) | 15 | 2 | 2 | 0 |
| Soy Sauce | 1 tbsp (0.6 oz) | 11 | 1 | 1 | 0 |
| ***Eden*** | | | | | |
| Organic Shoyu Reduced Sodium | 1 tbsp | 10 | 2 | 0 | 0 |
| Organic Tamari | 1 tbsp | 15 | 2 | 0 | 0 |
| Ponzu Sauce | 1 tbsp | 5 | 1 | 0 | 0 |
| Shoyu | 1 tbsp | 15 | 2 | 0 | 0 |
| ***Just Rite*** | | | | | |
| Soy Sauce | 1 tbsp (0.5 oz) | 11 | 1 | 1 | 0 |
| ***Kikkoman*** | | | | | |
| Lite | 1 tbsp (0.5 oz) | 10 | 1 | – | – |
| Soy Sauce | 1 tbsp (0.5 oz) | 10 | 0 | 0 | 0 |
| ***La Choy*** | | | | | |
| Lite | 1 tbsp (0.5 oz) | 15 | 2 | 2 | 0 |
| Soy Sauce | 1 tbsp (0.6 oz) | 11 | 1 | 1 | 0 |
| ***Tree Of Life*** | | | | | |
| Shoyu | 1 tbsp (0.5 oz) | 15 | 1 | 1 | – |
| Tamari Wheat Free | 1 tbsp (0.5 oz) | 15 | 1 | 1 | – |
| **SOYBEANS** | | | | | |
| dried cooked | 1 cup | 298 | 17 | – | – |
| dry roasted | ½ cup | 387 | 28 | – | – |
| green cooked | ½ cup | 127 | 10 | – | 4 |
| roasted | ½ cup | 405 | 29 | – | – |
| roasted & toasted | 1 oz | 129 | 9 | – | – |
| roasted & toasted | 1 cup | 490 | 33 | – | – |
| roasted & toasted salted | 1 cup | 490 | 33 | – | – |
| roasted & toasted salted | 1 oz | 129 | 9 | – | – |
| sprouts raw | ½ cup | 43 | 3 | – | – |

| FOOD | PORTION | CALS | CARB | SUGAR | FIBER |
|---|---|---|---|---|---|
| sprouts steamed | ½ cup | 38 | 3 | – | – |
| sprouts stir fried | 1 cup | 125 | 9 | – | – |
| ***Arrowhead*** | | | | | |
| Organic not prep | ¼ cup | 180 | 14 | 3 | 10 |
| ***Dakota Gourmet*** | | | | | |
| Soy Nuts | 1 oz | 129 | 9 | – | 1 |
| ***Eden*** | | | | | |
| Organic Black | ½ cup (4.6 oz) | 120 | 8 | 1 | 7 |
| ***Seapoint Farms*** | | | | | |
| Edamame Organic | ½ cup (2.6 oz) | 100 | 9 | 1 | 4 |
| Edamame In Pods frzn | ½ cup (2.6 oz) | 100 | 9 | 1 | 4 |
| Edamame Rice Bowl Kung Pao Vegetable | 1 pkg (12 oz) | 420 | 72 | 14 | 6 |
| Edamame Rice Bowl Szechwan Vegetables | 1 pkg (12 oz) | 420 | 80 | 22 | 6 |
| Edamame Rice Bowl Teriyaki Vegetable | 1 pkg (12 oz) | 430 | 83 | 21 | 5 |
| Edamame Rice Bowl Vegetable Fried Rice | 1 pkg (11 oz) | 220 | 31 | 6 | 1 |
| Edamame Shelled | ½ cup (2.6 oz) | 100 | 9 | 1 | 4 |

**SPAGHETTI** *(see* PASTA, PASTA DINNERS, PASTA SALAD, SPAGHETTI SAUCE*)*

## SPAGHETTI SAUCE

| FOOD | PORTION | CALS | CARB | SUGAR | FIBER |
|---|---|---|---|---|---|
| **JARRED** | | | | | |
| marinara sauce | 1 cup | 171 | 25 | – | – |
| spaghetti sauce | 1 cup | 272 | 40 | – | – |
| ***Amy's*** | | | | | |
| Family Marinara | ½ cup | 50 | 8 | 5 | 3 |
| Garlic Mushroom | ½ cup | 120 | 10 | 5 | 3 |
| Puttanesca | ½ cup | 40 | 5 | 2 | 1 |
| Tomato Basil | ½ cup | 80 | 11 | 6 | 3 |
| Wild Mushroom | ½ cup | 60 | 7 | 4 | 2 |
| ***Colavita*** | | | | | |
| Garden Style | ½ cup (4.4 oz) | 60 | 12 | 0 | 3 |
| ***Del Monte*** | | | | | |
| Chunky Garlic & Herb | ½ cup (4.4 oz) | 60 | 11 | 9 | 1 |
| Chunky Italian Herb | ½ cup (4.4 oz) | 60 | 12 | 8 | 1 |
| Tomato & Basil | ½ cup (4.4 oz) | 70 | 16 | 11 | 3 |
| Traditional | ½ cup (4.4 oz) | 60 | 15 | 10 | 3 |

| FOOD | PORTION | CALS | CARB | SUGAR | FIBER |
|---|---|---|---|---|---|
| With Garlic & Onion | ½ cup (4.4 oz) | 80 | 16 | 10 | 2 |
| With Green Peppers & Mushrooms | ½ cup (4.4 oz) | 80 | 16 | 10 | 3 |
| With Meat | ½ cup (4.4 oz) | 60 | 14 | 9 | 3 |
| With Mushrooms | ½ cup (4.4 oz) | 60 | 14 | 9 | 2 |
| ***Eden*** | | | | | |
| Organic Lightly Seasoned | ½ cup (4.4 oz) | 80 | 12 | 6 | 3 |
| ***Francesco Rinaldi*** | | | | | |
| Alfredo | ¼ cup (2.1 oz) | 70 | 4 | 1 | 0 |
| Chunky Garden Mushroom & Onion | ½ cup (4.4 oz) | 80 | 12 | 6 | 3 |
| Chunky Garden Tomato Garlic & Onion | ½ cup (4.4 oz) | 80 | 12 | 6 | 3 |
| Dolce Sweet & Tasty Tomato | ½ cup (4.4 oz) | 110 | 15 | 11 | 3 |
| Dolce Three Cheese | ½ cup (4.4 oz) | 90 | 15 | 11 | 3 |
| Dulce Super Mushroom | ½ cup (4.4 oz) | 110 | 15 | 11 | 3 |
| Hearty Diavolo | ½ cup (4.4 oz) | 70 | 7 | 4 | 3 |
| Hearty Mushroom Pepper & Onion | ½ cup (4.4 oz) | 80 | 10 | 7 | 3 |
| Hearty Tomato & Basil | ½ cup (4.4 oz) | 80 | 11 | 7 | 4 |
| Puttanesca | ½ cup (4.3 oz) | 70 | 8 | 7 | tr |
| Tomato Alfredo | ¼ cup (2.1 oz) | 60 | 4 | 4 | 0 |
| Traditional Meat Flavored | ½ cup (4.4 oz) | 90 | 11 | 7 | 3 |
| Traditional Mushroom | 1.2 cup (4.4 oz) | 90 | 11 | 7 | 3 |
| Traditional No Salt Added | ½ cup (4.4 oz) | 70 | 10 | 9 | tr |
| Traditional Original | ½ cup (4.4 oz) | 90 | 11 | 2 | 3 |
| Traditional Original | ½ cup (4.4 oz) | 90 | 11 | 7 | 3 |
| Vodka Sauce | ¼ cup (2.1 oz) | 60 | 4 | 4 | 0 |
| ***Healthy Choice*** | | | | | |
| Chunky Italian Vegetable | ½ cup (4.4 oz) | 40 | 9 | 7 | 2 |
| Chunky Mushroom | ½ cup (4.4 oz) | 42 | 9 | 8 | 2 |
| Garlic & Herbs | ½ cup (4.4 oz) | 49 | 10 | 7 | 2 |
| Garlic Lovers Garlic & Mushroom | ½ cup (4.4 oz) | 44 | 10 | 8 | 2 |
| Garlic Lovers Roasted Garlic | ½ cup (4.4 oz) | 52 | 12 | 8 | 3 |
| Garlic Lovers Roasted Garlic & Sun Dried Tomato | ½ cup (4.4 oz) | 52 | 11 | 8 | 3 |

| FOOD | PORTION | CALS | CARB | SUGAR | FIBER |
|---|---|---|---|---|---|
| Super Chunky Mushroom & Sweet Peppers | ½ cup (4.4 oz) | 43 | 9 | 6 | 2 |
| Super Chunky Tomato Mushroom & Garlic | ½ cup (4.4 oz) | 45 | 10 | 8 | 2 |
| Super Chunky Vegetable Primavera | ½ cup (4.4 oz) | 43 | 9 | 7 | 2 |
| Traditional | ½ cup (4.4 oz) | 48 | 11 | 8 | 2 |
| With Mushrooms | ½ cup (4.4 oz) | 48 | 11 | 8 | 2 |
| ***Hunt's*** | | | | | |
| Angela Mia Marinara | ¼ cup (2.2 oz) | 24 | 4 | 3 | 2 |
| Chunky | ½ cup (4.4 oz) | 38 | 8 | 7 | 2 |
| Chunky Italian Sausage | ½ cup (4.5 oz) | 72 | 45 | 8 | 3 |
| Chunky Italian Style Vegetable | ½ cup (4.4 oz) | 63 | 13 | 5 | 2 |
| Chunky Marinara | ½ cup (4.4 oz) | 61 | 12 | 5 | 2 |
| Chunky Tomato Garlic & Onion | ½ cup (4.4 oz) | 63 | 13 | 5 | 2 |
| Classic Four Cheese | ½ cup (4.4 oz) | 50 | 9 | 7 | 3 |
| Classic Garlic & Herb | ½ cup (4.4 oz) | 53 | 9 | 6 | 3 |
| Classic Parmesan | ½ cup (4.4 oz) | 49 | 8 | 6 | 3 |
| Classic Tomato & Basil | ½ cup (4.4 oz) | 48 | 9 | 7 | 2 |
| Family Favorites Seasoned Diced Tomato Sauce | ½ cup (4.3 oz) | 50 | 11 | 9 | 2 |
| Homestyle Meat Flavored | ½ cup (4.4 oz) | 51 | 9 | 5 | 3 |
| Homestyle Mushrooms | ½ cup (4.4 oz) | 48 | 9 | 7 | 3 |
| Homestyle Traditional | ½ cup (4.4 oz) | 49 | 9 | 7 | 3 |
| Light Meat Flavored | ½ cup (4.4 oz) | 45 | 8 | 6 | 3 |
| Light w/ Garlic & Herb | ½ cup (4.5 oz) | 40 | 7 | 5 | 3 |
| Original Meat Flavored | ½ cup (4.4 oz) | 68 | 12 | 9 | 3 |
| Original Traditional | ½ cup (4.4 oz) | 67 | 11 | 9 | 3 |
| Original w/ Mushrooms | ½ cup (4.4 oz) | 62 | 11 | 9 | 3 |
| Original w/ Italian Cheese & Garlic | ½ cup (4.5 oz) | 64 | 10 | 7 | 3 |
| Tomato Bits | ½ cup (4.5 oz) | 49 | 11 | 6 | 3 |
| Traditional Light | ½ cup (4.4 oz) | 40 | 7 | 6 | 1 |
| ***Muir Glen*** | | | | | |
| Organic Balsamic Roasted Onion | ½ cup (4.4 oz) | 50 | 10 | 5 | 0 |
| Organic Cabernet Marinara | ½ cup (4.4 oz) | 50 | 10 | 4 | 0 |
| Organic Chunky Herb | ½ cup (4.4 oz) | 50 | 10 | 5 | 0 |
| Organic Garden Vegetable | ½ cup (4.4 oz) | 50 | 10 | 4 | 0 |
| Organic Garlic & Onion | ½ cup (4.4 oz) | 55 | 10 | 5 | 0 |

| FOOD | PORTION | CALS | CARB | SUGAR | FIBER |
|---|---|---|---|---|---|
| Organic Garlic Roasted Garlic | ½ cup (4.4 oz) | 50 | 10 | 4 | 0 |
| Organic Green Olive | ½ cup (4.4 oz) | 60 | 10 | 4 | 0 |
| Organic Italian Herb | ½ cup (4.4 oz) | 55 | 10 | 5 | 0 |
| Organic Mushroom Marinara | ½ cup (4.4 oz) | 45 | 10 | 4 | 0 |
| Organic Portabello Mushroom | ½ cup (4.4 oz) | 50 | 10 | 4 | 0 |
| Organic Sun Dried Tomato | ½ cup (4.4 oz) | 55 | 10 | 4 | 1 |
| Organic Tomato Basil | ½ cup (4.4 oz) | 50 | 12 | 4 | 0 |
| ***Newman's Own*** | | | | | |
| Sockarooni | ½ cup (4.4 oz) | 60 | 9 | 7 | 3 |
| ***Prego*** | | | | | |
| Pasta Bake Sauce Tomato Garlic & Basil | 1 serv (3.4 oz) | 80 | 11 | 10 | 2 |
| Traditional | ½ cup (4.2 oz) | 140 | 23 | 15 | 2 |
| ***Progresso*** | | | | | |
| Marinara | ½ cup (4.3 oz) | 80 | 8 | 5 | 2 |
| Meat Flavored | ½ cup (4.4 oz) | 100 | 12 | 9 | 3 |
| Sauce | ½ cup (4.4 oz) | 100 | 12 | 8 | 2 |
| ***Ragu*** | | | | | |
| Chunky Garden Style Tomato Garlic & Onion | ½ cup (4.5 oz) | 110 | 18 | 13 | 2 |
| ***Sara Lee*** | | | | | |
| Chunky Garden Mushroom & Peppers | ½ cup (4.4 oz) | 80 | 12 | 6 | 3 |
| ***Tree Of Life*** | | | | | |
| Pasta Sauce | ½ cup (4 oz) | 50 | 9 | 8 | – |
| Pasta Sauce Fat Free Classic | ½ cup (3.9 oz) | 40 | 8 | 6 | 0 |
| Pasta Sauce Fat Free Mushroom & Basil | ½ cup (3.9 oz) | 30 | 7 | 6 | 0 |
| Pasta Sauce Fat Free Onion & Garlic | ½ cup (3.9 oz) | 30 | 7 | 6 | 0 |
| Pasta Sauce Fat Free Sweet Pepper | ½ cup (3.9 oz) | 30 | 7 | 6 | 0 |
| Pasta Sauce No Salt Added | ½ cup (3.9 oz) | 50 | 9 | 8 | – |
| ***Walden Farms*** | | | | | |
| Alfredo Sauce Calorie Free | ¼ cup | 0 | 0 | 0 | 0 |
| Marinara Calorie Free | ⅓ cup | 0 | 0 | 0 | 0 |

| FOOD | PORTION | CALS | CARB | SUGAR | FIBER |
|---|---|---|---|---|---|
| **MIX** | | | | | |
| ***Durkee*** | | | | | |
| Spaghetti Sauce as prep | ½ cup | 15 | 5 | 1 | 0 |
| With Mushrooms as prep | ½ cup | 15 | 4 | 2 | 0 |
| ***French's*** | | | | | |
| Italian as prep | ½ cup | 16 | 5 | 1 | 0 |
| Mushroom as prep | ½ cup | 20 | 4 | 1 | 0 |
| Thick as prep | ½ cup | 10 | 4 | 1 | 0 |
| ***McCormick*** | | | | | |
| Alfredo Pasta Blend as prep | ½ cup | 60 | 4 | 2 | 0 |
| Pasta Rosa Blend | 1 tbsp (10 g) | 40 | 4 | 2 | 0 |
| Pesto Pasta Sauce as prep | 2 tsp (4 g) | 10 | tr | – | – |
| Primavera Pasta Blend | 1 tbsp (7 g) | 30 | 4 | tr | – |
| Spaghetti Sauce | 1 tbsp (8 g) | 25 | 5 | 3 | – |
| **TAKE-OUT** | | | | | |
| bolognese | 5 oz | 195 | 4 | – | tr |

## SPANISH FOOD

| FOOD | PORTION | CALS | CARB | SUGAR | FIBER |
|---|---|---|---|---|---|
| **CANNED** | | | | | |
| ***Derby*** | | | | | |
| Tamales | 3 (6.5 oz) | 253 | 21 | 0 | 4 |
| ***Gebhardt*** | | | | | |
| Enchiladas | 2 (5.7 oz) | 258 | 20 | 0 | 3 |
| Tamales | 2 (5.7 oz) | 268 | 19 | 1 | 3 |
| Tamales Jumbo | 2 (6.9 oz) | 332 | 24 | 0 | 3 |
| ***Rosarita*** | | | | | |
| Enchilada Sauce Mild | ¼ cup (2.1 oz) | 23 | 3 | 3 | 0 |
| ***Van Camp*** | | | | | |
| Tamales | 2 (5 oz) | 210 | 20 | 1 | 3 |
| **FROZEN** | | | | | |
| ***Amy's*** | | | | | |
| Black Bean Vegetable Enchilada | 1 (4.75 oz) | 130 | 20 | 1 | 2 |
| Bowls Santa Fe Enchilada | 1 pkg (10 oz) | 340 | 47 | 5 | 10 |
| Burrito Bean & Cheese | 1 (6 oz) | 280 | 43 | 1 | 6 |
| Burrito Bean & Rice Non-Dairy | 1 (6 oz) | 270 | 48 | 2 | 5 |
| Burrito Black Bean Vegetable | 1 (6 oz) | 320 | 54 | 4 | 4 |
| Burrito Breakfast | 1 (6 oz) | 210 | 38 | 4 | 5 |
| Burrito Especial | 1 (6 oz) | 260 | 45 | 4 | 3 |
| Cheese Enchilada | 1 (4.75 oz) | 210 | 13 | 2 | 2 |
| Mexican Tamale Pie | 1 (8 oz) | 150 | 27 | 2 | 4 |

| FOOD | PORTION | CALS | CARB | SUGAR | FIBER |
|---|---|---|---|---|---|
| ***Banquet*** | | | | | |
| Chimichanga Meal | 1 meal (9.5 oz) | 500 | 56 | 9 | 9 |
| Enchilada Beef | 1 pkg (11 oz) | 370 | 54 | 7 | 6 |
| Enchilada Cheese | 1 pkg (11 oz) | 360 | 56 | 7 | 6 |
| Enchilada Chicken | 1 pkg (11 oz) | 350 | 54 | 7 | 9 |
| Enchilada Beef & Tamale Combo | 1 pkg (11 oz) | 450 | 50 | 7 | 9 |
| Mexican Style Enchilada Combo | 1 meal (11 oz) | 360 | 55 | 7 | 9 |
| ***Health Is Wealth*** | | | | | |
| Burrito Munchees | 10 (5 oz) | 310 | 53 | 2 | 6 |
| Mexican Munchees | 2 (1 oz) | 49 | 8 | 0 | 1 |
| ***Healthy Choice*** | | | | | |
| Chicken Enchilada Supreme | 1 meal (11.3 oz) | 300 | 46 | 8 | 4 |
| Chicken Enchiladas Suiz | 1 meal (10 oz) | 280 | 43 | 4 | 5 |
| Chicken Breast Con Queso Burrito | 1 meal (10.55 oz) | 350 | 60 | 11 | 6 |
| ***Lean Cuisine*** | | | | | |
| Everyday Favorites Chicken Enchilada Suiza | 1 pkg (9 oz) | 280 | 48 | 7 | 3 |
| ***Patio*** | | | | | |
| Beef & Cheese Enchiladas Chili 'N Beans | 1 meal (15.5 oz) | 670 | 80 | 6 | 12 |
| Beef Enchiladas Chili 'N Beans | 1 meal (15.5 oz) | 540 | 73 | 6 | 12 |
| Burrito Bean & Cheese | 1 (5 oz) | 300 | 45 | 4 | 4 |
| Burrito Beef & Bean Hot | 1 (5 oz) | 320 | 43 | 4 | 4 |
| Burrito Beef & Bean Mild | 1 (5 oz) | 330 | 45 | 3 | 4 |
| Burrito Chicken | 1 (5 oz) | 290 | 44 | 6 | 2 |
| Burritos Beef & Bean Medium | 1 (5 oz) | 310 | 45 | 5 | 4 |
| Burritos Beef & Bean Red Chili Pepper Red Hot | 1 (5 oz) | 320 | 42 | 4 | 4 |
| Enchilada Beef | 1 meal (12 oz) | 320 | 52 | 4 | 9 |
| Enchilada Cheese | 1 meal (12 oz) | 370 | 54 | 7 | 7 |

| FOOD | PORTION | CALS | CARB | SUGAR | FIBER |
|---|---|---|---|---|---|
| Enchilada Chicken | 1 meal (12 oz) | 400 | 60 | 6 | 8 |
| Fiesta | 1 meal (12 oz) | 350 | 53 | 5 | 7 |
| Mexican Style | 1 meal (13.25 oz) | 470 | 59 | 5 | 10 |
| ***Tyson*** | | | | | |
| Beef Fajita | 3½ pieces (12.5 oz) | 550 | 75 | 8 | 6 |
| Chicken Fajita | 3½ pieces (13.1 oz) | 460 | 61 | 10 | 6 |
| ***Weight Watchers*** | | | | | |
| Smart Ones Chicken Enchiladas Suiza | 1 pkg (9 oz) | 270 | 33 | 8 | 2 |
| Smart Ones Santa Fe Style Rice & Beans | 1 pkg (10 oz) | 290 | 43 | 6 | 6 |
| **MIX** | | | | | |
| ***Gebhardt*** | | | | | |
| Menudo Mix | ¼ tsp (0.4 g) | 1 | tr | tr | tr |
| ***McCormick*** | | | | | |
| Burrito Seasoning | 1 tbsp (8 g) | 25 | 5 | 1 | tr |
| Fajitas Marinade Mix | 2 tsp (4 g) | 15 | 2 | – | – |
| Taco Seasoning Hot | 2 tsp (6 g) | 20 | 3 | 1 | tr |
| Taco Seasoning Mild | 2 tsp (7 g) | 20 | 4 | 1 | tr |
| **READY-TO-EAT** | | | | | |
| taco shell baked | 1 med (0.5 oz) | 61 | 8 | – | tr |
| taco shell baked w/o salt | 1 med (½ oz) | 61 | 8 | – | tr |
| ***Gebhardt*** | | | | | |
| Taco Shells | 3 (1.1 oz) | 155 | 19 | 0 | 3 |
| ***La Mexicana*** | | | | | |
| Flour Burritos | 1 (1.6 oz) | 160 | 26 | 2 | 2 |
| ***Rosarita*** | | | | | |
| Taco Shells | 3 (1.1 oz) | 155 | 19 | 0 | 3 |
| Tostada Shells | 2 (1 oz) | 125 | 17 | tr | 0 |
| **TAKE-OUT** | | | | | |
| burrito w/ apple | 1 lg (5.4 oz) | 484 | 73 | – | – |
| burrito w/ apple | 1 sm (2.6 oz) | 231 | 35 | – | – |
| burrito w/ beans | 2 (7.6 oz) | 448 | 71 | – | – |

| FOOD | PORTION | CALS | CARB | SUGAR | FIBER |
|---|---|---|---|---|---|
| burrito w/ beans & cheese | 2 (6.5 oz) | 377 | 55 | – | – |
| burrito w/ beans & chili peppers | 2 (7.2 oz) | 413 | 58 | – | – |
| burrito w/ beans & meat | 2 (8.1 oz) | 508 | 66 | – | – |
| burrito w/ beans cheese & beef | 2 (7.1 oz) | 331 | 40 | – | – |
| burrito w/ beans cheese & chili peppers | 2 (11.8 oz) | 663 | 85 | – | – |
| burrito w/ beef | 2 (7.7 oz) | 523 | 59 | – | – |
| burrito w/ beef & chili peppers | 2 (7.1 oz) | 426 | 49 | – | – |
| burrito w/ beef cheese & chili peppers | 2 (10.7 oz) | 634 | 64 | – | – |
| burrito w/ cherry | 1 sm (2.6 oz) | 231 | 35 | – | – |
| burrito w/ cherry | 1 lg (5.4 oz) | 484 | 73 | – | – |
| chimichanga w/ beef | 1 (6.1 oz) | 425 | 43 | – | – |
| chimichanga w/ beef & cheese | 1 (6.4 oz) | 443 | 39 | – | – |
| chimichanga w/ beef & red chili peppers | 1 (6.7 oz) | 424 | 46 | – | – |
| chimichanga w/ beef cheese & red chili peppers | 1 (6.3 oz) | 364 | 38 | – | – |
| enchilada w/ cheese | 1 (5.7 oz) | 320 | 29 | – | – |
| enchilada w/ cheese & beef | 1 (6.7 oz) | 324 | 30 | – | – |
| enchirito w/ cheese beef & beans | 1 (6.8 oz) | 344 | 34 | – | – |
| frijoles w/ cheese | 1 cup (5.9 oz) | 226 | 29 | – | – |
| nachos w/ cheese | 6 to 8 (4 oz) | 345 | 36 | – | – |
| nachos w/ cheese & jalapeno peppers | 6 to 8 (7.2 oz) | 607 | 60 | – | – |
| nachos w/ cheese beans ground beef & peppers | 6 to 8 (8.9 oz) | 568 | 56 | – | – |
| nachos w/ cinnamon & sugar | 6 to 8 (3.8 oz) | 592 | 63 | – | – |
| taco | 1 sm (6 oz) | 370 | 27 | – | – |
| taco salad | 1 ½ cups | 279 | 24 | – | – |
| taco salad w/ chili con carne | 1 ½ cups | 288 | 27 | – | – |
| tostada w/ beans & cheese | 1 (5.1 oz) | 223 | 27 | – | – |
| tostada w/ beans beef & cheese | 1 (7.9 oz) | 334 | 30 | – | – |
| tostada w/ beef & cheese | 1 (5.7 oz) | 315 | 23 | – | – |
| tostada w/ guacamole | 2 (9.2 oz) | 360 | 32 | – | – |

**SPICES** *(see individual names,* HERBS/SPICES*)*

| FOOD | PORTION | CALS | CARB | SUGAR | FIBER |
|---|---|---|---|---|---|
| **SPINACH** | | | | | |
| **CANNED** | | | | | |
| spinach | ½ cup | 25 | 4 | – | – |
| ***Del Monte*** | | | | | |
| Chopped | ½ cup (4 oz) | 30 | 4 | 0 | 2 |
| No Salt Added | ½ cup (4 oz) | 30 | 4 | 0 | 2 |
| Whole Leaf | ½ cup (4 oz) | 30 | 4 | 0 | 2 |
| ***S&W*** | | | | | |
| Spinach | ½ cup (4.5 oz) | 30 | 4 | 1 | 2 |
| **FRESH** | | | | | |
| baby raw | 2 cups | 20 | 5 | 0 | 3 |
| cooked | ½ cup | 21 | 3 | – | 2 |
| malabar cooked | 1 cup (1.5 oz) | 10 | 1 | – | 1 |
| mustard chopped cooked | ½ cup | 14 | 3 | – | – |
| mustard raw chopped | ½ cup | 17 | 3 | – | – |
| new zealand chopped cooked | ½ cup | 11 | 2 | – | – |
| new zealand raw | ½ cup | 4 | 1 | – | – |
| raw chopped | ½ cup | 6 | 1 | – | 1 |
| raw chopped | 1 pkg (10 oz) | 46 | 7 | – | – |
| ***Dole*** | | | | | |
| Baby Spinach | 3½ cups (3 oz) | 35 | 9 | 0 | 4 |
| ***Fresh Express*** | | | | | |
| Baby Spinach | 3 cups | 20 | 3 | 0 | 2 |
| ***Ready Pac*** | | | | | |
| Baby | ½ cup | 20 | 3 | 0 | tr |
| **FROZEN** | | | | | |
| ***Fillo Factory*** | | | | | |
| cooked | ½ cup | 27 | 5 | – | – |
| Snacks Spinach Feta | 5-6 pieces | 170 | 24 | 3 | 2 |
| ***Birds Eye*** | | | | | |
| Creamed | ½ cup | 100 | 7 | 3 | 1 |
| Cut Leaf | 1 cup | 20 | 2 | 1 | 2 |
| ***Fresh Like*** | | | | | |
| Cut Leaf | 3.5 oz | 21 | 4 | – | 1 |
| ***Health Is Wealth*** | | | | | |
| Spinach Munchees | 2 (1 oz) | 60 | 9 | 0 | 1 |
| Spinach Feta Munchees | 2 (1 oz) | 70 | 9 | 0 | 1 |

| FOOD | PORTION | CALS | CARB | SUGAR | FIBER |
|---|---|---|---|---|---|
| ***Tree Of Life*** | | | | | |
| Organic | 1 cup (3 oz) | 20 | 2 | 1 | 2 |
| **SHELF-STABLE** | | | | | |
| ***TastyBite*** | | | | | |
| Kashmir Spinach | ½ pkg (5 oz) | 170 | 8 | 1 | 3 |
| **TAKE-OUT** | | | | | |
| indian saag | 1 serv | 28 | 2 | – | 1 |
| spanakopita spinach pie | 1 cup (6 oz) | 196 | 35 | 4 | 4 |
| **SPINACH JUICE** | | | | | |
| juice | 7 oz | 14 | 2 | – | – |
| **SPORTS DRINKS** *(see* ENERGY DRINKS*)* | | | | | |
| **SPOT** | | | | | |
| baked | 3 oz | 134 | 0 | 0 | 0 |
| **SPROUTS** | | | | | |
| kidney bean | ½ cup | 27 | 4 | – | – |
| kidney bean cooked | 1 lb | 152 | 21 | – | – |
| lentil sprouts | ½ cup | 40 | 8 | – | – |
| mung bean | ½ cup | 16 | 3 | – | – |
| mung bean canned | ½ cup | 8 | 1 | – | – |
| mung bean cooked | ½ cup | 13 | 3 | – | – |
| pea | ½ cup | 77 | 17 | – | – |
| pinto bean | 3½ oz | 62 | 12 | – | – |
| pinto bean cooked | 3½ oz | 22 | 4 | – | – |
| radish | ½ cup | 8 | 1 | – | – |
| ***Chun King*** | | | | | |
| Bean Sprouts | 1 cup (3 oz) | 11 | 1 | 0 | 1 |
| ***Fresh Alternatives*** | | | | | |
| BroccoSprouts | ½ cup (1 oz) | 10 | 1 | 0 | 1 |
| Deli Blend | ½ cup (1 oz) | 10 | 1 | 0 | tr |
| Salad Blend | ½ cup (1 oz) | 10 | 2 | 0 | tr |
| Sandwich Blend | ½ cup (1 oz) | 5 | 1 | 0 | tr |
| ***La Choy*** | | | | | |
| Bean Sprouts | 1 cup (2.9 oz) | 11 | 1 | 0 | 1 |
| **TAKE-OUT** | | | | | |
| mung bean stir fried | ½ cup | 31 | 7 | – | – |
| **SQUAB** | | | | | |
| boneless baked | 3.5 oz | 175 | 0 | 0 | 0 |

| FOOD | PORTION | CALS | CARB | SUGAR | FIBER |
|---|---|---|---|---|---|
| breast w/o skin raw | 1 (3.5 oz) | 135 | 0 | 0 | 0 |
| w/o skin raw | 1 squab (5.9 oz) | 239 | 0 | 0 | 0 |
| **SQUASH** *(see also* ZUCCHINI*)* | | | | | |
| **CANNED** | | | | | |
| crookneck sliced | ½ cup | 14 | 3 | – | – |
| **FRESH** | | | | | |
| acorn cooked mashed | ½ cup | 41 | 11 | – | 3 |
| acorn cubed baked | ½ cup | 57 | 15 | – | 2 |
| butternut baked | ½ cup | 41 | 11 | – | 2 |
| crookneck raw sliced | ½ cup | 12 | 3 | – | 1 |
| crookneck sliced cooked | ½ cup | 18 | 4 | – | 1 |
| hubbard baked | ½ cup | 51 | 11 | – | 3 |
| hubbard cooked mashed | ½ cup | 35 | 8 | – | 3 |
| scallop raw sliced | ½ cup | 12 | 3 | – | 1 |
| scallop sliced cooked | ½ cup | 14 | 3 | – | 1 |
| spaghetti cooked | ½ cup | 23 | 5 | – | 2 |
| **FROZEN** | | | | | |
| butternut cooked mashed | ½ cup | 47 | 12 | – | 3 |
| crookneck sliced cooked | ½ cup | 24 | 5 | – | – |
| ***Birds Eye*** | | | | | |
| Sliced Yellow | ⅔ cup | 15 | 2 | 1 | 1 |
| **SEEDS** | | | | | |
| dried | 1 cup | 747 | 25 | – | – |
| roasted | 1 cup | 1184 | 31 | – | – |
| roasted | 1 oz | 148 | 4 | – | – |
| salted & roasted | 1 oz | 148 | 4 | – | – |
| salted & roasted | 1 cup | 1184 | 31 | – | – |
| whole roasted | 1 cup | 285 | 34 | – | – |
| whole salted roasted | 1 cup | 285 | 34 | – | – |
| **SQUID** | | | | | |
| fried | 3 oz | 149 | 7 | – | – |
| raw | 3 oz | 78 | 3 | – | – |
| **SQUIRREL** | | | | | |
| roasted | 3 oz | 147 | 0 | 0 | 0 |
| **STARFRUIT** | | | | | |
| fresh | 1 | 42 | 10 | – | – |

| FOOD | PORTION | CALS | CARB | SUGAR | FIBER |
|---|---|---|---|---|---|
| **STRAWBERRIES** | | | | | |
| **CANNED** | | | | | |
| in heavy syrup | ½ cup | 117 | 30 | – | – |
| **FRESH** | | | | | |
| strawberries | 1 cup | 45 | 10 | – | 4 |
| strawberries | 1 pint | 97 | 22 | – | – |
| **FROZEN** | | | | | |
| sweetened sliced | 1 cup | 245 | 66 | – | – |
| sweetened sliced | 1 pkg (10 oz) | 273 | 74 | – | – |
| unsweetened | 1 cup | 52 | 14 | – | – |
| whole sweetened | 1 cup | 200 | 54 | – | – |
| whole sweetened | 1 pkg (10 oz) | 223 | 60 | – | – |
| ***Birds Eye*** | | | | | |
| In Syrup | ½ cup | 120 | 31 | 28 | 1 |
| Lite Syrup | 1 pkg (10 oz) | 120 | 31 | 28 | 1 |
| Whole | ½ cup | 100 | 25 | 23 | 1 |
| ***Tree Of Life*** | | | | | |
| Organic | ¾ cup (5 oz) | 50 | 13 | 8 | 2 |
| **STRAWBERRY JUICE** | | | | | |
| ***Squeezit*** | | | | | |
| Strawberry | 1 bottle (7 oz) | 110 | 29 | 27 | 0 |
| **STUFFING/DRESSING** | | | | | |
| bread as prep w/ water & fat | ½ cup | 251 | 25 | – | – |
| bread as prep w/ water egg & fat | ½ cup | 107 | 9 | – | – |
| bread dry as prep | ½ cup | 178 | 22 | – | 3 |
| cornbread as prep | ½ cup | 179 | 22 | – | – |
| ***Pepperidge Farm*** | | | | | |
| Corn Bread | ¾ cup (1.5 oz) | 170 | 33 | 2 | 2 |
| Herb Seasoned | ¾ cup (1.5 oz) | 170 | 33 | 2 | 3 |
| Herb Seasoned Cubed | ¾ cup (1.3 oz) | 140 | 28 | 2 | 2 |
| One Step Chicken | ½ cup (1.2 oz) | 140 | 23 | tr | tr |
| One Step Southwestern Corn Bread | ½ cup (1.2 oz) | 150 | 23 | 2 | tr |
| One Step Turkey | ½ cup (1.2 oz) | 150 | 22 | 3 | tr |
| **TAKE-OUT** | | | | | |
| bread | ½ cup (3½ oz) | 195 | 26 | – | 3 |

| FOOD | PORTION | CALS | CARB | SUGAR | FIBER |
|---|---|---|---|---|---|
| sausage | ½ cup | 292 | 40 | – | 1 |
| **STURGEON** | | | | | |
| cooked | 3 oz | 115 | 0 | 0 | 0 |
| roe raw | 1 oz | 59 | tr | – | – |
| smoked | 3 oz | 147 | 0 | 0 | 0 |
| smoked | 1 oz | 48 | 0 | 0 | 0 |
| **SUCKER** | | | | | |
| white baked | 3 oz | 101 | 0 | 0 | 0 |
| **SUGAR** | | | | | |
| brown packed | 1 cup (7.7 oz) | 828 | 214 | 214 | – |
| brown unpacked | 1 cup (5.1 oz) | 546 | 141 | – | – |
| maple | 1 piece (1 oz) | 100 | 26 | – | – |
| powdered | 1 tbsp (0.3 oz) | 31 | 8 | 8 | – |
| powdered unsifted | 1 cup (4.2 oz) | 467 | 119 | 115 | – |
| sugarcane stem | 3 oz | 54 | 14 | – | 3 |
| white | 1 cup (7 oz) | 773 | 200 | 200 | – |
| white | 1 tbsp | 45 | 12 | – | – |
| white | 1 packet (6 g) | 25 | 6 | – | – |
| white | 1 tsp (4 g) | 15 | 4 | 4 | – |
| ***Billington's*** | | | | | |
| Muscovado Light Brown | 1 tsp | 15 | 4 | 4 | – |
| ***Domino*** | | | | | |
| Dark Brown | 1 tsp | 15 | 4 | 4 | – |
| Light Brown | 1 tsp | 15 | 4 | 4 | – |
| White | 1 tsp | 16 | 4 | – | – |
| ***Maui Brand*** | | | | | |
| Raw Sugar | 1 tsp | 15 | 4 | 4 | – |
| ***Princess Of Yum*** | | | | | |
| Citrus Lemon | 2.5 tsp | 40 | 10 | 10 | – |
| French Vanilla | 2.5 tsp | 40 | 10 | 10 | – |
| **SUGAR SUBSTITUTES** | | | | | |
| ***Equal*** | | | | | |
| Packet | 1 pkg | 0 | tr | tr | – |
| ***Keto*** | | | | | |
| Sweet | ½ tsp | 0 | 0 | 0 | 0 |
| ***Lo Han*** | | | | | |
| Sweet | 2 scoops | 2 | 2 | 0 | tr |

| FOOD | PORTION | CALS | CARB | SUGAR | FIBER |
|---|---|---|---|---|---|
| ***SomerSweet*** | | | | | |
| Sweetener | ¼ tsp | 0 | tr | 0 | tr |
| ***Splenda*** | | | | | |
| Sweetener | 1 pkg | 0 | tr | tr | 0 |
| ***Steel's*** | | | | | |
| Brown | 1 tsp | 10 | 1 | 0 | 0 |
| Sugar Substitute | 1 tsp | 10 | 5 | 0 | – |
| ***Stevia*** | | | | | |
| Stevia Spoonable | ⅓ tsp | 0 | 0 | 0 | 0 |
| ***Sugar Twin*** | | | | | |
| Packets | 1 | 0 | tr | – | – |
| Spoonable Brown | 1 tsp | 0 | 0 | 0 | 0 |
| Spoonable White | 1 tsp | 0 | 0 | 0 | 0 |
| ***Weight Watchers*** | | | | | |
| Sweetener | 1 serv (1 g) | 5 | 1 | 1 | 0 |
| **SUGAR-APPLE** | | | | | |
| fresh | 1 | 146 | 37 | – | – |
| fresh cut up | 1 cup | 236 | 59 | – | – |
| **SUNCHOKE** | | | | | |
| fresh raw sliced | ½ cup | 57 | 13 | – | – |
| **SUNFISH** | | | | | |
| pumpkinseed baked | 3 oz | 97 | 0 | 0 | 0 |
| **SUNFLOWER** | | | | | |
| seeds dried | 1 oz | 162 | 5 | – | – |
| seeds dried | 1 cup | 821 | 27 | – | – |
| seeds dry roasted | 1 oz | 165 | 7 | – | – |
| seeds dry roasted | 1 cup | 745 | 31 | – | – |
| seeds dry roasted salted | 1 oz | 165 | 7 | – | – |
| seeds dry roasted salted | 1 cup | 745 | 31 | – | – |
| seeds oil roasted | 1 cup | 830 | 20 | – | – |
| seeds oil roasted salted | 1 oz | 175 | 4 | – | – |
| seeds oil roasted salted | 1 cup | 830 | 20 | – | – |
| seeds toasted | 1 oz | 176 | 6 | – | – |
| seeds toasted | 1 cup | 826 | 28 | – | – |
| seeds toasted salted | 1 cup | 826 | 28 | – | – |
| seeds toasted salted | 1 oz | 176 | 6 | – | – |
| sunflower butter | 1 tbsp | 93 | 4 | – | – |
| sunflower butter w/o salt | 1 tbsp | 93 | 4 | – | – |

| FOOD | PORTION | CALS | CARB | SUGAR | FIBER |
|---|---|---|---|---|---|
| ***Dakota Gourmet*** | | | | | |
| Honey Roasted Kernels | 1 pkg (1 oz) | 158 | 8 | 4 | 1 |
| Lightly Salted Kernels | 1 pkg (1 oz) | 168 | 5 | 1 | 2 |
| ***Frito Lay*** | | | | | |
| Seeds | 1 oz | 180 | 5 | tr | 2 |
| ***Lance*** | | | | | |
| Seeds In Shell | ⅔ cup (1.8 oz) | 160 | 5 | 1 | 2 |
| Seeds Roasted & Shelled | 1 pkg (1⅛ oz) | 190 | 6 | 1 | 2 |
| ***Maranatha*** | | | | | |
| Tamari Seeds | ¼ cup | 160 | 7 | 1 | 2 |
| ***SunGold*** | | | | | |
| SunButter | 2 tbsp | 200 | 7 | 3 | 4 |
| **SUSHI** | | | | | |
| **TAKE-OUT** | | | | | |
| california roll | 1 piece (0.8 oz) | 28 | 4 | tr | – |
| sashimi | 1 serv (6 oz) | 198 | 4 | 1 | – |
| tuna roll | 1 piece (0.7 oz) | 23 | 3 | tr | – |
| vegetable roll | 1 piece (1.2 oz) | 27 | 5 | tr | – |
| vinegared ginger | ⅓ cup (1.6 oz) | 48 | 12 | 4 | – |
| wasabi | 2 tsp (0.3 oz) | 5 | 1 | – | – |
| yellowtail roll | 1 piece (0.6 oz) | 25 | 3 | tr | – |
| **SWAMP CABBAGE** | | | | | |
| chopped cooked | ½ cup | 10 | 2 | – | – |
| raw chopped | 1 cup | 11 | 2 | – | – |
| **SWEET POTATO** *(see also* YAM*)* | | | | | |
| canned in syrup | ½ cup | 106 | 25 | – | – |
| canned pieces | 1 cup | 183 | 42 | – | – |
| frzn cooked | ½ cup | 88 | 21 | – | – |
| leaves cooked | ½ cup | 11 | 2 | – | – |
| mashed | ½ cup | 172 | 40 | – | 3 |
| **TAKE-OUT** | | | | | |
| candied | 3½ oz | 144 | 29 | – | – |
| **SWEETBREADS** | | | | | |
| beef braised | 3 oz | 230 | 0 | 0 | 0 |

| FOOD | PORTION | CALS | CARB | SUGAR | FIBER |
|---|---|---|---|---|---|
| lamb braised | 3 oz | 199 | 0 | 0 | 0 |
| veal braised | 3 oz | 218 | 0 | 0 | 0 |
| **SWISS CHARD** | | | | | |
| cooked | ½ cup | 18 | 4 | – | – |
| **SWORDFISH** | | | | | |
| cooked | 3 oz | 132 | 0 | 0 | 0 |
| **SYRUP** | | | | | |
| corn | 1 tbsp (0.7 oz) | 56 | 15 | 10 | – |
| corn dark | 1 cup (11.5 oz) | 925 | 251 | – | – |
| corn dark | 1 tbsp (0.7 oz) | 56 | 15 | – | – |
| corn light | 1 cup (11.5 oz) | 925 | 251 | 168 | – |
| date syrup | 1 tbsp | 63 | 15 | – | 0 |
| malt | 1 cup (13 oz) | 1222 | 274 | – | – |
| malt | 1 tbsp (0.8 oz) | 76 | 17 | – | – |
| maple | 1 cup (11.1 oz) | 824 | 212 | 191 | – |
| maple | 1 tbsp (0.8 oz) | 52 | 13 | 12 | – |
| raspberry | 1 oz | 76 | 19 | – | – |
| rose hip | 1 oz | 9 | 2 | 2 | 0 |
| sorghum | 1 cup (11.6 oz) | 957 | 247 | 247 | – |
| sorghum | 1 tbsp (0.7 oz) | 61 | 16 | 16 | – |
| ***DaVinci Gourmet*** | | | | | |
| Sugar Free All Flavors | 1 tbsp | 0 | 0 | 0 | 0 |
| ***Eden*** | | | | | |
| Organic Barley Malt | 1 tbsp | 60 | 14 | 8 | 0 |
| ***Estee*** | | | | | |
| Blueberry | ¼ cup | 80 | 20 | 20 | 0 |
| ***Hershey*** | | | | | |
| Strawberry | 2 tbsp (1.4 oz) | 100 | 26 | – | – |
| ***Karo*** | | | | | |
| Corn Syrup Light | 2 tbsp (1 oz) | 120 | 31 | 12 | – |
| ***Quik*** | | | | | |
| Strawberry | 2 tbsp (1.5 oz) | 110 | 27 | 26 | 0 |

| FOOD | PORTION | CALS | CARB | SUGAR | FIBER |
|---|---|---|---|---|---|
| ***Smucker's*** | | | | | |
| Apricot | ¼ cup | 210 | 52 | 52 | – |
| Blackberry | ¼ cup | 210 | 52 | 52 | – |
| Plate Scapers Kiwi Lime | 2 tbsp (1.3 oz) | 100 | 25 | 13 | – |
| Plate Scapers Mango Orange | 2 tbsp | 100 | 24 | 13 | – |
| Plate Scapers Raspberry | 2 tbsp (1.3 oz) | 100 | 25 | 13 | – |
| **TAHINI** *(see* SESAME*)* | | | | | |
| **TAMARIND** | | | | | |
| fresh | 1 | 5 | 1 | – | – |
| fresh cut up | 1 cup | 287 | 75 | – | – |
| **TANGERINE** | | | | | |
| **CANNED** | | | | | |
| in light syrup | ½ cup | 76 | 20 | – | – |
| juice pack | ½ cup | 46 | 12 | – | – |
| **FRESH** | | | | | |
| sections | 1 cup | 86 | 22 | – | – |
| tangerine | 1 | 37 | 9 | – | – |
| ***Chiquita*** | | | | | |
| Tangerine | 1 med (3.5 oz) | 50 | 15 | 12 | 2 |
| **TANGERINE JUICE** | | | | | |
| canned sweetened | 1 cup | 125 | 30 | – | – |
| fresh | 1 cup | 106 | 25 | – | – |
| frzn sweetened as prep | 1 cup | 110 | 27 | – | – |
| frzn sweetened not prep | 6 oz | 344 | 83 | – | – |
| ***Fresh Samantha*** | | | | | |
| Fresh Juice | 1 cup (8 oz) | 110 | 8 | – | 0 |
| ***Odwalla*** | | | | | |
| Juice | 8 fl oz | 110 | 25 | 24 | 0 |
| **TAPIOCA** | | | | | |
| pearl dry | ½ cup (2.7 oz) | 272 | 67 | – | 1 |
| starch | 1 oz | 98 | 24 | – | – |
| **TARO** | | | | | |
| chips | 1 oz | 141 | 19 | – | – |

| FOOD | PORTION | CALS | CARB | SUGAR | FIBER |
|---|---|---|---|---|---|
| chips | 10 (0.8 oz) | 115 | 16 | – | – |
| leaves cooked | ½ cup | 18 | 3 | – | – |
| shoots sliced cooked | ½ cup | 10 | 2 | – | – |
| sliced cooked | ½ cup (2.3 oz) | 94 | 23 | – | – |
| tahitian sliced cooked | ½ cup | 30 | 5 | – | – |
| **TARPON** | | | | | |
| fresh | 3 oz | 87 | 0 | 0 | 0 |
| **TARRAGON** | | | | | |
| ground | 1 tsp | 5 | 1 | – | – |
| **TEA/HERBAL TEA** *(see also* ICED TEA) | | | | | |
| **HERBAL** | | | | | |
| chamomile brewed | 1 cup | 2 | tr | 0 | 0 |
| ***Celestial Seasonings*** | | | | | |
| Mandarin Orange Spice | 1 tea bag | 0 | tr | 0 | – |
| ***Eden*** | | | | | |
| Organic Genmaicha Tea | 1 cup | 0 | 0 | 0 | 0 |
| Organic Kukicha Tea | 1 cup | 0 | 0 | 0 | 0 |
| ***Guayaki*** | | | | | |
| Yerba Mate Magical Mint | 1 tea bag | 5 | 1 | – | – |
| Yerba Mate Organic Chai Spice | 1 tea bag | 5 | 1 | – | – |
| Yerba Mate Organic Chocolatte | 1 tea bag | 5 | 1 | – | – |
| Yerba Mate Organic Orange Blossom | 1 tea bag | 5 | 1 | – | – |
| Yerba Mate Organic Rooiboost | 1 tea bag | 5 | 1 | 0 | – |
| Yerba Mate Organic Traditional | 1 tea bag | 5 | 1 | 0 | – |
| ***Lipton*** | | | | | |
| Bedtime Story | 1 tea bag | 0 | 1 | 0 | – |
| Cinnamon Apple | 1 tea bag | 0 | 1 | 0 | – |
| Ginger Twist | 1 tea bag | 0 | 0 | 0 | 0 |
| Lemon | 1 tea bag | 0 | 1 | 0 | – |
| Orange | 1 tea bag | 0 | 1 | 0 | – |
| Peppermint | 1 tea bag | 0 | 1 | 0 | – |
| Quietly Chamomile | 1 tea bag | 0 | 1 | 0 | – |
| ***Silk*** | | | | | |
| Chai | 1 cup | 140 | 19 | 14 | 0 |
| **REGULAR** | | | | | |
| brewed tea | 6 oz | 2 | 1 | – | 0 |

| FOOD | PORTION | CALS | CARB | SUGAR | FIBER |
|---|---|---|---|---|---|
| instant unsweetened as prep w/ water | 8 oz | 2 | tr | – | – |
| ***Activitea*** | | | | | |
| Green Tea | 1 cup | 36 | 3 | tr | – |
| ***Celestial Seasonings*** | | | | | |
| Green Tea Raspberry Garden as prep | 1 cup | 0 | 0 | 0 | 0 |
| Green Tea Honey Lemon Ginseng | 1 cup | 0 | 0 | 0 | 0 |
| Honey Darjeeling as prep | 1 cup | 0 | 0 | 0 | 0 |
| ***DaVinci Gourmet*** | | | | | |
| Sugar Free Tea Concentrate Green | 2 tbsp | 0 | 0 | 0 | 0 |
| Sugar Free Tea Concentrate Lemon | 2 tbsp | 0 | 0 | 0 | 0 |
| Sugar Free Tea Concentrate Spiced Chai | 1.5 tbsp | 0 | 0 | 0 | 0 |
| ***Guayaki*** | | | | | |
| Yerba Mate Organic Greener Green Tea | 1 tea bag | 5 | 1 | 0 | – |
| ***Lipton*** | | | | | |
| Green Tea | 1 tea bag | 0 | 0 | 0 | – |
| ***Pacific Chai*** | | | | | |
| All Flavors as prep | 1 serv | 93 | 18 | 11 | 0 |
| ***Paradise*** | | | | | |
| Tropical Tea | 8 fl oz | 1 | tr | 0 | 0 |
| Tropical Tea Decafe | 8 fl oz | 1 | tr | 0 | 0 |
| Tropical Tea Passion Fruit | 8 fl oz | 1 | tr | 0 | 0 |
| ***Salada*** | | | | | |
| Green Tea | 1 cup | 0 | 0 | 0 | 0 |
| Green Tea Decaffeinated | 1 tea bag | 0 | 0 | 0 | – |
| ***Tetley*** | | | | | |
| British Blend Round Teabags | 1 cup | 0 | 0 | 0 | 0 |
| Decaffeinated Tea Bag as prep | 1 | 0 | 0 | 0 | 0 |
| **TAKE-OUT** | | | | | |
| chai spiced latte decaf | 1 cup | 130 | 23 | 18 | 0 |

## TEMPEH

| | | | | | |
|---|---|---|---|---|---|
| tempeh | ½ cup | 165 | 14 | – | – |

| FOOD | PORTION | CALS | CARB | SUGAR | FIBER |
|---|---|---|---|---|---|
| ***Lightlife*** | | | | | |
| Garden Vege | 4 oz | 200 | 12 | 3 | 6 |
| Quinoa Sesame | 4 oz | 220 | 15 | 3 | 7 |
| Smokey Strips | 3 slices (2 oz) | 80 | 6 | 0 | 1 |
| Soy | 4 oz | 210 | 11 | 3 | 7 |
| Three Grain | 4 oz | 200 | 13 | 3 | 6 |
| Wild Rice | 4 oz | 190 | 13 | 3 | 6 |
| ***Turtle Island*** | | | | | |
| Five Grain | 3 oz | 190 | 20 | 0 | 6 |
| Low Fat Millet | 3 oz | 130 | 20 | 0 | 3 |
| Soy | 3 oz | 160 | 20 | 0 | 7 |
| Wild Rice Rhapsody | 3 oz | 160 | 20 | 0 | 7 |
| ***White Wave*** | | | | | |
| Five Grain | ⅓ block | 140 | 15 | 2 | 4 |
| Organic Original Soy | ⅓ block | 150 | 10 | 0 | 6 |
| Organic Sea Veggie | ⅓ block | 120 | 11 | 0 | 8 |
| Soy Rice | ⅓ block | 140 | 13 | 2 | 5 |
| **THYME** | | | | | |
| ground | 1 tsp | 4 | 1 | – | – |
| **TILEFISH** | | | | | |
| cooked | 3 oz | 125 | 0 | 0 | 0 |
| cooked | ½ fillet (5.3 oz) | 220 | 0 | 0 | 0 |
| **TOFU** | | | | | |
| firm | ¼ block (3 oz) | 118 | 3 | – | 1 |
| firm | ½ cup | 183 | 5 | – | 2 |
| fresh fried | 1 piece (0.5 oz) | 35 | 1 | – | tr |
| fuyu salted & fermented | 1 block (⅓ oz) | 13 | 1 | – | tr |
| koyadofu dried frozen | 1 piece (½ oz) | 82 | 2 | – | tr |
| okara | ½ cup | 47 | 8 | – | 1 |
| regular | ¼ block (4 oz) | 88 | 2 | – | 1 |
| regular | ½ cup | 94 | 2 | – | 1 |
| ***Azumaya*** | | | | | |
| Baked Chili Picante | 2 pieces | 200 | 9 | 3 | 2 |
| Baked Mesquite | 2 pieces | 100 | 6 | tr | 2 |

| FOOD | PORTION | CALS | CARB | SUGAR | FIBER |
|---|---|---|---|---|---|
| Baked Spicy Thai Peanut | 2 pieces | 190 | 6 | 2 | 2 |
| Baked Teriyaki | 2 pieces | 200 | 9 | 3 | 2 |
| Extra Firm | 1 serv (2.8 oz) | 70 | 2 | 0 | 1 |
| Firm | 1 serv (2.8 oz) | 70 | 2 | 0 | 0 |
| Lite Extra Firm | 1 serv (2.8 oz) | 60 | 3 | 0 | 1 |
| Lite Silken | 1 serv (3.2 oz) | 40 | 3 | 0 | 0 |
| Silken | 1 serv (3.2 oz) | 40 | 1 | tr | – |
| ***Galaxy*** | | | | | |
| Slices Hickory Smoked | 1 slice (1 oz) | 50 | 5 | 2 | 0 |
| Slices Italian Garlic Herb | 1 slice (1 oz) | 50 | 5 | 2 | 0 |
| Slices Original | 1 slice (1 oz) | 50 | 5 | 2 | 0 |
| Slices Savory | 1 slice (1 oz) | 50 | 5 | 2 | 0 |
| ***Hinoichi*** | | | | | |
| Firm | 1 inch slice (3 oz) | 60 | 2 | 0 | 1 |
| ***Nasoya*** | | | | | |
| 5 Spice | 1 serv (3 oz) | 70 | 0 | 1 | 0 |
| Baked Mesquite Smoke | 2 pieces | 220 | 17 | tr | 3 |
| Baked Teriyaki | 2 pieces | 230 | 21 | 3 | 3 |
| Baked TexMex | 2 pieces | 230 | 21 | 3 | 4 |
| Baked Thai Peanut | 2 pieces | 240 | 19 | 2 | 3 |
| Extra Firm | 1 serv (3 oz) | 90 | 3 | 0 | 0 |
| Firm | 1 serv (3 oz) | 70 | 2 | 0 | tr |
| Frim Enriched | 1 serv (3 oz) | 45 | 0 | 0 | 0 |
| Garlic & Onion | 1 serv (3 oz) | 70 | 1 | 1 | 0 |
| Silken | 1 serv (3.2 oz) | 45 | 2 | tr | 0 |
| Soft | 1 serv (3 oz) | 60 | 1 | 0 | 0 |
| TofuMate Breakfast Scramble | ¼ pkg | 15 | 3 | 0 | – |
| TofuMate Eggless Salad | ¼ pkg | 15 | 4 | 0 | – |
| TofuMate Mandarin Stirfry | ¼ pkg | 30 | 6 | 3 | – |
| TofuMate Mediterranean Herb | ¼ pkg | 15 | 3 | 1 | – |
| TofuMate Szechwan StirFry | ¼ pkg | 25 | 4 | 0 | – |
| TofuMate Texas Taco | ¼ pkg | 15 | 3 | 0 | 0 |
| ***Pete's Tofu*** | | | | | |
| Dessert Peach Mango | 1 serv (6 oz) | 120 | 20 | 17 | 0 |
| Dessert Very Berry | 1 serv (6 oz) | 120 | 17 | 14 | 0 |
| Medium Firm | 3 oz | 70 | 2 | 0 | 0 |
| Soft | 3 oz | 56 | 2 | 0 | 0 |
| Super Firm Italian Herb | 3 oz | 120 | 1 | 0 | tr |
| Super Firm | 3 oz | 130 | 2 | 0 | 0 |

| FOOD | PORTION | CALS | CARB | SUGAR | FIBER |
|---|---|---|---|---|---|
| Tofu 2 Go Lemon Pepper | 2 pieces + sauce | 160 | 9 | 7 | 2 |
| Tofu 2 Go Santa Fe | 2 pieces + sauce | 150 | 6 | 4 | 2 |
| Tofu 2 Go Sesame Ginger | 2 pieces + sauce | 160 | 7 | 4 | 2 |
| Tofu 2 Go Thai Tango | 2 pieces + sauce | 165 | 9 | 7 | 2 |
| ***Tree Of Life*** | | | | | |
| 30% Reduced Fat Firm | ⅕ block (3.2 oz) | 90 | 4 | 0 | 2 |
| Easymeal Pasta Primavera as prep | 1 serv | 460 | 54 | 4 | 3 |
| Easymeal Southwest Medley as prep | 1 serv | 380 | 44 | 4 | 3 |
| Easymeal Teriyaki Stir Fry as prep | 1 serv | 270 | 24 | 8 | 6 |
| Easymeal Thai Stir Fry as prep | 1 serv | 270 | 21 | 8 | 6 |
| Organic Baked | ⅓ block (2.7 oz) | 150 | 5 | 0 | 0 |
| Organic Baked Island Spice | ⅓ pkg (2.7 oz) | 130 | 3 | 0 | 0 |
| Organic Baked Oriental | ⅓ pkg (2.7 oz) | 130 | 5 | 2 | 0 |
| Organic Baked Savory | ⅓ block (2.7 oz) | 140 | 4 | 0 | 0 |
| Organic Firm | ⅕ block (3.2 oz) | 100 | 2 | 0 | 0 |
| Raw Firm | ⅕ block (3.2 oz) | 100 | 2 | 0 | 0 |
| ***White Wave*** | | | | | |
| Baked Garlic Herb Italian | 1 piece | 120 | 3 | 0 | 1 |
| Baked Hickory Smoke BBQ | 1 piece | 75 | 4 | 3 | 1 |
| Baked Roma Italian Basil | 1 piece | 100 | 3 | 1 | 2 |
| Baked Teriyaki Oriental | 1 piece | 120 | 3 | 0 | 1 |
| Baked Thai Style | 1 piece | 120 | 3 | 0 | 1 |
| Baked Zesty Lemon Pepper | 1 piece | 120 | 3 | 1 | 1 |
| Extra Firm | ¼ block | 80 | 1 | 0 | 1 |
| Organic Extra Firm | ⅕ block | 90 | 1 | 0 | 1 |

| FOOD | PORTION | CALS | CARB | SUGAR | FIBER |
|---|---|---|---|---|---|
| Organic Soft | ⅕ block | 90 | 1 | 0 | 1 |
| Reduced Fat | ⅕ block | 90 | 4 | 0 | 2 |
| **TOMATILLO** | | | | | |
| fresh | 1 (1.2 oz) | 11 | 2 | – | – |
| fresh chopped | ½ cup | 21 | 4 | – | – |
| **TOMATO** | | | | | |
| **CANNED** | | | | | |
| paste | ½ cup | 110 | 25 | – | 6 |
| puree | 1 cup | 102 | 25 | – | 6 |
| puree w/o salt | 1 cup | 102 | 25 | – | 6 |
| red whole | ½ cup | 24 | 5 | – | – |
| sauce | ½ cup | 37 | 9 | – | 2 |
| sauce spanish style | ½ cup | 40 | 9 | – | 2 |
| sauce w/ mushrooms | ½ cup | 42 | 10 | – | – |
| sauce w/ onion | ½ cup | 52 | 12 | – | – |
| stewed | ½ cup | 34 | 8 | – | – |
| w/ green chiles | ½ cup | 18 | 4 | – | – |
| wedges in tomato juice | ½ cup | 34 | 8 | – | – |
| ***Big R*** | | | | | |
| Cajun Stewed | ½ cup (4.2 oz) | 25 | 4 | 4 | 1 |
| Diced w/ Chilies | ½ cup (4.2 oz) | 25 | 4 | 3 | 1 |
| Mexican Stewed | ½ cups (4.2 oz) | 25 | 5 | 3 | 1 |
| Stewed | ½ cup (4.2 oz) | 25 | 5 | 3 | 1 |
| Whole | ½ cup (4.2 oz) | 25 | 5 | 3 | 1 |
| ***Claussen*** | | | | | |
| Halves | 1 serv (1 oz) | 5 | 1 | 0 | tr |
| ***Contadina*** | | | | | |
| Italian Pasta | 2 tbsp | 35 | 7 | 4 | 1 |
| Italian Paste Roasted Garlic | 2 tbsp | 35 | 6 | 1 | 1 |
| Paste | 2 tbsp (1.2 oz) | 30 | 6 | 3 | 1 |
| Puree | ¼ cup (2.2 oz) | 20 | 4 | 1 | tr |
| Recipe Ready Diced Roasted Garlic | ½ cup (4.3 oz) | 45 | 10 | 7 | tr |
| Stewed | ½ cup | 35 | 9 | 6 | 1 |
| Stewed w/ Celery & Green Peppers | ½ cup | 35 | 9 | 6 | 1 |
| ***Del Monte*** | | | | | |
| Chunky Chili Style | ½ cup (4.5 oz) | 30 | 8 | 6 | 2 |

| FOOD | PORTION | CALS | CARB | SUGAR | FIBER |
|---|---|---|---|---|---|
| Chunky Pasta Style | ½ cup (4.5 oz) | 45 | 11 | 8 | 2 |
| Crushed Italian Recipe | ½ cup (4.4 oz) | 45 | 9 | 5 | 1 |
| Crushed Original Recipe | ½ cup (4.4 oz) | 45 | 9 | 5 | 1 |
| Crushed w/ Garlic | ½ cup (4.4 oz) | 50 | 11 | 1 | 1 |
| Diced | ½ cup (4.4 oz) | 25 | 6 | 4 | 2 |
| Diced No Salt Added | ½ cup (4.4 oz) | 25 | 6 | 4 | 2 |
| Diced w/ Basil Garlic & Oregano | ½ cup | 50 | 11 | 8 | tr |
| Diced w/ Garlic & Onion | ½ cup (4.4 oz) | 40 | 8 | 6 | 1 |
| Diced w/ Green Pepper & Onion | ½ cup (4.4 oz) | 40 | 9 | 7 | 2 |
| Paste | 2 tbsp (1.2 oz) | 30 | 7 | 5 | 2 |
| Petite Cut Garlic & Olive Oil | ½ cup | 45 | 10 | 7 | 1 |
| Sauce | ¼ cup (2.1 oz) | 20 | 4 | 4 | 1 |
| Sauce No Salt Added | ¼ cup (2.1 oz) | 20 | 4 | 4 | 1 |
| Stewed Cajun Recipe | ½ cup (4.4 oz) | 35 | 9 | 7 | 2 |
| Stewed Italian Recipe | ½ cup (4.4 oz) | 30 | 8 | 6 | 2 |
| Stewed Mexican Recipe | ½ cup (4.4 oz) | 35 | 9 | 7 | 2 |
| Stewed Original | ½ cup (4.4 oz) | 35 | 9 | 7 | 2 |
| Stewed Original No Salt Added | ½ cup (4.4 oz) | 35 | 9 | 7 | 2 |
| Wedges | ½ cup (4.4 oz) | 35 | 9 | 7 | 2 |
| Zesty Diced w/ Mild Green Chilies | ½ cup (4.4 oz) | 30 | 6 | 3 | 1 |
| ***Eden*** | | | | | |
| Organic Diced | ½ cup | 30 | 6 | 4 | 2 |
| Organic Diced w/ Green Chilies | ½ cup | 30 | 5 | 3 | 2 |
| ***Hunt's*** | | | | | |
| Angela Mia Puree | ¼ cup (2.2 oz) | 16 | 3 | 3 | tr |
| Choice Cut | ½ cup (4.2 oz) | 23 | 5 | 5 | 1 |
| Choice Cut Diced Tomatoes & Italian Herb | ½ cup (4.2 oz) | 24 | 5 | 5 | 1 |
| Choice Cut Diced Tomatoes & Roasted Garlic | ½ cup (4.2 oz) | 24 | 5 | 5 | 1 |
| Choice Cut Diced Tomatoes w/ Red Pepper & Basil | ¼ cup (4.2 oz) | 27 | 6 | 5 | 1 |
| Crushed Pear Tomatoes | ½ cup (4.2 oz) | 29 | 7 | 6 | 2 |
| Diced In Juice | ½ cup | 20 | 5 | 4 | 1 |
| Diced In Puree | ½ cup (4.3 oz) | 23 | 5 | 5 | 1 |
| Diced W/ Green Chilies | 2 tbsp (0.4 oz) | 1 | tr | tr | tr |
| Paste | 2 tbsp (1.2 oz) | 30 | 6 | 4 | 2 |

| FOOD | PORTION | CALS | CARB | SUGAR | FIBER |
|---|---|---|---|---|---|
| Paste Italian | 2 tbsp (1.2 oz) | 27 | 6 | 4 | 2 |
| Paste No Salt Added | 2 tbsp (1.2 oz) | 30 | 6 | 4 | 2 |
| Paste With Garlic | 2 tbsp (1.2 oz) | 28 | 6 | 4 | 2 |
| Petite Diced | ½ cup | 20 | 5 | 3 | 1 |
| Petite Diced w/ Mushrooms | ½ cup | 45 | 6 | 5 | 1 |
| Puree | ¼ cup (2.2 oz) | 24 | 5 | 3 | 2 |
| Ready Sauce Chunky Chili | ¼ cup (2.2 oz) | 22 | 4 | 3 | 1 |
| Ready Sauce Chunky Italian | ¼ cup (2.2 oz) | 30 | 4 | 4 | 1 |
| Ready Sauce Chunky Mexican | ¼ cup (2.2 oz) | 21 | 4 | 3 | 1 |
| Ready Sauce Chunky Salsa | ¼ cup (2.2 oz) | 18 | 3 | 3 | 1 |
| Ready Sauce Chunky Tomato | ¼ cup (2.2 oz) | 15 | 3 | 2 | 1 |
| Ready Sauce Garlic & Herb | ¼ cup (2.2 oz) | 26 | 5 | 4 | 1 |
| Sauce | ¼ cup (2.2 oz) | 16 | 3 | 3 | 1 |
| Sauce Herb | ¼ cup (2.2 oz) | 32 | 5 | 5 | 1 |
| Sauce Italian | ¼ cup (2.2 oz) | 32 | 5 | 5 | 1 |
| Sauce Meatloaf Fixins | ¼ cup (2.2 oz) | 23 | 4 | 5 | 1 |
| Sauce No Salt Added | ¼ cup (2.2 oz) | 16 | 3 | 3 | 1 |
| Sauce Special | ¼ cup (2.2 oz) | 21 | 4 | 3 | 1 |
| Stewed | ½ cup (4.2 oz) | 33 | 7 | 6 | 2 |
| Stewed No Salt Added | ½ cup (4.2 oz) | 33 | 7 | 6 | 2 |
| Whole Peeled | 2 (5.2 oz) | 24 | 5 | 5 | 1 |
| Whole Peeled No Salt Added | 2 (4.8 oz) | 21 | 4 | 4 | 1 |
| ***Muir Glen*** | | | | | |
| Diced Fire Roasted | ¼ cup | 30 | 6 | 4 | 1 |
| Diced w/ Green Chilies | ½ cup (4.5 oz) | 25 | 4 | 4 | 1 |
| Organic Chunky Sauce | ¼ cup (2.3 oz) | 20 | 4 | 2 | 1 |
| Organic Crushed Fire Roasted | ¼ cup | 20 | 5 | 4 | 1 |
| Organic Diced | ½ cup (4.5 oz) | 25 | 4 | 4 | 1 |
| Organic Diced No Salt Added | ½ cup (4.5 oz) | 25 | 4 | 4 | 1 |
| Organic Diced w/ Basil & Garlic | ½ cup (4.5 oz) | 25 | 4 | 4 | 1 |
| Organic Diced w/ Italian Herbs | ½ cup (4.4 oz) | 25 | 4 | 4 | 1 |
| Organic Ground Peeled | ¼ cup (2.3 oz) | 10 | 2 | 2 | 1 |
| Organic Paste | 2 tbsp (1.2 oz) | 30 | 6 | 3 | 1 |
| Organic Puree | ¼ cup (2.2 oz) | 20 | 5 | 3 | 1 |
| Organic Sauce | ¼ cup (2.2 oz) | 20 | 5 | 3 | 1 |
| Organic Sauce No Salt Added | ¼ cup (2.2 oz) | 20 | 5 | 3 | 1 |
| Organic Stewed | ½ cup (4.5 oz) | 30 | 7 | 3 | tr |
| Organic Whole Peeled | ½ cup (4.6 oz) | 30 | 5 | 4 | 1 |
| Whole Peeled w/ Basil | ½ cup (4.6 oz) | 30 | 5 | 4 | 1 |

| FOOD | PORTION | CALS | CARB | SUGAR | FIBER |
|---|---|---|---|---|---|
| ***Progresso*** | | | | | |
| Crushed w/ Added Puree | ¼ cup (2.1 oz) | 20 | 3 | 2 | 0 |
| Italian Style Peeled | ½ cup (4.2 oz) | 20 | 4 | 3 | 1 |
| Paste | 2 tbsp (1.2 oz) | 30 | 6 | 3 | 1 |
| Puree | ¼ cup (2.2 oz) | 25 | 5 | 3 | 1 |
| Puree Thick Style | ¼ cup (2.2 oz) | 20 | 5 | 3 | 1 |
| Sauce | ¼ cup (2.1 oz) | 20 | 4 | 2 | 1 |
| Whole Peeled | ½ cup (4.2 oz) | 25 | 5 | 3 | 1 |
| ***Redpack*** | | | | | |
| Crushed In Puree | ¼ cup | 20 | 4 | 2 | 1 |
| **DRIED** | | | | | |
| sun dried | 1 piece | 5 | 1 | – | – |
| sun dried | 1 cup | 140 | 30 | – | – |
| sun dried in oil | 1 cup (4 oz) | 235 | 26 | – | – |
| sun dried in oil | 1 piece (3 g) | 6 | 1 | – | – |
| sun-dried | 5 pieces (0.5 oz) | 40 | 7 | 4 | 3 |
| **FRESH** | | | | | |
| cooked | ½ cup | 32 | 7 | – | – |
| grape tomatoes | 20 | 30 | 6 | 4 | 1 |
| green | 1 | 30 | 6 | – | – |
| red | 1 (4.5 oz) | 26 | 6 | – | 2 |
| red chopped | 1 cup | 35 | 8 | – | 2 |
| ***Chiquita*** | | | | | |
| Tomato | 1 med (5.2 oz) | 35 | 7 | 4 | 1 |
| **TAKE-OUT** | | | | | |
| stewed | 1 cup | 80 | 13 | – | – |

## TOMATO JUICE

| FOOD | PORTION | CALS | CARB | SUGAR | FIBER |
|---|---|---|---|---|---|
| beef broth & tomato | 5½ oz | 61 | 14 | – | – |
| clam & tomato | 1 can (5½ oz) | 77 | 18 | – | – |
| tomato juice | 6 oz | 32 | 8 | – | – |
| tomato juice | ½ cup | 21 | 5 | – | – |
| ***Campbell's*** | | | | | |
| Juice | 8 oz | 51 | 10 | 8 | 2 |
| ***Del Monte*** | | | | | |
| Juice | 8 fl oz | 50 | 10 | 7 | 1 |
| Snap-E-Tom Chile Cocktail | 6 fl oz | 40 | 8 | 4 | 1 |

| FOOD | PORTION | CALS | CARB | SUGAR | FIBER |
|---|---|---|---|---|---|
| ***Dole*** | | | | | |
| Juice | 1 bottle (12 oz) | 85 | 17 | – | 2 |
| ***Hunt's*** | | | | | |
| Juice | 1 can (6 oz) | 22 | 5 | 4 | 1 |
| No Salt Added | 8 fl oz | 34 | 8 | 7 | 2 |
| ***Mott's*** | | | | | |
| Tomato Juice | 8 fl oz | 40 | 9 | – | – |
| ***Muir Glen*** | | | | | |
| Organic | 5.5 oz | 40 | 8 | 3 | 4 |
| **TONGUE** | | | | | |
| beef simmered | 3 oz | 241 | tr | – | – |
| lamb braised | 3 oz | 234 | 0 | 0 | 0 |
| pork braised | 3 oz | 230 | 0 | 0 | 0 |
| **TORTILLA** | | | | | |
| corn | 1 (6 in diam) | 56 | 12 | – | 1 |
| corn w/o salt | 1-6 in diam (.9 oz) | 56 | 12 | – | 1 |
| flour w/o salt | 1-8 in diam (1.2 oz) | 114 | 20 | – | 1 |
| ***La Mexicana*** | | | | | |
| Corn | 1 (0.8 oz) | 50 | 10 | 0 | 1 |
| Flour | 1 (0.8 oz) | 80 | 13 | 1 | 1 |
| Tortillas de Trigo | 1 (1 oz) | 140 | 18 | 0 | 1 |
| ***La Tortilla Factory*** | | | | | |
| Low Carb Whole Wheat | 1 lg | 100 | 21 | 1 | 15 |
| Low Carb Whole Wheat | 1 reg | 60 | 12 | 0 | 9 |
| ***Mariachi*** | | | | | |
| Tortilla | 1 | 112 | 20 | – | – |
| ***Old El Paso*** | | | | | |
| Flour | 1 (1.4 oz) | 130 | 21 | 0 | 0 |
| ***Tyson*** | | | | | |
| Flour | 1 (1.7 oz) | 150 | 24 | 1 | 1 |
| Flour Heat Pressed | 2 (2 oz) | 170 | 30 | 1 | 2 |
| White Corn | 2 (1.8 oz) | 100 | 21 | 0 | 3 |
| Whole Wheat Heat Pressed | 1 (1.4 oz) | 120 | 20 | 2 | 3 |
| Yellow Corn | 3 (1.9 oz) | 140 | 27 | 0 | 3 |

**TORTILLA CHIPS** *(see* CHIPS)

| FOOD | PORTION | CALS | CARB | SUGAR | FIBER |
|---|---|---|---|---|---|
| **TREE FERN** | | | | | |
| chopped cooked | ½ cup | 28 | 8 | – | – |
| **TRITICALE** | | | | | |
| dry | 1 cup (6.7 oz) | 645 | 138 | – | – |
| triticale not prep | 1 oz | 94 | 18 | – | 2 |
| **TROUT** | | | | | |
| baked | 3 oz | 162 | 0 | 0 | 0 |
| rainbow cooked | 3 oz | 129 | 0 | 0 | 0 |
| seatrout baked | 3 oz | 113 | 0 | 0 | 0 |
| **TRUFFLES** | | | | | |
| fresh | 0.5 oz | 4 | 9 | – | 2 |
| **TUMERIC** | | | | | |
| ground | 1 tsp | 8 | 1 | – | – |
| **TUNA** | | | | | |
| **CANNED** | | | | | |
| light in oil | 1 can (6 oz) | 399 | 0 | 0 | 0 |
| light in oil | 3 oz | 169 | 0 | 0 | 0 |
| light in water | 3 oz | 99 | 0 | 0 | 0 |
| light in water | 1 can (5.8 oz) | 192 | 0 | 0 | 0 |
| white in oil | 1 can (6.2 oz) | 331 | 0 | 0 | 0 |
| white in oil | 3 oz | 158 | 0 | 0 | 0 |
| white in water | 1 can (6 oz) | 234 | 0 | 0 | 0 |
| white in water | 3 oz | 116 | 0 | 0 | 0 |
| ***Bumble Bee*** | | | | | |
| Chunk Light In Water | 2 oz | 60 | 0 | 0 | 0 |
| Chunk Light In Water Pouch | 2 oz | 60 | 0 | 0 | 0 |
| Chunk Light In Water Touch Of Lemon | 2 oz | 60 | 0 | 0 | 0 |
| Solid White Albacore in Water | 2 oz | 70 | 0 | 0 | 0 |
| Solid White In Water | 2 oz | 70 | 0 | 0 | 0 |
| ***Progresso*** | | | | | |
| In Olive Oil drained | ¼ cup (2 oz) | 160 | 0 | 0 | 0 |
| ***StarKist*** | | | | | |
| Chunk Light In Water | ¼ cup (2 oz) | 60 | 0 | 0 | 0 |
| Chunk Light No Drain Package | ¼ cup (2 oz) | 60 | 0 | 0 | 0 |
| Low Sodium Chunk White In Water | 2 oz | 60 | 0 | 0 | 0 |

| FOOD | PORTION | CALS | CARB | SUGAR | FIBER |
|---|---|---|---|---|---|
| Solid White Albacore In Spring Water | ¼ cup (2 oz) | 70 | 0 | 0 | 0 |
| Tuna Fillet In Spring Water | ¼ cup (2 oz) | 60 | 0 | 0 | 0 |
| **FRESH** | | | | | |
| bluefin cooked | 3 oz | 157 | 0 | 0 | 0 |
| bluefin raw | 3 oz | 122 | 0 | 0 | 0 |
| skipjack baked | 3 oz | 112 | 0 | 0 | 0 |
| yellowfin baked | 3 oz | 118 | 0 | 0 | 0 |

## TUNA DISHES

**MIX**

***Tuna Helper***

| FOOD | PORTION | CALS | CARB | SUGAR | FIBER |
|---|---|---|---|---|---|
| AuGratin 50% Less Fat Recipe as prep | 1 cup | 240 | 37 | 5 | 1 |
| AuGratin as prep | 1 cup | 300 | 37 | 5 | 1 |
| Cheesy Broccoli 50% Less Fat Recipe as prep | 1 cup | 240 | 38 | 6 | 1 |
| Cheesy Broccoli as prep | 1 cup | 290 | 38 | 6 | 1 |
| Cheesy Pasta 50% Less Fat Recipe as prep | 1 cup | 230 | 32 | 5 | tr |
| Cheesy Pasta as prep | 1 cup | 280 | 32 | 5 | tr |
| Creamy Broccoli 50% Less Fat Recipe as prep | 1 cup | 240 | 35 | 6 | 1 |
| Creamy Pasta 50% Less Fat Recipe as prep | 1 cup | 230 | 31 | 4 | 1 |
| Creamy Pasta as prep | 1 cup | 300 | 31 | 4 | 1 |
| Fettuccine Alfredo 50% Less Fat Recipe as prep | 1 cup | 240 | 32 | 6 | 1 |
| Fettuccine Alfredo as prep | 1 cup | 310 | 32 | 6 | 1 |
| Garden Cheddar 50% Less Fat Recipe as prep | 1 cup | 240 | 36 | 7 | 1 |
| Garden Cheddar as prep | 1 cup | 290 | 36 | 7 | 1 |
| Pasta Salad Low Fat Recipe as prep | ⅔ cup | 230 | 26 | 4 | 1 |
| Pasta Salad as prep | ⅔ cup | 380 | 26 | 4 | 1 |
| Tetrazzini 50% Less Fat Recipe as prep | 1 cup | 230 | 34 | 3 | 1 |
| Tetrazzini as prep | 1 cup | 300 | 34 | 3 | 1 |
| Tuna Melt Reduced Fat Recipe as prep | 1 cup | 240 | 34 | 9 | 1 |

| FOOD | PORTION | CALS | CARB | SUGAR | FIBER |
|---|---|---|---|---|---|
| Tuna Melt as prep | 1 cup | 300 | 34 | 9 | 1 |
| Tuna Pot Pie as prep | 1 cup | 440 | 40 | 9 | 1 |
| Tuna Romanoff 50% Less Fat Recipe as prep | 1 cup | 240 | 38 | 3 | 1 |
| Tuna Romanoff as prep | 1 cup | 280 | 38 | 3 | 1 |
| **READY-TO-EAT** | | | | | |
| ***Bumble Bee*** | | | | | |
| Tuna Salad Fat Free | 1 pkg (3.5 oz) | 190 | 25 | 7 | 0 |
| Tuna Salad Kit | 1 pkg (3.8 oz) | 250 | 15 | 2 | 0 |
| ***StarKist*** | | | | | |
| Lunch To-Go | 1 pkg | 310 | 26 | 11 | tr |
| Ready-Mixed Tuna Salad Kit | 1 pkg (3.5 oz) | 190 | 25 | 11 | 2 |
| Tuna Salad Lunch Kit | 1 pkg (4.3 oz) | 230 | 17 | 4 | 1 |
| ***Wampler*** | | | | | |
| Salad | ⅓ cup | 180 | 9 | – | – |
| Salad Chunky | ⅓ cup | 180 | 8 | – | – |
| **TAKE-OUT** | | | | | |
| tuna salad | 3 oz | 159 | 8 | – | – |
| tuna salad | 1 cup | 383 | 19 | – | – |

## TURBOT

| FOOD | PORTION | CALS | CARB | SUGAR | FIBER |
|---|---|---|---|---|---|
| european baked | 3 oz | 104 | 0 | 0 | 0 |

## TURKEY *(see also* TURKEY DISHES, TURKEY SUBSTITUTES*)*

| FOOD | PORTION | CALS | CARB | SUGAR | FIBER |
|---|---|---|---|---|---|
| **CANNED** | | | | | |
| w/ broth | ½ can (2.5 oz) | 116 | 0 | 0 | 0 |
| w/ broth | 1 can (5 oz) | 231 | 0 | 0 | 0 |
| **FRESH** | | | | | |
| back w/ skin roasted | ½ back (9 oz) | 637 | 0 | 0 | 0 |
| breast w/ skin roasted | 4 oz | 212 | 0 | 0 | 0 |
| dark meat w/ skin roasted | 3.6 oz | 230 | 0 | 0 | 0 |
| dark meat w/o skin roasted | 3 oz | 170 | 0 | 0 | 0 |
| dark meat w/o skin roasted | 1 cup (5 oz) | 262 | 0 | 0 | 0 |
| ground cooked | 3 oz | 188 | 0 | 0 | 0 |
| leg w/ skin roasted | 2.5 oz | 147 | 0 | 0 | 0 |
| leg w/ skin roasted | 1 (1.2 lbs) | 1133 | 0 | 0 | 0 |
| light meat w/ skin roasted | 4.7 oz | 268 | 0 | 0 | 0 |
| light meat w/ skin roasted | from ½ turkey (2.3 lbs) | 2069 | 0 | 0 | 0 |
| light meat w/o skin roasted | 4 oz | 183 | 0 | 0 | 0 |

| FOOD | PORTION | CALS | CARB | SUGAR | FIBER |
|---|---|---|---|---|---|
| neck simmered | 1 (5.3 oz) | 274 | 0 | 0 | 0 |
| skin roasted | 1 oz | 141 | 0 | 0 | 0 |
| skin roasted | from ½ turkey (9 oz) | 1096 | 0 | 0 | 0 |
| w/ skin roasted | ½ turkey (4 lbs) | 3857 | 0 | 0 | 0 |
| w/ skin roasted | 8.4 oz | 498 | 0 | 0 | 0 |
| w/ skin neck & giblets roasted | ½ turkey (8.8 lbs) | 4123 | 1 | – | – |
| w/o skin roasted | 7.3 oz | 354 | 0 | 0 | 0 |
| w/o skin roasted | 1 cup (5 oz) | 238 | 0 | 0 | 0 |
| wing w/ skin roasted | 1 (6.5 oz) | 426 | 0 | 0 | 0 |
| ***Jennie-O*** | | | | | |
| Ground | 4 oz | 160 | 0 | 0 | 0 |
| ***Perdue*** | | | | | |
| Breast Tenderloins Butter Garlic | 3 oz | 100 | 2 | – | – |
| Burger Cooked | 1 (4 oz) | 160 | 0 | – | – |
| Dark Cooked | 3 oz | 180 | 0 | – | – |
| Drumsticks Cooked | 1 (2.2 oz) | 110 | 0 | – | – |
| Ground Cooked | 3 oz | 160 | 0 | – | – |
| Tenderloins Black Pepper Cooked | 3 oz | 90 | 1 | – | – |
| Thighs Cooked | 1 (3.2 oz) | 240 | 0 | – | – |
| White Cooked | 3 oz | 150 | 0 | – | – |
| ***Shady Brook*** | | | | | |
| Ground Breast | 4 oz | 120 | 0 | – | – |
| ***Turkey Store*** | | | | | |
| Breakfast Sausage Patties Mild | 2 patties (2.3 oz) | 160 | 1 | – | – |
| Lean Ground Italian Style | 4 oz | 190 | 4 | – | – |
| ***Wampler*** | | | | | |
| Boneless Breast Roast | 4 oz | 160 | 0 | – | – |
| Breast Half | 4 oz | 160 | 0 | – | – |
| Breast Steaks | 4 oz | 120 | 0 | – | – |
| Drumsticks | 4 oz | 180 | 0 | – | – |
| Ground | 4 oz | 210 | 0 | – | – |
| Ground Breast | 4 oz | 130 | 0 | – | – |
| Ground Lean | 4 oz | 160 | 0 | – | – |
| Thighs | 4 oz | 170 | 0 | – | – |
| Wings | 4 oz | 220 | 0 | – | – |

| FOOD | PORTION | CALS | CARB | SUGAR | FIBER |
|---|---|---|---|---|---|
| Woodfire Grill Burger | 1 (3 oz) | 180 | 2 | – | – |
| **FROZEN** | | | | | |
| roast boneless seasoned light & dark meat roasted | 1 pkg (1.7 lbs) | 1213 | 24 | – | – |
| ***Wampler*** | | | | | |
| Burger BBQ | 1 (4 oz) | 240 | 3 | – | – |
| Burgers Cracked Peppercorn & Garlic | 1 (3 oz) | 170 | 0 | – | – |
| Seasoned Burgers Cracker Peppercorn & Garlic | 1 (3 oz) | 170 | 0 | – | – |
| **READY-TO-EAT** | | | | | |
| bologna | 1 oz | 57 | tr | – | – |
| breast | 1 slice (0.75 oz) | 23 | 0 | 0 | 0 |
| diced light & dark seasoned | 1 oz | 39 | tr | – | – |
| diced light & dark seasoned | ½ lb | 313 | 2 | – | – |
| ham thigh meat | 1 pkg (8 oz) | 291 | 1 | – | – |
| ham thigh meat | 2 oz | 73 | tr | – | – |
| pastrami | 1 pkg (8 oz) | 320 | 4 | – | – |
| pastrami | 2 oz | 80 | 1 | – | – |
| patties battered & fried | 1 (3.3 oz) | 266 | 15 | – | – |
| patties battered & fried | 1 (2.3 oz) | 181 | 10 | – | – |
| patties breaded & fried | 1 (3.3 oz) | 266 | 15 | – | – |
| patties breaded & fried | 1 (2.3 oz) | 181 | 10 | – | – |
| poultry salad sandwich spread | 1 oz | 238 | 2 | – | – |
| poultry salad sandwich spread | 1 tbsp | 109 | 1 | – | – |
| prebasted breast w/ skin roasted | ½ breast (1.9 lbs) | 1087 | 0 | 0 | 0 |
| prebasted breast w/ skin roasted | 1 breast (3.8 lbs) | 2175 | 0 | 0 | 0 |
| prebasted thigh w/ skin roasted | 1 thigh (11 oz) | 494 | 0 | 0 | 0 |
| roll light & dark meat | 1 oz | 42 | 1 | – | – |
| roll light meat | 1 oz | 42 | 2 | – | – |
| salami cooked | 1 pkg (8 oz) | 446 | 1 | – | – |
| salami cooked | 2 oz | 111 | tr | – | – |
| turkey loaf breast meat | 2 slices (1.5 oz) | 47 | 0 | 0 | 0 |
| turkey loaf breast meat | 1 pkg (6 oz) | 187 | 0 | 0 | 0 |

| FOOD | PORTION | CALS | CARB | SUGAR | FIBER |
|---|---|---|---|---|---|
| turkey sticks battered & fried | 1 stick (2.3 oz) | 178 | 11 | – | – |
| turkey sticks breaded & fried | 1 stick (2.3 oz) | 178 | 11 | – | – |
| ***Alpine Lace*** | | | | | |
| Breast Fat Free | 2 oz | 45 | 0 | 0 | 0 |
| ***Boar's Head*** | | | | | |
| Breast Cracked Pepper Smoked | 2 oz | 60 | 1 | 0 | 0 |
| Breast Golden Skin On | 2 oz | 60 | 0 | 0 | 0 |
| Breast Golden Skinless | 2 oz | 60 | tr | 0 | 0 |
| Breast Hickory Smoked | 2 oz | 70 | tr | 0 | 0 |
| Breast Low Sodium Skinless | 2 oz | 60 | tr | 0 | 0 |
| Breast Lower Sodium Skin On | 2 oz | 60 | tr | 0 | 0 |
| Breast Maple Glazed Honey Coat | 2 oz | 70 | 2 | 2 | 0 |
| Breast Ovengold Skin On | 2 oz | 60 | 1 | 0 | 0 |
| Breast Ovengold Skinless | 2 oz | 60 | 0 | 0 | 0 |
| Breast Roasted Mesquite Smoked Skinless | 2 oz | 60 | 0 | 0 | 0 |
| Breast Roasted Salsalito | 2 oz | 60 | 1 | 0 | 0 |
| Pastrami Seasoned | 2 oz | 60 | 1 | 0 | 0 |
| ***Carl Buddig*** | | | | | |
| Honey Roasted Turkey Breast | 1 pkg (2.5 oz) | 120 | 3 | 3 | – |
| Lean Slices Honey Roasted Breast | 1 pkg (2.5 oz) | 70 | 4 | 4 | – |
| Lean Slices Oven Roasted Breast | 1 pkg (2.5 oz) | 70 | 1 | 1 | – |
| Lean Slices Smoked Breast | 1 pkg (2.5 oz) | 70 | 1 | 1 | – |
| Oven Roasted Breast | 1 pkg (2.5 oz) | 110 | 1 | 1 | – |
| Smoked Breast | 1 pkg (2.5 oz) | 110 | 1 | 1 | – |
| Turkey Ham | 1 pkg (2.5 oz) | 100 | 1 | 1 | – |
| ***Jennie-O*** | | | | | |
| Turkey Breast Golden Roast | 3 oz | 100 | 2 | – | – |
| ***Oscar Mayer*** | | | | | |
| Lunchables Turkey Bagels | 1 pkg | 420 | 54 | 27 | 2 |
| ***Perdue*** | | | | | |
| Breast Sliced Cajun Style | 2 oz | 50 | 1 | – | – |
| Breast Sliced Honey Smoked | 2 oz | 50 | 2 | 2 | – |
| Breast Sliced Pan Roasted | 2 oz | 70 | 0 | – | – |

| FOOD | PORTION | CALS | CARB | SUGAR | FIBER |
|---|---|---|---|---|---|
| Ham Hickory Smoked | 2 oz | 60 | 1 | – | – |
| Healthsense Breast Sliced Oven Roasted | 2 oz | 60 | 3 | 1 | – |
| Pastrami Hickory Smoked | 2 oz | 70 | 2 | – | – |
| ***Shady Brook*** | | | | | |
| Meatballs Italian Style | 3 (3 oz) | 130 | 5 | 1 | 1 |
| ***Wampler*** | | | | | |
| Bologna | 2 oz | 130 | 1 | – | – |
| Dark Cured | 2 oz | 80 | 2 | – | – |
| Deli Roast Breast | 2 oz | 50 | 0 | – | – |
| Deli Roast Classic Spiced Breast | 2 oz | 70 | 1 | – | – |
| Deli Roast Pan Roasted Breast | 2 oz | 70 | 1 | – | – |
| Deli Roast Pan Roasted Skinless Breast | 2 oz | 50 | 1 | – | – |
| Deli Roast Peppered Breast | 21 oz | 40 | 1 | – | – |
| Deli Roast Rotisserie Breast | 2 oz | 50 | 1 | – | – |
| Pastrami | 2 oz | 90 | 1 | – | – |
| Salami | 2 oz | 90 | 1 | – | – |
| Turkey Ham | 2 oz | 60 | 0 | – | – |
| **TURKEY DISHES** | | | | | |
| gravy & turkey | 1 pkg (5 oz) | 95 | 7 | – | – |
| gravy & turkey | 1 cup (8.4 oz) | 160 | 11 | – | – |
| ***Banquet*** | | | | | |
| Sandwich Toppers Gravy & Sliced Turkey | 1 pkg (5 oz) | 160 | 6 | 1 | 0 |
| ***Jennie-O*** | | | | | |
| Stuffed Turkey Breast Pepper Cheese & Rice | 1 piece (6 oz) | 250 | 13 | 1 | 0 |
| Turkey Breast Roast In Homestyle Gravy | 1 serv (5 oz) | 110 | 3 | 1 | 0 |
| ***Mosey's*** | | | | | |
| Turkey Breast w/ Gravy | 1 serv (5 oz) | 140 | 4 | 0 | 0 |
| ***Wampler*** | | | | | |
| Turkey Ham Salad | ⅓ cup | 150 | 9 | – | – |
| **TAKE-OUT** | | | | | |
| boneless breast w/ cranberry apple stuffing | 1 serv (5 oz) | 260 | 10 | 2 | 1 |

| FOOD | PORTION | CALS | CARB | SUGAR | FIBER |
| --- | --- | --- | --- | --- | --- |
| **TURKEY SUBSTITUTES** | | | | | |
| ***Lightlife*** | | | | | |
| Smart Deli Turkey | 3 slices (1.5 oz) | 40 | 1 | 0 | 0 |
| ***Tofurkey*** | | | | | |
| Deli Slices Hickory | 1.5 oz | 120 | 14 | 0 | 2 |
| Deli Slices Original | 1.5 oz | 120 | 14 | 0 | 2 |
| Deli Slices Peppered | 1.5 oz | 120 | 14 | 0 | 2 |
| Drummettes | 1 (3 oz) | 105 | 11 | 2 | 4 |
| Giblet Gravy | 1 serv (3.5 oz) | 42 | 5 | 2 | 1 |
| Stuffed Tofu Roast | 1 serv (4 oz) | 193 | 10 | 1 | 2 |
| ***Yves*** | | | | | |
| Veggie Turkey Deli Slices | 1 serv (2.2 oz) | 85 | 4 | 2 | 1 |
| **TURNIPS** | | | | | |
| canned greens | ½ cup | 17 | 3 | – | – |
| cooked mashed | ½ cup (4.2 oz) | 47 | 10 | – | – |
| cubed cooked | ½ cup (3 oz) | 33 | 7 | – | – |
| frzn greens cooked | ½ cup | 24 | 4 | – | 2 |
| greens chopped cooked | ½ cup | 15 | 3 | – | 2 |
| greens raw chopped | ½ cup | 7 | 2 | – | 1 |
| ***Birds Eye*** | | | | | |
| Greens w/ Diced Turnip | 1 cup | 25 | 2 | 1 | 2 |
| **TURTLE** | | | | | |
| raw | 3.5 oz | 85 | 0 | 0 | 0 |
| **TUSK FISH** | | | | | |
| raw | 3.5 oz | 79 | 0 | 0 | 0 |
| **VANILLA** | | | | | |
| ***Steel's*** | | | | | |
| Sugar Free | 1 tbsp | 24 | 6 | 0 | 0 |
| **VEAL** *(see also* VEAL DISHES*)* | | | | | |
| cutlet lean only braised | 3 oz | 172 | 0 | 0 | 0 |
| cutlet lean only fried | 3 oz | 156 | 0 | 0 | 0 |
| ground broiled | 3 oz | 146 | 0 | 0 | 0 |
| loin chop w/ bone lean & fat braised | 1 chop (2.8 oz) | 227 | 0 | 0 | 0 |

| FOOD | PORTION | CALS | CARB | SUGAR | FIBER |
|---|---|---|---|---|---|
| loin chop w/ bone lean only braised | 1 chop (2.4 oz) | 155 | 0 | 0 | 0 |
| shoulder w/ bone lean only braised | 3 oz | 169 | 0 | 0 | 0 |
| sirloin w/ bone lean & fat roasted | 3 oz | 171 | 0 | 0 | 0 |
| sirloin w/ bone lean only roasted | 3 oz | 143 | 0 | 0 | 0 |
| **VEAL DISHES** | | | | | |
| **TAKE-OUT** | | | | | |
| parmigiana | 4.2 oz | 279 | 6 | – | 2 |
| **VEGETABLE JUICE** | | | | | |
| vegetable juice cocktail | 6 fl oz | 34 | 8 | – | – |
| vegetable juice cocktail | ½ cup | 22 | 6 | – | – |
| ***Dole*** | | | | | |
| Vegetable Blend | 1 bottle (12 oz) | 90 | 19 | – | 2 |
| ***Hunt's*** | | | | | |
| Cocktail | 1 can (6 oz) | 20 | 7 | 3 | 2 |
| ***Muir Glen*** | | | | | |
| Organic | 5.5 oz | 50 | 10 | 7 | 2 |
| ***V8*** | | | | | |
| Lightly Tangy | 8 oz | 58 | 11 | 9 | 2 |
| Low Sodium | 8 oz | 53 | 11 | 8 | 2 |
| Original | 8 oz | 51 | 10 | 8 | 2 |
| Picante Vegetable | 8 oz | 51 | 10 | 7 | 2 |
| Spicy Hot | 8 oz | 49 | 10 | 7 | 2 |
| **VEGETABLES MIXED** | | | | | |
| **CANNED** | | | | | |
| mixed vegetables | ½ cup | 39 | 8 | – | – |
| peas & carrots | ½ cup | 48 | 11 | – | – |
| peas & carrots low sodium | ½ cup | 48 | 11 | – | – |
| peas & onions | ½ cup | 30 | 5 | – | – |
| succotash | ½ cup | 102 | 23 | – | – |
| ***Chun King*** | | | | | |
| Chow Mein Vegetables | ⅔ cup (3 oz) | 14 | 3 | 0 | 1 |
| ***Del Monte*** | | | | | |
| Mixed | ½ cup (4.4 oz) | 40 | 8 | 3 | 2 |

| FOOD | PORTION | CALS | CARB | SUGAR | FIBER |
|---|---|---|---|---|---|
| Mixed No Salt Added | ½ cup (4.4 oz) | 40 | 8 | 3 | 2 |
| Peas And Carrots | ½ cup (4.5 oz) | 60 | 11 | 4 | 2 |
| ***La Choy*** | | | | | |
| Chop Suey Vegetables | ½ cup (2.2 oz) | 10 | 2 | 0 | 1 |
| ***S&W*** | | | | | |
| Mixed | ½ cup (4.4 oz) | 35 | 7 | 3 | 2 |
| Peas & Carrots | ½ cup (4.5 oz) | 60 | 11 | 4 | 2 |
| Peas & Onions | ½ cup (4.3 oz) | 40 | 11 | 1 | 3 |
| ***Veg-All*** | | | | | |
| Cajun Mixed | ½ cup | 50 | 10 | 2 | 3 |
| **FROZEN** | | | | | |
| mixed vegetables cooked | ½ cup | 54 | 12 | – | 2 |
| peas & carrots cooked | ½ cup | 38 | 8 | – | – |
| peas & onions cooked | ½ cup | 40 | 8 | – | – |
| succotash cooked | ½ cup | 79 | 17 | – | – |
| ***Birds Eye*** | | | | | |
| Baby Sweet Peas & Pearl Onions | ⅔ cup | 60 | 12 | 6 | 4 |
| Bavarian Vegetables | 1 cup (5.5 oz) | 150 | 15 | 3 | 3 |
| Broccoli Cauliflower & Carrots | ½ cup | 25 | 5 | 3 | 2 |
| Broccoli Cauliflower & Carrots In Cheese Sauce | ½ cup | 70 | 7 | 3 | 2 |
| Broccoli Cauliflower & Red Peppers | ½ cup | 20 | 5 | 3 | 2 |
| Broccoli & Cauliflower | ½ cup | 20 | 4 | 2 | 2 |
| Broccoli Carrots & Water Chestnuts | ½ cup | 30 | 7 | 3 | 3 |
| Broccoli Corn & Red Peppers | ½ cup | 50 | 12 | 3 | 3 |
| Broccoli Red Peppers Onions & Mushrooms | ½ cup | 25 | 5 | 3 | 2 |
| Brussels Sprouts Cauliflower & Carrots | ½ cup | 30 | 7 | 3 | 3 |
| California Style Vegetables | ½ cup | 100 | 9 | 4 | 3 |
| Cauliflower Nuggets Corn Carrots & Snow Pea pods | ½ cup | 30 | 6 | 3 | 2 |
| Gumbo Blend | ¾ cup | 40 | 10 | 3 | 2 |
| Italian Style Vegetables & Bow Tie Pasta | 1 cup | 150 | 13 | 3 | 2 |
| New England Style Vegetables & Pasta Shells | 1 pkg (9 oz) | 260 | 29 | 6 | 3 |

| FOOD | PORTION | CALS | CARB | SUGAR | FIBER |
|---|---|---|---|---|---|
| Oriental Style Vegetables | ½ cup | 60 | 4 | 3 | 2 |
| Peas & Pearl Onions | ⅔ cup | 90 | 18 | 9 | 5 |
| Peas & Potatoes In Real Cream Sauce | ½ cup | 90 | 13 | 5 | 2 |
| Radiatore Pasta & Vegetables | 1 cup | 200 | 27 | 5 | 1 |
| Roasted Potatoes & Broccoli | ⅔ cup (3.9 oz) | 100 | 15 | 2 | 1 |
| Roletti Pasta & Vegetables | 1 cup (4.4 oz) | 190 | 11 | 5 | 1 |
| Simply Grillin' Garden Herb | 1 cup | 140 | 19 | 6 | 4 |
| Stir Fry Asparagus | 2 cups | 90 | 16 | 4 | 3 |
| Stir Fry Broccoli | 1 cup | 30 | 5 | 3 | 2 |
| Stir Fry Pepper | 1 cup | 25 | 5 | 4 | 2 |
| Stir Fry Sugar Snap | ¾ cup | 35 | 5 | 3 | 1 |
| Stir Fry Whole Green Bean | 1¾ cup | 100 | 19 | 4 | 2 |
| Stir Fry Style Vegetables | ½ cup | 60 | 5 | 4 | 1 |
| Vegetables For Stew | ⅔ cup | 40 | 9 | 2 | 1 |
| Viola! Italian Pesto Chicken | 2 cups | 240 | 24 | 5 | 1 |
| Viola! Three Cheese Chicken | 1¾ cups | 220 | 24 | 6 | 1 |
| ***Fresh Like*** | | | | | |
| California Blend | 3.5 oz | 31 | 7 | – | 1 |
| Midwestern Blend | 3.5 oz | 42 | 9 | – | 1 |
| Mixed | 3.5 oz | 69 | 14 | – | 1 |
| Oriental Blend | 3.5 oz | 26 | 5 | – | 1 |
| Winter Blend | 3.5 oz | 26 | 5 | – | 1 |
| ***Green Giant*** | | | | | |
| Alfredo Vegetables | ¾ cup | 70 | 8 | 3 | 2 |
| Cheese Sauce Broccoli Cauliflower Carrots | 1 cup (4.1 oz) | 60 | 7 | 3 | 2 |
| ***Health Is Wealth*** | | | | | |
| Veggie Munchees | 2 (1 oz) | 50 | 9 | 0 | 1 |
| ***La Choy*** | | | | | |
| Fancy Chinese Mixed Vegetables | ½ cup (2.9 oz) | 9 | 1 | 0 | 1 |
| ***McKenzie's*** | | | | | |
| Gumbo Mixture | 1 serv (2.9 oz) | 35 | 8 | 3 | 2 |
| ***Tree Of Life*** | | | | | |
| Mixed | ½ cup (3 oz) | 65 | 13 | 3 | 3 |
| **SHELF-STABLE** | | | | | |
| ***TastyBite*** | | | | | |
| Curry Bangkok Red | ½ pkg (5.3 oz) | 88 | 7 | 0 | 1 |

| FOOD | PORTION | CALS | CARB | SUGAR | FIBER |
|---|---|---|---|---|---|
| Curry Patong Yellow | ½ pkg (5.3 oz) | 118 | 12 | 0 | 1 |
| Curry Siam Green | ½ pkg (5.3 oz) | 63 | 6 | 0 | 1 |
| Jaipur Vegetables | ½ pkg (5 oz) | 220 | 13 | 3 | 7 |
| Malabar Mixed | ½ pkg (5 oz) | 67 | 15 | 1 | 1 |
| **TAKE-OUT** | | | | | |
| buddha's delight | 1 serv (16 oz) | 174 | 17 | 8 | 3 |
| curry | 1 serv (7.7 oz) | 398 | 22 | – | – |
| gyoza potstickers vegetable | 8 (4.9 oz) | 210 | 34 | 7 | 5 |
| pakoras | 1 (2 oz) | 108 | 12 | – | 3 |
| ratatouille | 1 serv (3.5 oz) | 96 | 7 | 7 | 4 |
| samosa | 2 (4 oz) | 519 | 25 | – | 3 |
| succotash | ½ cup | 111 | 23 | – | – |
| tapenade grilled vegetables | ¼ cup | 40 | 4 | 2 | tr |
| **VENISON** | | | | | |
| roasted | 3 oz | 134 | 0 | 0 | 0 |
| **VINEGAR** | | | | | |
| cider | 1 tbsp | tr | 1 | – | – |
| ***Eden*** | | | | | |
| Organic Brown Rice | 1 tbsp | 2 | 0 | 0 | 0 |
| Ume Plum | 1 tsp | 2 | 0 | 0 | 0 |
| ***Progresso*** | | | | | |
| Balsamic | 2 tbsp (0.5 oz) | 10 | 2 | 2 | 0 |
| ***White House*** | | | | | |
| Apple Cider | 1 tbsp (0.5 oz) | 0 | 0 | 0 | 0 |
| White | 1 tbsp (0.5 oz) | 0 | 0 | 0 | – |
| ***Wild Thyme Farms*** | | | | | |
| Balsamic Red Raspberry | 1 tbsp | 13 | 3 | 3 | – |
| **WAFFLES** | | | | | |
| **FROZEN** | | | | | |
| buttermilk | 1 4 in sq (1.2 oz) | 88 | 14 | – | 1 |
| plain | 1 4 in sq (1.2 oz) | 88 | 14 | – | 1 |
| ***Kid Cuisine*** | | | | | |
| Wave Rider Waffle Sticks | 1 meal (6.6 oz) | 380 | 75 | 38 | 3 |

| FOOD | PORTION | CALS | CARB | SUGAR | FIBER |
|---|---|---|---|---|---|
| **MIX** | | | | | |
| plain | 1 7 in diam | 218 | 26 | – | 1 |
| as prep | (2.6 oz) | | | | |
| **READY-TO-EAT** | | | | | |
| ***Gol D Lite*** | | | | | |
| Low Carb Belgian Chocolate Covered | 1 (l.1 oz) | 130 | 18 | 0 | 1 |
| ***Kashi*** | | | | | |
| GoLean Blueberry | 2 | 170 | 33 | 4 | 6 |
| GoLean Original | 2 | 170 | 33 | 4 | 6 |
| ***Thomas'*** | | | | | |
| Buttermilk | 1 (1.6 oz) | 130 | 18 | 7 | tr |
| Homestyle | 1 (1.6 oz) | 140 | 19 | 7 | tr |
| **TAKE-OUT** | | | | | |
| plain | 1 (7 in diam) | 218 | 25 | – | – |

## WALNUTS

| FOOD | PORTION | CALS | CARB | SUGAR | FIBER |
|---|---|---|---|---|---|
| black dried chopped | 1 cup | 759 | 15 | – | – |
| english dried | 1 oz | 182 | 5 | – | 1 |
| english dried chopped | 1 cup | 770 | 22 | – | 6 |
| halves | 14 (1 oz) | 190 | 4 | 1 | 2 |
| ***Sweet Delights*** | | | | | |
| Walnut Roasters | ⅓ pkg (1 oz) | 210 | 3 | 0 | 2 |

## WASABI *(see* HORSERADISH*)*

## WATER

| FOOD | PORTION | CALS | CARB | SUGAR | FIBER |
|---|---|---|---|---|---|
| ice cubes | 3 | 0 | 0 | 0 | 0 |
| tap water | 8 oz | 0 | 0 | 0 | 0 |
| ***Absopure*** | | | | | |
| Natural Spring | 8 fl oz | 0 | 0 | 0 | 0 |
| ***Aquafina*** | | | | | |
| Essentials B-Power Wild Berry | 8 fl oz | 40 | 11 | 11 | – |
| Essentials Calcium + Tangerine Pineapple | 8 fl oz | 40 | 11 | 10 | – |
| Essentials Daily C Citrus | 8 fl oz | 40 | 11 | 11 | – |
| Essentials Multi-V Watermelon | 8 fl oz | 40 | 11 | 11 | – |
| Water | 8 fl oz | 0 | 0 | 0 | – |
| ***Aquess*** | | | | | |
| Purified Water w/ Soluble Fiber | 1 bottle (18 oz) | 30 | 8 | 2 | 5 |

| FOOD | PORTION | CALS | CARB | SUGAR | FIBER |
|---|---|---|---|---|---|
| ***Bong Water*** | | | | | |
| Chronic Tonic | 12 oz | 144 | 36 | 36 | – |
| Cottonmouth Quencher | 12 oz | 165 | 42 | 42 | – |
| Green Dreams | 12 oz | 165 | 42 | 42 | – |
| Purple Haze | 12 oz | 165 | 42 | 42 | – |
| ***Castellina*** | | | | | |
| Sparkling Spring | 8 fl oz | 0 | 0 | 0 | 0 |
| ***Crystal Geyser*** | | | | | |
| Spring Water | 8 fl oz | 0 | 0 | 0 | 0 |
| ***Dasani*** | | | | | |
| Purfied Water | 8 oz | 0 | 0 | 0 | – |
| ***Evamor*** | | | | | |
| Artesian Water | 8 fl oz | 0 | 0 | 0 | 0 |
| ***Evian*** | | | | | |
| Spring Water | 1 bottle (11.5 oz) | 0 | 0 | 0 | 0 |
| ***Ferrarelle*** | | | | | |
| Sparkling | 8 fl oz | 0 | 0 | 0 | 1 |
| ***Gerolsteiner*** | | | | | |
| Sparkling Mineral | 8 fl oz | 0 | 0 | 0 | 0 |
| ***Glaceau*** | | | | | |
| Smartwater | 8 oz | 0 | 0 | 0 | 0 |
| Vitamin Water Tropical Citrus | 1 cup (8 oz) | 40 | 9 | 8 | – |
| ***Hansen's*** | | | | | |
| Energy Water Lemon | 8 oz | 10 | 3 | 3 | – |
| ***Iceland Spring*** | | | | | |
| Spring Water | 1 liter | 0 | 0 | 0 | 0 |
| ***Meridian*** | | | | | |
| Clear All Flavors | 8 oz | 100 | 25 | 25 | – |
| ***Propel*** | | | | | |
| Fitness Water Berry | 8 fl oz | 10 | 3 | 2 | – |
| Fitness Water Black Cherry | 8 fl oz | 10 | 3 | 2 | – |
| ***Reebok*** | | | | | |
| Fitness Water Berry | 1 bottle (24 oz) | 30 | 0 | 0 | 0 |
| Fitness Water Natural | 1 bottle (24 oz) | 0 | 0 | 0 | 0 |
| ***Replenish*** | | | | | |
| Elements Enhanced Water Orange | 8 oz | 40 | 10 | 10 | – |

| FOOD | PORTION | CALS | CARB | SUGAR | FIBER |
|---|---|---|---|---|---|
| ***San Pellegrino*** | | | | | |
| Mineral Water | 1 liter (33.8 oz) | 0 | 0 | – | – |
| ***Saratoga*** | | | | | |
| Spring | 8 oz | 0 | 0 | – | – |
| ***Spa*** | | | | | |
| Mineral Water Reine | 1 bottle (17.5 oz) | 0 | 0 | – | – |
| ***Ty Nant*** | | | | | |
| Mineral Water | 1 liter | 0 | 0 | 0 | 0 |
| ***Veryfine*** | | | | | |
| Fruit 2 0 Lemon | 8 oz | 0 | 0 | 0 | – |
| Fruit 2 O Lemon Lime | 8 fl oz | 0 | 0 | 0 | – |
| Fruit 2 O Orange | 8 fl oz | 0 | 0 | 0 | – |
| Fruit 2 O Raspberry | 8 fl oz | 0 | 0 | 0 | – |
| ***Vittel*** | | | | | |
| Mineral Water | 1 bottle (18 oz) | 0 | 0 | – | – |
| ***Volvic*** | | | | | |
| Spring Water | 8 oz | 0 | 0 | 0 | 0 |
| **WATER CHESTNUTS** | | | | | |
| chinese sliced canned | ½ cup | 35 | 9 | – | – |
| fresh sliced | ½ cup | 66 | 15 | – | – |
| ***Chun King*** | | | | | |
| Sliced | 2 tbsp (0.8 oz) | 11 | 3 | tr | 1 |
| Whole | 2 (0.7 oz) | 10 | 2 | tr | 1 |
| ***La Choy*** | | | | | |
| Chopped | 2 tbsp (0.6 oz) | 9 | 2 | tr | 1 |
| Sliced | 2 tbsp (0.8 oz) | 11 | 3 | tr | 1 |
| Whole | 2 (0.7 oz) | 10 | 2 | tr | 1 |
| **WATERCRESS** | | | | | |
| fresh chopped | ½ cup | 2 | tr | – | tr |
| garden fresh | ½ cup | 8 | 1 | – | – |
| garden fresh cooked | ½ cup | 16 | 3 | – | – |
| **WATERMELON** | | | | | |
| cut up | 1 cup | 50 | 11 | – | 1 |
| seeds dried | 1 oz | 158 | 4 | – | – |
| seeds dried | 1 cup | 602 | 17 | – | – |

| FOOD | PORTION | CALS | CARB | SUGAR | FIBER |
|---|---|---|---|---|---|
| wedge | 1/16 | 152 | 35 | – | 2 |
| **WATERMELON JUICE** | | | | | |
| ***Squeezit*** | | | | | |
| Watermelon | 1 bottle (7 oz) | 110 | 28 | 27 | 0 |
| **WAX BEANS** | | | | | |
| **CANNED** | | | | | |
| ***Del Monte*** | | | | | |
| Cut Golden | ½ cup (4.2 oz) | 20 | 4 | 2 | 2 |
| ***S&W*** | | | | | |
| Cut | ½ cup (4.2 oz) | 20 | 4 | 2 | 2 |
| **WHALE** | | | | | |
| raw | 3.5 oz | 134 | 0 | 9 | 9 |
| **WHEAT** | | | | | |
| sprouted | 1 cup (3.8 oz) | 214 | 46 | – | 1 |
| starch | 3.5 oz | 348 | 86 | – | – |
| ***Bob's Red Mill*** | | | | | |
| Vital Wheat Gluten | ¼ cup | 120 | 6 | 0 | 0 |
| ***Lightlife*** | | | | | |
| Savory Seitan Barbecue | 4 oz | 160 | 12 | 3 | 0 |
| Savory Seitan Teriyaki | 4 oz | 160 | 10 | 2 | 0 |
| **WHEAT GERM** | | | | | |
| plain toasted | ¼ cup (1 oz) | 108 | 14 | – | 4 |
| plain toasted | 1 cup | 431 | 56 | – | – |
| w/ brown sugar & honey toasted | 1 oz | 107 | 17 | – | – |
| w/ brown sugar & honey toasted | 1 cup | 426 | 69 | – | – |
| ***Hodgson Mill*** | | | | | |
| Untoasted | 2 tbsp | 55 | 7 | 0 | 4 |
| ***Kretschmer*** | | | | | |
| Original Toasted | 2 tbsp (0.5 oz) | 50 | 6 | 1 | 2 |
| **WHEY** | | | | | |
| acid dry | 1 tbsp (3 g) | 10 | 2 | – | – |
| acid fluid | 1 cup (8 fl oz) | 59 | 13 | – | – |
| sweet dry | 1 tbsp (8 g) | 26 | 6 | – | – |

| FOOD | PORTION | CALS | CARB | SUGAR | FIBER |
|---|---|---|---|---|---|
| sweet fluid | 1 cup (8 fl oz) | 66 | 13 | – | – |
| whey cheese | 1 oz | 126 | 9 | 0 | 0 |
| **WHIPPED TOPPINGS** | | | | | |
| cream pressurized | 1 cup (2.1 oz) | 154 | 7 | – | – |
| cream pressurized | 1 tbsp (3 g) | 8 | tr | – | – |
| nondairy frzn | 1 tbsp | 13 | 1 | – | – |
| nondairy powdered as prep w/ whole milk | 1 cup | 151 | 13 | – | – |
| nondairy powdered as prep w/ whole milk | 1 tbsp (4 g) | 8 | 1 | – | – |
| nondairy pressurized | 1 tbsp (4 g) | 11 | 1 | – | – |
| nondairy pressurized | 1 cup | 184 | 11 | – | – |
| ***Estee*** | | | | | |
| Whipped Topping | 1 serv | 10 | 1 | 0 | 0 |
| **WHITE BEANS** | | | | | |
| canned | 1 cup | 306 | 58 | – | – |
| dried regular cooked | 1 cup | 249 | 45 | – | – |
| dried small cooked | 1 cup | 253 | 46 | – | – |
| ***Progresso*** | | | | | |
| Cannellini | ½ cup (4.6 oz) | 100 | 18 | 0 | 5 |
| **WHITEFISH** | | | | | |
| baked | 3 oz | 146 | 0 | 0 | 0 |
| smoked | 1 oz | 39 | 0 | 0 | 0 |
| smoked | 3 oz | 92 | 0 | 0 | 0 |
| **WHITING** | | | | | |
| cooked | 3 oz | 98 | 0 | 0 | 0 |
| **WILD RICE** | | | | | |
| cooked | 1 cup (5.7 oz) | 166 | 35 | – | 3 |
| ***Gourmet House*** | | | | | |
| Cracked not prep | ¼ cup | 170 | 35 | 0 | 2 |
| Hand Harvested not prep | ¼ cup | 170 | 35 | 0 | 2 |
| Quick Cooking not prep | ½ cup | 170 | 25 | 0 | 2 |
| White & Wild not prep | ¼ cup | 170 | 35 | 1 | 1 |
| Wild & Rice Garden Blend no prep | ¼ cup | 190 | 40 | 1 | 1 |
| **WINE** | | | | | |
| haiku | 1 serv | 93 | 3 | – | 0 |

| FOOD | PORTION | CALS | CARB | SUGAR | FIBER |
|---|---|---|---|---|---|
| japanese plum | 3 oz | 139 | 16 | – | 0 |
| japanese sake | 1 oz | 33 | 2 | – | 0 |
| kir | 1 serv | 78 | 3 | – | 0 |
| madeira | 3.5 oz | 169 | 10 | 10 | 0 |
| port | 3.5 oz | 156 | 11 | 11 | 0 |
| red | 1 serv (3.5 oz) | 74 | 2 | – | 0 |
| rose | 1 serv (3.5 oz) | 73 | 2 | – | 0 |
| sake screwdriver | 1 serv | 175 | 23 | – | tr |
| sangria | 1 serv | 88 | 6 | – | tr |
| sangria blanco | 1 serv | 155 | 24 | – | 3 |
| sherry | 2 oz | 84 | 5 | – | – |
| sweet dessert | 1 serv (3.5 oz) | 158 | 12 | – | 0 |
| vermouth dry | 3½ oz | 105 | 1 | – | – |
| vermouth sweet | 3½ oz | 167 | 12 | – | – |
| wassail wine | 1 serv | 142 | 22 | – | 2 |
| white | 1 serv (3.5 oz) | 70 | 1 | – | 0 |
| wine cooler | 1 serv | 218 | 8 | – | 0 |
| wine spritzer | 1 serv | 60 | 1 | – | 0 |
| ***Boone's*** | | | | | |
| Country Kwencher | 4 fl oz | 96 | 12 | – | – |
| Delicious Apple | 4 fl oz | 84 | 12 | – | – |
| Sangria | 4 fl oz | 88 | 12 | – | – |
| Snow Creek Berry | 4 fl oz | 72 | 12 | – | – |
| Strawberry Hill | 4 fl oz | 88 | 12 | – | – |
| Sun Peak Peach | 4 fl oz | 72 | 12 | – | – |
| Wild Island | 4 fl oz | 72 | 12 | – | – |
| ***Carlo Rossi*** | | | | | |
| Blush | 4 fl oz | 84 | 4 | – | – |
| Burgundy | 4 fl oz | 88 | tr | – | – |
| Chablis | 4 fl oz | 84 | tr | – | – |
| Paisano | 4 fl oz | 92 | tr | – | – |
| Red Sangria | 4 fl oz | 92 | 8 | – | – |
| Rhine | 4 fl oz | 84 | 4 | – | – |
| Vin Rose' | 4 fl oz | 84 | 4 | – | – |
| White Grenache | 4 fl oz | 80 | 4 | – | – |
| ***Eden*** | | | | | |
| Mirin Rice Cooking Wine | 1 tbsp | 25 | 7 | 4 | 0 |
| ***Fairbanks*** | | | | | |
| Cream Sherry | 4 fl oz | 168 | 16 | – | – |
| Port | 4 fl oz | 176 | 16 | – | – |

| FOOD | PORTION | CALS | CARB | SUGAR | FIBER |
|---|---|---|---|---|---|
| Sherry | 4 fl oz | 136 | 8 | – | – |
| White Port | 4 fl oz | 136 | 16 | – | – |
| ***Gallo*** | | | | | |
| Blush Chablis | 4 fl oz | 88 | 4 | – | – |
| Burgundy | 4 fl oz | 88 | tr | – | – |
| Cabernet Sauvignon | 4 fl oz | 88 | 0 | – | – |
| Chablis Blanc | 4 fl oz | 80 | tr | – | – |
| Chardonnay | 4 fl oz | 92 | tr | – | – |
| Classic Burgundy | 4 fl oz | 84 | 0 | – | – |
| French Colombard | 4 fl oz | 84 | 4 | – | – |
| Hearty Burgundy | 4 fl oz | 88 | tr | – | – |
| Pink Chablis | 4 fl oz | 80 | 4 | – | – |
| Red Rose' | 4 fl oz | 92 | 4 | – | – |
| Rhine | 4 fl oz | 88 | 4 | – | – |
| ***Sheffield Cellars*** | | | | | |
| Sherry | 4 fl oz | 136 | 16 | – | – |
| Tawny Port | 4 fl oz | 180 | 16 | – | – |
| Vermouth Extra Dry | 1 fl oz | 28 | 1 | – | – |
| Vermouth Sweet | 1 fl oz | 43 | 4 | – | – |
| Very Dry Sherry | 4 fl oz | 128 | 4 | – | – |
| **WINGED BEANS** | | | | | |
| dried cooked | 1 cup | 252 | 26 | – | – |
| **WOLFFISH** | | | | | |
| atlantic baked | 3 oz | 105 | 0 | 0 | 0 |
| **WRAPS** *(see* BREAD*)* | | | | | |
| **XANTHAN GUM** | | | | | |
| ***Bob's Red Mill*** | | | | | |
| Xanthan Gum | 1 tbsp | 8 | 9 | 0 | 8 |
| **YAM** *(see also* SWEET POTATO*)* | | | | | |
| **CANNED** | | | | | |
| ***S&W*** | | | | | |
| Candied | ½ cup (4.9 oz) | 170 | 46 | 21 | 4 |
| **FRESH** | | | | | |
| mountain yam hawaii cooked | ½ cup | 59 | 14 | – | – |
| yam cubed cooked | ½ cup | 79 | 19 | – | – |
| **YAMBEAN** | | | | | |
| cooked | ¾ cup | 38 | 9 | – | – |

| FOOD | PORTION | CALS | CARB | SUGAR | FIBER |
|---|---|---|---|---|---|
| **YARDLONG BEANS** | | | | | |
| dried cooked | 1 cup | 202 | 36 | – | – |
| **YAUTIA (TANNIER)** | | | | | |
| fresh sliced | 1 cup (4.7 oz) | 132 | 32 | – | 2 |
| root raw | 1 (10.7 oz) | 299 | 72 | – | 5 |
| **YEAST** | | | | | |
| baker's compressed | 1 cake (0.6 oz) | 18 | 3 | – | 2 |
| baker's dry | 1 pkg (¼ oz) | 21 | 3 | – | – |
| baker's dry | 1 tbsp | 35 | 5 | – | 3 |
| brewer's dry | 1 tbsp | 25 | 3 | – | – |
| ***Hodgson Mill*** | | | | | |
| Fast Rise | 1 tsp (9 g) | 25 | 4 | 0 | 1 |
| **YELLOW BEANS** | | | | | |
| canned | ½ cup | 13 | 3 | – | 1 |
| canned low sodium | ½ cup | 13 | 3 | – | 1 |
| dried cooked | 1 cup | 254 | 45 | – | – |
| fresh cooked | ½ cup | 22 | 5 | – | – |
| fresh raw | ½ cup | 17 | 4 | – | – |
| frozen cooked | ½ cup | 18 | 4 | – | – |
| **YELLOWTAIL** | | | | | |
| baked | 3 oz | 159 | 0 | 0 | 0 |
| **YOGURT** *(see also* YOGURT FROZEN*)* | | | | | |
| coffee lowfat | 8 oz | 194 | 31 | – | – |
| fruit lowfat | 4 oz | 113 | 21 | – | – |
| fruit lowfat | 8 oz | 225 | 42 | – | – |
| plain | 8 oz | 139 | 11 | – | – |
| plain lowfat | 8 oz | 144 | 16 | – | – |
| plain no fat | 8 oz | 127 | 17 | – | – |
| vanilla lowfat | 8 oz | 194 | 31 | – | – |
| ***Breyers*** | | | | | |
| Vanilla 98% Fat Free | ½ cup | 90 | 21 | 14 | 4 |
| ***Cabot*** | | | | | |
| Non Fat | 8 oz | 100 | 19 | 13 | 0 |
| Non Fat Berry Banana | 8 oz | 130 | 24 | 19 | 0 |
| Non Fat Blueberry | 8 oz | 130 | 24 | 19 | 0 |
| Non Fat Lemon | 8 oz | 130 | 24 | 19 | 0 |

| FOOD | PORTION | CALS | CARB | SUGAR | FIBER |
|---|---|---|---|---|---|
| Non Fat Raspberry | 8 oz | 130 | 24 | 19 | 0 |
| Non Fat Very Berry | 8 oz | 130 | 24 | 19 | 0 |
| ***Colombo*** | | | | | |
| Fat Free Plain | 8 oz | 100 | 16 | 10 | 0 |
| Fat Free Vanilla | 8 oz | 160 | 32 | 26 | 0 |
| French Vanilla | 8 oz | 180 | 42 | 32 | 0 |
| Fruit On The Bottom Strawberry Banana | 8 oz | 230 | 47 | 42 | 0 |
| Lowfat Plain | 8 oz | 130 | 16 | 10 | 0 |
| Multipack Blended All Flavors | 4 oz | 110 | 22 | 19 | 0 |
| Strawberry | 8 oz | 190 | 42 | 33 | – |
| ***Dannon*** | | | | | |
| Chunky Fruit Nonfat Apple Cinnamon | 6 oz | 160 | 33 | 29 | 0 |
| Chunky Fruit Nonfat Blueberry | 6 oz | 160 | 32 | 29 | 0 |
| Chunky Fruit Nonfat Cherry Vanilla | 6 oz | 160 | 31 | 28 | 0 |
| Chunky Fruit Nonfat Peach | 6 oz | 160 | 33 | 29 | 0 |
| Chunky Fruit Nonfat Strawberry | 6 oz | 160 | 32 | 28 | 0 |
| Chunky Fruit Nonfat Strawberry Banana | 6 oz | 160 | 32 | 28 | 0 |
| Danimals Lowfat Tropical Punch | 4.4 oz | 130 | 25 | 22 | 0 |
| Danimals Lowfat Blueberry | 4.4 oz | 130 | 24 | 21 | 0 |
| Danimals Lowfat Grape Lemonade | 4.4 oz | 120 | 22 | 20 | 0 |
| Danimals Lowfat Lemon Ice | 4.4 oz | 120 | 22 | 19 | 0 |
| Danimals Lowfat Orange Banana | 4.4 oz | 130 | 24 | 21 | 0 |
| Danimals Lowfat Strawberry | 4.4 oz | 130 | 24 | 21 | 0 |
| Danimals Lowfat Vanilla | 4.4 oz | 120 | 23 | 21 | 0 |
| Danimals Lowfat Wild Raspberry | 4.4 oz | 120 | 22 | 19 | 0 |
| Double Delights Banana Creme Strawberry | 6 oz | 160 | 32 | 28 | 0 |
| Double Delights Bavarian Creme Raspberry | 6 oz | 170 | 34 | 31 | 0 |
| Double Delights Cheesecake Cherry | 6 oz | 170 | 34 | 30 | 0 |
| Double Delights Cheesecake Strawberry | 6 oz | 170 | 33 | 39 | 0 |

| FOOD | PORTION | CALS | CARB | SUGAR | FIBER |
|---|---|---|---|---|---|
| Double Delights Chocolate Cheesecake | 6 oz | 220 | 45 | 42 | 0 |
| Double Delights Chocolate Dipped Strawberry | 6 oz | 210 | 45 | 41 | 0 |
| Double Delights Chocolate Eclair | 6 oz | 220 | 45 | 42 | 0 |
| Double Delights Vanilla Strawberry | 6 oz | 170 | 33 | 29 | 0 |
| Double Delights Vanilla Peach & Apricot | 6 oz | 170 | 33 | 29 | 0 |
| Fruit On The Bottom Lowfat Apple Cinnamon | 8 oz | 240 | 46 | 45 | 1 |
| Fruit On The Bottom Lowfat Blueberry | 8 oz | 240 | 46 | 44 | 1 |
| Fruit On The Bottom Lowfat Boysenberry | 8 oz | 240 | 45 | 42 | 1 |
| Fruit On The Bottom Lowfat Cherry | 8 oz | 240 | 46 | 44 | 1 |
| Fruit On The Bottom Lowfat Minipack Mixed Berry | 4.4 oz | 130 | 25 | 24 | tr |
| Fruit On The Bottom Lowfat Minipack Strawberry | 4.4 oz | 130 | 25 | 24 | tr |
| Fruit On The Bottom Lowfat Mixed Berries | 8 oz | 240 | 45 | 43 | 1 |
| Fruit On The Bottom Lowfat Orange | 8 oz | 240 | 45 | 44 | 0 |
| Fruit On The Bottom Lowfat Peach | 8 oz | 240 | 45 | 44 | 1 |
| Fruit On The Bottom Lowfat Raspberry | 8 oz | 240 | 45 | 43 | 1 |
| Fruit On The Bottom Lowfat Strawberry | 8 oz | 240 | 46 | 44 | 1 |
| Fruit On The Bottom Lowfat Strawberry Banana | 8 oz | 240 | 43 | 40 | 1 |
| La Creme Mousse French Vanilla | 1 pkg (2.6 oz) | 120 | 15 | 14 | – |
| LaCreme Vanilla | 1 pkg (4.4 oz) | 140 | 20 | 18 | – |
| Light 'N Crunchy Mint Chocolate Chip | 8 oz | 140 | 27 | 14 | 0 |

| FOOD | PORTION | CALS | CARB | SUGAR | FIBER |
|---|---|---|---|---|---|
| Light 'N Crunchy Nonfat Caramel Apple Crunch | 8 oz | 140 | 26 | 14 | 0 |
| Light 'N Crunchy Nonfat Lemon Blueberry Cobbler | 8 oz | 140 | 25 | 17 | 0 |
| Light 'N Crunchy Nonfat Mocha Cappuccino | 8 oz | 140 | 26 | 14 | 0 |
| Light 'N Crunchy Nonfat Raspberry w/ Granola | 8 oz | 140 | 26 | 13 | 2 |
| Light 'N Crunchy Nonfat Vanilla Chocolate Crunch | 8 oz | 130 | 23 | 13 | 0 |
| Light Duets Cherry Cheesecake | 6 oz | 90 | 18 | 12 | 0 |
| Light Duets Peaches N' Cream | 6 oz | 90 | 18 | 13 | 0 |
| Light Duets Raspberry Royale | 6 oz | 90 | 17 | 12 | 0 |
| Light Duets Strawberry Cheesecake | 6 oz | 90 | 18 | 12 | 0 |
| Light Nonfat Banana Cream Pie | 8 oz | 100 | 15 | 9 | 0 |
| Light Nonfat Blueberry | 8 oz | 100 | 18 | 12 | 0 |
| Light Nonfat Cappuccino | 8 oz | 100 | 16 | 9 | 0 |
| Light Nonfat Cherry Vanilla | 8 oz | 100 | 18 | 13 | 0 |
| Light Nonfat Coconut Cream Pie | 8 oz | 100 | 16 | 9 | 0 |
| Light Nonfat Creme Caramel | 8 oz | 100 | 15 | 9 | 0 |
| Light Nonfat Lemon Chiffon | 8 oz | 100 | 15 | 9 | 0 |
| Light Nonfat Mint Chocolate Cream Pie | 8 oz | 100 | 17 | 9 | 0 |
| Light Nonfat Peach | 8 oz | 100 | 16 | 11 | 0 |
| Light Nonfat Raspberry | 8 oz | 100 | 17 | 11 | 0 |
| Light Nonfat Strawberry | 8 oz | 100 | 16 | 10 | 0 |
| Light Nonfat Strawberry Banana | 8 oz | 100 | 17 | 11 | 0 |
| Light Nonfat Strawberry Kiwi | 8 oz | 100 | 16 | 10 | 0 |
| Light Nonfat Tangerine Chiffon | 8 oz | 100 | 15 | 9 | 0 |
| Light Nonfat Vanilla | 8 oz | 100 | 15 | 9 | 0 |
| Lowfat Coffee | 8 oz | 210 | 36 | 34 | 0 |
| Lowfat Cranberry Raspberry | 8 oz | 210 | 36 | 35 | 0 |
| Lowfat Lemon | 8 oz | 210 | 36 | 35 | 0 |
| Lowfat Vanilla | 8 oz | 210 | 36 | 34 | 0 |
| Minipack Blended Nonfat Blueberry | 4.4 oz | 120 | 25 | 22 | 0 |

| FOOD | PORTION | CALS | CARB | SUGAR | FIBER |
|---|---|---|---|---|---|
| Minipack Blended Nonfat Cherry | 4.4 oz | 110 | 24 | 20 | 0 |
| Minipack Blended Nonfat Peach | 4.4 oz | 120 | 23 | 21 | 0 |
| Minipack Blended Nonfat Raspberry | 4.4 oz | 120 | 24 | 21 | 0 |
| Minipack Blended Nonfat Strawberry | 4.4 oz | 120 | 23 | 20 | 0 |
| Minipack Blended Nonfat Strawberry Banana | 4.4 oz | 120 | 23 | 20 | 0 |
| Sprinkl'ins Cherry Vanilla | 1 (4.1 oz) | 130 | 24 | 20 | 0 |
| Sprinkl'ins Strawberry | 1 (4.1 oz) | 130 | 24 | 20 | 0 |
| Sprinkl'ins Strawberry Banana | 1 (4.1 oz) | 130 | 24 | 20 | 0 |
| Sprinkl'ins Vanilla w/ Cherry Crystals | 1 (4.1 oz) | 110 | 21 | 19 | 0 |
| Sprinkl'ins Vanilla w/ Orange Crystals | 1 (4.1 oz) | 110 | 21 | 19 | 0 |
| ***Horizon Organic*** | | | | | |
| Fat Free Apricot Mango | ¾ cup (6 oz) | 120 | 23 | 21 | 0 |
| Fat Free Honey | 1 cup (8 oz) | 160 | 32 | 31 | 0 |
| ***Oberweis*** | | | | | |
| Peach | 1 pkg (8 oz) | 210 | 39 | 35 | 0 |
| ***Pascual*** | | | | | |
| Nonfat Cherries & Berries | 1 pkg (4.4 oz) | 100 | 19 | 12 | 5 |
| Nonfat Peach | 1 pkg (4.4 oz) | 100 | 19 | 12 | 5 |
| ***Silk*** | | | | | |
| Organic Soy Strawberry | 1 pkg (6 oz) | 160 | 31 | 22 | 1 |
| Soy Apricot Mango | 1 pkg | 160 | 30 | 20 | 1 |
| Soy Banana Strawberry | 1 pkg | 160 | 30 | 20 | 1 |
| Soy Black Cherry | 1 pkg | 160 | 29 | 20 | 1 |
| Soy Blueberry | 1 pkg | 160 | 29 | 21 | 1 |
| Soy Key Lime | 1 pkg | 170 | 30 | 21 | 1 |
| Soy Lemon | 1 pkg | 160 | 31 | 22 | 1 |
| Soy Lemon Kiwi | 1 pkg | 150 | 29 | 21 | 1 |
| Soy Peach | 1 pkg | 170 | 32 | 25 | 1 |
| Soy Plain | 8 oz | 120 | 22 | 12 | 1 |
| Soy Raspberry | 1 pkg | 160 | 30 | 22 | 1 |
| Soy Vanilla | 1 pkg (8 oz) | 120 | 23 | 16 | 1 |
| ***Stonyfield Farm*** | | | | | |
| Creamy Maple | 1 pkg | 160 | 19 | 18 | 0 |

| FOOD | PORTION | CALS | CARB | SUGAR | FIBER |
|---|---|---|---|---|---|
| Mocho-Ccino | 1 pkg | 170 | 23 | 22 | 0 |
| Nonfat Apricot Mango | 1 pkg (8 oz) | 160 | 31 | 30 | tr |
| Nonfat Black Cherry | 1 pkg (8 oz) | 160 | 31 | 29 | tr |
| Nonfat Cappuccino | 1 pkg (8 oz) | 160 | 31 | 29 | 0 |
| Nonfat Cherry Vanilla | 1 pkg (8 oz) | 190 | 43 | 41 | tr |
| Nonfat Chocolate Underground | 1 pkg (8 oz) | 200 | 46 | 45 | tr |
| Nonfat French Vanilla | 1 pkg (8 oz) | 180 | 30 | 29 | 0 |
| Nonfat Lotsa Lemon | 1 pkg (8 oz) | 160 | 30 | 29 | 0 |
| Nonfat Peach | 1 pkg (8 oz) | 150 | 30 | 30 | tr |
| Nonfat Plain | 1 pkg (8 oz) | 100 | 15 | 15 | 0 |
| Nonfat Raspberry | 1 pkg (8 oz) | 160 | 31 | 28 | tr |
| Nonfat Strawberry | 1 pkg (8 oz) | 180 | 32 | 30 | tr |
| Organic French Vanilla | 1 pkg | 170 | 23 | 22 | 0 |
| Organic Wild Blueberry | 1 pkg | 160 | 22 | 21 | tr |
| Organic Lowfat Blueberry | 1 pkg (6 oz) | 130 | 23 | 22 | 1 |
| Organic Lowfat Luscious Lemon | 1 pkg (6 oz) | 130 | 23 | 22 | 1 |
| Organic Lowfat Maple Vanilla | 1 pkg (6 oz) | 120 | 19 | 19 | 0 |
| Organic Lowfat Mocha Latte | 1 pkg (6 oz) | 120 | 20 | 19 | 0 |
| Organic Lowfat Plain | 1 cup (8 oz) | 110 | 14 | 13 | 0 |
| Organic Lowfat Raspberry | 1 pkg (6 oz) | 130 | 23 | 21 | 1 |
| Organic Lowfat Strawberry | 1 pkg (6 oz) | 130 | 23 | 22 | 1 |
| Organic Lowfat Vanilla | 1 pkg (6 oz) | 120 | 20 | 20 | 0 |
| Strawberries & Cream | 1 pkg | 160 | 23 | 22 | tr |
| Vanilla Truffle | 1 pkg | 220 | 37 | 34 | tr |
| YoSelf Organic Chocolate | 1 (4 oz) | 110 | 21 | 19 | 2 |
| YoSelf Organic Creme Caramel | 1 (4 oz) | 110 | 21 | 19 | 2 |
| Yosqueeze Strawberry | 1 tube (2 oz) | 60 | 11 | 10 | 1 |
| ***Total*** | | | | | |
| Greek Yogurt | 1 pkg (5 oz) | 180 | 10 | 10 | 0 |
| Greek Yogurt 0% Fat | 1 pkg (5 oz) | 80 | 6 | 6 | 0 |
| Greek Yogurt 1% Fat | 1 pkg (5 oz) | 120 | 8 | 8 | 0 |
| ***Yoplait*** | | | | | |
| 99% Fat Free Blueberry | 6 oz | 180 | 34 | 31 | 0 |
| 99% Fat Free Boysenberry | 6 oz | 180 | 34 | 31 | 0 |
| 99% Fat Free Cherry | 6 oz | 180 | 34 | 31 | 0 |
| 99% Fat Free Harvest Peach | 6 oz | 120 | 23 | 20 | 0 |
| 99% Fat Free Harvest Peach | 6 oz | 180 | 34 | 31 | 0 |
| 99% Fat Free Key Lime Pie | 6 oz | 180 | 34 | 31 | 0 |
| 99% Fat Free Lemon | 6 oz | 180 | 34 | 31 | 0 |
| 99% Fat Free Mixed Berry | 6 oz | 180 | 34 | 31 | 0 |

| FOOD | PORTION | CALS | CARB | SUGAR | FIBER |
|---|---|---|---|---|---|
| 99% Fat Free Mixed Berry | 6 oz | 120 | 23 | 20 | 0 |
| 99% Fat Free Orange | 6 oz | 180 | 34 | 31 | 0 |
| 99% Fat Free Pina Colada | 6 oz | 180 | 34 | 31 | 0 |
| 99% Fat Free Pineapple | 6 oz | 180 | 34 | 31 | 0 |
| 99% Fat Free Raspberry | 6 oz | 180 | 34 | 31 | 0 |
| 99% Fat Free Strawberry | 6 oz | 120 | 23 | 20 | 0 |
| 99% Fat Free Strawberry | 6 oz | 180 | 43 | 31 | 0 |
| 99% Fat Free Strawberry Banana | 6 oz | 120 | 23 | 20 | 0 |
| 99% Fat Free Strawberry Banana | 6 oz | 180 | 34 | 31 | 0 |
| 99% Fat Free Strawberry Cheesecake | 6 oz | 180 | 34 | 31 | 0 |
| Custard Style Banana | 6 oz | 190 | 32 | 28 | 0 |
| Custard Style Blueberry | 6 oz | 190 | 32 | 28 | 0 |
| Custard Style Cherry Vanilla | 6 oz | 190 | 32 | 28 | 0 |
| Custard Style Key Lime Pie | 6 oz | 190 | 32 | 28 | 0 |
| Custard Style Lemon | 6 oz | 190 | 32 | 28 | 0 |
| Custard Style Peaches'n Cream | 6 oz | 190 | 32 | 28 | 0 |
| Custard Style Raspberry | 6 oz | 190 | 32 | 28 | 0 |
| Custard Style Raspberry Cheesecake | 6 oz | 190 | 32 | 28 | 0 |
| Custard Style Strawberry | 6 oz | 190 | 32 | 28 | 0 |
| Custard Style Strawberry Banana | 6 oz | 190 | 32 | 28 | 0 |
| Custard Style Strawberry Vanilla | 4 oz | 120 | 21 | 19 | 0 |
| Custard Style Vanilla | 6 oz | 190 | 32 | 27 | 0 |
| Go-Gurt Strawberry Banana Burst | 1 pkg (2.25 oz) | 80 | 12 | 10 | 0 |
| Go-Gurt Watermelon Meltdown | 1 pkg (2.25 oz) | 80 | 12 | 10 | 0 |
| Light Amaretto Cheesecake | 6 oz | 90 | 16 | 10 | 0 |
| Light Apricot Mango | 6 oz | 90 | 16 | 10 | 0 |
| Light Banana Cream | 6 oz | 90 | 16 | 0 | 0 |
| Light Blueberry | 6 oz | 90 | 16 | 10 | 0 |
| Light Boston Cream Pie | 6 oz | 90 | 16 | 10 | 0 |
| Light Caramel Apple | 6 oz | 90 | 16 | 10 | 0 |
| Light Cherry | 6 oz | 90 | 16 | 10 | 0 |
| Light Key Lime Pie | 6 oz | 90 | 16 | 10 | 0 |

| FOOD | PORTION | CALS | CARB | SUGAR | FIBER |
|---|---|---|---|---|---|
| Light Lemon Cream Pie | 6 oz | 90 | 16 | 10 | 0 |
| Light Peach | 6 oz | 90 | 16 | 10 | 0 |
| Light Peach Melba | 6 oz | 90 | 16 | 10 | 0 |
| Light Raspberry | 6 oz | 90 | 16 | 10 | 0 |
| Light Raspberry | 6 oz | 90 | 16 | 10 | 0 |
| Light Strawberry | 6 oz | 90 | 16 | 10 | 0 |
| Light Strawberry Banana | 6 oz | 90 | 16 | 10 | 0 |
| Light White Chocolate Strawberry | 6 oz | 90 | 16 | 10 | 0 |
| Original Cafe Au Lait | 6 oz | 170 | 31 | 27 | 0 |
| Original Coconut Cream Pie | 6 oz | 200 | 35 | 30 | 0 |
| Original French Vanilla | 6 oz | 180 | 34 | 30 | 0 |
| Trix Rainbow Punch | 6 oz | 190 | 36 | 31 | 0 |
| Trix Raspberry Rainbow | 6 oz | 190 | 36 | 31 | 0 |
| Trix Strawberry Banana Bash | 6 oz | 190 | 36 | 31 | 0 |
| Trix Strawberry Punch | 4 oz | 130 | 24 | 20 | 0 |
| Trix Triple Cherry | 6 oz | 190 | 36 | 31 | 0 |
| Trix Watermelon Burst | 4 oz | 130 | 24 | 20 | 0 |
| Trix Wild Berry Blue | 4 oz | 130 | 24 | 20 | 0 |
| Whips! Orange Creme | 1 pkg (4 oz) | 140 | 23 | 21 | – |
| Whips! Raspberry Mousse | 1 pkg (4 oz) | 140 | 23 | 21 | – |
| **YOGURT DRINKS** | | | | | |
| ***Dannon*** | | | | | |
| Frusion Smoothie Peach Passion Fruit | 1 bottle (10 oz) | 270 | 51 | 49 | 0 |
| Frusion Smoothie Tropical Fruit | 1 bottle (10 oz) | 270 | 52 | 49 | 0 |
| ***Yo-Goat*** | | | | | |
| Blueberry | 8 oz | 150 | 13 | 7 | – |
| ***Yoplait*** | | | | | |
| Nouriche All Flavors | 1 bottle (11 oz) | 290 | 60 | 46 | 6 |
| **YOGURT FROZEN** | | | | | |
| chocolate soft serve | ½ cup (4 fl oz) | 115 | 18 | – | – |
| vanilla soft serve | ½ cup (4 fl oz) | 114 | 17 | 16 | – |
| ***Breyers*** | | | | | |
| Chocolate | ½ cup | 150 | 23 | 17 | tr |
| Vanilla | ½ cup | 140 | 21 | 16 | 0 |
| Vanilla No Sugar Added | ½ cup | 100 | 13 | 6 | 0 |

| FOOD | PORTION | CALS | CARB | SUGAR | FIBER |
|---|---|---|---|---|---|
| ***Edy's*** | | | | | |
| Black Cherry Vanilla Swirl | ½ cup | 90 | 20 | 14 | – |
| Caramel Fudge Cosmo | ½ cup | 140 | 23 | 18 | – |
| Caramel Praline Crunch | ½ cup | 100 | 23 | 17 | – |
| Chocolate Decadence | ½ cup | 120 | 20 | 14 | – |
| Chocolate Fudge | ½ cup | 100 | 22 | 14 | – |
| Coffee Fudge Sundae | ½ cup | 100 | 22 | 15 | – |
| Cookies'N Cream | ½ cup | 120 | 19 | 14 | – |
| Heath Toffee Crunch | ½ cup | 120 | 18 | 15 | – |
| Raspberry | ½ cup | 90 | 16 | 13 | – |
| Ultimate Tin Roof Sundae | ½ cup | 130 | 20 | 15 | – |
| Vanilla | ½ cup | 90 | 19 | 13 | – |
| Vanilla Chocolate Swirl | ½ cup | 90 | 19 | 13 | – |
| ***Haagen-Dazs*** | | | | | |
| Lowfat Dulce De Leche | ½ cup | 190 | 35 | 25 | 0 |
| Nonfat Chocolate | ½ cup | 140 | 28 | 16 | tr |
| Nonfat Coffee | ½ cup | 140 | 29 | 16 | 0 |
| Nonfat Strawberry | ½ cup | 140 | 31 | 20 | 0 |
| Nonfat Vanilla | ½ cup | 140 | 29 | 16 | 0 |
| Nonfat Vanilla Raspberry Swirl | ½ cup | 130 | 29 | 20 | tr |
| Nonfat Vanilla Fudge | ½ cup | 160 | 34 | 21 | 0 |
| ***Turkey Hill*** | | | | | |
| Black Raspberry | ½ cup | 110 | 20 | – | – |
| Caramel Cashew Crunch | ½ cup | 160 | 18 | – | – |
| Chocolate Chip Cookie Dough | ½ cup | 140 | 23 | 21 | 0 |
| Chocolate Chip Cookie Dough | ½ cup | 190 | 23 | – | – |
| Clark Bar | ½ cup | 140 | 22 | – | – |
| Fat Free Chocolate Cherry Cordial | ½ cup | 100 | 24 | 21 | 0 |
| Fat Free Chocolate Marshmallow | ½ cup | 130 | 30 | 21 | 0 |
| Fat Free Mint Cookie 'N Cream | ½ cup | 110 | 24 | 18 | 0 |
| Fat Free Neapolitan | ½ cup | 100 | 22 | 19 | 0 |
| Fat Free Orange Swirl | ½ cup | 100 | 22 | – | – |
| Fat Free Vanilla Fudge | ½ cup | 110 | 24 | 21 | 0 |
| Peach Raspberry | ½ cup | 110 | 20 | 20 | 0 |
| Tin Roof Sundae | ½ cup | 140 | 21 | 20 | 0 |
| Vanilla & Chocolate | ½ cup | 110 | 19 | 18 | 0 |
| Vanilla Bean | ½ cup | 110 | 17 | 17 | 0 |

| FOOD | PORTION | CALS | CARB | SUGAR | FIBER |
|---|---|---|---|---|---|
| **ZUCCHINI** | | | | | |
| baby raw | 1 (0.5 oz) | 3 | 1 | – | tr |
| canned italian style | ½ cup | 33 | 8 | – | – |
| frzn cooked | ½ cup | 19 | 4 | – | – |
| raw sliced | ½ cup | 9 | 2 | – | 1 |
| sliced cooked | ½ cup | 14 | 4 | – | 1 |
| ***Progresso*** | | | | | |
| Italian Style | ½ cup (4.2 oz) | 50 | 7 | 4 | 2 |
| **TAKE-OUT** | | | | | |
| indian paalkora | 1 serv | 46 | 7 | – | 2 |

## PART TWO

# Restaurant Chains

| FOOD | PORTION | CALS | CARB | SUGAR | FIBER |
|---|---|---|---|---|---|
| **APPLEBEE'S** | | | | | |
| **DESSERTS** | | | | | |
| Apple Betty Cobbler Ala Mode | 1 serv | 598 | 94 | 57 | 2 |
| Fudge Brownie Sundae | 1 serv | 739 | 87 | 39 | 6 |
| Low Fat Bikini Banana Strawberry Shortcake | 1 serv | 248 | 48 | 27 | 2 |
| Low Fat Brownie Sundae | 1 serv | 415 | 82 | 57 | 3 |
| Low Fat Marble Cheesecake | 1 serv | 261 | 50 | 37 | 4 |
| **MAIN MENU SELECTIONS** | | | | | |
| Applebee's Burger w/ Fries | 1 serv | 1274 | 90 | 10 | 7 |
| Basic Hamburger w/ Fries | 1 serv | 980 | 86 | 8 | 6 |
| Beef Fajita Quesadilla | 1 serv | 1205 | 58 | 5 | 6 |
| Bourbon Street Steak w/ Fried New Potatoes | 1 serv | 1115 | 50 | 3 | – |
| Low Fat Asian Chicken Salad | 1 serv (5 oz) | 623 | 107 | – | 14 |
| Low Fat Asian Chicken Salad | 1 med serv (2.5 oz) | 370 | 64 | – | 7 |
| Low Fat Blackened Chicken Salad | 1 med serv (2.5 oz) | 287 | 27 | – | 6 |
| Low Fat Blackened Chicken Salad | 1 serv (5 oz) | 411 | 39 | – | 11 |
| Low Fat Garlic Chicken Pasta | 1 serv | 587 | 89 | 7 | 9 |
| Low Fat Lemon Chicken Pasta | 1 serv | 528 | 78 | 12 | 8 |
| Low Fat Quesadilla Chicken Fajita | 1 serv | 518 | 63 | 6 | 2 |
| Low Fat Quesadilla Veggie | 1 serv | 344 | 46 | 4 | 3 |
| Mozzarella Stix | 8 pieces | 963 | 74 | – | 1 |
| Quesadillas | 1 serv | 684 | 40 | 5 | 4 |
| Riblet Basket w/ Fries | 1 serv | 1317 | 45 | tr | 7 |
| Salad Dinner w/o Dressing | 1 serv | 303 | 13 | 4 | 3 |
| Salad Santa Fe Chicken | 1 med | 724 | 56 | 12 | 7 |
| Sandwich Bacon Cheese Chicken Grill w/o Fries | 1 | 746 | 36 | 1 | 1 |
| Sandwich Gyro | 1 | 880 | 44 | 5 | 3 |
| Stir Fry Chicken | 1 serv | 566 | 89 | 24 | 5 |
| **ARBY'S** | | | | | |
| **BEVERAGES** | | | | | |
| Chocolate Shake | 1 (14 oz) | 480 | 84 | – | 0 |
| Hot Chocolate | 1 serv (8.6 oz) | 110 | 23 | – | 0 |
| Jamocha Shake | 1 (14 oz) | 470 | 82 | – | 0 |

| FOOD | PORTION | CALS | CARB | SUGAR | FIBER |
|---|---|---|---|---|---|
| Milk | 1 serv (8 oz) | 120 | 12 | – | 0 |
| Orange Juice | 1 serv (10 oz) | 140 | 34 | – | 0 |
| Strawberry Shake | 1 (14 oz) | 500 | 87 | – | 0 |
| Vanilla Shake | 1 (14 oz) | 470 | 83 | – | 0 |
| **BREAKFAST SELECTIONS** | | | | | |
| Add Egg | 1 serv (2 oz) | 110 | 2 | – | 0 |
| Add Swiss Cheese Slice | 1 slice (0.5 oz) | 45 | 0 | – | 0 |
| Biscuit w/ Bacon | 1 (3.2 oz) | 320 | 27 | – | 1 |
| Biscuit w/ Butter | 1 (2.9 oz) | 280 | 27 | – | 1 |
| Biscuit w/ Ham | 1 (4.3 oz) | 330 | 28 | – | 1 |
| Biscuit w/ Sausage | 1 (4.2 oz) | 460 | 27 | – | 1 |
| Croissant w/ Bacon | 1 (2.5 oz) | 300 | 28 | – | 0 |
| Croissant w/ Ham | 1 (3.7 oz) | 310 | 29 | – | 0 |
| Croissant w/ Sausage | 1 (3.6 oz) | 420 | 28 | – | 0 |
| French Toast Syrup | 1 serv (0.5 oz) | 130 | 32 | – | 0 |
| Sourdough w/ Bacon | 1 (5 oz) | 380 | 29 | – | 2 |
| Sourdough w/ Ham | 1 (4 oz) | 220 | 30 | – | 1 |
| Sourdough w/ Sausage | 1 (4 oz) | 330 | 29 | – | 1 |
| Toastix w/o Syrup | 1 serv (4.4 oz) | 370 | 48 | – | 4 |
| **DESSERTS** | | | | | |
| Apple Turnover Iced | 1 (4.5 oz) | 420 | 65 | – | 2 |
| Cherry Turnover Iced | 1 (4.5 oz) | 410 | 63 | – | 1 |
| **MAIN MENU SELECTIONS** | | | | | |
| Arby's Sauce | 1 serv (0.5 oz) | 15 | 4 | – | 0 |
| Au Jus Sauce | 1 serv (3 oz) | 5 | 1 | – | tr |
| BBQ Dipping Sauce | 1 serv (1 oz) | 40 | 10 | – | 0 |
| Baked Potato Broccoli'N Cheddar | 1 (14 oz) | 540 | 71 | – | 7 |
| Baked Potato Deluxe | 1 (13 oz) | 650 | 67 | – | 6 |
| Baked Potato w/ Butter & Sour Cream | 1 (11.2 oz) | 500 | 65 | – | 6 |
| Bronco Berry Sauce | 1 serv (1.5 oz) | 90 | 23 | – | 0 |
| Chicken Finger 4-Pak | 1 serv (6.77 oz) | 640 | 42 | – | 0 |
| Chicken Finger Snack w/ Curly Fries | 1 serv (6.4 oz) | 580 | 55 | – | 3 |
| Curly Fries | 1 lg (7 oz) | 620 | 78 | – | 7 |
| Curly Fries | 1 med (4.5 oz) | 400 | 50 | – | 4 |

| FOOD | PORTION | CALS | CARB | SUGAR | FIBER |
|---|---|---|---|---|---|
| Curly Fries | 1 sm (3.8 oz) | 310 | 39 | – | 3 |
| Curly Fries Cheddar | 1 serv (6 oz) | 460 | 54 | – | 4 |
| German Mustard | 1 pkg (0.25 oz) | 5 | 0 | – | 0 |
| Homestyle Fries | 1 med (5 oz) | 370 | 53 | – | 4 |
| Homestyle Fries | 1 sm (4 oz) | 300 | 42 | – | 3 |
| Homestyle Fries | 1 lg (7.5 oz) | 560 | 79 | – | 6 |
| Homestyle Fries Child-Size | 1 serv (3 oz) | 220 | 32 | – | 3 |
| Honey Mustard | 1 serv (1 oz) | 130 | 5 | – | 0 |
| Horsey Sauce | 1 pkg (0.5 oz) | 60 | 3 | – | 0 |
| Jalapeno Bites | 1 serv (4 oz) | 330 | 30 | – | 2 |
| Ketchup | 1 pkg (0.3 oz) | 10 | 2 | – | 0 |
| Marinara Sauce | 1 serv (1.5 oz) | 35 | 4 | – | 0 |
| Mayonnaise | 1 pkg (0.4 oz) | 90 | 0 | – | 0 |
| Mayonnaise Light Cholesterol Free | 1 pkg (0.4 oz) | 20 | 1 | – | 0 |
| Mozzarella Sticks | 4 (4.8 oz) | 470 | 34 | – | 2 |
| Onion Petals | 1 serv (4 oz) | 410 | 43 | – | 2 |
| Potato Cakes | 2 (3.5 oz) | 250 | 26 | – | 3 |
| Sandwich Chicken Bacon'N Swiss | 1 (7.4 oz) | 610 | 49 | – | 2 |
| Sandwich Chicken Breast Fillet | 1 (7.2 oz) | 540 | 47 | – | 2 |
| Sandwich Chicken Cordon Bleu | 1 (8.4 oz) | 630 | 47 | – | 2 |
| Sandwich Grilled Chicken Deluxe | 1 (8.7 oz) | 450 | 37 | – | 2 |
| Sandwich Hot Ham 'N Swiss | 1 (5.9 oz) | 340 | 35 | – | 1 |
| Sandwich Market Fresh Roast Beef & Swiss | 1 (12.5 oz) | 810 | 73 | – | 5 |
| Sandwich Market Fresh Roast Beef Ranch & Bacon | 1 (13.5 oz) | 880 | 74 | – | 5 |
| Sandwich Market Fresh Roast Chicken Caesar | 1 (12.7 oz) | 820 | 75 | – | 5 |
| Sandwich Market Fresh Roast Ham & Swiss | 1 (12.5 oz) | 730 | 74 | – | 5 |
| Sandwich Market Fresh Roast Turkey & Swiss | 1 (12.5 oz) | 760 | 75 | – | 5 |
| Sandwich Market Fresh Ultimate BLT | 1 (10.5 oz) | 820 | 72 | – | 5 |
| Sandwich Roast Beef Arby-Q | 1 (6.4 oz) | 360 | 40 | – | 2 |

| FOOD | PORTION | CALS | CARB | SUGAR | FIBER |
|---|---|---|---|---|---|
| Sandwich Roast Beef Beef'N Cheddar | 1 (6.9 oz) | 480 | 43 | – | 2 |
| Sandwich Roast Beef Big Montana | 1 (11 oz) | 630 | 41 | – | 3 |
| Sandwich Roast Beef Giant | 1 (7.9 oz) | 480 | 41 | – | 3 |
| Sandwich Roast Beef Junior | 1 (4.4 oz) | 310 | 34 | – | 2 |
| Sandwich Roast Beef Melt w/ Cheddar | 1 (5.2 oz) | 340 | 36 | – | 2 |
| Sandwich Roast Beef Regular | 1 (5.4 oz) | 350 | 34 | – | 2 |
| Sandwich Roast Beef Super | 1 (8.5 oz) | 470 | 47 | – | 3 |
| Sandwich Roast Chicken Club | 1 (8.4 oz) | 520 | 38 | – | 2 |
| Sub Sandwich French Dip | 1 (10 oz) | 440 | 42 | – | 2 |
| Sub Sandwich Hot Ham'N Swiss | 1 (9.7 oz) | 530 | 45 | – | 3 |
| Sub Sandwich Italian | 1 (11 oz) | 780 | 49 | – | 3 |
| Sub Sandwich Philly Beef'N Swiss | 1 (10.8 oz) | 700 | 46 | – | 4 |
| Sub Sandwich Roast Beef | 1 (11.6 oz) | 760 | 47 | – | 3 |
| Sub Sandwich Roast Beef | 1 (11.6 oz) | 760 | 47 | – | 3 |
| Sub Sandwich Turkey | 1 (10.6 oz) | 630 | 51 | – | 2 |
| Tangy Southwest Sauce | 1 serv (1.5 oz) | 250 | 3 | – | 0 |
| **SALAD DRESSINGS** | | | | | |
| Bleu Cheese | 1 serv (2 oz) | 300 | 3 | – | 0 |
| Buttermilk Ranch | 1 serv (2 oz) | 290 | 3 | – | 0 |
| Buttermilk Ranch Light | 1 serv (2 oz) | 100 | 12 | – | 1 |
| Caesar | 1 serv (2 oz) | 310 | 1 | – | 0 |
| Honey French | 1 serv (2 oz) | 290 | 18 | – | tr |
| Italian Reduced Calorie | 1 serv (2 oz) | 25 | 3 | – | tr |
| Italian Parmesan | 1 serv (2 oz) | 240 | 4 | – | 0 |
| Thousand Island | 1 serv (2 oz) | 290 | 9 | – | 0 |
| **SALADS AND SALAD BARS** | | | | | |
| Caesar Side Salad | 1 (5 oz) | 45 | 4 | – | 2 |
| Caesar Salad w/o Dressing | 1 serv (8 oz) | 90 | 8 | – | 3 |
| Chicken Finger w/o Dressing | 1 serv (13 oz) | 570 | 39 | – | 3 |
| Croutons Seasoned | 1 serv (0.25 oz) | 30 | 5 | – | 1 |
| Croutons Cheese & Garlic | 1 serv (0.63 oz) | 100 | 10 | – | 0 |
| Garden Salad | 1 (12.3 oz) | 70 | 14 | – | 6 |
| Grilled Chicken | 1 serv (16.3 oz) | 210 | 14 | – | 6 |

| FOOD | PORTION | CALS | CARB | SUGAR | FIBER |
|---|---|---|---|---|---|
| Grilled Chicken Caesar w/o Dressing | 1 serv (12 oz) | 230 | 8 | – | 3 |
| Roast Chicken | 1 serv (14.8 oz) | 160 | 15 | – | 6 |
| Side Salad | 1 (5.7 oz) | 25 | 5 | – | 2 |
| Turkey Club Salad w/o Dressing | 1 serv (12 oz) | 350 | 9 | – | 3 |

## AU BON PAIN

### BAKED SELECTIONS

| FOOD | PORTION | CALS | CARB | SUGAR | FIBER |
|---|---|---|---|---|---|
| Bagel Cinnamon Crisp | 1 (6 oz) | 540 | 123 | 44 | 4 |
| Baguette | 1 loaf (10.6 oz) | 680 | 136 | 2 | 6 |
| Bread Stick | 1 (2.3 oz) | 200 | 37 | 3 | 2 |
| Cinnamon Roll | 1 (4 oz) | 300 | 60 | 25 | 2 |
| Cookie Chocolate Chip | 1 (2 oz) | 230 | 39 | 23 | 1 |
| Cookie Chocolate Chunk Macadamia | 1 (2 oz) | 250 | 31 | 17 | 1 |
| Cookie Gingerbread Man w/ Raisins & Icing | 1 (2.7 oz) | 280 | 52 | 28 | tr |
| Cookie Oatmeal Raisin | 1 (2 oz) | 210 | 38 | 13 | 2 |
| Cookie Peanut Butter | 1 (2 oz) | 240 | 21 | 16 | 2 |
| Cookie Shortbread | 1 (2.3 oz) | 240 | 44 | 12 | 1 |
| Cookie Walnut Raisin | 1 (2 oz) | 250 | 31 | 17 | 2 |
| Cookie English Toffee | 1 (2 oz) | 230 | 38 | 22 | tr |
| Creme De Fleur | 1 serv (5.55 oz) | 470 | 69 | 23 | 2 |
| Croissant Almond | 1 (4.7 oz) | 480 | 58 | 18 | 3 |
| Croissant Apple | 1 (3.5 oz) | 200 | 40 | 16 | 2 |
| Croissant Chocolate | 1 (3.1 oz) | 330 | 53 | 23 | 3 |
| Croissant Cinnamon Raisin | 1 (3.8 oz) | 300 | 60 | 13 | 2 |
| Croissant Raspberry Cheese | 1 (3.6 oz) | 290 | 47 | 17 | 1 |
| Croissant Sweet Cheese | 1 (3.6 oz) | 320 | 46 | 15 | 1 |
| Danish Cranberry | 1 (4.5 oz) | 350 | 59 | 25 | 2 |
| Danish Lemon | 1 (4.3 oz) | 340 | 59 | 23 | 5 |
| Danish Sweet Cheese | 1 (4.2 oz) | 390 | 55 | 21 | 1 |
| Focaccia | 1 piece (5.4 oz) | 430 | 61 | 2 | 3 |
| Four Grain Bread | 1 serv (4.7 oz) | 400 | 74 | 2 | 3 |
| French Roll | 1 (4.2 oz) | 260 | 53 | 0 | 2 |
| Hearth Roll | 1 (3 oz) | 210 | 38 | 1 | 2 |

| FOOD | PORTION | CALS | CARB | SUGAR | FIBER |
|---|---|---|---|---|---|
| Holiday Cookie w/ Icing & Sprinkles | 1 (1.6 oz) | 150 | 31 | 14 | 0 |
| Loaf Multigrain | 1 slice (1.8 oz) | 130 | 24 | 0 | 1 |
| Muffin Banana Walnut | 1 (5.4 oz) | 430 | 57 | 27 | 2 |
| Muffin Blueberry | 1 (5.6 oz) | 470 | 79 | 44 | 2 |
| Muffin Bran Raisin | 1 (5.5 oz) | 400 | 77 | 31 | 8 |
| Muffin Carrot | 1 (5.8 oz) | 520 | 67 | 38 | 4 |
| Muffin Corn | 1 (5.7 oz) | 390 | 56 | 26 | 2 |
| Muffin Cranberry Walnut | 1 (5.4 oz) | 500 | 57 | 26 | 3 |
| Muffin Milk Chocolate Chunk | 1 (5.3 oz) | 530 | 77 | 42 | 3 |
| Muffin Pumpkin | 1 (6 oz) | 510 | 74 | 38 | 3 |
| Muffin Low Fat 3 Berry | 1 (4.4 oz) | 270 | 58 | 29 | 2 |
| Muffin Low Fat Chocolate Cake | 1 (4.2 oz) | 470 | 117 | 113 | 0 |
| Parisienne Loaf | 1 loaf (19 oz) | 1210 | 244 | 2 | 11 |
| Petit Pain | 1 (2.9 oz) | 180 | 37 | 0 | 2 |
| Roll Braided w/ Topping | 1 (10 oz) | 430 | 63 | 8 | 3 |
| Roll Pecan | 1 (6 oz) | 620 | 94 | 40 | 3 |
| Sandwich Loaf Country White | 1 serv (1.75 oz) | 110 | 23 | 0 | 1 |
| Sandwich Loaf Tomato Herb | 1 serv (1.75 oz) | 120 | 27 | 0 | 1 |
| Scone Chocolate Walnut | 1 (4 oz) | 420 | 56 | 27 | 3 |
| Scone Cranberry Orange Almond | 1 (4 oz) | 400 | 60 | 26 | 3 |
| Scone Maple Oat Pecan Date | 1 (4 oz) | 410 | 58 | 27 | 3 |
| Scone Orange | 1 (4.2 oz) | 370 | 56 | 11 | 2 |
| Shortbread Heart ½ Chocolate | 1 (2.7 oz) | 290 | 51 | 13 | 1 |
| Shortbread Heart w/ Red Sugar | 1 (2.5 oz) | 270 | 51 | 19 | 1 |
| Sourdough Bagel Asiago Cheese | 1 (4.8 oz) | 340 | 57 | 5 | 2 |
| Sourdough Bagel Cheddar Scallion | 1 (4.1 oz) | 310 | 51 | 5 | 2 |
| Sourdough Bagel Cinnamon Crisp | 1 (4.6 oz) | 360 | 52 | 13 | 3 |
| Sourdough Bagel Cinnamon Raisin | 1 (4.5 oz) | 300 | 65 | 4 | 3 |
| Sourdough Bagel Cranberry Nut | 1 (4.7 oz) | 400 | 73 | 15 | 6 |
| Sourdough Bagel Cranberry Nut | 1 (4.7 oz) | 400 | 73 | 15 | 6 |

| FOOD | PORTION | CALS | CARB | SUGAR | FIBER |
|---|---|---|---|---|---|
| Sourdough Bagel Double Cheddar Jalapeno | 1 serv (4.1 oz) | 320 | 50 | 5 | 2 |
| Sourdough Bagel Dutch Apple | 1 (4.7 oz) | 380 | 80 | 22 | 4 |
| Sourdough Bagel Everything | 1 (4.4 oz) | 330 | 54 | 5 | 3 |
| Sourdough Bagel Focaccia | 1 (4.1 oz) | 320 | 61 | 5 | 3 |
| Sourdough Bagel Honey 9 Grain | 1 (4.8 oz) | 310 | 66 | 5 | 6 |
| Sourdough Bagel Plain | 1 (4 oz) | 300 | 61 | 5 | 3 |
| Sourdough Bagel Poppy Seed | 1 (4.4 oz) | 330 | 64 | 5 | 3 |
| Sourdough Bagel Sesame | 1 (4.4 oz) | 340 | 64 | 5 | 3 |
| Sourdough Bagel Wild Blueberry | 1 (4.1 oz) | 280 | 58 | 7 | 3 |
| Sourdough bagel Onion | 1 (4.4 oz) | 320 | 67 | 8 | 3 |
| Streudel Cherry | 1 serv (4 oz) | 380 | 37 | – | tr |
| Streudel Apple | 1 serv (4.35 oz) | 400 | 48 | 18 | tr |
| **SALADS AND SALAD BARS** | | | | | |
| Caesar w/o Dressing | 1 serv (7.8 oz) | 240 | 19 | 2 | 4 |
| Chef's | 1 serv (10.3 oz) | 290 | 11 | 7 | 3 |
| Chicken Caesar | 1 serv (10.2 oz) | 380 | 19 | 2 | 4 |
| Chicken Oriental | 1 serv (8.6 oz) | 220 | 16 | 8 | 5 |
| Chicken Pesto Salad | 1 serv (8 oz) | 400 | 7 | 2 | 2 |
| Garden | 1 serv (9.3 oz) | 160 | 26 | 5 | 5 |
| Garden Side | 1 serv (5.1 oz) | 90 | 14 | 3 | 3 |
| Gorgonzola & Walnut | 1 serv (5 oz) | 330 | 8 | 3 | 5 |
| Mozzarella & Red Pepper Salad | 1 serv (10.5 oz) | 360 | 10 | 6 | 2 |
| Tuna | 1 serv (13.2 oz) | 440 | 28 | 7 | 5 |
| **SANDWICHES AND FILLINGS** | | | | | |
| Club Hot Roasted Turkey | 1 (11.7 oz) | 630 | 53 | 3 | 3 |
| Cream Cheese Plain | 1 serv (2 oz) | 190 | 0 | 0 | 0 |
| Cream Cheese Reduced Fat Honey Walnut | 1 serv (2 oz) | 150 | 10 | 10 | 0 |
| Cream Cheese Reduced Fat Sundried Tomato | 1 serv (2 oz) | 140 | 3 | 2 | 0 |
| Cream Cheese Reduced Fat Veggie | 1 serv (2 oz) | 140 | 3 | 1 | 0 |

| FOOD | PORTION | CALS | CARB | SUGAR | FIBER |
|---|---|---|---|---|---|
| Croissant Spinach & Cheese | 1 (3.6 oz) | 220 | 29 | 4 | 2 |
| Croque Madame | 1 (11 oz) | 570 | 53 | 5 | 3 |
| Croque Monsieur | 1 (11 oz) | 590 | 53 | 5 | 3 |
| Egg On A Bagel | 1 serv (7.1 oz) | 500 | 64 | 6 | 4 |
| Egg On A Bagel w/ Bacon | 1 serv (7.6 oz) | 580 | 84 | 6 | 4 |
| Egg On A Bagel w/ Cheese | 1 serv (7.85 oz) | 590 | 84 | 6 | 4 |
| Egg On A Bagel w/ Cheese & Bacon | 1 serv (8.35 oz) | 670 | 84 | 6 | 4 |
| Fo-Ca-Cha-Cha Chicken | 1 serv (11.15 oz) | 730 | 75 | 5 | 9 |
| Focaccia Chicken & Mozzarella | 1 serv (13.75 oz) | 800 | 73 | 4 | 6 |
| Focaccia Chicken Tarragon w/ Field Greens | 1 (12.5 oz) | 870 | 54 | 3 | 4 |
| Focaccia Garden Vegetable Goat Cheese w/ Artichoke Spread | 1 (14.25 oz) | 570 | 75 | 5 | 5 |
| Focaccia Hickory Smoked Ham & Brie | 1 (13.3 oz) | 620 | 72 | 5 | 5 |
| Focaccia Smoked Turkey & Swiss w/ Cilantro | 1 (13.25 oz) | 810 | 68 | 4 | 4 |
| French Roll Ham | 1 (11 oz) | 390 | 58 | 3 | 3 |
| French Roll Hot Grilled Chicken | 1 (11 oz) | 620 | 57 | 1 | 3 |
| French Roll Hot Roast Turkey | 1 (11 oz) | 500 | 59 | 1 | 3 |
| French Roll Tuna | 1 (10.6 oz) | 550 | 58 | 3 | 4 |
| Hot Croissant Spinach & Cheese | 1 (4 oz) | 290 | 39 | 5 | 1 |
| Sandwich Arizona Chicken | 1 (12 oz) | 600 | 56 | 2 | 4 |
| Sandwich Cheese | 1 (7.2 oz) | 590 | 54 | 0 | 2 |
| Sandwich Fresh Mozzarella Tomato & Pesto | 1 (11 oz) | 790 | 60 | 4 | 3 |
| Sandwich Honey Dijon Chicken | 1 (13.6 oz) | 750 | 65 | 11 | 3 |
| Sandwich Thai Chicken | 1 (11.4 oz) | 550 | 62 | 4 | 3 |
| Wrap Chicken Caesar | 1 (10.5 oz) | 640 | 61 | 2 | 5 |
| Wrap Fields & Feta | 1 (13.5 oz) | 620 | 100 | 6 | 14 |
| Wrap Honey Smoked Turkey | 1 (15 oz) | 520 | 85 | 14 | 11 |
| Wrap Roast Beef & Brie | 1 (14 oz) | 570 | 64 | 3 | 6 |
| **SOUPS** | | | | | |
| Autumn Pumpkin | 1 serv (8 oz) | 170 | 18 | 2 | 5 |
| Black Bean | 1 serv (8 oz) | 180 | 33 | 2 | 18 |
| Chicken Florentine | 1 serv (8 oz) | 140 | 14 | 2 | 1 |

| FOOD | PORTION | CALS | CARB | SUGAR | FIBER |
|---|---|---|---|---|---|
| Chicken Noodle | 1 serv (8 oz) | 100 | 12 | 2 | 1 |
| Clam Chowder | 1 serv (8 oz) | 220 | 16 | 1 | 1 |
| Corn & Gree Chili Bisque | 1 serv (8 oz) | 200 | 21 | 4 | 2 |
| Corn Chowder | 1 serv (8 oz) | 270 | 28 | 4 | 2 |
| Curried Rice & Lentil | 1 serv (8 oz) | 140 | 24 | 2 | 5 |
| French Moroccan Tomato Lentil | 1 serv (8 oz) | 130 | 22 | 4 | 7 |
| Garden Vegetable | 1 serv (8 oz) | 50 | 8 | 3 | 2 |
| Low Sodium Mediterranean Pepper | 1 serv (12 oz) | 280 | 44 | 4 | 10 |
| Low Sodium Southwest Vegetable | 1 serv (12 oz) | 220 | 34 | 4 | 6 |
| Old Fashioned Tomato | 1 serv (8 oz) | 140 | 19 | 11 | 2 |
| Pasta E Fagioli | 1 serv (8 oz) | 240 | 36 | 3 | 7 |
| Potato Cheese | 1 serv (8 oz) | 190 | 21 | 2 | 1 |
| Potato Leek | 1 serv (8 oz) | 200 | 18 | 2 | 2 |
| Red Beans & Rice | 1 serv (8 oz) | 200 | 31 | 2 | 12 |
| Soup Bread Bowl | 1 (9.25 oz) | 600 | 118 | 3 | 5 |
| Southern Black Eyed Pea | 1 serv (8 oz) | 320 | 56 | 4 | 20 |
| Split Pea | 1 serv (8 oz) | 160 | 27 | 2 | 9 |
| Tomato Florentine | 1 serv (8 oz) | 120 | 17 | 5 | 2 |
| Tuscan Vegetable | 1 serv (8 oz) | 140 | 22 | 2 | 3 |
| Vegetable Beef Barley | 1 serv (8 oz) | 110 | 14 | 2 | 3 |
| Vegetarian Lentil | 1 serv (8 oz) | 120 | 21 | 2 | 8 |
| Vegetarian Chili | 1 serv (8 oz) | 170 | 31 | 3 | 15 |
| Vegetarian Chili | 1 serv (8 oz) | 170 | 31 | 3 | 15 |
| Wild Mushroom Bisque | 1 serv (8 oz) | 140 | 16 | 3 | 2 |

## AUNTIE ANNE'S

### BEVERAGES

| FOOD | PORTION | CALS | CARB | SUGAR | FIBER |
|---|---|---|---|---|---|
| Dutch Smoothie Pina Colada | 1 (14 oz) | 260 | 44 | 41 | 0 |
| Dutch Ice Blue Raspberry | 1 (14 oz) | 165 | 38 | 35 | 0 |
| Dutch Ice Grape | 1 (14 oz) | 180 | 43 | 41 | 0 |
| Dutch Ice Kiwi Banana | 1 (14 oz) | 190 | 44 | 41 | 0 |
| Dutch Ice Lemonade | 1 (14 oz) | 315 | 77 | 77 | 0 |
| Dutch Ice Mocha | 1 (14 oz) | 400 | 74 | 52 | 0 |
| Dutch Ice Orange Creme | 1 (14 oz) | 280 | 64 | 59 | 0 |
| Dutch Ice Pina Colada | 1 (14 oz) | 220 | 53 | 50 | 0 |
| Dutch Ice Strawberry | 1 (14 oz) | 220 | 50 | 48 | 0 |
| Dutch Ice Wild Cherry | 1 (14 oz) | 210 | 48 | 45 | 0 |
| Dutch Shake Chocolate | 1 (14 oz) | 580 | 75 | 67 | 0 |

| FOOD | PORTION | CALS | CARB | SUGAR | FIBER |
|---|---|---|---|---|---|
| Dutch Shake Coffee | 1 (14 oz) | 590 | 77 | 70 | 0 |
| Dutch Shake Strawberry | 1 (14 oz) | 610 | 78 | 74 | 0 |
| Dutch Shake Vanilla | 1 (14 oz) | 510 | 58 | 54 | 0 |
| Dutch Smoothie Blue Raspberry | 1 (14 oz) | 230 | 34 | 33 | 0 |
| Dutch Smoothie Grape | 1 (14 oz) | 230 | 36 | 35 | 0 |
| Dutch Smoothie Kiwi Banana | 1 (14 oz) | 240 | 38 | 35 | 0 |
| Dutch Smoothie Lemonade | 1 (14 oz) | 300 | 53 | 51 | 0 |
| Dutch Smoothie Mocha | 1 (14 oz) | 330 | 50 | 39 | 0 |
| Dutch Smoothie Orange Creme | 1 (14 oz) | 280 | 46 | 44 | 0 |
| Dutch Smoothie Strawberry | 1 (14 oz) | 250 | 40 | 39 | 0 |
| Dutch Smoothie Wild Cherry | 1 (14 oz) | 250 | 41 | 39 | 0 |
| Lemonade | 1 (22 oz) | 180 | 43 | 43 | 0 |
| Lemonade Strawberry | 1 (22 oz) | 190 | 48 | 48 | 0 |
| **DIPPING SAUCES** | | | | | |
| Caramel Dip | 1 serv (1.5 oz) | 135 | 27 | 21 | 0 |
| Cheese Sauce | 1 serv (1.25 oz) | 100 | 4 | 3 | 0 |
| Chocolate Dip | 1 serv (1.25 oz) | 130 | 24 | 12 | 1 |
| Cream Cheese Light | 1 serv (1.25 oz) | 70 | 1 | 1 | 0 |
| Cream Cheese Strawberry | 1 serv (1.25 oz) | 110 | 4 | 3 | 0 |
| Hot Salsa Cheese | 1 serv (1.25 oz) | 100 | 4 | 4 | 0 |
| Marinara Sauce | 1 serv (1.25 oz) | 10 | 4 | 2 | 0 |
| Sweet Mustard | 1 serv (1.25 oz) | 60 | 8 | 8 | 0 |
| **PRETZELS** | | | | | |
| Almond | 1 | 400 | 72 | 15 | 2 |
| Almond w/o Butter | 1 | 350 | 72 | 15 | 2 |
| Cinnamon Raisin w/o Butter | 1 | 350 | 74 | 16 | 2 |
| Cinnamon Sugar | 1 | 450 | 83 | 26 | 3 |
| Garlic | 1 | 350 | 68 | 9 | 2 |
| Garlic w/o Butter | 1 | 320 | 66 | 9 | 2 |
| Glazin' Raisin | 1 | 510 | 107 | 38 | 4 |
| Glazin' Raisin w/o Butter | 1 | 470 | 104 | 37 | 3 |
| Jalapeno | 1 | 310 | 59 | 9 | 2 |
| Jalapeno w/o Butter | 1 | 270 | 58 | 8 | 2 |

| FOOD | PORTION | CALS | CARB | SUGAR | FIBER |
|---|---|---|---|---|---|
| Maple Crumb | 1 | 550 | 112 | 42 | 3 |
| Maple Crumb w/o Butter | 1 | 520 | 112 | 42 | 3 |
| Original | 1 | 370 | 72 | 10 | 2 |
| Original w/o Butter | 1 | 340 | 72 | 10 | 3 |
| Parmesan Herb | 1 | 440 | 72 | 10 | 9 |
| Parmesan Herb w/o Butter | 1 | 390 | 74 | 10 | 4 |
| Sesame | 1 | 410 | 64 | 9 | 7 |
| Sesame w/o Butter | 1 | 350 | 63 | 9 | 3 |
| Sour Cream & Onion w/o Butter | 1 | 310 | 66 | 9 | 2 |
| Sour Cream & Onion | 1 | 340 | 66 | 10 | 2 |
| Stixs | 4 | 247 | 48 | 7 | 2 |
| Stixs w/o Butter | 4 | 227 | 48 | 7 | 2 |
| Whole Wheat | 1 | 370 | 72 | 10 | 7 |
| Whole Wheat w/o Butter | 1 | 350 | 72 | 10 | 7 |

## BAJA FRESH

### MAIN MENU SELECTIONS

| FOOD | PORTION | CALS | CARB | SUGAR | FIBER |
|---|---|---|---|---|---|
| Baja Burrito Chicken | 1 serv | 820 | 75 | – | 11 |
| Baja Burrito Steak | 1 serv | 920 | 75 | – | 9 |
| Black Beans | 1 serv | 360 | 61 | – | 26 |
| Burrito Bean & Cheese Chicken | 1 serv | 1000 | 104 | – | 21 |
| Burrito Bean & Cheese Steak | 1 serv | 1100 | 104 | – | 20 |
| Burrito Bean & Cheese Vegetarian | 1 serv | 870 | 104 | – | 20 |
| Burrito Dos Manos Chicken | 1 full serv | 1480 | 202 | – | 28 |
| Burrito Dos Manos Steak | 1 full serv | 1580 | 202 | – | 26 |
| Burrito Mexicano Chicken | 1 serv | 830 | 124 | – | 20 |
| Burrito Mexicano Steak | 1 serv | 920 | 124 | – | 19 |
| Burrito Ultimo Chicken | 1 serv | 860 | 90 | – | 10 |
| Burrito Ultimo Steak | 1 serv | 950 | 90 | – | 8 |
| Cebollitas | 1 serv | 40 | 5 | – | 3 |
| Chips & Salsa Baja | 1 serv | 1100 | 134 | – | 17 |
| Enchiladas Cheese | 1 serv | 850 | 92 | – | 19 |
| Enchiladas Chicken | 1 serv | 780 | 91 | – | 20 |
| Enchiladas Steak | 1 serv | 890 | 94 | – | 20 |
| Enchiladas Verde Cheese | 1 serv | 840 | 91 | – | 19 |
| Enchiladas Verde Chicken | 1 serv | 770 | 91 | – | 20 |
| Enchiladas Verde Vegetarian | 1 serv | 720 | 100 | – | 21 |
| Fajitas Chicken Corn Tortillas | 1 serv | 1200 | 164 | – | 36 |
| Fajitas Chicken Flour Tortillas | 1 serv | 1360 | 176 | – | 32 |

| FOOD | PORTION | CALS | CARB | SUGAR | FIBER |
|---|---|---|---|---|---|
| Fajitas Steak Corn Tortillas | 1 serv | 1360 | 164 | – | 33 |
| Fajitas Steak Flour Tortillas | 1 serv | 1530 | 176 | – | 30 |
| Grilled Vegetarian | 1 serv | 770 | 100 | – | 16 |
| Mini Quesa-Dita Cheese | 1 serv | 620 | 81 | – | 15 |
| Mini Quesa-Dita Chicken | 1 serv | 670 | 81 | – | 16 |
| Mini Quesa-Dita Steak | 1 serv | 700 | 81 | – | 15 |
| Mini Tosta-Dita Chicken | 1 serv | 570 | 67 | – | 13 |
| Mini Tosta-Dita Steak | 1 serv | 630 | 67 | – | 12 |
| Nachos Cheese | 1 serv | 1880 | 166 | – | 33 |
| Nachos Chicken | 1 serv | 2010 | 166 | – | 34 |
| Nachos Steak | 1 serv | 2100 | 166 | – | 33 |
| Pinto Beans | 1 serv | 320 | 56 | – | 21 |
| Quesadilla | 1 serv | 1180 | 92 | – | 12 |
| Quesadilla Cheese | 1 serv | 1130 | 80 | – | 9 |
| Quesadilla Chicken | 1 serv | 1260 | 80 | – | 10 |
| Quesadilla Steak | 1 serv | 1350 | 80 | – | 9 |
| Taco Baja Style Chicken | 1 serv | 190 | 26 | – | 4 |
| Taco Baja Style Steak | 1 serv | 220 | 26 | – | 3 |
| Taco Baja Style Wild Gulf Shrimp | 1 serv | 190 | 26 | – | 3 |
| Taco Chilio Chicken | 1 serv | 320 | 38 | – | 9 |
| Taco Chilito Steak | 1 serv | 340 | 38 | – | 8 |
| Taco Fish | 1 serv | 270 | 31 | – | 3 |
| Taco Mahi Mahi | 1 serv | 260 | 32 | – | 6 |
| Taquitos Chicken w/ Beans | 1 serv | 750 | 64 | – | 9 |
| Taquitos Chicken w/ Rice | 1 serv | 710 | 64 | – | 9 |
| Taquitos Steak w/ Beans | 1 serv | 820 | 69 | – | 20 |
| Taquitos Steak w/ Rice | 1 serv | 790 | 67 | – | 10 |
| Tostada Chicken | 1 serv | 1140 | 102 | – | 30 |
| Tostada Steak | 1 serv | 1230 | 102 | – | 28 |
| Tostada Vegetarian | 1 serv | 1010 | 102 | – | 28 |
| **SALAD DRESSINGS** | | | | | |
| Fat Free Salsa Verde | 1 serv (2.6 oz) | 15 | 3 | – | 0 |
| Guacamole | 2 oz | 70 | 5 | – | 4 |
| Olive Oil Vinaigrette | 1 serv (2.6 oz) | 230 | 1 | – | 0 |
| Pico De Gallo | 1 serv | 50 | 12 | – | 3 |
| Pronto Guacamole | 1 serv | 550 | 61 | – | 11 |
| Ranch | 1 serv (2.6 oz) | 220 | 6 | – | 0 |
| Salsa Baja | 1 serv | 70 | 7 | – | 4 |
| Salsa Roja | 1 serv | 70 | 13 | – | 4 |

| FOOD | PORTION | CALS | CARB | SUGAR | FIBER |
|---|---|---|---|---|---|
| Salsa Verde | 1 serv | 50 | 11 | – | 3 |
| Sour Cream | 1 oz | 60 | 2 | – | 0 |
| **SALADS AND SALAD BARS** | | | | | |
| Baja Ensalada Chicken | 1 serv | 310 | 17 | – | 7 |
| Baja Ensalada Fish | 1 serv | 360 | 27 | – | 10 |
| Baja Ensalada Steak | 1 serv | 460 | 17 | – | 5 |
| Side Salad | 1 serv | 70 | 10 | – | 3 |

## BASKIN-ROBBINS

| FOOD | PORTION | CALS | CARB | SUGAR | FIBER |
|---|---|---|---|---|---|
| **FROZEN YOGURT** | | | | | |
| Cafe Mocha Truly Free Soft Serve | 1 reg | 140 | 27 | 11 | – |
| Chocolate Nonfat Soft Serve | 1 reg | 190 | 39 | 36 | – |
| Lowfat Maui Brownie Madness | 1 reg | 250 | 34 | – | – |
| **ICE CREAM** | | | | | |
| Cappuccino Blast w/ Whipped Cream | 1 reg | 340 | 44 | 43 | – |
| Chocolate | 1 reg | 270 | 31 | 29 | - |
| Chocolate Chip | 1 reg | 270 | 26 | 25 | - |
| Espresso'n Cream Lowfat | 1 reg | 180 | 31 | 29 | – |
| Jamoca Almond Fudge | 1 reg | 280 | 30 | 29 | – |
| Peach Crumb Pie No Sugar Added | 1 reg | 180 | 27 | 7 | – |
| Pralines'n Cream | 1 reg | 280 | 33 | 32 | - |
| Shake Chocolate | 16 oz | 750 | 80 | 69 | – |
| Shake Vanilla | 16 oz | 630 | 69 | 61 | – |
| Smoothie Very Strawberry w/ Soft Serve Ice Cream | 1 reg | 320 | 70 | 47 | – |
| Thin Mint No Sugar Added | 1 reg | 160 | 27 | 7 | – |
| Vanilla | 1 reg | 270 | 24 | 23 | - |
| **ICES** | | | | | |
| Daiquiri Ice | 1 reg | 130 | 33 | 32 | - |
| Sherbet Rainbow | 1 reg | 160 | 34 | 32 | – |
| Sorbet Peachy Keen | 1 reg | 110 | 29 | 26 | – |

## BEN & JERRY'S

| FOOD | PORTION | CALS | CARB | SUGAR | FIBER |
|---|---|---|---|---|---|
| Sugar Cone | 1 | 48 | 10 | 3 | tr |
| **FROZEN YOGURT** | | | | | |
| Black Raspberry Low Fat | ½ cup | 140 | 28 | 21 | tr |
| Cherry Garcia | ½ cup | 170 | 32 | 27 | 0 |
| Chocolate Fudge Brownie | ½ cup | 190 | 36 | 31 | 1 |

| FOOD | PORTION | CALS | CARB | SUGAR | FIBER |
|---|---|---|---|---|---|
| Half Baked | ½ cup | 210 | 30 | 29 | tr |
| Phish Food | ½ cup | 230 | 42 | 30 | 1 |
| **ICE CREAM** | | | | | |
| Brownie Batter | ½ cup | 310 | 32 | 26 | 1 |
| Butter Pecan | ½ cup | 290 | 20 | 18 | 1 |
| Cherry Garcia | ½ cup | 250 | 26 | 23 | 0 |
| Chocolate Chip Cookie Dough | ½ cup | 280 | 31 | 24 | 0 |
| Chocolate Chocolate Cookie | ½ cup | 280 | 34 | 26 | 2 |
| Chocolate For A Change | ½ cup | 270 | 36 | 23 | 2 |
| Chocolate Fudge Brownie | ½ cup | 280 | 33 | 29 | 2 |
| Chubby Hubby | ½ cup | 330 | 32 | 24 | 1 |
| Chunky Monkey | ½ cup | 300 | 30 | 26 | 1 |
| Coffee For A Change | ½ cup | 240 | 21 | 19 | 0 |
| Coffee Heath Bar Crunch | ½ cup | 310 | 32 | 25 | 0 |
| Everything But The . . . | ½ cup | 320 | 30 | 27 | 1 |
| Fudge Central | ½ cup | 300 | 31 | 27 | 1 |
| Half Baked | ½ cup | 280 | 34 | 31 | 1 |
| Karamel Sutra | ½ cup | 290 | 33 | 27 | 1 |
| Makin' Whoopie Pie | ½ cup | 270 | 33 | 24 | 2 |
| Mint Chocolate Cookie | ½ cup | 270 | 26 | 22 | tr |
| New York Super Fudge Chunk | ½ cup | 270 | 30 | 25 | 2 |
| Oatmeal Cookie Chunk | ½ cup | 280 | 32 | 23 | 1 |
| One Sweet Whirled | ½ cup | 280 | 33 | 27 | 1 |
| Organic Chocolate Fudge Brownie | ½ cup | 260 | 30 | 25 | 2 |
| Organic Strawberry | ½ cup | 200 | 20 | 17 | 0 |
| Organic Sweet Cream & Cookies | ½ cup | 240 | 23 | 18 | 0 |
| Organic Vanilla | ½ cup | 220 | 18 | 16 | 0 |
| Peanut Butter Cup | ½ cup | 380 | 29 | 25 | 2 |
| Peanut Butter Me Up | ½ cup | 330 | 28 | 24 | 2 |
| Phish Food | ½ cup | 280 | 38 | 23 | 2 |
| Pistachio Pistachio | ½ cup | 280 | 21 | 18 | 0 |
| Uncanny Cashew | ½ cup | 290 | 27 | 22 | 0 |
| Vanilla Heath Bar Crunch | ½ cup | 300 | 29 | 27 | 0 |
| Vanilla For A Change | ½ cup | 240 | 21 | 19 | 0 |
| **SORBETS** | | | | | |
| Berry Berry Extraordinary | ½ cup | 100 | 25 | 22 | tr |
| Mango Lime | ½ cup | 100 | 27 | 22 | 0 |
| Strawberry Kiwi | ½ cup | 100 | 27 | 22 | tr |

| FOOD | PORTION | CALS | CARB | SUGAR | FIBER |
|---|---|---|---|---|---|
| **BLIMPIE** | | | | | |
| **COOKIES** | | | | | |
| Chocolate Chunk | 1 | 200 | 26 | 16 | 1 |
| Macadamia White Chunk | 1 | 210 | 26 | 15 | 1 |
| Oatmeal Raisin | 1 | 190 | 27 | 16 | 1 |
| Peanut Butter | 1 | 220 | 23 | 14 | 1 |
| Sugar | 1 | 330 | 24 | 24 | 0 |
| **SALAD DRESSINGS AND TOPPINGS** | | | | | |
| Caesar Dressing | 1 serv (1.5 oz) | 208 | 2 | 1 | 0 |
| Cracked Peppercorn Dressing | 1 serv (1.5 oz) | 237 | 2 | 2 | 0 |
| Frank's Red Hot Buffalo Sauce | 1 serv (1 oz) | 13 | 2 | 1 | tr |
| French's Honey Mustard | 1 tbsp | 5 | 1 | 1 | 0 |
| GourMayo Chipotle Chili | 1 tbsp | 50 | 1 | 0 | 0 |
| GourMayo Sun Dried Tomato | 1 tbsp | 50 | 1 | 0 | 0 |
| GourMayo Wasabi Horseradish | 1 tbsp | 50 | 1 | 0 | 0 |
| Guacamole | 1 serv (1.5 oz) | 194 | 7 | 6 | 1 |
| Oil & Vinegar | 1 serv | 36 | 1 | 0 | 0 |
| Pesto Dressing | 1 serv (1 oz) | 132 | 1 | 0 | 0 |
| **SALADS AND SALAD BARS** | | | | | |
| Antipasto | 1 reg serv | 244 | 10 | 6 | 3 |
| Chef | 1 reg serv | 212 | 9 | 5 | 3 |
| Chili Ole | 1 reg serv | 480 | 42 | 2 | 3 |
| Grilled Chicken w/ Caesar Dressing | 1 reg serv | 347 | 9 | 5 | 3 |
| Grilled Chicken w/o Dressing | 1 serv | 139 | 7 | 4 | 3 |
| Roast Beef 'N Blue | 1 reg serv | 390 | 29 | 0 | 0 |
| Seafood | 1 reg serv | 122 | 16 | 5 | 3 |
| Tuna | 1 reg serv | 261 | 8 | 3 | 3 |
| Zesto Pesto Turkey | 1 reg serv | 370 | 31 | 1 | 0 |
| **SANDWICHES** | | | | | |
| 6 Inch Hot Sub BLT | 1 | 588 | 49 | 8 | 3 |
| 6 Inch Hot Sub Buffalo Chicken | 1 | 400 | 50 | 7 | 3 |
| 6 Inch Hot Sub Buffalo Chicken w/o Cheese | 1 | 320 | 50 | 7 | 3 |
| 6 Inch Hot Sub ChiliMax | 1 | 511 | 71 | 10 | 8 |
| 6 Inch Hot Sub Grilled Chicken | 1 | 373 | 50 | 8 | 3 |
| 6 Inch Hot Sub Meatball | 1 | 572 | 55 | 12 | 2 |
| 6 Inch Hot Sub MexiMelt | 1 | 425 | 65 | 9 | 7 |
| 6 Inch Hot Sub Pastrami | 1 | 507 | 53 | 11 | 3 |

| FOOD | PORTION | CALS | CARB | SUGAR | FIBER |
|---|---|---|---|---|---|
| 6 Inch Hot Sub Steak & Onion Melt | 1 | 440 | 49 | 9 | 3 |
| 6 Inch Hot Sub VegiMax | 1 | 395 | 60 | 8 | 8 |
| 6 Inch Sub Blimpie Best | 1 | 476 | 52 | 10 | 2 |
| 6 Inch Sub Club | 1 | 440 | 51 | 9 | 3 |
| 6 Inch Sub Ham & Cheese | 1 | 436 | 52 | 10 | 3 |
| 6 Inch Sub Roast Beef | 1 | 468 | 49 | 7 | 3 |
| 6 Inch Sub Roast Beef w/o Cheese | 1 | 388 | 49 | 7 | 3 |
| 6 Inch Sub Seafood | 1 | 355 | 58 | 9 | 4 |
| 6 Inch Sub Tuna | 1 | 493 | 51 | 7 | 3 |
| 6 Inch Sub Turkey w/o Cheese | 1 | 344 | 49 | 7 | 3 |
| 6 inch Sub Turkey | 1 | 424 | 49 | 7 | 3 |
| Cheddar | 1 slice | 52 | 0 | 0 | 0 |
| Grilled Subs Beef Turkey & Cheddar | 1 | 600 | 49 | 9 | 3 |
| Grilled Subs Cuban | 1 | 462 | 50 | 9 | 3 |
| Grilled Subs Pastrami | 1 | 462 | 52 | 11 | 3 |
| Grilled Subs Reuben | 1 | 630 | 55 | 15 | 2 |
| Provolone | 1 slice | 80 | 0 | 0 | 0 |
| Swiss | 1 slice | 80 | 0 | 0 | 0 |
| Wraps Southwestern | 1 | 674 | 54 | 4 | 3 |
| Wraps Beef & Cheddar | 1 | 714 | 57 | 5 | 3 |
| Wraps Chicken Caesar | 1 | 646 | 56 | 6 | 3 |
| Wraps Steak & Onions | 1 | 716 | 64 | 7 | 3 |
| Wraps Ultimate BLT | 1 | 831 | 60 | 7 | 3 |
| Wraps Zesty Italian | 1 | 638 | 74 | 13 | 3 |
| **SIDE ORDERS** | | | | | |
| Cole Slaw | 1 serv (5 oz) | 180 | 13 | 13 | 1 |
| Macaroni Salad | 1 serv (5 oz) | 360 | 25 | 6 | 1 |
| Mustard Potato Salad | 1 serv (5 oz) | 160 | 21 | 13 | 1 |
| Potato Chips Cheddar & Sour Cream | 1 bag | 210 | 25 | 0 | 1 |
| Potato Chips Jalapeño | 1 bag | 210 | 25 | 0 | 2 |
| Potato Chips Lea & Perrins Barbecue | 1 bag | 210 | 25 | 2 | 2 |
| Potato Chips Regular | 1 bag | 210 | 25 | 0 | 2 |
| Potato Chips Romano & Garlic | 1 bag | 210 | 25 | 0 | 2 |
| Potato Chips Sour Cream & Onion | 1 bag | 210 | 25 | 1 | 1 |

| FOOD | PORTION | CALS | CARB | SUGAR | FIBER |
|---|---|---|---|---|---|
| Potato Salad | 1 serv (5 oz) | 270 | 19 | 10 | 1 |
| **SOUPS** | | | | | |
| Chicken w/ White & Wild Rice | 1 serv (8 oz) | 230 | 21 | 2 | 2 |
| Cream Of Broccoli & Cheese | 1 serv (8 oz) | 190 | 15 | 5 | 3 |
| Cream Of Potato | 1 serv (8 oz) | 190 | 24 | 3 | 3 |
| Garden Vegetable | 1 serv (8 oz) | 80 | 14 | 5 | 3 |
| Grande Chili w/ Beans & Beef | 1 serv (8 oz) | 250 | 30 | 7 | 18 |
| Homestyle Chicken Noodle | 1 serv (8 oz) | 120 | 18 | 4 | 1 |
| Vegetable Beef | 1 serv (8 oz) | 80 | 13 | 3 | 2 |

## BOJANGLES

| FOOD | PORTION | CALS | CARB | SUGAR | FIBER |
|---|---|---|---|---|---|
| Biscuit | 1 | 243 | 29 | – | 2 |
| Biscuit + Bacon | 1 | 290 | 26 | – | 1 |
| Biscuit + Bacon Egg Cheese | 1 | 550 | 27 | – | 1 |
| Biscuit + Cajun Fillet | 1 | 454 | 46 | – | 1 |
| Biscuit + Country Ham | 1 | 270 | 26 | – | 1 |
| Biscuit + Egg | 1 | 400 | 26 | – | 1 |
| Biscuit + Sausage | 1 | 350 | 26 | – | 1 |
| Biscuit + Smoked Sausage | 1 | 380 | 27 | – | 1 |
| Biscuit + Steak | 1 | 649 | 37 | – | 1 |
| Botato Rounds | 1 serv | 235 | 31 | – | 3 |
| Buffalo Bites | 1 serv | 180 | 5 | – | 0 |
| Cajun Pintos | 1 serv | 110 | 18 | – | 6 |
| Cajun Spiced Breast | 1 serv | 278 | 12 | – | tr |
| Cajun Spiced Leg | 1 serv | 284 | 11 | – | tr |
| Cajun Spiced Thigh | 1 serv | 310 | 11 | – | tr |
| Cajun Spiced Wing | 1 serv | 355 | 11 | – | tr |
| Chicken Supremes | 1 serv | 337 | 26 | – | 1 |
| Corn On The Cob | 1 serv | 140 | 34 | – | 2 |
| Dirty Rice | 1 serv | 166 | 24 | – | 1 |
| Green Beans | 1 serv | 25 | 5 | – | 2 |
| Macaroni & Cheese | 1 serv | 198 | 12 | – | tr |
| Marinated Cole Slaw | 1 serv | 136 | 26 | – | 3 |
| Potatoes w/o Gravy | 1 serv | 80 | 16 | – | 1 |
| Sandwich Cajun Filet w/o Mayo | 1 | 337 | 41 | – | 3 |
| Sandwich Cajun Filet w/ Mayo | 1 | 437 | 41 | – | 3 |
| Sandwich Grilled Filet w/ Mayo | 1 | 335 | 25 | – | 2 |
| Sandwich Grilled Filet w/o Mayo | 1 serv | 235 | 25 | – | 2 |
| Seasoned Fries | 1 serv | 344 | 39 | – | 4 |
| Southern Style Breast | 1 serv | 261 | 12 | – | tr |

| FOOD | PORTION | CALS | CARB | SUGAR | FIBER |
|---|---|---|---|---|---|
| Southern Style Leg | 1 serv | 254 | 11 | – | tr |
| Southern Style Thigh | 1 serv | 308 | 14 | – | tr |
| Southern Style Wing | 1 serv | 337 | 19 | – | tr |
| Sweet Biscuit Bo Berry | 1 | 220 | 29 | – | 1 |
| Sweet Biscuit Cinnamon | 1 | 320 | 37 | – | 1 |
| **BOSTON MARKET** | | | | | |
| **BAKED SELECTIONS** | | | | | |
| Brownie | 1 (3.3 oz) | 450 | 47 | 32 | 3 |
| Cinnamon Apple Pie | ⅕ pie (4.8 oz) | 390 | 46 | 2 | 2 |
| Cookie Chocolate Chip | 1 (2.8 oz) | 340 | 48 | 29 | 1 |
| **MAIN MENU SELECTIONS** | | | | | |
| ½ Chicken w/ Skin | 1 serv (9.7 oz) | 590 | 4 | 4 | 0 |
| ¼ Dark Meat Chicken No Skin | 1 serv (3.3 oz) | 190 | 1 | 1 | 0 |
| ¼ Dark Meat Chicken w/ Skin | 1 serv (4.4 oz) | 320 | 2 | 2 | 0 |
| ¼ White Meat Chicken No Skin Or Wing | 1 serv (4.9 oz) | 170 | 2 | 1 | 0 |
| ¼ White Meat Chicken w/ Skin And Wing | 1 serv (5.3 oz) | 280 | 2 | 2 | 0 |
| BBQ Baked Beans | ¾ cup (7.1 oz) | 270 | 48 | 20 | 12 |
| BBQ Chicken Sandwich | 1 (9.9 oz) | 540 | 84 | 33 | 3 |
| Baked Sweet Potato Low Fat | 1 (12.5 oz) | 460 | 94 | 49 | 10 |
| Black Beans And Rice | 1 cup (8 oz) | 300 | 45 | 3 | 5 |
| Boston Hearth Ham Lean | 1 serv (5 oz) | 210 | 9 | 7 | 0 |
| Broccoli Cauliflower Au Gratin | ¾ cup (6.1 oz) | 200 | 14 | 4 | 3 |
| Broccoli Rice Casserole | ¾ cup (6 oz) | 240 | 26 | 2 | 2 |
| Broccoli With Red Peppers | ¾ cup (3.4 oz) | 60 | 5 | 1 | 3 |
| Butternut Squash Low Fat | ¾ cup (6.8 oz) | 160 | 25 | 13 | 3 |
| Chicken Gravy | 1 serv (1 oz) | 15 | 2 | 0 | 0 |
| Chicken Salad Sandwich | 1 (11.5 oz) | 680 | 63 | 12 | 4 |
| Chicken Sandwich w/ Cheese & Sauce | 1 (12.4 oz) | 750 | 72 | 13 | 5 |
| Chicken Sandwich w/o Cheese & Sauce Low Fat | 1 (10 oz) | 430 | 62 | 12 | 4 |
| Chunky Chicken Salad | ¾ cup (5.5 oz) | 370 | 3 | 1 | 1 |
| Chunky Cinnamon Apple Sauce No Fat | ¾ cup (6.4 oz) | 250 | 62 | 55 | 2 |
| Cole Slaw | ¾ cup (6.5 oz) | 300 | 30 | 26 | 3 |
| Corn Bread | 1 (2.4 oz) | 200 | 33 | 13 | 1 |
| Coyote Bean Salad | ¾ cup (5.3 oz) | 190 | 24 | 2 | 9 |

| FOOD | PORTION | CALS | CARB | SUGAR | FIBER |
|---|---|---|---|---|---|
| Cranberry Relish Low Fat | ¾ cup (7.9 oz) | 370 | 84 | 72 | 5 |
| Creamed Spinach | ¾ cup (6.4 oz) | 260 | 11 | 2 | 2 |
| Fruit Salad Low Fat | ¾ cup (5.5 oz) | 70 | 15 | 14 | 1 |
| Green Bean Casserole | ¾ cup (6 oz) | 130 | 10 | 3 | 2 |
| Green Beans | ¾ cup (3 oz) | 80 | 5 | 2 | 3 |
| Ham Sandwich w/ Cheese & Sauce | 1 (11.8 oz) | 760 | 72 | 20 | 5 |
| Ham Sandwich w/o Cheese & Sauce | 1 (9.3 oz) | 440 | 66 | 16 | 4 |
| Homestyle Mashed Potatoes & Gravy | ¾ cup (6.6 oz) | 210 | 26 | 4 | 1 |
| Honey Glazed Carrots | ¾ cup (5.4 oz) | 280 | 35 | 9 | 4 |
| Hot Cinnamon Apples | ¾ cup (6.4 oz) | 250 | 56 | 48 | 3 |
| Macaroni & Cheese | ¾ cup (6.7 oz) | 280 | 32 | 8 | 1 |
| Mashed Potatoes | ⅔ cup (5.6 oz) | 190 | 24 | 4 | 1 |
| Meat Loaf & Brown Gravy | 1 serv (7 oz) | 390 | 19 | 4 | 1 |
| Meat Loaf & Chunky Tomato Sauce | 1 serv (8 oz) | 370 | 22 | 5 | 2 |
| Meat Loaf Sandwich w/ Cheese | 1 (13.8 oz) | 860 | 95 | 21 | 6 |
| Meat Loaf Sandwich w/o Cheese | 1 (12.3 oz) | 690 | 86 | 21 | 6 |
| New Potatoes Low Fat | ¾ cup (4.6 oz) | 130 | 25 | 2 | 2 |
| Old Fashioned Potato Salad | ¾ cup (6.2 oz) | 340 | 30 | 8 | 2 |
| Open Face Turkey Sandwich | 1 (13.4 oz) | 500 | 61 | 13 | 3 |
| Original Chicken Pot Pie | 1 pie (14.9 oz) | 780 | 61 | 5 | 4 |
| Oven Roasted Potato Planks Low Fat | 5 pieces (5.8 oz) | 180 | 32 | 3 | 3 |
| Pastry Sandwich BBQ Chicken | 1 (7.2 oz) | 640 | 56 | 13 | 1 |
| Pastry Sandwich Broccoli Chicken Cheddar | 1 (7.2 oz) | 690 | 45 | 2 | 2 |
| Pastry Sandwich Ham & Cheddar | 1 (6.6 oz) | 640 | 47 | 5 | 1 |
| Pastry Sandwich Italian Chicken | 1 (7.2 oz) | 630 | 43 | 3 | 2 |
| Red Beans And Rice Low Fat | 1 cup (8 oz) | 260 | 45 | 2 | 4 |
| Rice Pilaf | ⅔ cup (5.1 oz) | 180 | 32 | 0 | 2 |
| Rotisserie Turkey Breast Skinless Low Fat | 1 serv (5 oz) | 170 | 1 | 0 | 0 |
| Savory Stuffing | ¾ cup (6.1 oz) | 310 | 44 | 3 | 3 |
| Southwest Savory Chicken | 1 serv (9.6 oz) | 400 | 26 | 4 | 4 |
| Squash Casserole | ¾ cup (6.6 oz) | 330 | 20 | 8 | 3 |

| FOOD | PORTION | CALS | CARB | SUGAR | FIBER |
|---|---|---|---|---|---|
| Steamed Vegetables Low Fat | ⅔ cup (3.7 oz) | 35 | 7 | 3 | 3 |
| Sweet Potato Casserole | ¾ cup (6.4 oz) | 280 | 39 | 23 | 2 |
| Tabasco BBQ Drumstick | 1 (2.4 oz) | 130 | 4 | 4 | 0 |
| Tabasco BBQ Wing | 1 (1.8 oz) | 110 | 4 | 4 | 0 |
| Teriyaki Chicken ¼ White w/ Skin | 1 serv (6.8 oz) | 340 | 17 | 14 | 0 |
| Teriyaki Chicken ¼ w/ Skin | 1 serv (5.9 oz) | 380 | 17 | 15 | 0 |
| Triple Topped Chicken | 1 serv (9.2 oz) | 470 | 20 | 5 | 1 |
| Turkey Club Sandwich | 1 (11.1 oz) | 650 | 64 | 16 | 4 |
| Turkey Sandwich w/ Cheese & Sauce | 1 (11.8 oz) | 710 | 68 | 17 | 4 |
| Turkey Sandwich w/o Cheese & Sauce | 1 (9.3 oz) | 400 | 61 | 12 | 4 |
| Whole Kernel Corn | ¾ cup (5.8 oz) | 180 | 30 | 13 | 2 |
| Zucchini Marinara Low Fat | ¾ cup (6.6 oz) | 60 | 7 | 3 | 2 |
| **SALADS AND SALAD BARS** | | | | | |
| Caesar Salad Entree | 1 serv (10 oz) | 510 | 17 | 5 | 3 |
| Caesar Salad w/o Dressing | 1 serv (8 oz) | 230 | 14 | 4 | 3 |
| Caesar Side Salad | 1 (4 oz) | 200 | 7 | 2 | 1 |
| Chicken Caesar Salad | 1 serv (13 oz) | 650 | 17 | 5 | 3 |
| Tossed Salad w/ Caesar Dressing | 1 serv (8 oz) | 380 | 18 | 6 | 3 |
| Tossed Salad w/ Fat Free Ranch | 1 serv (8 oz) | 160 | 29 | 9 | 4 |
| Tossed Salad w/ Old Venice Dressing | 1 serv (8 oz) | 340 | 20 | 6 | 3 |
| **SOUPS** | | | | | |
| Chicken Chili | 1 cup (8.7 oz) | 220 | 21 | 4 | 6 |
| Chicken Noodle | 1 cup (8.4 oz) | 130 | 12 | 2 | 2 |
| Chicken Tortilla | 1 cup (8.4 oz) | 220 | 19 | 2 | 2 |
| Potato | 1 cup (8 oz) | 270 | 24 | 5 | 2 |
| Tomato Bisque | 1 cup (8 oz) | 280 | 16 | 12 | 2 |

## BOSTON PIZZA

| | | | | | |
|---|---|---|---|---|---|
| **CHILDREN'S MENU SELECTIONS** | | | | | |
| Corkscrews n' Cheese | 1 serv | 870 | 112 | – | – |
| Dino Fingers & Fries w/ Ketchup | 1 serv | 680 | 87 | – | – |
| Grill Cheese Sandwich w/ Fries & Ketchup | 1 serv | 770 | 103 | – | – |
| Mini Lasagna | 1 serv | 400 | 48 | – | – |
| Pint Sized Ham Pizza | 1 serv | 430 | 66 | – | – |

| FOOD | PORTION | CALS | CARB | SUGAR | FIBER |
|---|---|---|---|---|---|
| Potato Smiles | 1 serv | 580 | 84 | – | – |
| Stuffed Pizza w/ Fries & Ketchup | 1 serv | 850 | 124 | – | – |
| Super Spaghetti | 1 serv | 340 | 61 | – | – |
| **MAIN MENU SELECTIONS** | | | | | |
| BBQ Ribs w/ Fries | 1 serv | 2220 | 140 | – | – |
| BBQ Ribs w/ Garlic Mashed Potatoes | 1 serv | 1760 | 94 | – | – |
| BBQ Ribs w/ Spaghetti | 1 serv | 1870 | 113 | – | – |
| Baked Onion Soup | 1 serv | 210 | 28 | – | – |
| Bayou Chicken Strips w/ Dipping Sauce | 1 serv | 370 | 6 | – | – |
| Boston's Extreme Double Order | 1 serv | 1660 | 15 | – | – |
| Boston's Extreme Starter Order | 1 serv | 940 | 10 | – | – |
| Bruschetta | 1 serv | 640 | 55 | – | – |
| Buffalo Chicken Fingers w/ Caesar Salad | 1 serv | 650 | 42 | – | – |
| Buffalo Chicken Fingers w/ Fries | 1 serv | 1430 | 122 | – | – |
| Buffalo Chicken Fingers w/ Light Ranch | 1 serv | 600 | 40 | – | – |
| Cactus Cuts & Dip | 1 serv | 1380 | 136 | – | – |
| Carne Amore | 1 full order | 1250 | 144 | – | – |
| Cheese Toast | 1 basket | 800 | 64 | – | – |
| Cheese Toast | 1 serv | 400 | 32 | – | – |
| Chicken & Rib Combo | 1 serv | 1470 | 94 | – | – |
| Chicken & Rib Combo w/ Fries | 1 serv | 1920 | 140 | – | – |
| Chicken & Rib Combo w/ Spaghetti | 1 serv | 1590 | 113 | – | – |
| Chicken Fingers w/ Caesar Salad | 1 serv | 640 | 38 | – | – |
| Chicken Fingers w/ Fries | 1 serv | 1420 | 118 | – | – |
| Chicken Fingers w/ Light Ranch | 1 serv | 590 | 36 | – | – |
| Chips & Salsa | 1 serv | 830 | 109 | – | – |
| Deluxe Cheese Bread | 1 basket | 890 | 84 | – | – |
| Deluxe Cheese Toast | 1 serv | 420 | 35 | – | – |
| Fettuccini Cajun Shrimp | 1 full order | 1200 | 144 | – | – |
| Fettuccini Four Cheese | 1 full order | 1370 | 140 | – | – |
| Fettuccini Jambalaya | 1 full order | 1360 | 151 | – | – |
| Fettuccini Spicy Chicken & Spinach | 1 full order | 1330 | 146 | – | – |
| Fries | 1 serv | 700 | 87 | – | – |

| FOOD | PORTION | CALS | CARB | SUGAR | FIBER |
|---|---|---|---|---|---|
| Garlic Toast w/ Garlic Margarine | 1 slice | 170 | 22 | – | – |
| Garlic Twist Bread | 1 serv | 540 | 84 | – | – |
| Garlic Twist Bread | 1 basket | 1080 | 168 | – | – |
| Homestyle Macaroni | 1 full order | 1490 | 119 | – | – |
| Italian Pizza Bread w/ Dip | 1 serv | 1000 | 98 | – | – |
| Ketchup | 1 serv (2 oz) | 20 | 16 | – | – |
| Lasagna Boston's | 1 full order | 820 | 95 | – | – |
| Lasagna Mediterranean | 1 full order | 870 | 97 | – | – |
| Lasagna Seafood | 1 full order | 970 | 95 | – | – |
| Linguini Chicken & Mushroom | 1 full order | 1320 | 144 | – | – |
| Mashed Potatoes | 1 serv | 240 | 41 | – | – |
| Mexican Beef w/ Sour Cream | 1 serv | 970 | 66 | – | – |
| Mini Tortellini | 1 serv | 490 | 73 | – | – |
| NY Steak Sandwich w/ Fries | 1 serv | 1580 | 118 | – | – |
| Nachos | 1 full order | 1540 | 127 | – | – |
| Nachos Beef | 1 full order | 1760 | 129 | – | – |
| Nachos Chicken | 1 full order | 1630 | 129 | – | – |
| Penne Baked 3 Cheese | 1 full order | 990 | 118 | – | – |
| Penne Italiano | 1 full order | 1160 | 137 | – | – |
| Penne Pisa Pesto | 1 full order | 1270 | 110 | – | – |
| Penne Roast Veggie | 1 full order | 900 | 146 | – | – |
| Pizza Bread w/o Meat Sauce | 1 serv | 520 | 84 | – | – |
| Plain Pasta w/ Alfredo Sauce | 1 full order | 1200 | 141 | – | – |
| Plain Pasta w/ Creamy Tomato Sauce | 1 full order | 1070 | 142 | – | – |
| Plain Pasta w/ Marinara Sauce | 1 full order | 870 | 144 | – | – |
| Plain Pasta w/ Meatsauce | 1 full order | 910 | 142 | – | – |
| Plain Pasta w/ Seafood Sauce | 1 full order | 1050 | 141 | – | – |
| Plain Pasta w/ Spicy Tomato Sauce | 1 full order | 880 | 145 | – | – |
| Plain Pasta w/ Tex Mex Sauce | 1 full order | 940 | 141 | – | – |
| Potato Skins | 1 full order | 860 | 70 | – | – |
| Quesadilla Chicken w/ Sour Cream | 1 serv | 770 | 67 | – | – |
| Quesadilla Garden Veggie w/ Sour Cream | 1 serv | 750 | 70 | – | – |
| Quesadilla Sundried Tomato w/ Sour Cream | 1 serv | 890 | 39 | – | – |
| Shrimp Dinner w/ Fries | 1 serv | 1510 | 135 | – | – |

| FOOD | PORTION | CALS | CARB | SUGAR | FIBER |
|---|---|---|---|---|---|
| Shrimp Dinner w/ Garlic Mashed Potatoes | 1 serv | 1050 | 89 | – | – |
| Shrimp Dinner w/ Spaghetti | 1 serv | 1180 | 108 | – | – |
| Side Tossed Salad w/ House Dressing | 1 serv | 170 | 10 | – | – |
| Sirloin Steak Dinner w/ Fries | 1 serv | 1910 | 117 | – | – |
| Sirloin Steak Dinner w/ Garlic Mashed Potatoes | 1 serv | 1450 | 71 | – | – |
| Sirloin Steak Dinner w/ Spaghetti | 1 serv | 1580 | 90 | – | – |
| Smokey Mountain Spaghetti | 1 full order | 1860 | 211 | – | – |
| Spaghetti w/ Meatsauce | 1 serv | 370 | 60 | – | – |
| Spinach & Artichoke Dip w/ Tortilla Chips | 1 serv | 890 | 81 | – | – |
| Steak & Shrimp Dinner w/ Fries | 1 serv | 1760 | 129 | – | – |
| Steak & Shrimp Dinner w/ Garlic Mashed Potatoes | 1 serv | 1310 | 83 | – | – |
| Steak & Shrimp Dinner w/ Spaghetti | 1 serv | 1430 | 102 | – | – |
| The Ribber w/ Fries | 1 serv | 1470 | 121 | – | – |
| The Ribber w/ Garlic Mashed Potatoes | 1 serv | 1010 | 74 | – | – |
| The Ribber w/ Spaghetti | 1 serv | 1140 | 94 | – | – |
| Tortellini w/ Alfredo Sauce | 1 full order | 1220 | 165 | – | – |
| Tortellini w/ Creamy Tomato Sauce | 1 full order | 1370 | 166 | – | – |
| Tortellini w/ Marinara Sauce | 1 full order | 1180 | 167 | – | – |
| Tortellini w/ Meatsauce | 1 full order | 1500 | 164 | – | – |
| Tortellini w/ Seafood Sauce | 1 full order | 1360 | 164 | – | – |
| Tortellini w/ Spicy Tomato Sauce | 1 full order | 1180 | 168 | – | – |
| Tortellini w/ Tex Mex Sauce | 1 full order | 1240 | 164 | – | – |
| Veal Pamigan w/ Fries | 1 serv | 1550 | 138 | – | – |
| Veal Parmigan w/ Garlic Mashed Potatoes | 1 serv | 1090 | 92 | – | – |
| Veal Parmigan w/ Spaghetti | 1 serv | 1220 | 112 | – | – |
| Wings BBQ Double Order | 1 serv | 1700 | 26 | – | – |
| Wings BBQ Starter Size | 1 serv | 960 | 13 | – | – |
| Wings Cajun Double Order | 1 serv | 1610 | 5 | – | – |
| Wings Cajun Starter Size | 1 serv | 910 | 3 | – | – |

| FOOD | PORTION | CALS | CARB | SUGAR | FIBER |
|---|---|---|---|---|---|
| Wings Honey Garlic Double Order | 1 serv | 1720 | 32 | – | – |
| Wings Honey Garlic Starter Size | 1 serv | 970 | 17 | – | – |
| Wings Screamin' Hot Double Order | 1 serv | 1630 | 10 | – | – |
| Wings Screamin' Hot Starter Size | 1 serv | 920 | 5 | – | – |
| Wings Teriyaki Double Order | 1 serv | 1690 | 21 | – | – |
| Wings Teriyaki Starter Size | 1 serv | 950 | 11 | – | – |
| Wings Thai Double Order | 1 serv | 1870 | 27 | – | – |
| Wings Thai Starter Size | 1 serv | 1040 | 14 | – | – |
| **PIZZA** | | | | | |
| Bacon Double Cheeseburger Individual | 1 pie | 1210 | 94 | – | – |
| Bacon Double Cheeseburger Large | 1 slice | 350 | 30 | – | – |
| Bacon Double Cheeseburger Medium | 1 slice | 300 | 25 | – | – |
| Boston Royal Individual | 1 pie | 770 | 96 | – | – |
| Boston Royal Large | 1 slice | 230 | 31 | – | – |
| Boston Royal Medium | 1 slice | 200 | 26 | – | – |
| Cajun Chicken Individual | 1 pie | 780 | 99 | – | – |
| Cajun Chicken Large | 1 slice | 250 | 31 | – | – |
| Cajun Chicken Medium | 1 slice | 200 | 26 | – | – |
| Californian Individual | 1 pie | 580 | 109 | – | – |
| Californian Large | 1 slice | 190 | 35 | – | – |
| Californian Medium | 1 slice | 160 | 30 | – | – |
| Four Cheese Individual | 1 pie | 800 | 89 | – | – |
| Four Cheese Large | 1 slice | 260 | 29 | – | – |
| Four Cheese Medium | 1 slice | 240 | 24 | – | – |
| Great White Individual | 1 pie | 880 | 89 | – | – |
| Great White Large | 1 slice | 260 | 29 | – | – |
| Great White Medium | 1 slice | 220 | 24 | – | – |
| Hawaiian Individual | 1 pie | 690 | 97 | – | – |
| Hawaiian Large | 1 slice | 220 | 31 | – | – |
| Hawaiian Medium | 1 slice | 180 | 26 | – | – |
| Meat Lovers Individual | 1 pie | 1120 | 89 | – | – |
| Meat Lovers Large | 1 slice | 330 | 28 | – | – |
| Meat Lovers Medium | 1 slice | 280 | 24 | – | – |
| Pepperoni Individual | 1 pie | 760 | 89 | – | – |

| FOOD | PORTION | CALS | CARB | SUGAR | FIBER |
|---|---|---|---|---|---|
| Pepperoni Large | 1 slice | 240 | 28 | – | – |
| Pepperoni Medium | 1 slice | 200 | 24 | – | – |
| Pepperoni & Mushroom Individual | 1 pie | 760 | 40 | – | – |
| Pepperoni & Mushroom Large | 1 slice | 250 | 29 | – | – |
| Pepperoni & Mushroom Medium | 1 slice | 200 | 24 | – | – |
| Perogy Individual | 1 pie | 1010 | 102 | – | – |
| Perogy Large | 1 slice | 330 | 33 | – | – |
| Perogy Medium | 1 slice | 280 | 28 | – | – |
| Popeye Individual | 1 pie | 730 | 94 | – | – |
| Popeye Large | 1 slice | 240 | 30 | – | – |
| Popeye Medium | 1 slice | 200 | 26 | – | – |
| Rustic Italian Individual | 1 pie | 940 | 102 | – | – |
| Rustic Italian Large | 1 slice | 310 | 33 | – | – |
| Rustic Italian Medium | 1 slice | 250 | 28 | – | – |
| Sante Fe Chicken Individual | 1 pie | 800 | 94 | – | – |
| Sante Fe Chicken Large | 1 slice | 260 | 30 | – | – |
| Sante Fe Chicken Medium | 1 slice | 220 | 25 | – | – |
| Super Veggie Individual | 1 pie | 850 | 108 | – | – |
| Super Veggie Large | 1 slice | 280 | 35 | – | – |
| Super Veggie Medium | 1 slice | 230 | 30 | – | – |
| Thai Chicken Individual | 1 pie | 870 | 106 | – | – |
| Thai Chicken Large | 1 slice | 280 | 34 | – | – |
| Thai Chicken Medium | 1 slice | 240 | 29 | – | – |
| The Basic Individual | 1 pie | 620 | 89 | – | – |
| The Basic Large | 1 slice | 200 | 28 | – | – |
| The Basic Medium | 1 slice | 160 | 24 | – | – |
| The Deluxe Individual | 1 pie | 780 | 92 | – | – |
| The Deluxe Large | 1 slice | 240 | 30 | – | – |
| The Deluxe Medium | 1 slice | 190 | 25 | – | – |
| Tropical Chicken Individual | 1 pie | 1060 | 94 | – | – |
| Tropical Chicken Large | 1 slice | 340 | 30 | – | – |
| Tropical Chicken Medium | 1 slice | 280 | 25 | – | – |
| Tuscan Individual | 1 pie | 900 | 108 | – | – |
| Tuscan Large | 1 slice | 290 | 35 | – | – |
| Tuscan Medium | 1 slice | 240 | 30 | – | – |
| Vegetarian Individual | 1 pie | 670 | 100 | – | – |
| Vegetarian Large | 1 slice | 220 | 31 | – | – |
| Vegetarian Medium | 1 slice | 170 | 26 | – | – |

| FOOD | PORTION | CALS | CARB | SUGAR | FIBER |
|---|---|---|---|---|---|
| Zorba The Greek Individual | 1 pie | 810 | 99 | – | – |
| Zorba The Greek Large | 1 slice | 270 | 32 | – | – |
| Zorba The Greek Medium | 1 slice | 220 | 27 | – | – |
| **SALADS AND SALAD BARS** | | | | | |
| Boston's Cobb Salad | 1 serv | 1100 | 66 | – | – |
| Caesar Salad | 1 reg | 260 | 15 | – | – |
| Caesar Salad Meal Sized | 1 serv | 690 | 52 | – | – |
| Greek Salad | 1 serv | 500 | 19 | – | – |
| Greek Salad Meal Sized | 1 serv | 1110 | 53 | – | – |
| House Dressing | 1 serv (2 oz) | 136 | 4 | – | – |
| Spinach Salad | 1 serv | 190 | 6 | – | – |
| Spinach Salad Meal Sized | 1 serv | 500 | 32 | – | – |
| Taco Salad Beef w/ Sour Cream & Salsa | 1 serv | 640 | 40 | – | – |
| Taco Salad Chicken w/ Sour Cream & Salsa | 1 serv | 520 | 39 | – | – |
| Thai Chicken Salad | 1 serv | 730 | 90 | – | – |
| Tossed Garden Greens w/ House Dressing | 1 serv | 170 | 10 | – | – |
| Veggie Plate w/ Low Fat Ranch Dressing | 1 serv | 180 | 26 | – | – |
| **SANDWICHES** | | | | | |
| BBQ Beef w/ Fries | 1 serv | 1580 | 179 | – | – |
| Beef Dip w/ Fries & Au Jus | 1 serv | 1560 | 151 | – | – |
| Boston Cheesesteak w/ Fries & Au Jus | 1 serv | 1790 | 172 | – | – |
| Boston Brute w/ Fries | 1 serv | 1420 | 163 | – | – |
| Buffalo Chicken w/ Fries | 1 serv | 1720 | 187 | – | – |
| Chicken Foccacia w/ Fries | 1 serv | 1350 | 140 | – | – |
| Spicy Italian Sausage w/ Caesar Salad | 1 serv | 1070 | 104 | – | – |
| Stromboli Chicken w/ Caesar Salad | 1 serv | 1020 | 101 | – | – |
| Stromboli Perogy w/ Caesar Salad | 1 serv | 1120 | 109 | – | – |
| Stromboli Sante Fe w/ Caesar Salad | 1 serv | 1000 | 104 | – | – |
| Super Ham & Cheese w/ Fries | 1 serv | 1370 | 137 | – | – |
| Tango Chicken Wrap w/ Caesar Salad | 1 serv | 740 | 55 | – | – |

| FOOD | PORTION | CALS | CARB | SUGAR | FIBER |
|---|---|---|---|---|---|
| **BRUEGGER'S BAGELS** | | | | | |
| **BAGELS** | | | | | |
| Blueberry | 1 | 330 | 68 | 14 | 4 |
| Chocolate Chip | 1 | 310 | 69 | 19 | 4 |
| Cinnamon Raisin | 1 | 320 | 68 | 16 | 4 |
| Cinnamon Sugar | 1 | 340 | 71 | 15 | 6 |
| Everything | 1 | 310 | 62 | 8 | 4 |
| Garlic | 1 | 310 | 62 | 7 | 4 |
| Honey Grain | 1 | 330 | 64 | 10 | 5 |
| Jalapeno Bagel | 1 | 310 | 63 | 7 | 4 |
| Onion | 1 | 310 | 62 | 8 | 4 |
| Orange Cranberry | 1 | 330 | 68 | 17 | 4 |
| Plain | 1 | 300 | 61 | 7 | 4 |
| Poppy Seed | 1 | 310 | 61 | 7 | 4 |
| Pumpernickel | 1 | 320 | 64 | 11 | 5 |
| Rosemary Olive Oil | 1 | 350 | 62 | 10 | 4 |
| Salt | 1 | 300 | 61 | 7 | 4 |
| Sesame | 1 | 320 | 61 | 7 | 4 |
| Sun Dried Tomato | 1 | 320 | 65 | 11 | 4 |
| **DESSERTS** | | | | | |
| Blondies | 1 | 370 | 42 | 29 | 2 |
| Brownie Chocolate Chunk | 1 | 330 | 39 | 26 | 2 |
| Brownie Mint | 1 | 300 | 34 | 27 | 0 |
| Bruegger Bar | 1 | 420 | 47 | 31 | 3 |
| Cappuccino Bar | 1 | 420 | 45 | 32 | 1 |
| Luscious Lemon Bar | 1 | 350 | 39 | 24 | 0 |
| Oatmeal Cranberry Mountains | 1 | 430 | 49 | 22 | 3 |
| Raspberry Sammies | 1 | 270 | 36 | 18 | 1 |
| **SANDWICH FILLINGS** | | | | | |
| Atlantic Smoked Salmon | 2 oz | 90 | tr | tr | 0 |
| Cream Cheese Bacon Scallion | 2 tbsp | 100 | 4 | 1 | 0 |
| Cream Cheese Chive | 2 tbsp | 100 | 2 | 1 | 0 |
| Cream Cheese Garden Veggie | 2 tbsp | 90 | 3 | 2 | 0 |
| Cream Cheese Garden Veggie Light | 2 tbsp | 60 | 2 | 1 | 0 |
| Cream Cheese Herb Garlic Light | 2 tbsp | 70 | 3 | 2 | 0 |
| Cream Cheese Honey Walnut | 2 tbsp | 110 | 5 | 2 | 0 |
| Cream Cheese Jalapeno | 2 tbsp | 100 | 3 | 2 | 0 |
| Cream Cheese Light Strawberry | 2 tbsp | 70 | 4 | 3 | 0 |
| Cream Cheese Olive Pimento | 2 tbsp | 100 | 2 | 1 | 0 |

| FOOD | PORTION | CALS | CARB | SUGAR | FIBER |
|---|---|---|---|---|---|
| Cream Cheese Plain | 2 tbsp | 90 | 4 | 1 | 0 |
| Cream Cheese Plain Light | 2 tbsp | 70 | 3 | 2 | 0 |
| Cream Cheese Wildberry | 2 tbsp | 100 | 4 | 2 | 0 |
| Hummus | 2 tbsp | 60 | 4 | 0 | 2 |
| Tuna Salad | 1 serv (2.5 oz) | 180 | 6 | 4 | 0 |
| **SANDWICHES** | | | | | |
| Chicken Breast | 1 | 440 | 62 | 7 | 4 |
| Chicken Salad w/ Mayo | 1 | 460 | 67 | 11 | 4 |
| Deli-Style Ham w/ Honey Mustard | 1 | 440 | 77 | 21 | 4 |
| Egg Cheese | 1 | 480 | 66 | 10 | 4 |
| Egg Cheese Sausage | 1 | 680 | 66 | 11 | 4 |
| Egg Cheese Bacon | 1 | 560 | 66 | 10 | 4 |
| Egg Cheese Ham | 1 | 520 | 66 | 10 | 4 |
| Garden Veggie | 1 | 390 | 80 | 15 | 7 |
| Leonardo Da Veggie | 1 | 460 | 69 | 11 | 4 |
| Santa Fe Turkey | 1 | 480 | 71 | 13 | 4 |
| Turkey w/ Mayo | 1 | 480 | 65 | 10 | 4 |
| Chicken Fajita | 1 | 500 | 74 | 15 | 5 |

## BURGER KING

| FOOD | PORTION | CALS | CARB | SUGAR | FIBER |
|---|---|---|---|---|---|
| **BEVERAGES** | | | | | |
| Cocoa Cola Classic | 1 med (22 fl oz) | 280 | 70 | 70 | 0 |
| Coffee | 1 serv (12 oz) | 5 | 1 | 0 | 0 |
| Diet Coke | 1 med (22 fl oz) | 1 | tr | tr | 0 |
| Milk 2% | 1 (8 oz) | 130 | 12 | 12 | 0 |
| Shake Chocolate | 1 med (13.9 oz) | 440 | 75 | 67 | 4 |
| Shake Chocolate | 1 sm (10.7 oz) | 330 | 58 | 51 | 3 |
| Shake Chocolate Syrup Added | 1 med (15.9 oz) | 570 | 105 | 96 | 3 |
| Shake Chocolate Syrup Added | 1 sm (11.7 oz) | 390 | 72 | 66 | 2 |
| Shake Strawberry Syrup Added | 1 med (15.9 oz) | 550 | 104 | 96 | 2 |
| Shake Strawberry Syrup Added | 1 sm (11.7 oz) | 390 | 72 | 66 | 1 |

| FOOD | PORTION | CALS | CARB | SUGAR | FIBER |
|---|---|---|---|---|---|
| Shake Vanilla | 1 med (13.9 oz) | 430 | 73 | 66 | 2 |
| Shake Vanilla | 1 sm (10.7 oz) | 330 | 56 | 51 | 1 |
| Sprite | 1 med (22 fl oz) | 260 | 66 | 66 | 0 |
| Tropicana Orange Juice | 1 serv (10 oz) | 140 | 33 | 28 | 0 |
| **BREAKFAST SELECTIONS** | | | | | |
| AM Express Dip | 1 serv (1 oz) | 80 | 21 | – | – |
| AM Express Grape Jam | 1 serv (0.4 oz) | 30 | 7 | – | – |
| AM Express Strawberry Jam | 1 serv (0.4 oz) | 30 | 8 | – | – |
| Bacon | 3 strips (0.3 oz) | 40 | 0 | – | – |
| Biscuit | 1 (3.3 oz) | 300 | 35 | 3 | 1 |
| Biscuit w/ Bacon Egg & Cheese | 1 (6.6 oz) | 620 | 37 | 4 | 1 |
| Biscuit w/ Egg | 1 (4.6 oz) | 380 | 37 | 3 | tr |
| Biscuit w/ Sausage | 1 (4.6 oz) | 490 | 36 | 3 | 1 |
| Cini-minis w/o Icing | 4 (3.8 oz) | 440 | 51 | 20 | 1 |
| Croissan'wich Sausage Egg & Cheese | 1 (5.3 oz) | 530 | 23 | 4 | 1 |
| Croissan'wich w/ Sausage & Cheese | 1 (3.7 oz) | 450 | 21 | 3 | 1 |
| French Toast Sticks | 5 sticks (4 oz) | 440 | 51 | 12 | 3 |
| Ham | 1 serv (1.2 oz) | 35 | 0 | – | – |
| Hash Browns | 1 sm (2.6 oz) | 240 | 25 | 0 | 2 |
| Land O'Lakes Whipped Classic Blend | 1 serv (0.4 oz) | 65 | 0 | – | – |
| Vanilla Icing Cini-Minis | 1 serv (1 oz) | 110 | 20 | – | – |
| **MAIN MENU SELECTIONS** | | | | | |
| American Cheese | 2 slices (0.9 oz) | 90 | 0 | – | – |
| BK Big Fish Sandwich | 1 (8.8 oz) | 720 | 59 | 4 | 3 |
| BK Broiler Chicken Breast Patty | 1 (3.5 oz) | 140 | 4 | – | – |
| BK Broiler Chicken Sandwich | 1 (8.7 oz) | 530 | 45 | 5 | 2 |
| BK Broiler Chicken Sandwich w/o Mayo | 1 (8.7 oz) | 370 | 45 | 5 | 2 |
| Bacon Cheeseburger | 1 (4.9 oz) | 400 | 27 | 4 | 1 |
| Bacon Double Cheeseburger | 1 (7.2 oz) | 630 | 28 | 5 | 1 |
| Big King Sandwich | 1 (7.6 oz) | 640 | 28 | 4 | 1 |
| Bull's Eye Barbecue Sauce | 1 serv (0.5 oz) | 20 | 5 | 5 | – |
| Cheeseburger | 1 (4.7 oz) | 360 | 27 | 4 | 1 |

| FOOD | PORTION | CALS | CARB | SUGAR | FIBER |
|---|---|---|---|---|---|
| Chick'N Crisp Sandwich | 1 (4.9 oz) | 460 | 37 | 3 | 3 |
| Chick'N Crisp Sandwich w/o Mayo | 1 (4.9 oz) | 360 | 37 | 3 | 3 |
| Chicken Sandwich | 1 (8 oz) | 710 | 54 | 4 | 2 |
| Chicken Sandwich w/o Mayo | 1 (8 oz) | 500 | 54 | 4 | 2 |
| Chicken Tenders | 4 (2.2 oz) | 180 | 9 | 0 | 0 |
| Chicken Tenders | 8 (4.3 oz) | 350 | 17 | 0 | 1 |
| Chicken Tenders | 5 (2.7 oz) | 230 | 11 | 0 | tr |
| Dipping Sauce Barbecue | 1 serv (1 oz) | 35 | 9 | – | – |
| Dipping Sauce Honey | 1 serv (1 oz) | 90 | 23 | – | – |
| Dipping Sauce Honey Mustard | 1 serv (1 oz) | 90 | 10 | – | – |
| Dipping Sauce Ranch | 1 serv (1 oz) | 170 | 2 | – | – |
| Dipping Sauce Sweet & Sour | 1 serv (1 oz) | 45 | 11 | – | – |
| Double Cheeseburger | 1 (6.9 oz) | 580 | 27 | 5 | 1 |
| Double Whopper | 1 (12.2 oz) | 920 | 47 | 8 | 3 |
| Double Whopper w/ Cheese | 1 (13.1 oz) | 1010 | 47 | 8 | 3 |
| Double Whopper w/ Mayo | 1 (13.1 oz) | 850 | 47 | 8 | 3 |
| Double Whopper w/o Mayo | 1 (12.2 oz) | 760 | 47 | 8 | 3 |
| Dutch Apple Pie | 1 serv (4 oz) | 300 | 39 | 22 | 2 |
| French Fries No Salt | 1 king size (6 oz) | 590 | 74 | 0 | 5 |
| French Fries No Salt | 1 sm (2.6 oz) | 250 | 32 | 0 | 2 |
| French Fries No Salt | 1 med (4.1 g) | 400 | 50 | 0 | 4 |
| French Fries Salted | 1 sm (2.6 oz) | 250 | 32 | 0 | 2 |
| French Fries Salted | 1 med (4.1 oz) | 400 | 50 | 0 | 4 |
| French Fries Salted | 1 king size (6 oz) | 590 | 74 | 0 | 5 |
| Hamburger | 1 (4.2 oz) | 320 | 27 | 4 | 1 |
| Hamburger Bun | 1 (4.6 oz) | 130 | 24 | – | – |
| Hamburger Patty | 1 (1.9 oz) | 170 | 0 | – | – |
| Hash Browns | 1 lg (4.5 oz) | 410 | 42 | 0 | 4 |
| Ketchup | 1 serv (0.5 oz) | 15 | 4 | – | – |
| King Sauce | 1 serv (0.5 oz) | 70 | 2 | – | – |
| Lettuce | 1 leaf (0.7 oz) | 0 | 0 | – | – |
| Mustard | 1 serv (3 g) | 0 | 0 | – | – |
| Onion | 1 serv (0.5 oz) | 5 | 1 | – | – |
| Onion Rings | 1 med serv (3.3 oz) | 380 | 46 | 4 | 4 |
| Onion Rings | 1 king serv (5.3 oz) | 600 | 74 | 7 | 6 |

| FOOD | PORTION | CALS | CARB | SUGAR | FIBER |
|---|---|---|---|---|---|
| Pickles | 4 slices (0.5 oz) | 0 | 0 | – | – |
| Tartar Sauce | 1 serv (1.5 oz) | 260 | 0 | – | – |
| Tomato | 2 slices (1 oz) | 5 | 1 | – | – |
| Whopper | 1 (9.5 oz) | 660 | 47 | 8 | 3 |
| Whopper Bun | 1 (2.7 oz) | 220 | 39 | – | – |
| Whopper Jr. | 1 (5.5 oz) | 400 | 28 | 5 | 2 |
| Whopper Jr. w/ Cheese | 1 (6 oz) | 450 | 28 | 5 | 2 |
| Whopper Jr. w/ Cheese w/o Mayo | 1 (6 oz) | 370 | 28 | 5 | 2 |
| Whopper Jr. w/o Mayo | 1 (5.5 oz) | 320 | 28 | 5 | 2 |
| Whopper Patty | 1 (2.8 oz) | 250 | 0 | – | – |
| Whopper w/ Cheese | 1 (10.4 oz) | 760 | 47 | 8 | 3 |
| Whopper w/ Cheese w/o Mayo | 1 (10.4 oz) | 600 | 47 | 8 | 3 |
| Whopper w/o Mayo | 1 (9.5 oz) | 510 | 47 | 8 | 3 |
| **CARL'S JR.** | | | | | |
| **BAKED SELECTIONS** | | | | | |
| Cheese Danish | 1 | 400 | 49 | 21 | 1 |
| Cheesecake Strawberry Swirl | 1 serv | 290 | 30 | 20 | 2 |
| Chocolate Cake | 1 serv | 300 | 48 | 37 | 1 |
| Chocolate Chip Cookie | 1 | 350 | 46 | 27 | 1 |
| Muffin Blueberry | 1 | 340 | 49 | 29 | 1 |
| Muffin Bran Raisin | 1 | 370 | 61 | 35 | 6 |
| **BEVERAGES** | | | | | |
| Coca-Cola Classic | 1 reg (21 oz) | 220 | 54 | 54 | 0 |
| Coffee | 1 reg (12 oz) | 2 | tr | 0 | 0 |
| Diet Coke | 1 reg (21 oz) | tr | tr | 0 | 0 |
| Dr. Pepper | 1 reg (21 oz) | 200 | 53 | 53 | 0 |
| Hot Chocolate | 1 serv (12 oz) | 120 | 22 | 21 | 1 |
| Iced Tea | 1 reg (12 oz) | 5 | 0 | 0 | 0 |
| Lemonade Minute Maid Orange | 1 reg (21 oz) | 200 | 52 | 52 | 0 |
| Milk 1% | 1 (10 fl oz) | 150 | 18 | 18 | 0 |
| Minute Maid Orange Soda | 1 reg (21 oz) | 200 | 52 | 52 | 0 |
| Nestea Raspberry | 1 reg (21 oz) | 160 | 42 | 42 | 0 |
| Orange Juice | 1 (10 oz) | 150 | 37 | 35 | 0 |
| Ramblin' Root Beer | 1 reg (21 oz) | 220 | 60 | 60 | 0 |
| Shake Chocolate | 1 reg (32 oz) | 770 | 140 | 121 | tr |

| FOOD | PORTION | CALS | CARB | SUGAR | FIBER |
|---|---|---|---|---|---|
| Shake Strawberry | 1 reg (32 oz) | 750 | 133 | 117 | 0 |
| Shake Vanilla | 1 reg (32 oz) | 700 | 115 | 98 | 0 |
| Sprite | 1 reg (21 oz) | 200 | 52 | 52 | 0 |
| **BREAKFAST SELECTIONS** | | | | | |
| Bacon | 2 strips | 45 | 0 | 0 | 0 |
| Breakfast Burrito | 1 | 560 | 36 | 2 | 1 |
| Breakfast Quesadilla | 1 | 370 | 36 | 3 | 1 |
| English Muffin w/ Margarine | 1 | 210 | 28 | 2 | 2 |
| French Toast Dips w/o Syrup | 1 serv | 370 | 42 | 11 | 1 |
| Grape Jelly | 1 serv (0.5 oz) | 40 | 9 | 7 | 0 |
| Hash Brown Nuggets | 1 serv | 330 | 32 | 1 | 2 |
| Sausage | 1 patty | 190 | 2 | 0 | 0 |
| Scrambed Eggs | 1 serv | 180 | 1 | 1 | 0 |
| Sourdough Breakfast | 1 serv | 410 | 33 | 4 | 1 |
| Strawberry Jam | 1 serv (0.5 oz) | 40 | 9 | 7 | 0 |
| Sunrise Sandwich w/o Meat | 1 | 360 | 28 | 5 | tr |
| Table Syrup | 1 serv (1 oz) | 90 | 21 | 16 | 0 |
| **MAIN MENU SELECTIONS** | | | | | |
| American Cheese | 1 sm | 50 | 1 | 1 | 0 |
| BBQ Sauce | 1 serv (1.1 oz) | 50 | 11 | 7 | 0 |
| Breadstick | 1 (0.3 oz) | 35 | 7 | 0 | tr |
| Carl's Famous Star | 1 | 590 | 50 | 8 | 3 |
| Chicken Stars | 6 pieces | 260 | 14 | 1 | tr |
| CrissCut Fries | 1 serv | 410 | 43 | 0 | 4 |
| Croutons | 1 serv (0.5 oz) | 30 | 5 | 0 | 0 |
| Double Sourdough Bacon Cheeseburger | 1 | 880 | 37 | 7 | 2 |
| Double Western Bacon Cheeseburger | 1 | 920 | 65 | 15 | 3 |
| Famous Bacon Cheeseburger | 1 | 700 | 51 | 9 | 3 |
| French Fries | 1 med | 460 | 59 | 1 | 5 |
| French Fries | 1 kid size | 250 | 32 | tr | 2 |
| Hamburger | 1 | 280 | 36 | 5 | 1 |
| Honey Sauce | 1 serv (1 oz) | 90 | 22 | 20 | 0 |
| Mustard Sauce | 1 serv (1 oz) | 50 | 11 | 8 | 0 |
| Onion Rings | 1 serv | 430 | 53 | 5 | 3 |
| Potato Bacon & Cheese | 1 | 640 | 75 | 7 | 6 |
| Potato Broccoli & Cheese | 1 serv | 530 | 76 | 6 | 6 |
| Potato Plain w/o Margarine | 1 | 290 | 68 | 4 | 6 |
| Potato Sour Cream & Chives | 1 | 430 | 70 | 6 | 6 |

| FOOD | PORTION | CALS | CARB | SUGAR | FIBER |
|---|---|---|---|---|---|
| Salsa | 1 serv (0.9 oz) | 10 | 2 | 1 | 0 |
| Sandwich Bacon Swiss Crispy Chicken | 1 | 760 | 72 | 8 | 3 |
| Sandwich Carl's Catch Fish | 1 | 530 | 55 | 8 | 2 |
| Sandwich Charbroiled Sirloin Stead | 1 | 550 | 52 | 6 | 2 |
| Sandwich Chargrilled Chicken Club | 1 | 470 | 37 | 6 | 2 |
| Sandwich Chargrilled Santa Fe Chicken | 1 | 540 | 37 | 7 | 2 |
| Sandwich Chargrilled BBQ Chicken | 1 | 290 | 41 | 9 | 2 |
| Sandwich Ranch Crispy Chicken | 1 | 660 | 71 | 8 | 3 |
| Sandwich Southwest Spicy Chicken | 1 | 620 | 48 | 7 | 2 |
| Sandwich Spicy Chicken | 1 | 480 | 47 | 6 | 2 |
| Sandwich Western Bacon Crispy Chicken | 1 | 750 | 91 | 15 | 3 |
| Sourdough Bacon Cheeseburger | 1 | 640 | 37 | 6 | 2 |
| Sourdough Ranch Bacon Cheeseburger | 1 | 720 | 43 | 5 | 3 |
| Super Star | 1 | 790 | 51 | 9 | 3 |
| Sweet N'Sour Sauce | 1 serv (1 oz) | 50 | 12 | 9 | 0 |
| Swiss Cheese | 1 serv | 50 | 0 | 0 | 0 |
| Western Bacon Cheeseburger | 1 | 660 | 64 | 15 | 3 |
| Zucchini | 1 serv | 320 | 31 | 3 | 2 |
| **SALAD DRESSINGS** | | | | | |
| 1000 Island | 1 serv (2 oz) | 230 | 5 | 3 | 0 |
| Blue Cheese | 1 serv (2 oz) | 320 | 1 | 1 | 0 |
| French Fat Free | 1 serv (2 oz) | 60 | 16 | 12 | tr |
| House | 1 serv (2 oz) | 220 | 1 | 2 | 0 |
| Italian Fat Free | 1 serv (2 oz) | 15 | 4 | 2 | 0 |
| **SALADS AND SALAD BARS** | | | | | |
| Salad-To-Go Charbroiled Chicken | 1 serv | 200 | 12 | 3 | 4 |
| Salad-To-Go Garden | 1 | 50 | 4 | 2 | 2 |

| FOOD | PORTION | CALS | CARB | SUGAR | FIBER |
|---|---|---|---|---|---|
| **CARVEL** | | | | | |
| **BEVERAGES** | | | | | |
| Carvelanche w/ Topping | 1 (16 oz) | 600 | 71 | – | tr |
| Regular Fizzlers | 1 (16 oz) | 340 | 75 | – | 1 |
| Thick Shake Reduced Fat Chocolate | 1 (16 oz) | 520 | 100 | – | tr |
| Thick Shake Reduced Fat Vanilla | 1 (16 oz) | 460 | 84 | – | tr |
| **ICE CREAM** | | | | | |
| Cake Butterscotch Dream | 1 slice (4 oz) | 260 | 37 | – | 0 |
| Cake Celebration | 1 slice (4 oz) | 200 | 24 | – | tr |
| Cake Cookies & Cream | 1 serv (4 oz) | 240 | 29 | – | 1 |
| Cake Fudge Drizzle | 1 slice (4 oz) | 240 | 32 | – | 1 |
| Cake Fudge Drizzle | 1 slice (4 oz) | 240 | 32 | – | 1 |
| Cake Game Ball | 1 slice (4 oz) | 330 | 41 | – | 1 |
| Cake Holiday | 1 slice (4 oz) | 200 | 24 | – | tr |
| Cake Lil'Love | 1 piece (4 oz) | 200 | 24 | – | tr |
| Cake Lil'Love All Vanilla | 1 piece (4.4 oz) | 330 | 41 | 27 | tr |
| Cake Sinfully Chocolate | 1 slice (4 oz) | 240 | 34 | – | 1 |
| Cake Strawberries & Cream | 1 slice (4 oz) | 270 | 40 | – | 1 |
| Chocolate | 4 oz | 190 | 22 | 19 | 0 |
| Chocolate No Fat | 4 oz | 120 | 28 | 25 | 0 |
| Flying Saucer 98% Fat Free Black Raspberry | 1 | 170 | 40 | 24 | tr |
| Flying Saucer 98% Fat Free Chocolate | 1 | 170 | 34 | 17 | 1 |
| Flying Saucer 98% Fat Free Coffee | 1 | 190 | 40 | 26 | tr |
| Flying Saucer 98% Fat Free Maple | 1 | 190 | 40 | 26 | tr |
| Flying Saucer 98% Fat Free Mint | 1 | 190 | 40 | 26 | tr |
| Flying Saucer 98% Fat Free Pistachio | 1 | 190 | 40 | 26 | tr |
| Flying Saucer 98% Fat Free Strawberry | 1 | 190 | 40 | 27 | 1 |
| Flying Saucer 98% Fat Free Vanilla | 1 | 190 | 40 | 26 | tr |
| Flying Saucer Chocolate | 1 | 230 | 33 | 19 | 2 |

| FOOD | PORTION | CALS | CARB | SUGAR | FIBER |
|---|---|---|---|---|---|
| Flying Saucer Vanilla | 1 | 240 | 33 | 19 | 1 |
| Vanilla | 4 oz | 200 | 21 | 19 | 0 |
| Vanilla No Fat | 4 oz | 120 | 25 | 22 | 0 |
| Vanilla No Sugar Added | 4 oz | 130 | 25 | 7 | 0 |
| **ICES** | | | | | |
| Italian Ice Blue Raspberry | 4 oz | 70 | 19 | 18 | 0 |
| Italian Ice Bubble Gum | 4 oz | 70 | 19 | 18 | 0 |
| Italian Ice Cherry | 4 oz | 100 | 25 | 21 | 0 |
| Italian Ice Chocolate Ice Cream | 4 oz | 90 | 20 | 19 | 0 |
| Italian Ice Cotton Candy | 4 oz | 70 | 19 | 18 | 0 |
| Italian Ice Lemon | 4 oz | 70 | 19 | 18 | 0 |
| Italian Ice Mango | 4 oz | 70 | 27 | 22 | 0 |
| Italian Ice Orange | 4 oz | 70 | 19 | 18 | 0 |
| Italian Ice Vanilla Ice Cream | 4 oz | 90 | 20 | 20 | 0 |
| Italian Ice Watermelon | 4 oz | 70 | 19 | 18 | 0 |
| Sherbet All Flavors | 4 oz | 140 | 31 | 24 | 0 |

## CHICK-FIL-A

| FOOD | PORTION | CALS | CARB | SUGAR | FIBER |
|---|---|---|---|---|---|
| **BEVERAGES** | | | | | |
| Coca-Cola Classic | 1 sm | 110 | 28 | 28 | 0 |
| Diet Coke | 1 sm | 0 | 0 | 0 | 0 |
| Diet Lemonade | 1 sm | 25 | 5 | 3 | 0 |
| Ice Tea Sweetened | 1 sm | 80 | 19 | 19 | 0 |
| Iced Tea Unsweetened | 1 serv | 0 | 0 | 0 | 0 |
| Lemonade | 1 sm | 170 | 41 | 40 | 0 |
| **DESSERTS** | | | | | |
| Cheesecake w/ Blueberry Topping | 1 slice | 370 | 39 | 32 | 2 |
| Cheesecake w/ Strawberry Topping | 1 slice | 360 | 38 | 31 | 2 |
| Fudge Nut Brownie | 1 | 330 | 45 | 29 | 2 |
| IceDream Cup | 1 sm | 230 | 39 | 38 | 0 |
| Icedream Cone | 1 sm | 160 | 28 | 24 | 0 |
| Lemon Pie | 1 slice | 320 | 51 | 39 | 3 |
| **MAIN MENU SELECTIONS** | | | | | |
| Barbecue Sauce | 1 pkg | 45 | 11 | 9 | 0 |
| Carrot & Raisin Salad | 1 sm | 130 | 22 | 15 | 2 |
| Chargrilled Chicken Caesar Salad | 1 serv | 240 | 6 | 3 | 2 |

| FOOD | PORTION | CALS | CARB | SUGAR | FIBER |
|---|---|---|---|---|---|
| Chargrilled Chicken Club Sandwich w/o Sauce | 1 | 360 | 31 | 5 | 2 |
| Chargrilled Chicken Deluxe Sandwich | 1 | 280 | 30 | 5 | 2 |
| Chargrilled Chicken Fillet | 1 | 100 | 1 | 1 | 0 |
| Chargrilled Chicken Sandwich | 1 | 280 | 29 | 4 | 1 |
| Chargrilled Chicken Sandwich w/o Butter | 1 | 240 | 28 | 4 | 1 |
| Chick-N-Strips | 4 | 250 | 12 | 2 | 0 |
| Chicken Deluxe Sandwich | 1 | 420 | 39 | 5 | 2 |
| Chicken Sandwich | 1 | 410 | 38 | 5 | 1 |
| Chicken Sandwich w/o Butter | 1 | 380 | 37 | 5 | 1 |
| Chicken Filet | 1 | 230 | 10 | 2 | 0 |
| Chicken Salad Sandwich On Whole Wheat | 1 | 350 | 32 | 6 | 5 |
| Cole Slaw | 1 sm | 210 | 14 | 9 | 2 |
| Cool Wrap Chargrilled Chicken | 1 | 390 | 53 | 6 | 3 |
| Cool Wrap Chicken Caesar | 1 | 460 | 51 | 5 | 3 |
| Cool Wrap Spicy Chicken | 1 | 390 | 51 | 5 | 3 |
| Dijon Honey Mustard Sauce | 1 pkg | 50 | 2 | 2 | 0 |
| Hearty Breast of Chicken Soup | 1 cup | 100 | 13 | 2 | 1 |
| Honey Mustard Sauce | 1 pkg | 45 | 10 | 10 | 0 |
| Nuggets | 8 | 260 | 12 | 3 | tr |
| Polynesian Sauce | 1 pkg | 110 | 13 | 13 | 0 |
| Waffle Fries w/o Salt | 1 sm | 280 | 36 | 0 | 4 |
| Waffle Potato Fries | 1 sm | 280 | 37 | 0 | 5 |
| **SALAD DRESSINGS** | | | | | |
| Basil Vinaigrette | 1 pkg | 210 | 4 | 4 | 0 |
| Blue Cheese | 1 pkg | 190 | 2 | 1 | 0 |
| Buttermilk Ranch | 1 pkg | 190 | 2 | 1 | 0 |
| Caesar | 1 pkg | 200 | 1 | 0 | 0 |
| Fat Free Dijon Honey Mustard | 1 pkg | 60 | 14 | 11 | 0 |
| Light Italian | 1 pkg | 20 | 3 | 2 | 0 |
| Spicy | 1 pkg | 210 | 2 | 1 | 0 |
| Thousand Island | 1 pkg | 170 | 6 | 5 | 0 |
| **SALADS AND SALAD BARS** | | | | | |
| Chargrilled Chicken Garden Salad | 1 serv | 180 | 8 | 4 | 3 |
| Chick-N-Strips Salad | 1 serv | 340 | 19 | 5 | 3 |
| Croutons Garlic & Butter | 1 pkg | 90 | 11 | 0 | 0 |

| FOOD | PORTION | CALS | CARB | SUGAR | FIBER |
|---|---|---|---|---|---|
| Roasted Sunflower Kernels Unsalted | 1 pkg | 80 | 3 | 1 | tr |
| Side Salad | 1 serv | 80 | 6 | 3 | 2 |
| **CHURCH'S CHICKEN** | | | | | |
| **DESSERTS** | | | | | |
| Apple Pie | 1 pie | 280 | 41 | 13 | 1 |
| Edward's Double Lemon Pie | 1 pie | 300 | 39 | 29 | 0 |
| Edward's Strawberry Cream Cheese Pie | 1 pie | 280 | 32 | 22 | 2 |
| **MAIN MENU SELECTIONS** | | | | | |
| Breast | 1 serv | 200 | 4 | 0 | 0 |
| Cajun Rice | 1 reg | 130 | 16 | 0 | tr |
| Chicken Fried Steak w/ White Gravy | 1 serv | 470 | 36 | 4 | 1 |
| Cole Slaw | 1 reg | 92 | 8 | 6 | 2 |
| Collard Greens | 1 reg | 25 | 5 | 0 | 2 |
| Corn On The Cob | 1 ear | 139 | 24 | 2 | 9 |
| French Fries | 1 reg | 210 | 29 | 0 | 2 |
| Honey Butter Biscuit | 1 | 250 | 26 | 3 | 1 |
| Jalapeno Cheese Bombers | 4 pieces | 240 | 29 | 5 | 3 |
| Krispy Tender Strips | 1 piece | 137 | 11 | 0 | tr |
| Leg | 1 serv | 140 | 2 | 0 | 0 |
| Macaroni & Cheese | 1 reg | 210 | 23 | 6 | 1 |
| Mashed Potatoes & Gravy | 1 reg | 90 | 14 | 2 | 1 |
| Okra | 1 reg | 210 | 19 | tr | 4 |
| Sweet Corn Nuggets | 1 reg | 250 | 30 | 6 | 2 |
| Tender Crunchers | 6-8 pieces | 411 | 32 | 0 | 1 |
| Thigh | 1 serv | 230 | 5 | 0 | 0 |
| Whole Jalapeno Peppers | 2 | 10 | 2 | tr | 1 |
| Wing | 1 serv | 250 | 8 | 0 | 0 |
| **SAUCES** | | | | | |
| BBQ | 1 pkg | 29 | 7 | 2 | 0 |
| Creamy Jalapeño | 1 pkg | 102 | 1 | 0 | 0 |
| Purple Pepper | 1 pkg | 21 | 12 | 6 | 0 |
| Sweet & Sour | 1 pkg | 31 | 8 | 2 | 0 |
| **CINNABON** | | | | | |
| Caramel Pecanbon | 1 | 890 | – | 48 | – |
| Cinnabon | 1 reg | 670 | – | 49 | – |

| FOOD | PORTION | CALS | CARB | SUGAR | FIBER |
|---|---|---|---|---|---|
| **COLOMBO FROZEN YOGURT** | | | | | |
| Strawberry Lowfat | ½ cup | 110 | 21 | 16 | 0 |
| Strawberry Nonfat | ½ cup | 100 | 20 | 16 | 0 |
| **D'ANGELO'S SANDWICH SHOP** | | | | | |
| **CHILDREN'S MENU SELECTIONS** | | | | | |
| D'Lite Turkey | 1 kidz | 217 | 30 | 2 | 3 |
| Sub Ham & Cheese | 1 kidz | 214 | 31 | 2 | 1 |
| Sub Meatball | 1 kidz | 330 | 37 | 5 | 4 |
| Sub Tuna | 1 kidz | 450 | 30 | 2 | 1 |
| **SALAD DRESSINGS AND TOPPINGS** | | | | | |
| Bleu Cheese | 1 serv (1 oz) | 152 | 3 | 2 | 0 |
| Caesar | 1 serv (1 oz) | 140 | 2 | 2 | 0 |
| Caesar Fat Free | 1 serv (1 oz) | 20 | 3 | 3 | 0 |
| Creamy Italian | 1 serv (1 oz) | 122 | 3 | 2 | 0 |
| Cucumbers | 3 slices | 2 | 0 | 0 | tr |
| Greek Dressing w/ Feta | 1 serv (3 oz) | 227 | 6 | 3 | 0 |
| Honey Mustard Dressing | 1 serv (1 oz) | 150 | 7 | 6 | 0 |
| Hot Peppers | 1 serv | 0 | 1 | 1 | 0 |
| Olive Oil Vinaigrette | 1 serv (3 oz) | 170 | 9 | 6 | 0 |
| Ranch Lite | 1 serv (3 oz) | 240 | 6 | 4 | 1 |
| Sesame Ginger | 1 serv (1 oz) | 170 | 10 | 10 | 0 |
| **SALADS** | | | | | |
| Antipasto Salad w/o Dressing | 1 serv | 275 | 15 | 5 | 6 |
| Asian Chicken w/o Dressing | 1 serv | 224 | 23 | 7 | 6 |
| Caesar w/ Dressing | 1 serv | 474 | 20 | 2 | 3 |
| Chef w/o Dressing | 1 serv | 273 | 17 | 5 | 4 |
| Chicken Caesar w/ Dressing | 1 serv | 532 | 13 | 2 | 3 |
| Chicken Stir Fry w/o Dressing | 1 serv | 166 | 10 | 5 | 4 |
| Cobb w/o Dressing | 1 serv | 289 | 9 | 5 | 4 |
| Greek w/o Dressing | 1 serv | 298 | 16 | 6 | 4 |
| Lobster w/o Dressing | 1 serv | 385 | 11 | 4 | 4 |
| Roast Beef w/o Dressing | 1 serv | 146 | 9 | 4 | 4 |
| Tossed Garden w/o Dressing | 1 serv | 47 | 9 | 4 | 4 |
| Turkey w/o Dressing | 1 serv | 157 | 9 | 4 | 4 |
| **SANDWICHES** | | | | | |
| D'Lite Chicken Stir Fry | 1 sm | 426 | 57 | 8 | 7 |
| D'Lite Fresh Veggie | 1 | 348 | 62 | 14 | 7 |
| D'Lite Grilled Chicken Breast | 1 sm | 387 | 52 | 5 | 6 |
| D'Lite Ham & Cheese | 1 sm | 351 | 52 | 5 | 2 |

| FOOD | PORTION | CALS | CARB | SUGAR | FIBER |
|---|---|---|---|---|---|
| D'Lite Roast Beef | 1 sm | 353 | 51 | 5 | 6 |
| D'Lite Turkey | 1 sm | 364 | 51 | 5 | 6 |
| D'Lite Turkey Cranberry | 1 sm | 460 | 75 | 22 | 6 |
| Pokket Caesar Salad | 1 sm | 643 | 55 | 1 | 2 |
| Pokket Capacola & Cheese | 1 sm | 426 | 52 | 5 | 6 |
| Pokket Cheeseburger | 1 sm | 481 | 37 | 2 | 1 |
| Pokket Chicken Caesar Salad | 1 sm | 701 | 48 | 2 | 2 |
| Pokket Chicken Club | 1 sm | 559 | 47 | 2 | 1 |
| Pokket Chicken Honey Dijon | 1 sm | 527 | 45 | 5 | 1 |
| Pokket Chicken Salad | 1 sm | 705 | 39 | 1 | 1 |
| Pokket Chicken Stir Fry | 1 sm | 425 | 45 | 4 | 1 |
| Pokket Classic Veggie No Cheese | 1 sm | 238 | 50 | 6 | 4 |
| Pokket Greek | 1 sm | 812 | 54 | 6 | 3 |
| Pokket Grilled Chicken | 1 sm | 328 | 41 | 1 | 1 |
| Pokket Ham & Cheese | 1 sm | 349 | 41 | 2 | 1 |
| Pokket Ham & Salami | 1 sm | 412 | 39 | 2 | 1 |
| Pokket Hamburger | 1 sm | 422 | 35 | 1 | 1 |
| Pokket Italian | 1 sm | 574 | 42 | 2 | 1 |
| Pokket Lobster | 1 sm | 568 | 39 | 0 | 1 |
| Pokket Meatball | 1 sm | 600 | 56 | 9 | 3 |
| Pokket Mortadella & Cheese | 1 sm | 505 | 42 | 2 | 1 |
| Pokket Seafood Salad | 1 sm | 532 | 56 | 5 | 2 |
| Pokket Steak | 1 sm | 335 | 29 | 0 | 0 |
| Pokket Steak & Cheese | 1 sm | 407 | 31 | 1 | 0 |
| Pokket Tuna | 1 sm | 791 | 28 | 38 | 1 |
| Sub Cheeseburger | 1 sm | 542 | 47 | 5 | 5 |
| Sub Chicken Club | 1 sm | 619 | 52 | 5 | 6 |
| Sub Chicken Honey Dijon | 1 sm | 587 | 56 | 8 | 6 |
| Sub Chicken Salad | 1 sm | 769 | 50 | 4 | 6 |
| Sub Chicken Stir Fry | 1 sm | 487 | 57 | 8 | 6 |
| Sub Classic Veggie | 1 sm | 465 | 64 | 11 | 8 |
| Sub Grilled Chicken | 1 sm | 387 | 52 | 5 | 6 |
| Sub Ham & Cheese | 1 sm | 412 | 53 | 5 | 2 |
| Sub Ham & Salami | 1 sm | 474 | 51 | 5 | 2 |
| Sub Hamburger | 1 sm | 482 | 45 | 4 | 5 |
| Sub Italian | 1 sm | 637 | 54 | 5 | 3 |
| Sub Lobster | 1 sm | 628 | 50 | 3 | 5 |
| Sub Meatball | 1 sm | 663 | 70 | 13 | 8 |
| Sub Mortadella & Cheese | 1 sm | 568 | 54 | 5 | 6 |

| FOOD | PORTION | CALS | CARB | SUGAR | FIBER |
|---|---|---|---|---|---|
| Sub Number 9 | 1 sm | 475 | 44 | 6 | 5 |
| Sub Pastrami | 1 sm | 526 | 51 | 3 | 5 |
| Sub Pepperoni | 1 sm | 614 | 53 | 5 | 6 |
| Sub Roast Beef | 1 sm | 350 | 50 | 4 | 5 |
| Sub Salad | 1 sm | 298 | 60 | 10 | 9 |
| Sub Salami & Cheese | 1 sm | 597 | 51 | 5 | 6 |
| Sub Seafood Salad | 1 | 595 | 67 | 9 | 7 |
| Sub Steak | 1 sm | 383 | 37 | 2 | 4 |
| Sub Steak & Cheese | 1 sm | 455 | 40 | 4 | 4 |
| Sub Steak Tip | 1 sm | 486 | 63 | 13 | 3 |
| Sub Stuffed Turkey | 1 sm | 1036 | 136 | 18 | 10 |
| Sub Tuna | 1 sm | 853 | 49 | 4 | 2 |
| Sub Turkey | 1 sm | 361 | 50 | 4 | 5 |
| Sub Turkey Club | 1 sm | 360 | 37 | 4 | 3 |
| Wrap Asian Chicken Salad | 1 | 914 | 105 | 26 | 9 |
| Wrap BLT & Cheese | 1 | 500 | 58 | 5 | 3 |
| Wrap Buffalo Chicken Salad | 1 | 778 | 71 | 7 | 3 |
| Wrap Caesar Salad | 1 | 669 | 64 | 3 | 4 |
| Wrap Capacola & Cheese | 1 | 451 | 57 | 4 | 3 |
| Wrap Cheese | 1 | 631 | 63 | 7 | 3 |
| Wrap Cheeseburger | 1 | 569 | 52 | 4 | 3 |
| Wrap Chef | 1 | 832 | 82 | 18 | 5 |
| Wrap Chicken Caesar Salad | 1 | 788 | 65 | 4 | 4 |
| Wrap Chicken Cobb | 1 | 855 | 69 | 17 | 4 |
| Wrap Chicken Filet & Bacon | 1 | 643 | 57 | 3 | 3 |
| Wrap Chicken Honey Dijon | 1 | 619 | 63 | 8 | 4 |
| Wrap Chicken Salad | 1 | 780 | 55 | 3 | 3 |
| Wrap Chicken Stir Fry | 1 | 511 | 61 | 7 | 3 |
| Wrap Classic Veggie | 1 | 490 | 69 | 10 | 6 |
| Wrap Greek | 1 | 761 | 43 | 6 | 4 |
| Wrap Grilled Chicken | 1 | 420 | 56 | 4 | 4 |
| Wrap Ham & Cheese | 1 | 436 | 58 | 4 | 3 |
| Wrap Ham & Salami | 1 | 499 | 56 | 4 | 3 |
| Wrap Hamburger | 1 | 509 | 50 | 3 | 3 |
| Wrap Italian | 1 | 654 | 59 | 4 | 3 |
| Wrap Lobster | 1 | 766 | 56 | 2 | 3 |
| Wrap Meatball | 1 | 687 | 75 | 11 | 5 |
| Wrap Mortadella & Cheese | 1 | 592 | 58 | 4 | 3 |
| Wrap Number 9 | 1 | 494 | 48 | 5 | 3 |
| Wrap Pastrami | 1 | 550 | 55 | 2 | 2 |

| FOOD | PORTION | CALS | CARB | SUGAR | FIBER |
|---|---|---|---|---|---|
| Wrap Pepperoni | 1 | 638 | 58 | 4 | 3 |
| Wrap Roast Beef | 1 | 374 | 55 | 3 | 3 |
| Wrap Salad | 1 | 322 | 65 | 8 | 6 |
| Wrap Salami & Cheese | 1 | 605 | 56 | 4 | 3 |
| Wrap Steak | 1 | 402 | 41 | 2 | 2 |
| Wrap Steak & Cheese | 1 | 474 | 43 | 3 | 2 |
| Wrap Steak Tip | 1 | 374 | 40 | 11 | 2 |
| Wrap Tuna | 1 | 881 | 55 | 3 | 3 |
| Wrap Turkey | 1 | 385 | 55 | 3 | 3 |
| Wrap Turkey Club | 1 | 435 | 52 | 4 | 3 |
| **SOUPS** | | | | | |
| #9 Steak & Cheese | 1 sm | 280 | 11 | 2 | 1 |
| Chicken Noodle | 1 sm | 130 | 8 | 5 | 1 |
| Hearty Vegetable | 1 sm | 40 | 7 | 4 | 2 |
| Lobster Bisque | 1 sm | 360 | 16 | 3 | 0 |
| New England Clam Chowder | 1 sm | 270 | 15 | 2 | 1 |
| Santa Fe Chipotle Vegetable | 1 sm | 130 | 22 | 3 | 8 |
| Shrimp & Roasted Corn | 1 sm | 250 | 23 | 6 | 2 |
| Thanksgiving Everyday | 1 sm | 250 | 18 | 4 | 2 |

## DAIRY QUEEN

| FOOD | PORTION | CALS | CARB | SUGAR | FIBER |
|---|---|---|---|---|---|
| **FOOD SELECTIONS** | | | | | |
| Chicken Breast Fillet Sandwich | 1 (6.7 oz) | 430 | 37 | 5 | 2 |
| Chicken Strip Basket | 1 serv (14.5 oz) | 1000 | 102 | 3 | 5 |
| Chili 'n' Cheese Dog | 1 (5 oz) | 330 | 22 | 4 | 2 |
| DQ Homestyle Bacon Double Cheeseburger | 1 (8.9 oz) | 610 | 31 | 6 | 2 |
| DQ Homestyle Cheeseburger | 1 (5.3 oz) | 340 | 29 | 5 | 2 |
| DQ Homestyle Double Cheeseburger | 1 (7.7 oz) | 540 | 30 | 5 | 2 |
| DQ Homestyle Hamburger | 1 (4.8 oz) | 290 | 29 | 5 | 2 |
| DQ Ultimate Burger | 1 (9.4 oz) | 670 | 29 | 6 | 2 |
| French Fries | 1 sm (4 oz) | 350 | 42 | tr | 3 |
| French Fries | 1 med (3.9 oz) | 440 | 53 | tr | 4 |
| Grilled Chicken Sandwich | 1 (6.5 oz) | 310 | 30 | 5 | 3 |
| Hot Dog | 1 (3.5 oz) | 240 | 19 | 4 | 1 |
| Onion Rings | 1 serv (4 oz) | 320 | 39 | 4 | 3 |

| FOOD | PORTION | CALS | CARB | SUGAR | FIBER |
|---|---|---|---|---|---|
| The Great Steakmelt Basket | 1 serv (13.2 oz) | 770 | 72 | 7 | 5 |
| **ICE CREAM** | | | | | |
| Banana Split | 1 (12.9 oz) | 510 | 96 | 82 | 3 |
| Blizzard Chocolate Sandwich Cookie | 1 med (11.4 oz) | 640 | 97 | 74 | 1 |
| Blizzard Chocolate Sandwich Cookie | 1 sm (12 oz) | 520 | 79 | 61 | 1 |
| Blizzard Chocolate Chip Cookie Dough | 1 med (15.4 oz) | 950 | 143 | 106 | 2 |
| Blizzard Chocolate Chip Cookie Dough | 1 sm (12 oz) | 660 | 99 | 74 | 1 |
| Breeze Heath | 1 sm (10.2 oz) | 470 | 85 | 70 | 1 |
| Breeze Heath | 1 med (14.2 oz) | 710 | 123 | 103 | 1 |
| Breeze Strawberry | 1 sm (12 oz) | 320 | 68 | 54 | 1 |
| Breeze Strawberry | 1 med (13.4 oz) | 460 | 99 | 79 | 1 |
| Buster Bar | 1 (5.2 oz) | 450 | 41 | 33 | 2 |
| Chocolate Malt | 1 sm (14.7 oz) | 650 | 111 | 95 | 0 |
| Chocolate Malt | 1 med (19.9 oz) | 880 | 153 | 131 | 0 |
| Cone Chocolate | 1 sm (5 oz) | 240 | 37 | 25 | 0 |
| Cone Chocolate | 1 med (6.9 oz) | 340 | 53 | 34 | 0 |
| Cone Vanilla | 1 lg (8.9 oz) | 410 | 65 | 49 | 0 |
| Cone Vanilla | 1 med (6.9 oz) | 330 | 53 | 38 | 0 |
| Cone Vanilla | 1 sm (5 oz) | 230 | 38 | 27 | 0 |
| Cone Yogurt | 1 med (6.9 oz) | 260 | 56 | 36 | 0 |
| Cone Dipped | 1 med (7.7 oz) | 490 | 59 | 43 | 1 |
| Cone Dipped | 1 sm (5.5 oz) | 340 | 42 | 31 | 1 |
| Cup Of Yogurt | 1 med (6.7 oz) | 230 | 48 | 36 | 0 |
| DQ 8 Inch Round Cake Undecorated | ⅛ of cake (6.2 oz) | 340 | 56 | 42 | 1 |
| DQ Fudge Bar No Sugar Added | 1 (2.3 oz) | 50 | 13 | 3 | 0 |

| FOOD | PORTION | CALS | CARB | SUGAR | FIBER |
|---|---|---|---|---|---|
| DQ Lemon Freez'r | ½ cup (3.2 oz) | 80 | 20 | 20 | 0 |
| DQ Nonfat Frozen Yogurt | ½ cup (3 oz) | 100 | 21 | 16 | 0 |
| DQ Sandwich | 1 (2.1 oz) | 200 | 31 | 18 | 1 |
| DQ Soft Serve Chocolate | ½ cup (3.3 oz) | 150 | 22 | 17 | 0 |
| DQ Soft Serve Vanilla | ½ cup (3.3 oz) | 140 | 22 | 19 | 0 |
| DQ Treatzza Pizza Heath | ⅛ of pie (2.3 oz) | 180 | 28 | 18 | 1 |
| DQ Treatzza Pizza M&M | ⅛ of pie (2.4 oz) | 190 | 29 | 20 | 1 |
| DQ Vanilla Orange Bar No Sugar Added | 1 (2.3 oz) | 60 | 17 | 2 | 0 |
| Dilly Bar Chocolate | 1 (3 oz) | 210 | 21 | 17 | 0 |
| Frozen Hot Chocolate | 1 (20.9 oz) | 860 | 127 | 109 | 3 |
| Misty Slush | 1 sm (15.9 oz) | 220 | 56 | 56 | 0 |
| Misty Slush | 1 med (20.9 oz) | 290 | 74 | 74 | 0 |
| Peanut Buster Parfait | 1 (10.7 oz) | 730 | 99 | 85 | 2 |
| Pecan Mudslide Treat | 1 (4.6 oz) | 650 | 85 | 70 | 2 |
| S'more Galore Parfait | 1 (10.7 oz) | 730 | 111 | 86 | 3 |
| Shake Chocolate | 1 med (18.9 oz) | 770 | 130 | 113 | 0 |
| Shake Chocolate | 1 sm (13.9 oz) | 560 | 94 | 81 | 0 |
| Starkiss | 1 (3 oz) | 80 | 21 | 21 | 0 |
| Strawberry Shortcake | 1 (8.5 oz) | 430 | 70 | 57 | 1 |
| Sundae Chocolate | 1 med (8.2 oz) | 400 | 71 | 61 | 0 |
| Sundae Chocolate | 1 sm (5.7 oz) | 280 | 49 | 42 | 0 |
| Yogurt Sundae Strawberry | 1 med (8.2 oz) | 280 | 61 | 49 | 1 |

## DELTACO

### BEVERAGES

| | | | | | |
|---|---|---|---|---|---|
| Coffee | 1 serv (8 oz) | 0 | 1 | 0 | 0 |
| Coke Classic | 1 med (12 oz) | 150 | 37 | 37 | 0 |
| Coke Classic | 1 sm (10 oz) | 120 | 29 | 29 | 0 |
| Coke Classic | 1 lg (20 oz) | 230 | 59 | 59 | 0 |
| Coke Classic Best Value | 1 serv (27 oz) | 320 | 81 | 81 | 0 |
| Diet Coke | 1 med (12 oz) | 0 | 0 | 0 | 0 |
| Diet Coke | 1 lg (20 oz) | 5 | 1 | 0 | 0 |
| Diet Coke | 1 sm (10 oz) | 0 | 0 | 0 | 0 |

| FOOD | PORTION | CALS | CARB | SUGAR | FIBER |
|---|---|---|---|---|---|
| Diet Coke Best Value | 1 serv (27 oz) | 10 | 1 | 0 | 0 |
| Iced Tea | 1 med (12 oz) | 0 | 1 | 0 | 0 |
| Iced Tea | 1 sm (10 oz) | 0 | 0 | 0 | 0 |
| Iced Tea | 1 lg (20 oz) | 5 | 2 | 0 | 0 |
| Iced Tea Best Value | 1 serv (27 oz) | 10 | 2 | 0 | 0 |
| Milk 1% Lowfat | 1 serv (11 oz) | 130 | 15 | 15 | 0 |
| Mr Pibb | 1 lg (20 oz) | 230 | 59 | 59 | 0 |
| Mr Pibb | 1 sm (10 oz) | 120 | 29 | 29 | 0 |
| Mr Pibb | 1 med (12 oz) | 150 | 37 | 37 | 0 |
| Mr Pibb Best Value | 1 serv (27 oz) | 320 | 81 | 81 | 0 |
| Orange Juice | 1 serv (11 oz) | 140 | 34 | 33 | 1 |
| Shake Chocolate | 1 lg (15 oz) | 680 | 117 | 101 | 1 |
| Shake Chocolate | 1 sm (11.4 oz) | 520 | 89 | 77 | 1 |
| Shake Strawberry | 1 lg (15 oz) | 540 | 100 | 85 | 1 |
| Shake Strawberry | 1 sm (11.4 oz) | 410 | 76 | 65 | 1 |
| Shake Vanilla | 1 lg (15 oz) | 550 | 97 | 81 | 0 |
| Shake Vanilla | 1 sm (11.4 oz) | 420 | 75 | 62 | 0 |
| Sprite | 1 sm (10 oz) | 110 | 29 | 29 | 0 |
| Sprite | 1 med (12 oz) | 140 | 37 | 37 | 0 |
| Sprite | 1 lg (20 oz) | 230 | 59 | 59 | 0 |
| Sprite Best Value | 1 serv (27 oz) | 310 | 81 | 81 | 0 |
| **BREAKFAST SELECTIONS** | | | | | |
| Burrito Breakfast | 1 (3.8 oz) | 250 | 24 | 2 | 1 |
| Burrito Egg & Cheese | 1 (7.5 oz) | 450 | 39 | 2 | 3 |
| Burrito Macho Bacon & Egg | 1 (15.9 oz) | 1030 | 82 | 6 | 6 |
| Burrito Steak & Egg | 1 (9 oz) | 580 | 41 | 2 | 3 |
| Quesadilla Bacon & Egg | 1 (6.1 oz) | 450 | 40 | 2 | 2 |
| Side of Bacon | 2 strips (0.3 oz) | 50 | 0 | 0 | 0 |
| **MAIN MENU SELECTIONS** | | | | | |
| Beans 'n Cheese Cup | 1 serv (7.7 oz) | 260 | 44 | 4 | 16 |
| Burrito Combo | 1 (8.2 oz) | 490 | 53 | 3 | 8 |
| Burrito Del Beef | 1 (8 oz) | 550 | 42 | 2 | 3 |
| Burrito Del Classic Chicken | 1 (8.5 oz) | 580 | 42 | 4 | 3 |
| Burrito Deluxe Combo | 1 (10.7 oz) | 530 | 56 | 5 | 9 |
| Burrito Deluxe Del Beef | 1 (10.5 oz) | 590 | 45 | 4 | 4 |
| Burrito Green | 1 (5 oz) | 280 | 38 | 2 | 6 |
| Burrito Macho Beef | 1 (18.9 oz) | 1170 | 89 | 8 | 7 |
| Burrito Macho Combo | 1 (19.4 oz) | 1050 | 113 | 9 | 17 |
| Burrito Red | 1 (5 oz) | 270 | 38 | 2 | 6 |

| FOOD | PORTION | CALS | CARB | SUGAR | FIBER |
|---|---|---|---|---|---|
| Burrito Red Regular | 1 (7.5 oz) | 390 | 59 | 3 | 11 |
| Burrito Regular Green | 1 (7.5 oz) | 400 | 59 | 3 | 10 |
| Burrito Spicy Chicken | 1 (8.7 oz) | 480 | 65 | 3 | 8 |
| Burrito The Works | 1 (10.2 oz) | 480 | 69 | 5 | 9 |
| Cheeseburger | 1 (4.6 oz) | 330 | 37 | 4 | 3 |
| Del Cheeseburger | 1 (5.6 oz) | 430 | 35 | 3 | 4 |
| Double Del Cheeseburger | 1 (7.1 oz) | 560 | 35 | 4 | 4 |
| Fries | 1 sm (3 oz) | 210 | 20 | 0 | 2 |
| Fries | 1 reg (5 oz) | 350 | 34 | 1 | 3 |
| Fries Best Value | 1 serv (7 oz) | 490 | 47 | 1 | 5 |
| Fries Chili Cheese | 1 serv (10.5 oz) | 670 | 51 | 2 | 5 |
| Fries Deluxe Chili Cheese | 1 serv (11.9 oz) | 710 | 53 | 4 | 6 |
| Get A Lot Meals #1 Combo Burrito Fries Drink | 1 meal | 980 | 124 | 41 | 11 |
| Get A Lot Meals #2 Del Classic Chicken Burrito Fries Drink | 1 meal | 1080 | 113 | 42 | 7 |
| Get A Lot Meals #3 Regular Red Burrito Fries Drink | 1 meal | 890 | 130 | 41 | 14 |
| Get A Lot Meals #4 Two Chicken Soft Tacos Fries Drink | 1 meal | 910 | 102 | 39 | 5 |
| Get A Lot Meals #5 Taco Combo Burrito Drink | 1 meal | 790 | 101 | 40 | 9 |
| Get A Lot Meals #6 Two Tacos Quesadilla Drink | 1 meal | 960 | 98 | 40 | 3 |
| Get A Lot Meals #7 Macho Combo Burrito Fries Drink | 1 meal | 1530 | 183 | 47 | 20 |
| Get A Lot Meals #8 Two Big Fat Tacos Fries Drink | 1 meal | 802 | 148 | 44 | 10 |
| Get A Lot Meals #9 Double Del Cheeseburger Fries Drink | 1 meal | 1050 | 106 | 41 | 7 |
| Nachos | 1 serv (4 oz) | 380 | 40 | 1 | 2 |
| Nachos Macho | 1 serv (17 oz) | 1200 | 130 | 7 | 16 |
| Quesadilla Chicken | 1 (6.8 oz) | 580 | 41 | 2 | 2 |
| Quesadilla Regular | 1 (5.3 oz) | 500 | 39 | 2 | 2 |
| Quesadilla Spicy Jack Chicken | 1 (6.8 oz) | 570 | 40 | 1 | 2 |
| Quesadilla Spicy Jack Regular | 1 (5.3 oz) | 490 | 38 | 1 | 2 |
| Rice Cup | 1 serv (4 oz) | 150 | 28 | 2 | 1 |
| Soft Taco | 1 (2.8 oz) | 160 | 16 | 1 | 1 |

| FOOD | PORTION | CALS | CARB | SUGAR | FIBER |
|---|---|---|---|---|---|
| Soft Taco Chicken | 1 (3.3 oz) | 210 | 16 | 1 | 1 |
| Taco | 1 (2.2 oz) | 160 | 11 | 1 | 1 |
| Taco Big Fat | 1 (5.4 oz) | 320 | 39 | 3 | 3 |
| Taco Big Fat Chicken | 1 (5.4 oz) | 340 | 38 | 3 | 3 |
| Taco Big Fat Steak | 1 (5.4 oz) | 390 | 38 | 3 | 3 |
| Taco Salad Deluxe | 1 (18.8 oz) | 760 | 76 | 10 | 14 |
| Tostada Salad | 1 (4.5 oz) | 210 | 24 | 2 | 6 |
| **DONATOS PIZZA** | | | | | |
| **PIZZA** | | | | | |
| Dessert Apple | ¼ pie | 722 | 137 | 66 | 15 |
| Dessert Cherry | ¼ pie | 818 | 149 | 70 | 13 |
| Original | ¼ pie | 660 | 58 | 6 | 6 |
| Original Chicken Vegy Medley | ¼ pie | 500 | 56 | 6 | 11 |
| Original Chicken Vegy Medly No Cheese | ¼ pie | 392 | 54 | 6 | 11 |
| Original Founders | ¼ pie | 737 | 71 | 6 | 10 |
| Original Hawaiian | ¼ pie | 620 | 58 | 16 | 4 |
| Original Hawaiian No Cheese | ¼ pie | 411 | 58 | 10 | 11 |
| Original Mariachi Beef | ¼ pie | 613 | 56 | 6 | 11 |
| Original Mariachi Chicken | ¼ pie | 580 | 56 | 6 | 11 |
| Original Serious Cheese | ¼ pie | 640 | 62 | 4 | 6 |
| Original Serious Meat | ¼ pie | 817 | 68 | 6 | 10 |
| Original Vegy | ¼ pie | 564 | 60 | 8 | 12 |
| Original Vegy No Cheese | ¼ pie | 370 | 59 | 7 | 12 |
| Original Works | ¼ pie | 729 | 75 | 6 | 12 |
| Traditional Chicken Vegy Medley | ¼ pie | 647 | 90 | 8 | 4 |
| Traditional Founders | ¼ pie | 900 | 107 | 11 | 3 |
| Traditional Hawaiian | ¼ pie | 794 | 98 | 17 | 4 |
| Traditional Mariachi Beef | ¼ pie | 797 | 95 | 11 | 4 |
| Traditional Mariachi Chicken | ¼ pie | 770 | 95 | 11 | 4 |
| Traditional Serious Meat | ¼ pie | 977 | 104 | 11 | 3 |
| Traditional Vegy | ¼ pie | 752 | 98 | 12 | 5 |
| Traditional Works | ¼ pie | 892 | 111 | 11 | 5 |
| Tradtional Original | ¼ pie | 928 | 89 | 11 | 9 |
| Tradtional Serious Cheese | ¼ pie | 830 | 123 | 8 | 12 |
| **SALAD DRESSINGS** | | | | | |
| Italian | 1 serv (1.5 oz) | 230 | 1 | 1 | 0 |
| Italian Lite | 1 serv (1.5 oz) | 20 | 2 | 0 | 0 |

| FOOD | PORTION | CALS | CARB | SUGAR | FIBER |
|---|---|---|---|---|---|
| **SALADS** | | | | | |
| Grilled Chicken w/o Dressing | 1 serv | 314 | 12 | 8 | 5 |
| Italian Chef w/o Dressing | 1 serv | 338 | 13 | 8 | 5 |
| Side w/o Dressing | 1 serv | 106 | 6 | 4 | 2 |
| **SIDE ORDERS** | | | | | |
| Breadsticks | 2 | 220 | 29 | 1 | 0 |
| Chicken Wings Hot | 5 | 449 | 6 | – | tr |
| Chicken Wings Mild | 5 | 451 | 6 | – | tr |
| Three Cheese Garlic Bread | 1 bun | 605 | 66 | 3 | 3 |
| **SUBS** | | | | | |
| Big Don Italian | 1 serv | 705 | 68 | 6 | 3 |
| Big Don Lite Italian | 1 serv | 631 | 69 | 6 | 3 |
| Grilled Chicken | 1 serv | 786 | 68 | 5 | 3 |
| Ham & Cheese Italian | 1 serv | 609 | 70 | 8 | 3 |
| Ham & Cheese Lite Italian | 1 serv | 534 | 70 | 8 | 3 |
| Southwest Turkey | 1 serv | 710 | 74 | 12 | 3 |
| Steak & Cheese | 1 serv | 929 | 107 | 4 | 3 |
| Vegy Italian | 1 serv | 730 | 75 | 8 | 6 |
| Vegy Lite Italian | 1 serv | 661 | 78 | 6 | 6 |
| **DUNKIN' DONUTS** | | | | | |
| **BAGELS AND CREAM CHEESE** | | | | | |
| Bagel Blueberry | 1 | 340 | 75 | 7 | tr |
| Bagel Cinnamon Raisin | 1 | 340 | 74 | 11 | 1 |
| Bagel Egg | 1 | 350 | 72 | 3 | 0 |
| Bagel Everything | 1 | 360 | 74 | 3 | 0 |
| Bagel Garlic | 1 | 360 | 76 | 4 | 0 |
| Bagel Onion | 1 | 330 | 70 | 3 | 0 |
| Bagel Plain | 1 | 340 | 73 | 3 | 0 |
| Bagel Poppyseed | 1 | 360 | 74 | 3 | tr |
| Bagel Pumpernickel | 1 | 350 | 75 | 6 | 2 |
| Bagel Salt | 1 | 340 | 73 | 3 | 0 |
| Bagel Sesame | 1 | 380 | 74 | 3 | 0 |
| Bagel Wheat | 1 | 330 | 73 | 6 | 4 |
| Cream Cheese Chive | 1 pkg | 190 | 3 | 3 | tr |
| Cream Cheese Garden Vegetable | 1 pkg | 180 | 3 | 2 | tr |
| Cream Cheese Lite | 1 pkg | 130 | 3 | 2 | 0 |
| Cream Cheese Plain | 1 pkg | 200 | 3 | 2 | 0 |
| Cream Cheese Salmon | 1 pkg | 180 | 2 | 2 | 0 |

| FOOD | PORTION | CALS | CARB | SUGAR | FIBER |
|---|---|---|---|---|---|
| **BAKED SELECTIONS** | | | | | |
| Bow Tie Donut | 1 | 300 | 34 | 10 | tr |
| Cake Donut Blueberry | 1 | 290 | 35 | 16 | tr |
| Cake Donut Butternut | 1 | 300 | 36 | 16 | tr |
| Cake Donut Chocolate Coconut | 1 | 300 | 31 | 12 | 1 |
| Cake Donut Chocolate Frosted | 1 | 300 | 38 | 18 | tr |
| Cake Donut Chocolate Glazed | 1 | 290 | 33 | 14 | 1 |
| Cake Donut Cinnamon | 1 | 270 | 31 | 12 | tr |
| Cake Donut Coconut | 1 | 290 | 33 | 13 | tr |
| Cake Donut Double Chocolate | 1 | 310 | 37 | 18 | 2 |
| Cake Donut Glazed | 1 | 270 | 33 | 14 | tr |
| Cake Donut Old Fashioned | 1 | 250 | 26 | 7 | tr |
| Cake Donut Powdered | 1 | 270 | 32 | 13 | tr |
| Cake Donut Toasted Coconut | 1 | 300 | 35 | 16 | tr |
| Cake Donut Whole Wheat Glazed | 1 | 310 | 32 | 14 | 2 |
| Chocolate Frosted Donut | 1 | 200 | 29 | 10 | tr |
| Chocolate Kreme Filled Donut | 1 | 270 | 35 | 16 | tr |
| Cinnamon Bun | 1 | 510 | 85 | 42 | 0 |
| Coffee Roll | 1 | 270 | 33 | 10 | 1 |
| Coffee Roll Chocolate Frosted | 1 | 290 | 36 | 12 | 1 |
| Coffee Roll Maple Frosted | 1 | 290 | 36 | 13 | 1 |
| Coffee Roll Vanilla Frosted | 1 | 290 | 36 | 13 | 1 |
| Cookie Chocolate Chocolate Chunk | 1 | 210 | 26 | 16 | 2 |
| Cookie Chocolate Chunk | 1 | 220 | 28 | 17 | 1 |
| Cookie Chocolate Chunk w/ Nut | 1 | 230 | 27 | 16 | 1 |
| Cookie Chocolate White Chocolate Chunk | 1 | 230 | 28 | 19 | 1 |
| Cookie Oatmeal Raisin Pecan | 1 | 220 | 29 | 18 | 1 |
| Cookie Peanut Butter Chocolate Chunk w/ Nuts | 1 | 240 | 24 | 16 | 2 |
| Cookie Peanut Butter w/ Nuts | 1 | 240 | 24 | 15 | 1 |
| Croissant Almond | 1 | 350 | 34 | 13 | 2 |
| Croissant Chocolate | 1 | 400 | 37 | 15 | 2 |
| Croissant Plain | 1 | 290 | 26 | 3 | tr |
| Cruller Glazed | 1 | 290 | 37 | 18 | tr |
| Cruller Glazed Chocolate | 1 | 280 | 35 | 16 | 1 |
| Cruller Plain | 1 | 240 | 25 | 6 | tr |

| FOOD | PORTION | CALS | CARB | SUGAR | FIBER |
|---|---|---|---|---|---|
| Cruller Powdered | 1 | 270 | 30 | 11 | tr |
| Cruller Sugar | 1 | 250 | 27 | 8 | tr |
| Donut Apple Crumb | 1 | 230 | 34 | 12 | tr |
| Donut Apple N' Spice | 1 | 200 | 29 | 7 | tr |
| Donut Bavarian Kreme | 1 | 210 | 30 | 9 | tr |
| Donut Black Raspberry | 1 | 210 | 32 | 10 | tr |
| Donut Blueberry Crumb | 1 | 240 | 36 | 15 | tr |
| Donut Boston Kreme | 1 | 240 | 36 | 14 | tr |
| Donut Chocolate Iced Bismark | 1 | 340 | 50 | 31 | tr |
| Dunkin' Donut | 1 | 240 | 25 | 6 | tr |
| Eclair Donut | 1 | 270 | 39 | 17 | tr |
| Fritter Glazed | 1 | 260 | 31 | 7 | 1 |
| Glazed Donut | 1 | 180 | 25 | 6 | tr |
| Jelly Filled Donut | 1 | 210 | 32 | 14 | tr |
| Jelly Stick | 1 | 290 | 44 | 24 | tr |
| Lemon Donut | 1 | 200 | 28 | 8 | tr |
| Maple Frosted Donut | 1 | 210 | 30 | 12 | tr |
| Marble Frosted Donut | 1 | 200 | 29 | 11 | tr |
| Muffin Apple Cinnamon Pecan | 1 | 510 | 74 | 41 | 1 |
| Muffin Apple N'Spice | 1 | 350 | 57 | 29 | 2 |
| Muffin Banana Nut | 1 | 360 | 52 | 29 | 3 |
| Muffin Blueberry | 1 (4 oz) | 320 | 49 | 27 | 3 |
| Muffin Blueberry | 1 (6 oz) | 490 | 78 | 41 | 2 |
| Muffin Bran | 1 | 390 | 60 | 34 | 3 |
| Muffin Cherry | 1 | 340 | 53 | 29 | 2 |
| Muffin Chocolate Hazelnut | 1 | 610 | 87 | 52 | 3 |
| Muffin Chocolate Chip | 1 (6 oz) | 590 | 88 | 50 | 3 |
| Muffin Chocolate Chip | 1 (4 oz) | 400 | 58 | 36 | 4 |
| Muffin Corn | 1 (4 oz) | 390 | 57 | 22 | 2 |
| Muffin Corn | 1 (6 oz) | 500 | 78 | 34 | 1 |
| Muffin Cranberry Orange | 1 | 470 | 76 | 41 | 2 |
| Muffin Cranberry Orange Nut | 1 | 350 | 52 | 27 | 3 |
| Muffin Lemon Poppyseed | 1 | 360 | 56 | 27 | 1 |
| Muffin Oat Bran | 1 | 370 | 55 | 29 | 3 |
| Muffin Lowfat Apple & Spice | 1 | 240 | 54 | 32 | tr |
| Muffin Lowfat Banana | 1 | 250 | 57 | 35 | tr |
| Muffin Lowfat Blueberry | 1 | 250 | 55 | 33 | 1 |
| Muffin Lowfat Bran | 1 | 240 | 57 | 32 | 4 |
| Muffin Lowfat Cherry | 1 | 250 | 56 | 34 | tr |
| Muffin Lowfat Chocolate | 1 | 250 | 53 | 29 | 2 |

| FOOD | PORTION | CALS | CARB | SUGAR | FIBER |
|---|---|---|---|---|---|
| Muffin Lowfat Corn | 1 | 240 | 52 | 20 | 0 |
| Muffin Lowfat Cranberry Orange | 1 | 240 | 55 | 32 | 1 |
| Muffin Reduced Fat Blueberry | 1 | 450 | 77 | 42 | 2 |
| Muffin Reduced Fat Corn | 1 | 460 | 79 | 35 | 1 |
| Munchkins Chocolate Cake Glazed | 3 | 200 | 26 | 13 | tr |
| Munchkins Cake Butternut | 3 | 200 | 25 | 12 | tr |
| Munchkins Cake Cinnamon | 4 | 250 | 29 | 13 | tr |
| Munchkins Cake Coconut | 3 | 200 | 23 | 10 | tr |
| Munchkins Cake Glazed | 3 | 200 | 27 | 14 | 0 |
| Munchkins Cake Plain | 4 | 220 | 22 | 6 | tr |
| Munchkins Cake Powdered | 4 | 250 | 29 | 12 | tr |
| Munchkins Cake Sugared | 4 | 240 | 28 | 12 | tr |
| Munchkins Cake Toasted Coconut | 3 | 200 | 24 | 11 | tr |
| Munchkins Yeast Glazed | 5 | 200 | 27 | 12 | tr |
| Munchkins Yeast Jelly Filled | 5 | 210 | 30 | 15 | tr |
| Munchkins Yeast Lemon Filled | 4 | 170 | 23 | 9 | 0 |
| Munchkins Yeast Sugar Raised | 7 | 220 | 26 | 5 | tr |
| Strawberry Frosted Donut | 1 | 210 | 30 | 12 | tr |
| Strawberry Donut | 1 | 210 | 32 | 11 | tr |
| Sugar Raised Donut | 1 | 170 | 22 | 4 | tr |
| Sugared Cake Donut | 1 | 250 | 27 | 9 | tr |
| Vanilla Frosted Donut | 1 | 210 | 30 | 12 | tr |
| Vanilla Kreme Filled Donut | 1 | 270 | 36 | 17 | tr |
| **BEVERAGES** | | | | | |
| Coffee Coolatta w/ 2% Milk | 1 (16 oz) | 240 | 52 | 51 | 0 |
| Coffee Coolatta w/ Cream | 1 (16 oz) | 410 | 51 | 50 | 0 |
| Coffee Coolatta w/ Milk | 1 (16 oz) | 260 | 52 | 51 | 0 |
| Coffee Coolatta w/ Skim Milk | 1 (16 oz) | 230 | 52 | 51 | 0 |
| Coolatta Orange Mango Fruit | 1 (16 oz) | 290 | 71 | 63 | tr |
| Coolatta Pink Lemonade Fruit | 1 (16 oz) | 350 | 88 | 63 | 0 |
| Coolatta Raspberry Lemonade | 1 (16 oz) | 280 | 68 | 64 | 0 |
| Coolatta Strawberry Fruit | 1 (16 oz) | 280 | 70 | 63 | 1 |
| Coolatta Vanilla | 1 (16 oz) | 450 | 94 | 80 | 0 |
| Dunkaccino | 1 (20 oz) | 510 | 71 | 50 | 1 |
| Dunkaccino | 1 (18.75 oz) | 480 | 67 | 48 | 1 |
| Dunkaccino | 1 (10 oz) | 250 | 34 | 25 | tr |
| Dunkaccino | 1 (14 oz) | 360 | 51 | 36 | 1 |

| FOOD | PORTION | CALS | CARB | SUGAR | FIBER |
|---|---|---|---|---|---|
| Hot Cocoa | 1 (10 oz) | 230 | 38 | 29 | 2 |
| Hot Cocoa | 1 (14 oz) | 330 | 57 | 43 | 2 |
| Hot Cocoa | 1 (18.75 oz) | 440 | 75 | 57 | 3 |
| Hot Cocoa | 1 (20 oz) | 470 | 79 | 61 | 3 |
| **SANDWICHES** | | | | | |
| Breakfast Sandwich Ham Egg Cheese | 1 | 320 | 31 | 3 | 2 |
| Omwich Bagel Bacon Cheddar | 1 | 600 | 79 | 5 | tr |
| Omwich Bagel Spanish Cheese | 1 | 570 | 79 | 5 | tr |
| Omwich Bagel Three Cheese | 1 | 610 | 78 | 5 | tr |
| Omwich Croissant Spanish Cheese | 1 | 530 | 33 | 5 | 1 |
| Omwich Croissant Bacon Cheddar | 1 | 560 | 33 | 5 | 1 |
| Omwich Croissant Three Cheese | 1 | 560 | 33 | 5 | 1 |
| Omwich English Muffin Bacon Cheddar | 1 | 400 | 33 | 4 | 2 |
| Omwich English Muffin Spanish Cheese | 1 | 370 | 34 | 4 | 2 |
| Omwich English Muffin Three Cheese | 1 | 400 | 33 | 4 | 2 |

## EINSTEIN BROS BAGELS

| FOOD | PORTION | CALS | CARB | SUGAR | FIBER |
|---|---|---|---|---|---|
| **BAGELS AND BREADS** | | | | | |
| Bagel Asiago Cheese | 1 | 360 | 71 | 4 | 2 |
| Bagel Egg | 1 | 340 | 69 | 5 | 2 |
| Bagel Honey Whole Wheat | 1 | 320 | 71 | 11 | 3 |
| Bagel Jalapeno | 1 | 330 | 71 | 4 | 2 |
| Bagel Lucky Gree | 1 | 320 | 71 | 4 | 2 |
| Bagel Mango | 1 | 360 | 80 | 14 | 2 |
| Bagel Power | 1 | 410 | 81 | 18 | 4 |
| Bagel Pumpkin | 1 | 330 | 72 | 6 | 3 |
| Bagel Spicy Nacho | 1 | 450 | 77 | 5 | 3 |
| Bagel Spinach Florentine | 1 | 410 | 72 | 5 | 3 |
| Bagel Croutons | ¼ cup | 25 | 4 | 0 | 0 |
| Bagel Twist | 1 | 220 | 39 | 3 | 1 |
| Chocolate Chip | 1 | 370 | 76 | 10 | 3 |
| Chopped Garlic | 1 | 380 | 79 | 3 | 4 |
| Chopped Onion | 1 | 330 | 71 | 4 | 2 |

| FOOD | PORTION | CALS | CARB | SUGAR | FIBER |
|---|---|---|---|---|---|
| Cinnamon Raisin Swirl | 1 | 350 | 78 | 14 | 2 |
| Cinnamon Sugar | 1 | 330 | 74 | 10 | 2 |
| Dark Pumpernickel | 1 | 320 | 68 | 3 | 3 |
| Everything | 1 | 340 | 75 | 5 | 2 |
| Focaccia Pepperoni Pizza | 1 serv | 590 | 76 | 6 | 3 |
| Nutty Banana | 1 | 360 | 74 | 5 | 2 |
| Plain | 1 | 320 | 71 | 4 | 2 |
| Poppy Dip'd | 1 | 350 | 74 | 3 | 2 |
| Roll Challah | 1 | 300 | 55 | 7 | 2 |
| Salt | 1 | 330 | 73 | 3 | 2 |
| Sesame Dip'd | 1 | 380 | 75 | 3 | 3 |
| Sun Dried Tomato | 1 | 320 | 69 | 3 | 3 |
| Wild Blueberry | 1 | 350 | 77 | 9 | 3 |
| **BEVERAGES** | | | | | |
| Americano | 1 reg | 1 | 0 | 0 | 0 |
| Cafe Latte | 1 reg | 140 | 13 | 13 | 0 |
| Cafe Latte Nonfat | 1 reg | 100 | 14 | 12 | 0 |
| Cappuccino | 1 reg | 90 | 9 | 8 | 0 |
| Cappuccino Nonfat | 1 reg | 60 | 9 | 8 | 0 |
| Chai 2% Milk | 1 reg | 210 | 41 | 41 | 0 |
| Chai Skim Milk | 1 reg | 190 | 41 | 41 | 0 |
| Coffee | 1 reg | 0 | 0 | 0 | 0 |
| Espresso | 1 reg | 1 | 0 | 0 | 0 |
| Half & Half | 2 tbsp | 40 | 1 | 1 | – |
| Hot Chocolate | 1 reg | 290 | 39 | 33 | 0 |
| Hot Chocolate Lower Fat | 1 reg | 260 | 39 | 33 | 0 |
| Hot Tea All Flavors | 1 cup | 0 | 0 | 0 | 0 |
| Iced Americano | 1 serv | 1 | 0 | 0 | 0 |
| Iced Coffee | 1 serv | 0 | 0 | 0 | 0 |
| Iced Latte | 1 serv | 120 | 12 | 11 | 0 |
| Iced Latte Nonfat | 1 serv | 90 | 12 | 11 | 0 |
| Iced Mocha | 1 serv | 210 | 33 | 31 | 0 |
| Iced Mocha Low Fat | 1 serv | 180 | 32 | 30 | 0 |
| Mocha | 1 reg | 230 | 34 | 32 | 0 |
| Mocha Low Fat | 1 reg | 190 | 34 | 31 | 0 |
| **DESSERTS** | | | | | |
| Brownie Iced | 1 | 550 | 81 | 56 | 3 |
| Brownie Iced w/ Walnuts | 1 | 600 | 82 | 57 | 4 |
| Cherry Figure 8 | 1 | 400 | 51 | 26 | 1 |
| Cinnamon Roll | 1 | 810 | 118 | 50 | 4 |

| FOOD | PORTION | CALS | CARB | SUGAR | FIBER |
|---|---|---|---|---|---|
| Cookie Chocolate Chunk | 1 | 640 | 87 | 48 | 3 |
| Cookie Oatmeal Raisin | 1 | 600 | 82 | 40 | 2 |
| Cookie Peanut Butter | 1 | 640 | 75 | 36 | 3 |
| Muffin Blueberry | 1 | 540 | 80 | 35 | 1 |
| Muffin Chocolate Chip | 1 | 620 | 89 | 48 | 3 |
| Pound Cake Lemon Iced | 1 slice | 540 | 74 | 50 | 0 |
| Pound Cake Marble | 1 slice | 460 | 57 | 33 | 1 |
| Rice Krispy Bar | 1 | 420 | 83 | 29 | 1 |
| Scone Blueberry w/ Icing | 1 | 450 | 64 | 21 | 2 |
| Scone Lemon Currant | 1 | 430 | 69 | 25 | 4 |
| Strudel Cinnamon Walnut | 1 piece | 550 | 63 | 25 | 3 |
| Sweetie Pie | 1 | 620 | 106 | 72 | 1 |
| **SALAD DRESSINGS** | | | | | |
| Asian Sesame | 2 tbsp | 80 | 16 | 13 | 0 |
| Caesar | 2 tbsp | 150 | 1 | 1 | 0 |
| Chipotle Vinaigrette | 2 tbsp | 110 | 5 | 4 | 0 |
| Horseradish Sauce | 2 tbsp | 170 | 1 | 0 | 0 |
| Raspberry Vinaigrette | 2 tbsp | 160 | 8 | 8 | 0 |
| Thousand Island | 2 tbsp | 110 | 5 | 4 | 0 |
| **SALADS** | | | | | |
| Asian Chicken Salad | 1 serv (14.5 oz) | 550 | 88 | 23 | 5 |
| Bros Bistro | 1 serv (9.5 oz) | 520 | 25 | 18 | 2 |
| Chicken Caesar | 1 serv (12.5 oz) | 750 | 26 | 8 | 2 |
| Chicken Chipotle Salad | 1 serv | 710 | 48 | 18 | 13 |
| Chicken Salad On Greens | 1 serv (10.5 oz) | 210 | 11 | 6 | 3 |
| Egg Salad | 1 serv (4 oz) | 200 | 5 | 2 | 0 |
| Fresh Fruit Cup | 1 serv (8 oz) | 110 | 25 | 24 | 2 |
| Mixed Greens | 1 serv (3.5 oz) | 228 | 13 | 4 | 1 |
| Potato | ½ cup | 290 | 21 | 1 | 2 |
| Tuna Salad On Greens | 1 serv (10.5 oz) | 170 | 10 | 6 | 3 |
| **SANDWICHES** | | | | | |
| 12 Grain Bread Deli Chicken Salad | 1 | 440 | 55 | 8 | 6 |
| 12 Grain Bread Deli Egg Salad | 1 | 490 | 57 | 8 | 5 |
| 12 Grain Bread Deli Ham | 1 | 560 | 55 | 8 | 5 |

| FOOD | PORTION | CALS | CARB | SUGAR | FIBER |
|---|---|---|---|---|---|
| 12 Grain Bread Deli Roast Beef | 1 | 560 | 56 | 8 | 5 |
| 12 Grain Bread Deli Smoked Turkey | 1 | 530 | 56 | 9 | 5 |
| 12 Grain Bread Deli Tuna Salad | 1 | 440 | 56 | 8 | 6 |
| 12 Grain Bread Deli Turkey Pastrami | 1 | 540 | 55 | 9 | 5 |
| 12 Grain Bread Ultimate Toasted Cheese w/ Tomato | 1 | 870 | 77 | 7 | 2 |
| Bagel Chicken Salad | 1 | 500 | 78 | 8 | 4 |
| Bagel Egg Bacon | 1 | 580 | 74 | 6 | 2 |
| Bagel Egg Ham | 1 | 530 | 74 | 6 | 2 |
| Bagel Egg Salad | 1 | 560 | 79 | 7 | 3 |
| Bagel Egg Sausage | 1 | 550 | 74 | 6 | 2 |
| Bagel Ham | 1 | 450 | 74 | 6 | 3 |
| Bagel Holey Cow | 1 | 900 | 77 | 6 | 3 |
| Bagel Hummus & Feta | 1 | 540 | 89 | 10 | 5 |
| Bagel Hummus & Feta | 1 | 540 | 89 | 10 | 5 |
| Bagel New York Lox | 1 | 660 | 79 | 10 | 3 |
| Bagel Original | 1 | 480 | 74 | 6 | 2 |
| Bagel Roast Beef | 1 | 460 | 76 | 6 | 3 |
| Bagel Rueben Deli | 1 | 660 | 83 | 8 | 4 |
| Bagel Salmon & Shmear | 1 | 650 | 82 | 10 | 2 |
| Bagel Smoked Turkey | 1 | 420 | 75 | 6 | 3 |
| Bagel Tasty Turkey | 1 | 570 | 83 | 9 | 4 |
| Bagel The Veg Out | 1 | 490 | 77 | 11 | 3 |
| Bagel Tuna Salad | 1 | 470 | 77 | 7 | 4 |
| Bagel Turkey Pastrami | 1 | 440 | 76 | 7 | 3 |
| Challah Club Mex | 1 | 750 | 47 | 3 | 2 |
| Challah Cobbie | 1 | 630 | 45 | 5 | 4 |
| Challah Deli Chicken Salad | 1 | 480 | 62 | 11 | 4 |
| Challah Deli Egg Salad | 1 | 430 | 45 | 7 | 2 |
| Challah Deli Pastrami | 1 | 480 | 43 | 8 | 2 |
| Challah Deli Roasted Beef | 1 | 500 | 44 | 7 | 2 |
| Challah Deli Smoked Turkey | 1 | 470 | 44 | 8 | 2 |
| Challah Deli Tuna Salad | 1 | 370 | 42 | 6 | 2 |
| Challah Deli Turkey Ham | 1 | 500 | 43 | 7 | 2 |
| Challah EBBQ Chicken | 1 | 380 | 52 | 17 | 2 |
| Challah Roasted Chicken & Smoked Gouda | 1 | 440 | 47 | 10 | 2 |
| Chicago Bagel Dog Asiago | 1 | 740 | 78 | 6 | 2 |

| FOOD | PORTION | CALS | CARB | SUGAR | FIBER |
|---|---|---|---|---|---|
| Chicago Bagel Dog Chili Cheese | 1 | 810 | 83 | 9 | 4 |
| Chicago Bagel Dog Everything | 1 | 730 | 80 | 6 | 3 |
| Chicago Bagel Dog Onion w/o Cheese | 1 | 680 | 78 | 6 | 2 |
| Country White Deli Chicken Salad | 1 | 540 | 75 | 8 | 4 |
| Country White Deli Egg Salad | 1 | 590 | 77 | 8 | 3 |
| Country White Deli Ham | 1 | 660 | 75 | 8 | 3 |
| Country White Deli Roast Beef | 1 | 660 | 76 | 8 | 3 |
| Country White Deli Smoked Turkey | 1 | 630 | 76 | 9 | 3 |
| Country White Deli Tuna Salad | 1 | 510 | 74 | 7 | 4 |
| Country White Deli Turkey Pastrami | 1 | 640 | 75 | 9 | 3 |
| Country White Ultimate Toasted Cheese w/ Tomato | 1 | 870 | 73 | 7 | 2 |
| Panini Cali Club | 1 | 730 | 90 | 15 | 9 |
| Panini Cuban Ham | 1 | 700 | 68 | 2 | 4 |
| Panini Denver Omelet Breakfast | 1 | 740 | 70 | 4 | 3 |
| Panini Italian Chicken | 1 | 770 | 69 | 3 | 4 |
| Panini Ultimate Toasted Cheese | 1 | 900 | 96 | 19 | 7 |
| Roll Ups Albuquerque Turkey | 1 | 790 | 81 | 28 | 5 |
| Roll Ups Thai Vegetable w/ Chicken | 1 | 670 | 99 | 26 | 4 |
| Roll Ups Thai Vegetables | 1 | 630 | 97 | 17 | 5 |
| **SOUPS** | | | | | |
| Broccoli Sharp Cheddar | 1 cup | 230 | 13 | 8 | 1 |
| Chicken & Wild Rice | 1 cup | 190 | 29 | 3 | 2 |
| Chicken Noodle | 1 cup | 220 | 17 | 2 | 2 |
| Clam Chowda | 1 cup | 160 | 11 | 1 | 0 |
| Minestroni Low Fat | 1 cup | 180 | 32 | 7 | 5 |
| Tomato Bisque | 1 cup | 190 | 23 | 9 | 3 |
| Tortilla | 1 cup | 90 | 14 | 5 | 2 |
| Turkey Chili | 1 cup | 140 | 14 | 4 | 2 |
| **SPREADS** | | | | | |
| Butter | 1 tbsp | 100 | 0 | 0 | 0 |
| Butter & Margarine Blend | 1 tbsp | 60 | 0 | 0 | 0 |
| Cream Cheese Blueberry | 1 tbsp | 70 | 6 | 5 | 0 |
| Cream Cheese Cappuccino | 2 tbsp | 70 | 4 | 4 | 0 |

| FOOD | PORTION | CALS | CARB | SUGAR | FIBER |
|---|---|---|---|---|---|
| Cream Cheese Garden Vegetable | 2 tbsp | 60 | 2 | 1 | 0 |
| Cream Cheese Honey Almond Reduced Fat | 2 tbsp | 70 | 5 | 4 | 0 |
| Cream Cheese Jalapeno Salsa | 1 tbsp | 60 | 3 | 1 | 0 |
| Cream Cheese Maple Walnut Raisin | 2 tbsp | 60 | 4 | 3 | 0 |
| Cream Cheese Plain Reduced Fat | 2 tbsp | 60 | 2 | 1 | 0 |
| Cream Cheese Pumpkin | 2 tbsp | 100 | 6 | 5 | 0 |
| Cream Cheese Smoked Salmon | 2 tbsp | 60 | 3 | 1 | 0 |
| Cream Cheese Strawberry | 2 tbsp | 70 | 5 | 4 | 0 |
| Cream Cheese Sun Dried Tomato & Basil | 2 tbsp | 60 | 2 | 1 | 0 |
| Fruit Spread Strawberry | 1 serv (1 oz) | 75 | 19 | 0 | 0 |
| Honey Butter | 1 tbsp | 90 | 4 | 3 | 0 |
| Hummus | 1 serv | 110 | 9 | 2 | 2 |
| Mayo Ancho Lime | 1 tbsp | 50 | 1 | 0 | 0 |
| Mustard French Dijon | 1 tsp | 10 | 0 | 0 | 0 |
| Mustard Grain Dijon | 1 tsp | 5 | 0 | 0 | 0 |
| Mustard Honey | 1 tsp | 15 | 2 | 0 | 0 |
| Mustard Raspberry | 2 tbsp | 50 | 7 | 5 | 0 |
| Mustard Yellow | 1 tbsp | 5 | 0 | 0 | 0 |
| Peanut Butter | 2 tbsp | 190 | 8 | 3 | 2 |
| Salsa Ancho Lime | ¼ cup | 20 | 3 | 0 | 0 |
| **EL POLLO LOCO** | | | | | |
| **DESSERTS** | | | | | |
| Churro | 1 | 179 | 18 | 0 | 1 |
| Fosters Freeze Soft Serve | 1 cup | 180 | 30 | 26 | 0 |
| **MAIN MENU SELECTIONS** | | | | | |
| Bowl Chicken Caesar | 1 serv | 535 | 46 | 4 | 4 |
| Bowl Pollo | 1 serv | 545 | 84 | 1 | 12 |
| Bowl Veggie | 1 serv | 570 | 91 | 3 | 16 |
| Bowl Veggie w/o Cheese | 1 serv | 529 | 91 | 3 | 16 |
| Burrito Classic Chicken | 1 | 580 | 66 | 1 | 6 |
| Burrito Twice Grilled | 1 serv | 835 | 60 | 3 | 2 |
| Burrito BRC | 1 serv | 530 | 79 | 1 | 6 |
| Burrito Caesar | 1 serv | 895 | 76 | 3 | 4 |
| Burrito Chicken Lover's | 1 serv | 525 | 55 | 2 | 2 |

| FOOD | PORTION | CALS | CARB | SUGAR | FIBER |
|---|---|---|---|---|---|
| Burrito Spicy | 1 serv | 555 | 64 | 2 | 9 |
| Burrito Ultimate Chicken | 1 serv | 685 | 84 | 2 | 6 |
| Chicken Breast | 1 piece | 153 | 0 | 0 | 0 |
| Chicken Leg | 1 piece | 86 | 0 | 0 | 0 |
| Chicken Thigh | 1 piece | 120 | 0 | 0 | 0 |
| Chicken Wing | 1 | 83 | 0 | 0 | 0 |
| Cole Slaw | 1 serv | 206 | 12 | 5 | 2 |
| Corn Cobbette | 1 serv | 80 | 18 | 4 | 1 |
| French Fries | 1 serv | 444 | 61 | 0 | 0 |
| Fresh Vegetables | 1 serv | 70 | 6 | 2 | 4 |
| Gravy | 1 serv (1 oz) | 107 | 15 | 4 | 0 |
| Mashed Potatoes | 1 serv | 97 | 21 | 1 | 2 |
| Nachos Chicken | 1 serv | 1420 | 105 | 6 | 15 |
| Pinto Beans | 1 serv | 165 | 26 | 0 | 10 |
| Popcorn Chicken | 1 serv | 226 | 15 | 0 | 0 |
| Potato Salad | 1 serv | 256 | 30 | 6 | 3 |
| Quesadilla Cheese | 1 serv | 495 | 45 | 2 | 2 |
| Quesadilla Chicken | 1 serv | 593 | 48 | 2 | 0 |
| Smokey Black Beans | 1 serv | 306 | 35 | 19 | 5 |
| Spanish Rice | 1 serv | 165 | 34 | 0 | 1 |
| Taco Al Carbon Chicken | 1 serv | 135 | 18 | 0 | 1 |
| Taco Soft Chicken | 1 | 237 | 15 | 1 | 0 |
| Taquitos Chicken | 2 | 370 | 43 | 2 | 3 |
| Tortilla Chips | 1 serv | 426 | 48 | 1 | 4 |
| Tortilla Corn | 1 (6 inches) | 70 | 14 | 0 | 1 |
| Tortilla Corn | 1 (4.5 inch) | 40 | 8 | 0 | 1 |
| Tortilla Flour | 1 (6.5 inch) | 110 | 13 | 0 | 0 |
| Tortilla Flour | 1 (12 inches) | 325 | 51 | 1 | 2 |
| Tortilla Spicy Tomato | 1 (12 inches) | 270 | 43 | 1 | 2 |
| Tostada Salad | 1 serv | 700 | 76 | 8 | 10 |
| **SALAD DRESSINGS AND TOPPINGS** | | | | | |
| Bleu Cheese | 1 serv (1.5 oz) | 230 | 2 | 2 | 0 |
| Buttermilk Ranch | 1 serv (1.5 oz) | 220 | 2 | 2 | 0 |
| Creamy Chipotle | 1 (0.5 oz) | 75 | 1 | 0 | 0 |
| Creamy Cilantro | 1 serv (0.5 oz) | 80 | 0 | 0 | 0 |
| Guacamole | 1 serv (1 oz) | 30 | 3 | 0 | 0 |
| Hot Sauce Jalapeno | 1 pkg (0.5 oz) | 5 | 1 | 0 | 0 |
| Light Italian | 1 serv (1.5 oz) | 20 | 2 | 2 | 0 |
| Salsa Avocado | 1 serv (1 oz) | 20 | 1 | 0 | 0 |
| Salsa House | 1 serv (1 oz) | 6 | 1 | 1 | 0 |

| FOOD | PORTION | CALS | CARB | SUGAR | FIBER |
|---|---|---|---|---|---|
| Salsa Spicy Chipotle | 1 serv (1 oz) | 7 | 1 | 1 | 0 |
| Sour Cream | 1 serv (1 oz) | 60 | 1 | 1 | 0 |
| Thousand Island | 1 serv (1.5 oz) | 220 | 7 | 7 | 0 |
| **SALADS** | | | | | |
| Caesar | 1 serv | 565 | 18 | 5 | 3 |
| Ceasar w/o Dressing | 1 serv | 250 | 16 | 4 | 3 |
| Fiesta Salad | 1 serv | 755 | 28 | 6 | 4 |
| Fiesta Salad w/o Dressing | 1 serv | 450 | 25 | 5 | 4 |
| Garden Salad | 1 serv | 110 | 8 | 2 | 2 |
| Tostada Salad w/o Shell | 1 serv | 360 | 34 | 3 | 6 |

## FAZOLI'S

| FOOD | PORTION | CALS | CARB | SUGAR | FIBER |
|---|---|---|---|---|---|
| **DESSERTS** | | | | | |
| Cheesecake | 1 slice | 290 | 17 | 17 | 0 |
| Cheesecake Turtle | 1 slice | 420 | 24 | 21 | 2 |
| Cookie Milk Chocolate Chunk | 1 | 360 | 54 | 33 | 0 |
| Lemon Ice | 1 serv | 190 | 45 | 44 | 0 |
| Specialty Cheesecake | 1 serv | 300 | 22 | 19 | 1 |
| Strawberry Topping | 1 serv | 35 | 8 | 8 | 0 |
| **MAIN MENU SELECTIONS** | | | | | |
| Baked Chicken Parmesan | 1 serv | 740 | 99 | 10 | 6 |
| Baked Spaghetti Parmesan | 1 serv | 700 | 76 | 8 | 5 |
| Baked Ziti | 1 sm | 490 | 56 | 7 | 4 |
| Baked Ziti | 1 reg | 750 | 87 | 11 | 6 |
| Breadstick | 1 | 140 | 18 | 1 | 1 |
| Breadstick Dry | 1 | 90 | 17 | 1 | 1 |
| Broccoli Fettuccine Alfredo | 1 sm | 560 | 85 | 5 | 6 |
| Broccoli Fettuccine Alfredo | 1 reg | 830 | 125 | 5 | 6 |
| Cheese Ravioli w/ Marinara Sauce | 1 serv | 480 | 65 | 9 | 4 |
| Cheese Ravioli w/ Meat Sauce | 1 serv | 510 | 65 | 8 | 4 |
| Classic Sampler | 1 serv | 710 | 97 | 9 | 6 |
| Fettuccine Alfredo | 1 sm | 530 | 80 | 3 | 3 |
| Fettuccine Alfredo | 1 reg | 800 | 119 | 5 | 5 |
| Fettuccine w/ Shrimp & Scallop | 1 serv | 590 | 81 | 3 | 3 |
| Homestyle Lasagna | 1 serv | 440 | 41 | 7 | 4 |
| Homestyle Lasagna w/ Broccoli | 1 serv | 420 | 45 | 4 | 5 |
| Minestrone Soup | 1 serv | 120 | 23 | 8 | 8 |
| Peppery Chicken Alfredo | 1 serv | 610 | 80 | 3 | 3 |
| Pizza Cheese | 1 serv | 460 | 58 | 6 | 2 |

| FOOD | PORTION | CALS | CARB | SUGAR | FIBER |
|---|---|---|---|---|---|
| Pizza Combination Double Slice | 1 serv | 570 | 63 | 7 | 3 |
| Pizza Pepperoni | 1 serv | 530 | 61 | 6 | 2 |
| Pizza Baked Spaghetti | 1 serv | 750 | 78 | 8 | 5 |
| Spaghetti w/ Marinara Sauce | 1 sm | 420 | 74 | 8 | 5 |
| Spaghetti w/ Marinara Sauce | 1 reg | 620 | 111 | 12 | 7 |
| Spaghetti w/ Meat Sauce | 1 reg | 670 | 111 | 11 | 8 |
| Spaghetti w/ Meat Sauce | 1 sm | 450 | 74 | 8 | 5 |
| Spaghetti w/ Meatballs | 1 reg | 1020 | 119 | 13 | 8 |
| Spaghetti w/ Meatballs | 1 sm | 730 | 80 | 9 | 6 |
| **SALAD DRESSINGS** | | | | | |
| Honey French | 1 serv | 150 | 9 | 9 | 0 |
| House Italian | 1 serv | 110 | 5 | 5 | 0 |
| Ranch | 1 serv | 150 | 1 | 1 | 0 |
| Reduced Calorie Italian | 1 serv | 50 | 3 | 2 | 0 |
| Thousand Island | 1 serv | 130 | 4 | 4 | 0 |
| **SALADS AND SALAD BARS** | | | | | |
| Caesar Side Salad | 1 | 220 | 13 | 3 | 3 |
| Chicken & Pasta Caesar Salad | 1 | 500 | 35 | 8 | 4 |
| Chicken Caesar Salad | 1 | 420 | 17 | 5 | 4 |
| Chicken Finger Salad | 1 | 190 | 8 | 4 | 2 |
| Chicken Finger Salad w/ Bacon & Honey Mustard | 1 | 400 | 17 | 13 | 2 |
| Garden Salad | 1 | 25 | 4 | 3 | 1 |
| Garden Salad w/ Balsamic Vinaigrette | 1 | 120 | 10 | 8 | 1 |
| Italian Chef Salad | 1 | 260 | 13 | 3 | 3 |
| Pasta Salad | 1 serv | 590 | 70 | 13 | 5 |
| **SANDWICHES** | | | | | |
| Panini Chicken Caesar Club | 1 | 660 | 51 | 1 | 3 |
| Panini Chicken Pesto | 1 | 510 | 51 | 1 | 3 |
| Panini Four Cheese & Tomato | 1 | 720 | 55 | 3 | 3 |
| Panini Ham & Swiss | 1 | 600 | 53 | 4 | 2 |
| Panini Italian Club | 1 | 670 | 54 | 3 | 3 |
| Panini Italian Deli | 1 | 660 | 61 | 1 | 4 |
| Panini Smoked Turkey | 1 | 710 | 57 | 3 | 3 |
| Submarinos Club | half | 1100 | 121 | 8 | 7 |
| Submarinos Ham & Swiss | 1 | 1000 | 120 | 8 | 7 |
| Submarinos Meatball | half | 1260 | 128 | 10 | 8 |
| Submarinos Original | half | 1160 | 124 | 8 | 8 |
| Submarinos Pepperoni Pizza | half | 1060 | 133 | 11 | 6 |

| FOOD | PORTION | CALS | CARB | SUGAR | FIBER |
|---|---|---|---|---|---|
| Submarinos Turkey | half | 990 | 121 | 8 | 7 |
| **FRULLATI CAFE** | | | | | |
| **BEVERAGES** | | | | | |
| Smoothie | 1 serv (14 oz) | 195 | 41 | 27 | tr |
| **HÄAGEN-DAZS** | | | | | |
| **FROZEN YOGURT** | | | | | |
| Pinapple Coconut | ½ cup | 230 | 25 | 24 | 0 |
| Soft Serve Nonfat Chocolate | ½ cup | 110 | 23 | 20 | 0 |
| Soft Serve Nonfat Chocolate Mousse | ½ cup | 80 | 24 | 7 | 1 |
| Soft Serve Nonfat Coffee | ½ cup | 110 | 22 | 21 | 0 |
| Soft Serve Nonfat Strawberry | ½ cup | 110 | 24 | 23 | 0 |
| Soft Serve Nonfat Vanilla | ½ cup | 110 | 22 | 21 | 0 |
| Soft Serve Nonfat Vanilla Mousse | ½ cup | 70 | 23 | 7 | 0 |
| Soft Serve Nonfat White Chocolate | ½ cup | 110 | 22 | 21 | 0 |
| Vanilla Fudge | ½ cup | 160 | 34 | 22 | 0 |
| Vanilla Raspberry Swirl | ½ cup | 130 | 29 | 20 | tr |
| **ICE CREAM** | | | | | |
| Bailey's Irish Cream | ½ cup | 270 | 23 | 22 | 0 |
| Bar Chocolate | 1 (2.7 oz) | 200 | 16 | 15 | tr |
| Bar Chocolate & Dark Chocolate | 1 (3.6 oz) | 350 | 28 | 24 | 2 |
| Bar Coffee | 1 (2.7 oz) | 190 | 15 | 15 | 0 |
| Bar Coffee & Almond Crunch | 1 (3.7 oz) | 370 | 27 | 26 | tr |
| Bar Vanilla | 1 (2.7 oz) | 190 | 15 | 15 | 0 |
| Bar Vanilla & Almonds | 1 (3.7 oz) | 380 | 26 | 24 | 1 |
| Bar Vanilla & Milk Chocolate | 1 (3.5 oz) | 340 | 25 | 24 | tr |
| Belgian Chocolate Chocolate | ½ cup | 330 | 29 | 26 | 2 |
| Brownies A La Mode | ½ cup | 280 | 28 | 23 | tr |
| Butter Pecan | ½ cup | 300 | 20 | 17 | tr |
| Cappuccino Commotion | ½ cup | 310 | 25 | 23 | 1 |
| Chocolate | ½ cup | 269 | 21 | 20 | 1 |
| Chocolate Chocolate Chip | ½ cup | 300 | 26 | 23 | 2 |
| Chocolate Chocolate Mint | ½ cup | 300 | 25 | 22 | 1 |
| Chocolate Swiss Almond | ½ cup | 300 | 24 | 21 | 2 |
| Coffee | ½ cup | 250 | 20 | 20 | 0 |
| Coffee Mocha Chip | ½ cup | 270 | 24 | 21 | tr |
| Cookie Dough Dynamo | ½ cup | 310 | 29 | 24 | 0 |

| FOOD | PORTION | CALS | CARB | SUGAR | FIBER |
|---|---|---|---|---|---|
| Cookies & Cream | ½ cup | 270 | 23 | 21 | 0 |
| Cookies & Fudge | ½ cup | 180 | 33 | 20 | tr |
| Deep Chocolate Peanut Butter | ½ cup | 350 | 26 | 21 | 4 |
| Dulce De Leche Caramel | ½ cup | 270 | 27 | 27 | 0 |
| Lowfat Coffee Fudge | ½ cup | 170 | 32 | 22 | 0 |
| Macadamia Brittle | ½ cup | 280 | 24 | 23 | 0 |
| Macadamia Nut | ½ cup | 320 | 20 | 19 | 0 |
| Mint Chip | ½ cup | 280 | 25 | 22 | tr |
| Pistachio | ½ cup | 280 | 21 | 18 | tr |
| Pralines & Cream | ½ cup | 280 | 28 | 26 | 0 |
| Rum Raisin | ½ cup | 260 | 21 | 20 | 0 |
| Strawberry | ½ cup | 250 | 22 | 21 | tr |
| Vanilla | ½ cup | 250 | 20 | 20 | 0 |
| Vanilla Chocolate Chip | ½ cup | 290 | 25 | 22 | tr |
| Vanilla Swiss Almond | ½ cup | 290 | 23 | 20 | tr |
| **SORBET** | | | | | |
| Bar Raspberry & Vanilla | 1 (2.5 oz) | 90 | 21 | 15 | tr |
| Mango | ½ cup | 120 | 31 | 29 | tr |
| Orange | ½ cup | 120 | 30 | 24 | tr |
| Raspberry | ½ cup | 120 | 30 | 26 | 2 |
| Soft Serve Raspberry | ½ cup | 110 | 28 | 25 | 2 |
| Strawberry | ½ cup | 120 | 30 | 27 | 1 |
| Zesty Lemon | ½ cup | 120 | 31 | 27 | tr |

## HUNGRY HOWIE'S

| FOOD | PORTION | CALS | CARB | SUGAR | FIBER |
|---|---|---|---|---|---|
| **MAIN MENU SELECTIONS** | | | | | |
| Howie Wings | 6 (3 oz) | 180 | 0 | – | 0 |
| Three Cheeser Bread | 1 serv | 370 | 47 | – | 1 |
| **PIZZA** | | | | | |
| Large Cheese | 1 slice | 175 | 24 | – | 1 |
| Large Cheese + Bacon | 1 slice | 208 | 25 | – | 1 |
| Large Cheese + Beef | 1 slice | 197 | 24 | – | 1 |
| Large Cheese + Black Olives | 1 slice | 181 | 24 | – | 1 |
| Large Cheese + Green Olives | 1 slice | 181 | 24 | – | 1 |
| Large Cheese + Green Peppers | 1 slice | 175 | 24 | – | 1 |
| Large Cheese + Ham | 1 slice | 179 | 24 | – | 1 |
| Large Cheese + Mushrooms | 1 slice | 175 | 24 | – | 1 |
| Large Cheese + Onions | 1 slice | 175 | 24 | – | 1 |
| Large Cheese + Pepperoni | 1 slice | 191 | 24 | – | 1 |
| Large Cheese + Pineapple | 1 slice | 388 | 25 | – | 1 |

| FOOD | PORTION | CALS | CARB | SUGAR | FIBER |
|---|---|---|---|---|---|
| Large Cheese + Sausage | 1 slice | 195 | 24 | – | 1 |
| Medium Cheese | 1 slice | 153 | 21 | – | 1 |
| Medium Cheese + Bacon | 1 slice | 179 | 21 | – | 1 |
| Medium Cheese + Beef | 1 slice | 177 | 21 | – | 1 |
| Medium Cheese + Black Olives | 1 slice | 159 | 21 | – | 1 |
| Medium Cheese + Green Olives | 1 slice | 159 | 21 | – | 1 |
| Medium Cheese + Green Peppers | 1 slice | 155 | 21 | – | 1 |
| Medium Cheese + Ham | 1 slice | 159 | 21 | – | 1 |
| Medium Cheese + Mushrooms | 1 slice | 155 | 21 | – | 1 |
| Medium Cheese + Onions | 1 slice | 155 | 21 | – | 1 |
| Medium Cheese + Pepperoni | 1 slice | 171 | 21 | – | 1 |
| Medium Cheese + Pineapple | 1 slice | 158 | 22 | – | 1 |
| Medium Cheese + Sausage | 1 slice | 175 | 21 | – | 1 |
| Small Cheese | 1 slice | 121 | 37 | – | 1 |
| Small Cheese + Bacon | 1 slice | 138 | 17 | – | 1 |
| Small Cheese + Beef | 1 slice | 137 | 17 | – | 1 |
| Small Cheese + Black Olives | 1 slice | 125 | 17 | – | 1 |
| Small Cheese + Green Olives | 1 slice | 125 | 17 | – | 1 |
| Small Cheese + Green Peppers | 1 slice | 122 | 17 | – | 1 |
| Small Cheese + Ham | 1 slice | 126 | 17 | – | 1 |
| Small Cheese + Mushrooms | 1 slice | 123 | 17 | – | 1 |
| Small Cheese + Onions | 1 slice | 122 | 17 | – | 1 |
| Small Cheese + Pepperoni | 1 slice | 136 | 17 | – | 1 |
| Small Cheese + Pineapple | 1 slice | 124 | 18 | – | 1 |
| Small Cheese + Sausage | 1 slice | 136 | 17 | – | 1 |
| **SALADS AND SALAD BARS** | | | | | |
| Antipasto Salad w/o Dressing | 1 lg | 101 | 3 | – | 1 |
| Chef Salad w/o Dressing | 1 lg | 99 | 4 | – | 2 |
| Garden Salad w/o Dressing | 1 lg | 17 | 3 | – | 2 |
| Greek Salad w/o Dressing | 1 lg | 109 | 7 | – | 2 |
| **SANDWICHES** | | | | | |
| Sub Deluxe Italian | ½ sub | 506 | 61 | – | 2 |
| Sub Ham & Cheese | ½ sub | 475 | 61 | – | 2 |
| Sub Pizza | ½ sub | 689 | 67 | – | 3 |
| Sub Pizza Special | ½ sub | 606 | 68 | – | 3 |
| Sub Steak Cheese Mushroom | ½ sub | 491 | 64 | – | 2 |
| Sub Turkey | ½ sub | 466 | 63 | – | 2 |
| Sub Turkey Club | ½ sub | 556 | 62 | – | 2 |
| Sub Vegetarian | ½ sub | 530 | 64 | – | 3 |

| FOOD | PORTION | CALS | CARB | SUGAR | FIBER |
|---|---|---|---|---|---|
| **JACK IN THE BOX** | | | | | |
| **BEVERAGES** | | | | | |
| Barq's Root Beer | 1 serv (20 oz) | 180 | 50 | 50 | 0 |
| Coca-Cola Classic | 1 serv (20 oz) | 170 | 46 | 46 | 0 |
| Coffee | 1 serv (12 oz) | 5 | 1 | 0 | 0 |
| Diet Coke | 1 serv (20 oz) | 0 | 0 | 0 | 0 |
| Dr Pepper | 1 serv (20 oz) | 190 | 50 | 50 | 0 |
| Ice Cream Shake Caramel | 1 serv (16 oz) | 660 | 86 | 74 | 0 |
| Ice Cream Shake Chocolate | 1 (16 oz) | 660 | 89 | 79 | 1 |
| Ice Cream Shake Oreo | 1 serv (16 oz) | 670 | 81 | 62 | 1 |
| Ice Cream Shake Strawberry | 1 serv (16 oz) | 640 | 84 | 71 | 0 |
| Ice Cream Shake Strawberry Banana | 1 serv (16 oz) | 700 | 100 | 67 | 0 |
| Ice Cream Shake Vanilla | 1 (16 oz) | 570 | 65 | 54 | 0 |
| Iced Tea | 1 serv (20 oz) | 0 | 0 | 0 | 0 |
| Lowfat Milk 2% | 1 serv (8 oz) | 140 | 14 | 13 | 0 |
| Orange Juice | 1 serv (10 oz) | 140 | 32 | 27 | 2 |
| Sprite | 1 serv (20 oz) | 160 | 41 | 41 | 0 |
| **BREAKFAST SELECTIONS** | | | | | |
| Breakfast Sandwich Sourdough | 1 | 440 | 36 | 3 | 2 |
| Breakfast Sandwich Ultimate | 1 | 730 | 66 | 9 | 2 |
| Breakfast Jack | 1 | 310 | 33 | 4 | 1 |
| Croissant Sausage | 1 | 680 | 41 | 5 | 2 |
| Croissant Supreme | 1 | 570 | 41 | 5 | 1 |
| French Toast Sticks | 4 pieces | 430 | 57 | 11 | 2 |
| Hash Brown | 1 serv | 150 | 13 | 0 | 2 |
| Sandwich Extreme Sausage | 1 | 720 | 35 | 5 | 2 |
| **DESSERTS** | | | | | |
| Cheesecake | 1 serv | 310 | 34 | 23 | 0 |
| Double Fudge Cake | 1 serv | 310 | 49 | 37 | 4 |
| **MAIN MENU SELECTIONS** | | | | | |
| American Cheese | 1 slice | 45 | 1 | 0 | 0 |
| Bacon Cheddar Potato Wedges | 1 serv | 770 | 52 | 2 | 4 |
| Cheeseburger Bacon Bacon | 1 | 910 | 58 | 10 | 3 |
| Cheeseburger Bacon Ultimate | 1 | 1120 | 59 | 12 | 2 |
| Cheeseburger Junior Bacon | 1 | 540 | 31 | 6 | 1 |
| Cheeseburger Ultimate | 1 | 990 | 59 | 12 | 2 |
| Chicken Breast Pieces | 4 | 360 | 24 | 0 | 1 |
| Chicken Breast Strips | 1 serv | 500 | 36 | 1 | 3 |
| Chicken Fajita Pita | 1 | 330 | 35 | 4 | 3 |

| FOOD | PORTION | CALS | CARB | SUGAR | FIBER |
|---|---|---|---|---|---|
| Chicken Sandwich | 1 | 410 | 39 | 4 | 2 |
| Dipping Sauce Barbeque | 1 serv (1.6 oz) | 45 | 11 | 4 | 0 |
| Egg Rolls | 1 | 130 | 15 | 1 | 2 |
| Fish & Chips | 1 serv | 610 | 66 | 0 | 5 |
| French Fries | 1 lg | 580 | 77 | 0 | 6 |
| French Fries | 1 med | 410 | 55 | 0 | 4 |
| French Fries | 1 sm | 330 | 44 | 0 | 3 |
| Hamburger | 1 | 310 | 30 | 6 | 1 |
| Hamburger w/ Cheese | 1 | 360 | 31 | 6 | 1 |
| Jumbo Jack | 1 | 600 | 58 | 12 | 3 |
| Jumbo Jack w/ Cheese | 1 | 690 | 61 | 13 | 3 |
| Onion Rings | 1 serv | 500 | 51 | 3 | 3 |
| Philly Cheesesteak | 1 | 580 | 55 | 6 | 3 |
| Salsa | 1 serv (1 oz) | 10 | 2 | 1 | 0 |
| Sandwich Roasted Turkey | 1 | 580 | 50 | 5 | 3 |
| Sandwich Ultimate Club | 1 | 640 | 51 | 7 | 3 |
| Seasoned Curly Fries | 1 serv | 400 | 45 | 1 | 5 |
| Sour Cream | 1 serv (1 oz) | 60 | 2 | 0 | 0 |
| Sourdough Grilled Chicken Club | 1 | 520 | 33 | 5 | 3 |
| Sourdough Jack | 1 | 700 | 36 | 7 | 3 |
| Spicy Crispy Chicken | 1 | 730 | 69 | 9 | 4 |
| Stuffed Jalapeno | 3 pieces | 230 | 22 | 2 | 2 |
| Swiss Style Cheese | 1 slice | 40 | 1 | 0 | 0 |
| Taco | 1 | 170 | 15 | 2 | 2 |
| Taco Monster | 1 | 260 | 21 | 4 | 3 |
| Turkey Jack | 1 | 700 | 69 | 18 | 4 |
| **SALAD DRESSINGS AND TOPPINGS** | | | | | |
| Almonds Roasted Silvered | 1 serv (0.7 oz) | 130 | 4 | 1 | 2 |
| Asian Sesame | 1 serv (2.5 oz) | 230 | 20 | 13 | 0 |
| Bacon Ranch | 1 serv (2.5 oz) | 320 | 5 | 2 | 0 |
| Balsamic Vinaigrette Low Fat | 1 serv (2.5 oz) | 40 | 6 | 3 | 0 |
| Country Crock Spread | 1 pkg | 25 | 0 | 0 | 0 |
| Creamy Southwest Dressing | 1 serv (2.5 oz) | 270 | 7 | 2 | 0 |
| Dipping Sauce Buttermilk House | 1 serv (0.9 oz) | 130 | 3 | 0 | 0 |
| Dipping Sauce Frank's Red Hot Buffalo | 1 serv (1 oz) | 10 | 2 | 0 | 0 |
| Dipping Sauce Sweet & Sour | 1 serv (1 oz) | 45 | 11 | 6 | 0 |
| Grape Jelly | 1 serv (0.5 oz) | 35 | 9 | 9 | 0 |
| Herb Mayo Sauce Low Fat | 1 serv (1.5 oz) | 45 | 3 | 1 | 1 |

| FOOD | PORTION | CALS | CARB | SUGAR | FIBER |
|---|---|---|---|---|---|
| Ketchup | 1 pkg (0.3 oz) | 10 | 2 | 2 | 0 |
| Marinara Sauce | 1 serv (0.9 oz) | 15 | 3 | 3 | 0 |
| Mustard | 1 pkg | 0 | 0 | 0 | 0 |
| Ranch | 1 serv (2.5 oz) | 390 | 4 | 2 | 0 |
| Ranch Lite | 1 serv (2.5 oz) | 190 | 3 | 2 | 0 |
| Soy Sauce | 1 serv (0.3 oz) | 5 | 1 | 0 | 0 |
| Syrup | 1 serv (1.5 oz) | 130 | 32 | 27 | 0 |
| Taco Sauce | 1 serv (0.3 oz) | 0 | 0 | 0 | 0 |
| Tartar Sauce | 1 serv (1.5 oz) | 210 | 2 | 1 | 0 |
| Thousand Island | 1 serv (2 oz) | 160 | 12 | 10 | 0 |
| Vinegar | 1 serv | 0 | 0 | 0 | 0 |
| Wonton Strips | 1 serv (0.7 oz) | 110 | 13 | 1 | 2 |
| **SALADS** | | | | | |
| Asian Salad | 1 serv | 140 | 18 | 11 | 6 |
| Chicken Club Salad | 1 serv | 290 | 12 | 5 | 5 |
| Side Salad | 1 serv | 50 | 4 | 2 | 2 |
| Southwest Chicken | 1 serv | 320 | 28 | 6 | 8 |
| **JAMBA JUICE** | | | | | |
| Jambolas Honey Nut Energy | 1 serv | 192 | – | - | 2 |
| Jambolas Mighty Multi Grain | 1 serv | 208 | – | - | 5 |
| Jambolas Mind Over Blueberry | 1 serv | 170 | – | - | 2 |
| Jambolas Pizza Protein | 1 serv | 199 | – | - | 3 |
| Mango-A-Go-Go | 1 reg (24 oz) | 460 | – | - | 3 |
| Orchard Oasis | 1 reg (24 oz) | 440 | – | - | 4 |
| Protein Berry Pizazz | 1 reg (24 oz) | 470 | – | - | 6 |
| Razzmatazz | 1 reg (24 oz) | 440 | – | - | 4 |
| **JERSEY MIKE'S** | | | | | |
| Ham On Wheat | 1 | 240 | 31 | – | 2 |
| Ham/Turkey Wheat | 1 | 230 | 32 | – | 1 |
| Ham/Turkey White | 1 | 240 | 32 | – | 2 |
| Roast Beef Wheat | 1 | 290 | 30 | – | 2 |
| Roast Beef White | 1 | 280 | 30 | – | 0 |
| Turkey On White | 1 | 230 | 18 | – | 1 |
| Veggie On Wheat | 1 | 170 | 32 | – | 2 |
| Veggie On White | 1 | 170 | 31 | – | 2 |
| **KOO-KOO-ROO** | | | | | |
| Original Breast | 1 piece | 187 | tr | – | 0 |
| Original Chicken Dark | 3 pieces | 320 | 5 | – | 0 |

| FOOD | PORTION | CALS | CARB | SUGAR | FIBER |
|---|---|---|---|---|---|
| Rotisserie Chicken Breast & Wing | 1 serv | 355 | 1 | – | tr |
| Rotisserie Chicken Leg & Thigh | 1 serv | 300 | 1 | – | tr |
| Rotisserie Half Chicken | 1 serv | 655 | 2 | – | tr |
| Sandwich BBQ Chicken | 1 | 562 | 71 | – | 3 |
| Sandwich Chicken Caesar | 1 | 781 | 63 | – | 2 |
| Sandwich Original Chicken | 1 | 661 | 63 | – | 3 |
| Traditional Turkey Dinner | 1 serv | 692 | 67 | – | 8 |
| Turkey Pot Pie | 1 serv | 883 | 83 | – | 6 |
| Turkey Sandwich Hand Carved | 1 | 599 | 31 | – | 5 |
| Wrap Caesar Chicken | 1 | 757 | 59 | – | 4 |
| Wrap Chipotle Chicken | 1 | 924 | 89 | – | 6 |
| **KRISPY KREME** | | | | | |
| Chocolate Iced | 1 (2 oz) | 260 | 30 | 24 | 1 |
| Chocolate Iced Cake | 1 (2 oz) | 230 | 28 | 11 | tr |
| Chocolate Iced Creme Filled | 1 (2.3 oz) | 270 | 32 | 19 | 2 |
| Chocolate Iced Cruller | 1 (1.7 oz) | 240 | 26 | 8 | tr |
| Chocolate Iced Custard Filled | 1 (2.7 oz) | 250 | 38 | 26 | 3 |
| Chocolated Iced w/ Sprinkles | 1 (2 oz) | 220 | 31 | 19 | tr |
| Cinnamon Apple Filled | 1 (2.3 oz) | 210 | 29 | 11 | 3 |
| Cinnamon Bun | 1 (2.1 oz) | 220 | 26 | 7 | 4 |
| Glazed Blueberry | 1 (2.4 oz) | 300 | 37 | 29 | 1 |
| Glazed Creme Filled | 1 (2.3 oz) | 270 | 32 | 19 | 2 |
| Glazed Cruller | 1 (1.5 oz) | 220 | 22 | 5 | 0 |
| Glazed Devil's Food | 1 (1.9 oz) | 240 | 29 | 20 | 3 |
| Lemon Filled | 1 (2.2 oz) | 210 | 28 | 14 | tr |
| Maple Iced | 1 (1.8 oz) | 200 | 28 | 18 | 2 |
| Original Glazed | 1 (1.3 oz) | 180 | 17 | 7 | tr |
| Powdered Blueberry Filled | 1 (2.1 oz) | 200 | 26 | 9 | 2 |
| Powdered Cake | 1 (1.8 oz) | 220 | 26 | 10 | 0 |
| Raspberry Filled | 1 (2 oz) | 210 | 27 | 16 | 3 |
| Traditional Cake | 1 (1.7 oz) | 200 | 22 | 7 | tr |
| **MAUI WOWI** | | | | | |
| Smoothie Rip Sticks All Flavors | 1 | 88 | 22 | 17 | 0 |
| **MAX & ERMA'S** | | | | | |
| Black Bean Roll Up | 1 serv | 401 | 71 | – | 8 |
| Black Bean Salsa | ½ cup | 215 | 17 | – | 5 |

| FOOD | PORTION | CALS | CARB | SUGAR | FIBER |
|---|---|---|---|---|---|
| Fruit Smoothie | 1 serv | 124 | 29 | – | 1 |
| Garden Grill Sandwich w/ Tex Mex Dressing | 1 | 569 | 101 | – | 14 |
| Garlic Breadstick | 1 | 156 | 21 | – | 0 |
| Hula Bowl w/ Fat Free Honey Mustard Dressing w/o Breadsticks | 1 serv | 583 | 73 | – | 5 |
| Salad Dressing Fat Free French | 2 tbsp | 126 | 31 | – | 2 |
| Salad Dressing Fat Free Honey Mustard | 2 tbsp | 60 | 14 | – | 0 |
| Salad Dressing Tex Mex | 2 tbsp | 33 | 2 | – | tr |
| Sugar Snap Peas w/ Lemon Pepper Butter | 1 serv (4 oz) | 106 | 8 | – | 3 |
| **McDONALD'S** | | | | | |
| **BAKED SELECTIONS** | | | | | |
| Apple Pie Baked | 1 (2.7 oz) | 260 | 34 | 13 | tr |
| Cinnamon Roll | 1 (3.5 oz) | 340 | 52 | 28 | 3 |
| Cookie Chocolate Chip | 1 (1.4 oz) | 170 | 23 | 14 | tr |
| McDonaldland Cookies | 1 pkg (2 oz) | 230 | 38 | 12 | 1 |
| **BEVERAGES** | | | | | |
| Coca-Cola Classic | 1 sm (16 oz) | 150 | 40 | 40 | 0 |
| Coca-Cola Classic | 1 lg (32 oz) | 310 | 86 | 86 | 0 |
| Coffee | 1 sm (8 oz) | 0 | tr | 0 | 0 |
| Coffee | 1 lg (16 oz) | 10 | 2 | 0 | 0 |
| Diet Coke | 1 sm (16 oz) | 0 | 0 | 0 | 0 |
| Diet Coke | 1 lg (32 oz) | 0 | 0 | 0 | 0 |
| Half & Half Creamer | 1 pkg | 15 | 0 | 0 | 0 |
| Hi-C Orange | 1 sm (16 oz) | 160 | 44 | 44 | 0 |
| Hi-C Orange | 1 lg (32 oz) | 350 | 94 | 94 | 0 |
| Iced Tea | 1 lg (32 oz) | 0 | tr | 0 | 0 |
| Iced Tea | 1 sm (16 oz) | 0 | 0 | 0 | 0 |
| Milk Lowfat 1% | 1 serv (8 oz) | 100 | 13 | 13 | 0 |
| Orange Juice | 1 (12 oz) | 140 | 33 | 29 | 0 |
| Shake Strawberry | 1 (12 oz) | 420 | 67 | 59 | tr |
| Sprite | 1 sm (16 oz) | 150 | 39 | 39 | 0 |
| Sprite | 1 lg (32 oz) | 310 | 83 | 83 | – |
| Triple Shake Chocolate | 1 (12 oz) | 430 | 70 | 61 | 1 |
| Triple Shake Vanilla | 1 (12 oz) | 430 | 67 | 57 | 0 |

| FOOD | PORTION | CALS | CARB | SUGAR | FIBER |
|---|---|---|---|---|---|
| **BREAKFAST SELECTIONS** | | | | | |
| Bagel Ham Egg Cheese | 1 (7.7 oz) | 550 | 58 | 10 | 2 |
| Bagel Spanish Omelet | 1 (9.1 oz) | 710 | 59 | 10 | 3 |
| Bagel Steak Egg Cheese | 1 (8.5 oz) | 640 | 57 | 9 | 2 |
| Big Breakfast | 1 serv (9.4 oz) | 710 | 45 | 3 | 3 |
| Biscuit | 1 (2.4 oz) | 240 | 30 | 1 | 1 |
| Biscuit Bacon Egg Cheese | 1 (5.4 oz) | 480 | 31 | 3 | 1 |
| Biscuit Sausage | 1 (4 oz) | 410 | 30 | 2 | 1 |
| Biscuit Sausage w/ Egg | 1 (5.7 oz) | 490 | 31 | 2 | 1 |
| Breakfast Burrito Sausage | 1 (4 oz) | 290 | 24 | 2 | 2 |
| English Muffin | 1 (2 oz) | 150 | 27 | 2 | 2 |
| Hash Browns | 1 serv (1.9 oz) | 130 | 14 | 0 | 1 |
| Hotcakes Margarine & Syrup | 1 serv (8 oz) | 600 | 104 | 40 | 0 |
| McGriddles Bacon Egg & Cheese | 1 (5.9 oz) | 450 | 43 | 16 | 1 |
| McGriddles Sausage Egg Cheese | 1 (7 oz) | 550 | 43 | 16 | 1 |
| McMuffin Sausage | 1 (4 oz) | 370 | 28 | 2 | 2 |
| McMuffin Sausage w/ Egg | 1 (5.8 oz) | 450 | 29 | 3 | 2 |
| McMuffin Egg | 1 (4.9 oz) | 300 | 29 | 3 | 2 |
| Sausage | 1 (1.5 oz) | 170 | 0 | 0 | 0 |
| Scrambled Eggs | 2 (3.6 oz) | 160 | 1 | 1 | 0 |
| **DESSERTS** | | | | | |
| Fruit 'n Yogurt Parfait | 1 snack size (5.3 oz) | 160 | 30 | 21 | tr |
| Fruit 'n Yogurt Parfait | 1 serv (11.9 oz) | 380 | 76 | 49 | 2 |
| Fruit 'n Yogurt Parfait w/o Granola | 1 serv (5 oz) | 130 | 25 | 19 | 0 |
| Fruit 'n Yogurt Parfait w/o Granola | 1 serv (10.9 oz) | 280 | 53 | 40 | tr |
| Kiddo Cone | 1 (1 oz) | 45 | 7 | 6 | 0 |
| McDonaldland Chocolate Chip Cookies | 1 pkg (2 oz) | 280 | 37 | 20 | 1 |
| McFlurry Butterfinger | 1 (12 oz) | 620 | 90 | 76 | tr |
| McFlurry M&M | 1 (12 oz) | 630 | 90 | 81 | 1 |
| McFlurry Nestle Crunch | 1 (12 oz) | 630 | 89 | 78 | tr |
| McFlurry Oreo | 1 (12 oz) | 570 | 82 | 69 | tr |
| Nuts For Sundaes | 1 serv (7 g) | 40 | 2 | 0 | tr |

| FOOD | PORTION | CALS | CARB | SUGAR | FIBER |
|---|---|---|---|---|---|
| Reduced Fat Ice Cream Cone Vanilla | 1 (3.2 oz) | 150 | 23 | 17 | 0 |
| Sundae Hot Caramel | 1 (6.4 oz) | 360 | 61 | 47 | 0 |
| Sundae Hot Fudge | 1 (6.3 oz) | 340 | 52 | 47 | 1 |
| Sundae Strawberry | 1 (6.3 oz) | 290 | 50 | 46 | tr |
| Triple Shake Chocolate | 1 (32 oz) | 1150 | 187 | 163 | 3 |
| Triple Shake Raspberry | 1 (12 oz) | 420 | 67 | 58 | tr |
| Triple Shake Raspberry | 1 (32 oz) | 1120 | 179 | 154 | 2 |
| Triple Shake Strawberry | 1 (32 oz) | 1120 | 178 | 158 | 2 |
| Triple Shake Vanilla | 1 (32 oz) | 1140 | 178 | 152 | tr |
| **MAIN MENU SELECTIONS** | | | | | |
| Barbeque Sauce | 1 pkg (1 oz) | 45 | 10 | 10 | 0 |
| Big Mac | 1 (7.6 oz) | 560 | 47 | 7 | 3 |
| Big N' Tasty | 1 (8.2 oz) | 530 | 37 | 8 | 2 |
| Big N' Tasty w/ Cheese | 1 (8.7 oz) | 580 | 38 | 8 | 2 |
| Cheeseburger | 1 (4.2 oz) | 330 | 35 | 7 | 2 |
| Cheeseburger Double | 1 (6.1 oz) | 480 | 37 | 7 | 2 |
| Chicken McNuggets | 4 pieces (2.5 oz) | 210 | 12 | 0 | 1 |
| Chicken McNuggets | 6 pieces (3.8 oz) | 310 | 18 | 0 | 2 |
| Chicken McNuggets | 20 pieces (12.7 oz) | 1030 | 61 | 0 | 5 |
| Chicken McNuggets | 10 pieces (6.3 oz) | 510 | 30 | 0 | 3 |
| Chicken McGrill | 1 (7.5 oz) | 400 | 37 | 6 | 2 |
| Crispy Chicken | 1 serv (7.7 oz) | 500 | 46 | 6 | 2 |
| Filet-O-Fish | 1 (5.5 oz) | 470 | 45 | 5 | 1 |
| French Fries | 1 sm (2.4 oz) | 210 | 26 | 0 | 2 |
| French Fries | 1 lg (6.2 oz) | 540 | 68 | 0 | 6 |
| French Fries | 1 med (5.2 oz) | 450 | 57 | 0 | 5 |
| French Fries | 1 McValue (3.7 oz) | 320 | 40 | 0 | 4 |
| Hamburger | 1 (3.7 oz) | 280 | 35 | 7 | 2 |
| Honey | 1 pkg (0.5 oz) | 45 | 12 | 11 | 0 |
| Honey Mustard | 1 pkg (0.5 oz) | 50 | 3 | 3 | 0 |
| Hot Mustard | 1 pkg (0.5 oz) | 60 | 7 | 6 | tr |
| Light Mayonnaise | 1 pkg (0.4 oz) | 40 | tr | 0 | 0 |
| McChicken | 1 (5.2 oz) | 430 | 41 | 6 | 3 |

| FOOD | PORTION | CALS | CARB | SUGAR | FIBER |
|---|---|---|---|---|---|
| McChicken Hot 'n Spicy | 1 (5.1 oz) | 450 | 39 | 5 | 1 |
| Quarter Pounder | 1 (6.1 oz) | 420 | 36 | 8 | 2 |
| Quarter Pounder Double w/ Cheese | 1 (9.9 oz) | 760 | 38 | 9 | 2 |
| Quarter Pounder w/ Cheese | 1 (7 oz) | 530 | 38 | 9 | 2 |
| Sweet 'N Sour Sauce | 1 pkg (1 oz) | 50 | 11 | 10 | 0 |
| **SALAD DRESSINGS** | | | | | |
| Newman's Own Cobb | 1 pkg (2 oz) | 120 | 9 | 5 | 0 |
| Newman's Own Creamy Caesar | 1 pkg (2 oz) | 190 | 4 | 2 | 0 |
| Newman's Own Low Fat Balsamic Vinaigrette | 1 pkg (1.5 oz) | 40 | 4 | 3 | 0 |
| Newman's Own Ranch | 1 pkg (2 oz) | 290 | 4 | 3 | 0 |
| **SALADS AND SALAD BARS** | | | | | |
| Bacon Ranch w/o Chicken | 1 serv (7.1 oz) | 140 | 7 | 3 | 3 |
| Caesar w/o Chicken | 1 serv (7.1 oz) | 90 | 7 | 3 | 3 |
| California Cobb w/o Chicken | 1 serv (7.6 oz) | 160 | 7 | 4 | 3 |
| Crispy Chicken Bacon Ranch | 1 serv (10.4 oz) | 370 | 20 | 4 | 3 |
| Crispy Chicken Caesar | 1 serv (10 oz) | 310 | 20 | 4 | 3 |
| Crispy Chicken California Cobb | 1 serv (10.9 oz) | 380 | 20 | 4 | 3 |
| Croutons Butter Garlic | 1 pkg (0.5 oz) | 50 | 8 | 0 | 0 |
| Grilled Chicken Bacon Ranch | 1 serv (10.2 oz) | 270 | 11 | 4 | 3 |
| Grilled Chicken Caesar | 1 serv (9.8 oz) | 210 | 11 | 3 | 3 |
| Grilled Chicken California Cobb | 1 serv (10.7 oz) | 280 | 11 | 4 | 3 |
| Side Salad | 1 (3.1 oz) | 15 | 3 | 1 | 1 |
| **MR. HERO** | | | | | |
| **DESSERTS** | | | | | |
| Cheesecake | 1 serv | 350 | 26 | – | – |
| Cheesecake w/ Cherries | 1 serv | 385 | 35 | – | – |
| **MAIN MENU SELECTIONS** | | | | | |
| Breadsticks w/ Sauce | 1 serv | 291 | 47 | – | – |
| Cheddar Cheese Sauce | 1 serv | 60 | 5 | – | – |
| Onion Rings | 1 serv | 564 | 64 | – | – |
| Potato Waffers | 1 serv | 334 | 42 | – | – |
| Spaghetti Dinner | 1 serv | 606 | 112 | – | – |

| FOOD | PORTION | CALS | CARB | SUGAR | FIBER |
|---|---|---|---|---|---|
| Spaghetti w/ Meatballs | 1 serv | 846 | 116 | – | – |
| **SALAD DRESSINGS** | | | | | |
| Buttermilk | 1 serv (2 oz) | 290 | 6 | – | – |
| Creamy Italian | 1 serv (2 oz) | 190 | 11 | – | – |
| Fat Free Ranch | 1 serv (2 oz) | 70 | 18 | – | – |
| Fat Free Ranch | 1 serv (2 oz) | 70 | 16 | – | – |
| **SALADS AND SALAD BARS** | | | | | |
| Croutons | 1 serv | 59 | 9 | – | – |
| Garden Salad | 1 serv | 36 | 7 | – | – |
| Grilled Chicken | 1 serv | 225 | 7 | – | – |
| Seafood Crab | 1 serv | 452 | 18 | – | – |
| Side Salad | 1 serv | 27 | 6 | – | – |
| Tuna | 1 serv | 745 | 8 | – | – |
| **SANDWICHES** | | | | | |
| Cheesesteaks Grilled Steak Pill | 7 inch | 450 | 48 | – | – |
| Cheesesteaks Hot Buttered Deluxe | 7 inch | 566 | 48 | – | – |
| Cold Subs Classic Italian | 7 inch | 586 | 50 | – | – |
| Cold Subs Tuna & Cheese | 7 inch | 666 | 47 | – | – |
| Cold Subs Turkey & Cheese | 7 inch | 453 | 46 | – | – |
| Cold Subs Ultimate Italian | 7 inch | 608 | 51 | – | – |
| Hot Subs Grilled Chicken Philly | 7 inch | 438 | 48 | – | – |
| Hot Subs Meatball | 7 inch | 620 | 53 | – | – |
| Hot Subs Romanburger | 7 inch | 717 | 49 | – | – |
| Round Bacon Cheeseburger | 1 | 352 | 23 | – | – |
| Round Chicken | 1 | 420 | 23 | – | – |
| Round Fish | 1 | 412 | 31 | – | – |
| Round Tuna | 1 | 302 | 23 | – | – |

## MR. PITA

| FOOD | PORTION | CALS | CARB | SUGAR | FIBER |
|---|---|---|---|---|---|
| Cranberry Turkey | 1 reg | 424 | 77 | 17 | 3 |
| Grilled Raspberry Chicken | 1 reg | 342 | 56 | 5 | 1 |
| Grilled Chicken & Broccoli | 1 reg | 373 | 57 | 4 | 2 |
| Grilled Chicken Caesar | 1 reg | 353 | 50 | 3 | 1 |
| Grilled Hawaiian Chicken | 1 reg | 375 | 57 | 5 | 1 |
| Ultra Combo | 1 reg | 354 | 56 | 4 | 2 |
| Ultra Grilled Chicken | 1 reg | 367 | 56 | 5 | 2 |
| Ultra Supreme | 1 reg | 350 | 56 | 5 | 1 |
| Ultra Turkey | 1 reg | 343 | 56 | 4 | 2 |

| FOOD | PORTION | CALS | CARB | SUGAR | FIBER |
|---|---|---|---|---|---|
| **MRS. FIELDS** | | | | | |
| Stokabunga Energy Cookie | 1 (5 oz) | 750 | 74 | 46 | 5 |
| **P.J. CHANG'S CHINA BISTRO** | | | | | |
| Cantonese Scallops | 1 serv | 305 | 15 | – | – |
| Chicken w/ Black Bean Sauce | 1 serv | 426 | 19 | – | – |
| Pin Rice Noodles | 1 serv | 270 | 55 | – | – |
| Vegetable Chow Fun | 1 serv | 677 | 112 | – | – |
| **PANERA BREAD** | | | | | |
| **BAGELS AND SPREADS** | | | | | |
| Bagel Asiago Cheese | 1 | 330 | 58 | 5 | 2 |
| Bagel Blueberry | 1 | 320 | 67 | 11 | 3 |
| Bagel Cinnamon Crunch | 1 | 490 | 91 | 35 | 3 |
| Bagel Dutch Apple & Raisin | 1 | 340 | 70 | 21 | 3 |
| Bagel Everything | 1 | 290 | 58 | 4 | 2 |
| Bagel French Toast | 1 | 340 | 65 | 16 | 2 |
| Bagel Mochachip Swirl | 1 | 340 | 68 | 13 | 3 |
| Bagel Nine Grain | 1 | 290 | 58 | 4 | 3 |
| Bagel Peanut Butter Crunch | 1 | 400 | 77 | 27 | 3 |
| Bagel Plain | 1 | 280 | 57 | 4 | 2 |
| Bagel Sesame | 1 | 310 | 60 | 4 | 3 |
| Cream Cheese Hazelnut Reduced Fat | 1 serv (2 oz) | 150 | 6 | 6 | tr |
| Cream Cheese Honey Walnut Reduced Fat | 1 serv (2 oz) | 150 | 9 | 6 | tr |
| Cream Cheese Mocha Reduced Fat | 1 serv (2 oz) | 160 | 10 | 8 | 1 |
| Cream Cheese Plain | 1 serv (2 oz) | 190 | 2 | 1 | 0 |
| Cream Cheese Plain Reduced Fat | 1 serv (2 oz) | 130 | 2 | 1 | tr |
| Cream Cheese Raspberry Reduced Fat | 1 serv (2 oz) | 120 | 3 | 2 | 0 |
| Cream Cheese Smoked Salmon Reduced Fat | 1 serv (2 oz) | 120 | 2 | 1 | 0 |
| Cream Cheese Sun Dried Tomato Reduced Fat | 1 serv (2 oz) | 140 | 4 | 2 | tr |
| Cream Cheese Veggie Reduced Fat | 1 serv (2 oz) | 130 | 4 | 2 | 1 |
| Hummus Roasted Garlic | 1 serv (2 oz) | 100 | 11 | 7 | 4 |

| FOOD | PORTION | CALS | CARB | SUGAR | FIBER |
|---|---|---|---|---|---|
| **BEVERAGES** | | | | | |
| Caffe Mocha | 1 serv (11.5 oz) | 360 | 47 | 39 | 2 |
| Homestyle Lemonade | 1 serv (16 oz) | 80 | 19 | – | 0 |
| Hot Chocolate | 1 serv (11 oz) | 350 | 45 | 38 | 2 |
| IC Cappuccino Chip | 1 serv (16 oz) | 590 | 64 | 56 | 0 |
| IC Caramel | 1 serv (16 oz) | 550 | 76 | 63 | 0 |
| IC Honeydew Green Tea | 1 serv (16 oz) | 270 | 36 | 31 | 0 |
| IC Mocha | 1 serv (16 oz) | 520 | 70 | 56 | 2 |
| IC Spice | 1 serv (16 oz) | 470 | 66 | 56 | 0 |
| Iced Green Tea | 1 serv (16 oz) | 60 | 15 | 14 | 0 |
| Latte Caffe | 1 serv (8.5 oz) | 120 | 12 | 11 | 0 |
| Latte Caramel | 1 serv (11 oz) | 400 | 54 | 46 | 0 |
| Latte Chai Tea | 1 serv (10 oz) | 210 | 37 | 33 | 0 |
| Latte House | 1 serv (10.8 oz) | 320 | 43 | 39 | 0 |
| Sierra Turkey | 1 | 950 | 71 | 4 | 4 |
| **BREADS** | | | | | |
| Artisan Country | 1 slice | 120 | 25 | 1 | 1 |
| Artisan French | 1 slice (2 oz) | 110 | 23 | 1 | tr |
| Artisan Kalamata Olive | 1 slice (2 oz) | 140 | 26 | 1 | 1 |
| Artisan Multigrain | 1 slice (2 oz) | 120 | 24 | 1 | 1 |
| Artisan Raisin Pecan | 1 slice (2 oz) | 140 | 25 | 5 | 1 |
| Artisan Sesame Semolina | 1 slice (2 oz) | 120 | 24 | 1 | 4 |
| Artisan Stone Milled Rye | 1 slice (2 oz) | 110 | 22 | 1 | 2 |
| Artisan Three Cheese | 1 slice (2 oz) | 120 | 21 | 1 | tr |
| Artisan Three Seed | 1 slice | 130 | 23 | 1 | 1 |
| Ciabatta | 1 (6 oz) | 430 | 70 | 2 | 3 |
| Cinnamon Raisin | 1 slice (2 oz) | 160 | 31 | 12 | 1 |
| Focaccia Asiago Cheese | 1 slice (2 oz) | 150 | 19 | 1 | 1 |
| Focaccia Basil Pesto | 1 slice (2 oz) | 150 | 19 | 1 | 1 |
| Focaccia Rosemary & Onion | 1 slice (2 oz) | 140 | 19 | 1 | 1 |
| French | 1 slice (2 oz) | 130 | 24 | 1 | 1 |
| French Roll | 1 (2.25 oz) | 140 | 28 | 1 | 1 |
| Holiday | 1 slice (2 oz) | 150 | 33 | 23 | tr |
| Honey Wheat | 1 slice (2 oz) | 140 | 25 | 3 | 1 |
| Nine Grain | 1 slice (2 oz) | 150 | 26 | 3 | 2 |
| Rye | 1 slice (2 oz) | 140 | 25 | 3 | 1 |
| Sourdough | 1 slice (2 oz) | 120 | 25 | 1 | 1 |
| Sourdough Roll | 1 (2.5 oz) | 160 | 32 | 1 | 1 |

| FOOD | PORTION | CALS | CARB | SUGAR | FIBER |
|---|---|---|---|---|---|
| Sourdough Soup Bowl | 1 serv (8 oz) | 500 | 102 | 2 | 4 |
| Sunflower | 1 slice (2 oz) | 160 | 24 | 4 | 1 |
| Tomato Basil | 1 slice (2 oz) | 130 | 27 | 1 | 1 |
| **DESSERTS** | | | | | |
| Bear Claw | 1 | 380 | 37 | 14 | 1 |
| Brownie Caramel Pecan | 1 | 470 | 60 | 47 | 2 |
| Brownie Chocolate Raspberry | 1 | 370 | 47 | 37 | 2 |
| Brownie Very Chocolate | 1 | 460 | 62 | 47 | 2 |
| Cinnamon Roll | 1 | 560 | 64 | 21 | 3 |
| Cobblestone | 1 | 560 | 100 | 42 | 4 |
| Coffee Cake Cherry Cheese | 1 | 190 | 21 | 11 | 1 |
| Cookie Chocolate Chipper | 1 | 420 | 51 | 21 | 2 |
| Cookie Chocolate Duet w/ Walnuts | 1 | 410 | 47 | 24 | 3 |
| Cookie Nutty Chocolate Chipper | 1 | 440 | 46 | 20 | 3 |
| Cookie Nutty Oatmeal Raisin | 1 | 350 | 51 | 22 | 5 |
| Cookie Shortbread | 1 | 340 | 36 | 11 | 1 |
| Croissant Apple | 1 | 260 | 34 | 17 | 1 |
| Croissant Cheese | 1 | 300 | 34 | 11 | 1 |
| Croissant Chocolate | 1 | 440 | 56 | 27 | 4 |
| Croissant French | 1 | 265 | 28 | 3 | 1 |
| Croissant Raspberry Cheese | 1 | 280 | 37 | 14 | 1 |
| Danish Apple | 1 | 510 | 50 | 17 | 2 |
| Danish Cheese | 1 | 590 | 55 | 25 | 1 |
| Danish Cherry | 1 | 520 | 60 | 31 | 1 |
| Danish Georgia Peach | 1 | 580 | 67 | 28 | 2 |
| Danish German Chocolate | 1 | 770 | 83 | 37 | 4 |
| Macaroon Chocolate Hazelnut | 1 | 270 | 30 | 18 | 3 |
| Mini Bundt Cake Carrot Walnut | 1 | 430 | 51 | 31 | 2 |
| Mini Bundt Cake Lemon Poppyseed | 1 | 460 | 62 | 33 | 1 |
| Mini Bundt Cake Pineapple Upside Down | 1 | 450 | 64 | 36 | 2 |
| Muffin Banana Nut | 1 | 260 | 34 | 15 | 3 |
| Muffin Chocolate Chip | 1 | 240 | 36 | 18 | 2 |
| Muffin Pumpkin | 1 | 270 | 43 | 26 | 1 |
| Muffin Banana Nut | 1 | 470 | 57 | 31 | 5 |
| Muffin Blueberry | 1 | 450 | 73 | 33 | 4 |
| Muffin Chocolate Chip | 1 | 540 | 83 | 42 | 5 |

| FOOD | PORTION | CALS | CARB | SUGAR | FIBER |
|---|---|---|---|---|---|
| Muffin Pumpkin | 1 | 510 | 80 | 48 | 1 |
| Muffin Low Fat Tripleberry | 1 | 300 | 63 | 28 | 3 |
| Pecan Roll | 1 | 520 | 60 | 26 | 2 |
| Scone Cinnamon Chip | 1 | 560 | 70 | 23 | 2 |
| Scone Orange | 1 | 530 | 67 | 22 | 3 |
| Strudel Apple Raisin | 1 | 390 | 40 | 18 | 1 |
| Strudel Cherry | 1 | 400 | 38 | 20 | 1 |
| **SALADS** | | | | | |
| Asian Sesame Chicken | 1 serv | 370 | 45 | 19 | 5 |
| Caesar | 1 serv | 350 | 15 | 1 | 3 |
| Caesar Grilled Chicken | 1 serv | 470 | 22 | 1 | 3 |
| Classic Cafe | 1 serv | 380 | 15 | 10 | 4 |
| Fandango | 1 serv | 400 | 21 | 15 | 6 |
| Greek | 1 serv | 520 | 17 | 4 | 5 |
| **SANDWICHES** | | | | | |
| Asiago Roast Beef | 1 | 730 | 54 | 4 | 2 |
| Bacon Turkey Bravo | 1 | 770 | 84 | 6 | 5 |
| Chicken Salad On Artison Sesame Semolina | 1 | 730 | 80 | 12 | 6 |
| Chicken Salad On Nine Grain | 1 | 640 | 56 | 15 | 4 |
| Garden Veggie | 1 | 570 | 74 | 6 | 5 |
| Italian Combo | 1 | 1050 | 80 | 5 | 5 |
| Panini Coronado Carnitas | 1 | 810 | 77 | 4 | 3 |
| Panini Frontega Chicken | 1 | 860 | 71 | 5 | 5 |
| Panini Portobello & Mozzarella | 1 | 650 | 73 | 7 | 8 |
| Panini Turkey Artichoke | 1 | 810 | 76 | 10 | 6 |
| Peanut Butter & Jelly On French | 1 | 450 | 63 | 23 | 3 |
| Smoked Ham On Artisan Stone Milled Rye | 1 | 930 | 106 | 6 | 6 |
| Smoked Ham On Rye | 1 | 650 | 47 | 7 | 4 |
| Smoked Turkey Breast On Artisan Country | 1 | 590 | 73 | 4 | 5 |
| Smoked Turkey On Sourdough | 1 | 440 | 44 | 4 | 3 |
| Tuna Salad On Artisan Multigrain | 1 | 830 | 78 | 7 | 5 |
| Tuna Salad On Honey Wheat | 1 | 720 | 50 | 10 | 4 |
| Turkey Fresco | 1 | 580 | 74 | 5 | 4 |
| Tuscan Chicken | 1 | 950 | 76 | 8 | 6 |

| FOOD | PORTION | CALS | CARB | SUGAR | FIBER |
|---|---|---|---|---|---|
| **SOUPS** | | | | | |
| Baked Potato | 1 serv | 260 | 23 | 2 | 1 |
| Boston Clam Chowder | 1 serv | 210 | 19 | 2 | tr |
| Broccoli Cheddar | 1 serv | 230 | 13 | 4 | 1 |
| Cream Of Chicken & Wild Rice | 1 serv | 200 | 19 | 2 | tr |
| Forest Mushroom | 1 serv | 140 | 15 | 3 | 2 |
| French Onion | 1 serv | 220 | 23 | 6 | 2 |
| Low Fat Chicken Noodle | 1 serv | 100 | 15 | 1 | 1 |
| Low Fat Vegetarian Garden Vegetable | 1 serv | 90 | 17 | 4 | 2 |
| Low Fat Vegetarian Black Bean | 1 serv | 100 | 29 | 2 | 17 |
| Vegetarian Santa Fe Roasted Corn | 1 serv | 130 | 22 | 4 | 3 |
| **PAPA MURPHY'S** | | | | | |
| **MAIN MENU SELECTIONS** | | | | | |
| Calzone Combo | 1/8 pie | 450 | 45 | 2 | 2 |
| Calzone Italian | 1/8 pie | 480 | 46 | 1 | 2 |
| Calzone Veggie | 1/8 pie | 410 | 46 | 1 | 3 |
| Cheesy Bread | 1 serv | 180 | 23 | 0 | tr |
| **PIZZA** | | | | | |
| Deeper Dish Traditional | 1/8 pie | 440 | 34 | 1 | 2 |
| Gourmet Family Size Chicken Garlic | 1/12 pie | 320 | 30 | 1 | 1 |
| Gourmet Family Size Classic Italian | 1/12 pie | 360 | 30 | 1 | 2 |
| Gourmet Family Size Veggie | 1/12 pie | 300 | 31 | 1 | 2 |
| Papa's Family Size All Meat | 1/12 pie | 370 | 31 | 1 | 2 |
| Papa's Family Size Cheese | 1/12 pie | 270 | 29 | 1 | 2 |
| Papa's Family Size Cowboy | 1/12 pie | 370 | 31 | 1 | 2 |
| Papa's Family Size Hawaiian | 1/12 pie | 290 | 34 | 4 | 2 |
| Papa's Family Size Murphy's Combo | 1/12 pie | 480 | 32 | 2 | 2 |
| Papa's Family Size Pepperoni | 1/12 pie | 310 | 29 | 1 | 2 |
| Papa's Family Size Perfect | 1/12 pie | 300 | 32 | 4 | 2 |
| Papa's Family Size Rancher | 1/12 pie | 330 | 31 | 2 | 2 |
| Papa's Family Size Specialty | 1/12 pie | 340 | 31 | 1 | 2 |
| Papa's Family Size Veggie Combo | 1/12 pie | 300 | 32 | 2 | 2 |

| FOOD | PORTION | CALS | CARB | SUGAR | FIBER |
| --- | --- | --- | --- | --- | --- |
| Stuffed Big Murphy | ⅛ pie | 380 | 39 | 1 | 2 |
| Stuffed Chicago Style | ⅛ pie | 370 | 39 | 2 | 2 |
| Stuffed Chicken & Bacon | 1/16 pie | 370 | 38 | 1 | 2 |
| **SALADS** | | | | | |
| Chicken & Bacon w/o Dressing | 1 serv | 370 | 9 | 2 | 3 |
| Italian Salad w/o Dressing | 1 serv | 260 | 6 | 1 | 3 |
| Veggie Salad w/o Dressing | 1 serv | 140 | 7 | 3 | 4 |
| **PIZZA HUT** | | | | | |
| **APPETIZERS** | | | | | |
| Breadstick Cheese | 1 | 200 | 21 | 4 | tr |
| Hot Wings | 2 pieces | 110 | 1 | 0 | 0 |
| Mild Wings | 2 pieces | 110 | tr | 0 | 0 |
| Wing Blue Cheese Dipping Sauce | 1 serv (1.5 oz) | 230 | 2 | 2 | 0 |
| Wing Ranch Dipping Sauce | 1 serv (1.5 oz) | 210 | 4 | 2 | 0 |
| **BEVERAGES** | | | | | |
| Diet Pepsi | 1 med (14 oz) | 0 | 0 | 0 | 0 |
| Mt. Dew | 1 med (14 oz) | 190 | 54 | 54 | 0 |
| Pepsi | 1 med (14 oz) | 180 | 47 | 47 | 0 |
| **DESSERTS** | | | | | |
| Apple Pizza | 1 slice | 260 | 53 | 14 | 1 |
| Cherry Pizza | 1 slice | 240 | 47 | 24 | 1 |
| Cinnamon Sticks | 2 | 170 | 27 | 10 | tr |
| White Icing Dipping Cup | 1 serv (2 oz) | 170 | 46 | 39 | 0 |
| **MAIN MENU SELECTIONS** | | | | | |
| Breadstick | 1 | 150 | 20 | 4 | tr |
| Breadstick Dipping Sauce | 1 serv (3 oz) | 50 | 11 | 6 | 2 |
| **PIZZA** | | | | | |
| Fit 'N Delicious Diced Chicken Mushroom Jalapeno | 1 med slice | 170 | 22 | 5 | 2 |
| Fit 'N Delicious Diced Chicken Red Onion Green Pepper | 1 med slice | 170 | 23 | 6 | 2 |
| Fit 'N Delicious Green Pepper Red Onion Diced Red Tomato | 1 med slice | 150 | 24 | 6 | 2 |
| Fit 'N Delicious Ham Pineapple Diced Red Tomato | 1 med slice | 160 | 24 | 7 | 2 |
| Fit 'N Delicious Ham Red Onion Mushroom | 1 med slice | 160 | 22 | 6 | 2 |

| FOOD | PORTION | CALS | CARB | SUGAR | FIBER |
|---|---|---|---|---|---|
| Fit 'N Delicious Tomato Mushroom Jalapeno | 1 med slice | 150 | 22 | 5 | 2 |
| Hand Tossed Cheese | 1 med slice | 240 | 30 | 5 | 2 |
| Hand Tossed Chicken Supreme | 1 slice | 230 | 30 | 6 | 2 |
| Hand Tossed Ham | 1 med slice | 220 | 29 | 5 | 2 |
| Hand Tossed Meat Lover's | 1 med slice | 300 | 29 | 6 | 2 |
| Hand Tossed Pepperoni | 1 med slice | 250 | 29 | 6 | 2 |
| Hand Tossed Pepperoni Lover's | 1 med slice | 300 | 30 | 6 | 2 |
| Hand Tossed Sausage Lover's | 1 med slice | 280 | 30 | 8 | 2 |
| Hand Tossed Super Supreme | 1 med slice | 300 | 30 | 6 | 2 |
| Hand Tossed Supreme | 1 med slice | 270 | 30 | 6 | 2 |
| Hand Tossed Veggie Lover's | 1 med slice | 220 | 31 | 6 | 2 |
| Marinara Dipping Sauce | 1 serv (3 oz) | 45 | 9 | 6 | 2 |
| Pan Cheese | 1 med slice | 280 | 29 | 6 | 1 |
| Pan Chicken Supreme | 1 med slice | 280 | 30 | 7 | 2 |
| Pan Ham | 1 med slice | 260 | 29 | 6 | 1 |
| Pan Meat Lover's | 1 med slice | 340 | 29 | 6 | 2 |
| Pan Pepperoni | 1 med slice | 290 | 29 | 6 | 2 |
| Pan Pepperoni Lover's | 1 med slice | 340 | 29 | 6 | 2 |
| Pan Sausage Lover's | 1 med slice | 330 | 29 | 6 | 2 |
| Pan Super Supreme | 1 med slice | 340 | 30 | 7 | 2 |
| Pan Supreme | 1 med slice | 320 | 30 | 7 | 2 |
| Pizone Classic | 1 | 1220 | 142 | 18 | 6 |
| Pizone Pepperoni | 1 | 1220 | 138 | 16 | 6 |
| Thin'N Crispy Cheese | 1 med slice | 200 | 27 | 4 | 1 |
| Thin'N Crispy Chicken Supreme | 1 med slice | 200 | 23 | 6 | 2 |
| Thin'N Crispy Ham | 1 med slice | 180 | 21 | 5 | 1 |
| Thin'N Crispy Meat Lover's | 1 med slice | 270 | 21 | 5 | 2 |
| Thin'N Crispy Pepperoni | 1 med slice | 170 | 21 | 5 | 1 |
| Thin'N Crispy Pepperoni Lover's | 1 med slice | 260 | 21 | 5 | 2 |
| Thin'N Crispy Super Supreme | 1 med slice | 260 | 23 | 6 | 2 |
| Thin'N Crispy Supreme | 1 med slice | 240 | 22 | 5 | 2 |
| Thin'N Crispy Veggie Lover's | 1 med slice | 180 | 23 | 5 | 2 |
| **QUIZNO'S** | | | | | |
| Cookie Oatmeal Chocolate Chip | 1 | 360 | 48 | 23 | 1 |
| Cookie w/ Reese's Pieces | 1 | 360 | 48 | 22 | 1 |
| Sub Honey Bourbon Chicken | 1 sm | 329 | 45 | – | 3 |
| Sub Turkey Lite | 1 sm | 334 | 52 | – | 3 |

| FOOD | PORTION | CALS | CARB | SUGAR | FIBER |
|---|---|---|---|---|---|
| Sub Tuscan Chicken Salad | 1 sm | 326 | 45 | – | 4 |
| **RANCH 1** | | | | | |
| **MAIN MENU SELECTIONS** | | | | | |
| Baked Potato w/ Broccoli | 1 serv | 510 | 117 | 8 | 12 |
| Baked Potato w/ Cheese | 1 serv | 790 | 118 | 9 | 11 |
| Baked Potato w/ Chicken | 1 serv | 610 | 114 | 7 | 11 |
| Chicken Tenders | 1 serv | 370 | 7 | 0 | 0 |
| Fijita Grilled Chicken | 1 | 330 | 25 | 4 | 4 |
| Fruit Cup | 1 serv | 90 | 21 | 18 | 2 |
| Hot Pasta Grilled Chicken | 1 serv | 590 | 86 | 7 | 6 |
| Platter Grilled Chicken & Vegetables | 1 serv | 790 | 129 | 12 | 16 |
| Ranch Fries | 1 reg | 350 | 51 | 1 | 5 |
| Ranch Fries | 1 lg | 420 | 62 | 2 | 7 |
| Sandwich American Rancher | 1 | 390 | 51 | 4 | 3 |
| Sandwich Grilled Chicken Philly | 1 | 450 | 53 | 4 | 3 |
| Sandwich Ranch Classic | 1 | 370 | 53 | 4 | 3 |
| Sandwich Spicy Grilled Chicken | 1 | 420 | 58 | 7 | 3 |
| Sandwich Club | 1 | 470 | 53 | 4 | 3 |
| **SALADS** | | | | | |
| Gourmet Greens | 1 serv | 220 | 31 | 7 | 5 |
| Gourmet Greens w/ Chicken | 1 serv | 350 | 31 | 7 | 5 |
| Zesty Caesar | 1 serv | 180 | 31 | 4 | 4 |
| Zesty Chicken Caesar | 1 serv | 290 | 31 | 4 | 4 |
| **RUBY TUESDAY'S** | | | | | |
| Cajun Chicken Salad w/ Ranch Dressing | 1 serv | 636 | 16 | – | – |
| Peppercorn Mushroom Sirloin | 1 serv | 947 | 19 | – | – |
| **SBARRO** | | | | | |
| Pizza Veggie Slice | 1 serv (10 oz) | 490 | 75 | 3 | 1 |
| **SEE'S CANDIES** | | | | | |
| Bridge Mix | 14 pieces (1.4 oz) | 200 | 24 | 19 | 1 |
| Dark Chocolate Bordeaux | 2 (1.4 oz) | 170 | 27 | 25 | 1 |
| Dark Chocolates | 2 (1.2 oz) | 160 | 19 | 15 | 2 |
| Lollypop Butterscotch | 1 | 90 | 17 | 12 | 0 |
| Lollypop Cafe Latte | 1 | 90 | 16 | 8 | 0 |
| Lollypop Chocolate | 1 | 90 | 14 | 9 | tr |

| FOOD | PORTION | CALS | CARB | SUGAR | FIBER |
|---|---|---|---|---|---|
| Lollypop Peanut Butter | 1 | 90 | 14 | 8 | 0 |
| Marshmints | 3 (1.4 oz) | 140 | 27 | 21 | tr |
| Milk Chocolate Bordeaux | 2 (1.4 oz) | 170 | 27 | 25 | tr |
| Milk Chocolate Butter | 2 (1.4 oz) | 190 | 27 | 24 | tr |
| Milk Chocolate Buttercreams | 2 (1.4 oz) | 180 | 27 | 25 | 0 |
| Milk Chocolate California Brittle | 2 (1.3 oz) | 220 | 19 | 17 | 0 |
| Milk Chocolate Nuts & Chews | 3 (1.7 oz) | 250 | 26 | 19 | 2 |
| Milk Chocolate Peanuts | 3 (1.5 oz) | 230 | 18 | 14 | 2 |
| Milk Chocolate Soft Centers | 2 (1.4 oz) | 170 | 25 | 21 | tr |
| Milk Chocolates | 2 (1.2 oz) | 160 | 20 | 17 | tr |
| Nuts & Chews | 3 (1.6 oz) | 240 | 25 | 18 | 2 |
| P-Nut Crunch | 2 (1.4 oz) | 220 | 21 | 17 | 1 |
| Peanut Brittle | 1.5 oz | 230 | 21 | 15 | 0 |
| Pecan Buds | 3 (1.7 oz) | 270 | 22 | 16 | tr |
| Red Hot Swamp Goo | 3 pieces (1.4 oz) | 140 | 27 | 21 | tr |
| Soft Centers | 2 (1.4 oz) | 170 | 25 | 21 | tr |
| Truffles Black or Gold | 2 (1.4 oz) | 180 | 22 | 13 | 1 |
| Truffles Mint | 3 (1.6 oz) | 200 | 26 | 22 | tr |
| Victoria Toffee | 1.5 oz | 250 | 19 | 15 | 1 |
| **SMOOTHIE KING** | | | | | |
| Activator Chocolate | 1 (20 oz) | 429 | 90 | – | 4 |
| Activator Strawberry | 1 (20 oz) | 559 | 123 | – | 5 |
| Activator Vanilla | 1 (20 oz) | 429 | 90 | – | 4 |
| Banana Boat | 1 (20 oz) | 520 | 93 | – | 5 |
| Coconut Surprise | 1 (20 oz) | 457 | 99 | – | 5 |
| Coffee Smoothie Hazelnut | 1 (20 oz) | 118 | 23 | – | tr |
| Coffee Smoothies Amaretto | 1 (20 oz) | 118 | 23 | – | tr |
| Coffee Smoothies French Roast | 1 (20 oz) | 164 | 35 | – | tr |
| Coffee Smoothies French Vanilla | 1 (20 oz) | 118 | 23 | – | tr |
| Coffee Smoothies Irish Creme | 1 (20 oz) | 118 | 23 | – | tr |
| Coffee Smoothies Mocha | 1 (20 oz) | 206 | 42 | – | 1 |
| HeaterZ Banana Nut | 1 | 400 | 67 | – | 3 |
| HeaterZ Blueberry Muffin | 1 | 370 | 15 | – | 9 |
| HeaterZ Chocolate Peanut Butter Cup | 1 | 380 | 48 | – | 6 |
| HeaterZ Cinnamon Oatmeal Raisin | 1 | 420 | 36 | – | 9 |
| HeaterZ Coconut | 1 | 440 | 3 | – | 3 |

| FOOD | PORTION | CALS | CARB | SUGAR | FIBER |
|---|---|---|---|---|---|
| HeaterZ Coffee Amaretto | 1 (12 oz) | 177 | 34 | – | 4 |
| HeaterZ Coffee French Roast | 1 (12 oz) | 172 | 33 | – | 4 |
| HeaterZ Coffee French Vanilla | 1 (12 oz) | 177 | 34 | – | 4 |
| HeaterZ Coffee Hazelnut | 1 (12 oz) | 177 | 34 | – | 4 |
| HeaterZ Coffee Irish Creme | 1 (12 oz) | 177 | 34 | – | 4 |
| HeaterZ Coffee Mocha | 1 (12 oz) | 266 | 55 | – | 5 |
| High Protein Almond Mocha | 1 (20 oz) | 402 | 45 | – | 4 |
| High Protein Banana | 1 (20 oz) | 412 | 44 | – | 6 |
| High Protein Chocolate | 1 (20 oz) | 401 | 45 | – | 4 |
| High Protein Lemon | 1 (20 oz) | 390 | 41 | – | 3 |
| High Protein Pineapple | 1 (20 oz) | 380 | 41 | – | 7 |
| Hot Coffee Amaretto | 1 (12 oz) | 168 | 35 | – | tr |
| Hot Coffee French Roast | 1 (12 oz) | 164 | 35 | – | tr |
| Hot Coffee French Vanilla | 1 (12 oz) | 168 | 35 | – | tr |
| Hot Coffee Hazelnut | 1 (12 oz) | 168 | 35 | – | tr |
| Hot Coffee Irish Creme | 1 (12 oz) | 168 | 35 | – | tr |
| Hot Coffee Mocha | 1 (12 oz) | 209 | 44 | – | 1 |
| Iced Coffee Amaretto | 1 (20 oz) | 168 | 35 | – | tr |
| Iced Coffee French Roast | 1 (20 oz) | 164 | 35 | – | tr |
| Iced Coffee French Vanilla | 1 (20 oz) | 168 | 35 | – | tr |
| Iced Coffee Hazelnut | 1 (20 oz) | 168 | 35 | – | tr |
| Iced Coffee Irish Creme | 1 (20 oz) | 168 | 35 | – | tr |
| Iced Coffee Mocha | 1 (20 oz) | 209 | 44 | – | 1 |
| Kid Cup Berry Interesting | 1 | 150 | 37 | – | 2 |
| Kid Cup Choc-A-Laka | 1 | 210 | 44 | – | 2 |
| Kid Cup Gimmi Grape | 1 | 170 | 42 | – | 1 |
| Kid Cup Smarti Tarti | 1 | 150 | 36 | – | 0 |
| Low Carb All Flavors | 1 (20 oz) | 225 | 4 | – | 2 |
| Low Fat Angel Food | 1 (20 oz) | 330 | 79 | – | 4 |
| Low Fat Blackberry Dream | 1 (20 oz) | 343 | 86 | – | 3 |
| Low Fat Carribean Way | 1 (20 oz) | 392 | 96 | – | 5 |
| Low Fat Celestial Cherry High | 1 (20 oz) | 285 | 69 | – | 4 |
| Low Fat Cherry Picker | 1 (20 oz) | 360 | 98 | – | 2 |
| Low Fat Cranberry Supreme | 1 (20 oz) | 577 | 139 | – | 3 |
| Low Fat Cranberry Cooler | 1 (20 oz) | 538 | 132 | – | 3 |
| Low Fat Great Expectations | 1 (20 oz) | 399 | 96 | – | 2 |
| Low Fat Grape Expectations II | 1 (20 oz) | 529 | 129 | – | 4 |
| Low Fat Hearthy Apple | 1 (20 oz) | 380 | 81 | – | 2 |
| Low Fat Immune Builder | 1 (20 oz) | 333 | 80 | – | 4 |
| Low Fat Instant Vigor | 1 (20 oz) | 359 | 87 | – | 2 |

| FOOD | PORTION | CALS | CARB | SUGAR | FIBER |
|---|---|---|---|---|---|
| Low Fat Island Treat | 1 (20 oz) | 334 | 81 | – | 5 |
| Low Fat Lemon Twist Banana | 1 (20 oz) | 339 | 82 | – | 2 |
| Low Fat Lemon Twist Strawberry | 1 (20 oz) | 399 | 97 | – | 2 |
| Low Fat Light & Fluffy | 1 (20 oz) | 389 | 98 | – | 4 |
| Low Fat Mangofest | 1 (20 oz) | 320 | 78 | – | 2 |
| Low Fat Muscle Punch | 1 (20 oz) | 339 | 80 | – | 4 |
| Low Fat Muscle Punch Plus | 1 (20 oz) | 340 | 80 | – | 5 |
| Low Fat Orange Ka-BAM | 1 (20 oz) | 320 | 104 | – | 3 |
| Low Fat Peach Slice | 1 (20 oz) | 341 | 80 | – | 3 |
| Low Fat Peg Upper | 1 (20 oz) | 334 | 80 | – | 5 |
| Low Fat Pineapple Pleasure | 1 (20 oz) | 331 | 76 | – | 4 |
| Low Fat Pineapple Surf | 1 (20 oz) | 440 | 104 | – | 4 |
| Low Fat Raspberry Sunrise | 1 (20 oz) | 335 | 85 | – | 4 |
| Low Fat Strawberry X-Treme | 1 (20 oz) | 370 | 91 | – | 4 |
| Low Fat Strawberry Kiwi Breeze | 1 (20 oz) | 300 | 70 | – | 2 |
| Low Fat Youth Mountain | 1 (20 oz) | 267 | 65 | – | 5 |
| Malts | 1 (20 oz) | 887 | 119 | – | tr |
| Mo'cuccino | 1 (20 oz) | 420 | 71 | – | 1 |
| Peanut Power | 1 (20 oz) | 502 | 72 | – | 4 |
| Peanut Power Plus Grape | 1 (20 oz) | 703 | 119 | – | 4 |
| Peanut Power Plus Strawberry | 1 (20 oz) | 632 | 104 | – | 5 |
| Pina Colada Island | 1 (20 oz) | 550 | 102 | – | 6 |
| Power Punch | 1 (20 oz) | 430 | 102 | – | 4 |
| Power Punch Plus | 1 (20 oz) | 499 | 113 | – | 4 |
| Shakes | 1 (20 oz) | 875 | 117 | – | 0 |
| Slim-N-Trim Chocolate | 1 (20 oz) | 270 | 55 | – | 3 |
| Slim-N-Trim Orange Vanilla | 1 (20 oz) | 199 | 43 | – | 1 |
| Slim-N-Trim Strawberry | 1 (20 oz) | 357 | 79 | – | 3 |
| Slim-N-Trim Vanilla | 1 (20 oz) | 227 | 51 | – | 2 |
| Super Punch | 1 (20 oz) | 425 | 95 | – | 6 |
| Super Punch Plus | 1 (20 oz) | 516 | 118 | – | 6 |
| The Hulk Chocolate | 1 (20 oz) | 846 | 129 | – | 6 |
| The Hulk Strawberry | 1 (20 oz) | 953 | 156 | – | 6 |
| The Hulk Vanilla | 1 (20 oz) | 846 | 129 | – | 5 |
| Yogurt D-Lite | 1 (20 oz) | 335 | 58 | – | 0 |
| **SONIC DRIVE-IN** | | | | | |
| **ADD-ONS** | | | | | |
| Bacon | 1 serv (0.5 oz) | 80 | 0 | 0 | 0 |

| FOOD | PORTION | CALS | CARB | SUGAR | FIBER |
|---|---|---|---|---|---|
| Cheddar Cheese Shredded | 1 serv (0.5 oz) | 104 | 1 | 0 | 0 |
| Cheese | 1 serv (0.7 oz) | 70 | 1 | 0 | 0 |
| Chili | 1 serv (1 oz) | 52 | 1 | 0 | 0 |
| Cone Coat Chocolate | 1 serv (1 oz) | 143 | 16 | 15 | 1 |
| Green Chilies | 1 serv (1 oz) | 10 | 3 | 0 | 0 |
| Hickory Barbecue Sauce | 1 serv (1 oz) | 41 | 10 | 1 | – |
| Honey Mustard Dressing | 1 serv (1.1 oz) | 110 | 9 | 7 | 0 |
| Jalapenos Nachos Sliced | 1 serv (1 oz) | 5 | 1 | 0 | 1 |
| Malt | 1 serv ( 1oz) | 104 | 22 | – | – |
| Maraschino Cherry | 1 serv (8 g) | 10 | 3 | 3 | 0 |
| Marinara Sauce | 1 serv (1 oz) | 15 | 3 | 2 | 1 |
| Ranch Dressing | 1 serv (1 oz) | 147 | 2 | 1 | 0 |
| Slaw | 1 serv (0.9 oz) | 45 | 4 | 3 | 1 |
| Sweet Pickle Relish | 1 serv (1.1 oz) | 40 | 11 | 10 | 0 |
| Syrup Blue Coconut | 1 serv (1 oz) | 65 | 16 | 15 | 0 |
| Syrup Cherry | 1 serv (1 oz) | 64 | 16 | 16 | 0 |
| Syrup Chocolate | 1 serv (1 oz) | 74 | 16 | 16 | 0 |
| Syrup Grape | 1 serv (1 oz) | 63 | 16 | 15 | 0 |
| Syrup Grape | 1 serv (1 oz) | 61 | 15 | 13 | 0 |
| Syrup Vanilla | 1 serv (1 oz) | 61 | 15 | – | 0 |
| Syrup Watermelon | 1 serv (1 oz) | 71 | 18 | 12 | 0 |
| Thousand Island Dressing | 1 serv (1 oz) | 150 | 3 | 3 | 0 |
| Topping Pineapple | 1 serv (1.5 oz) | 108 | 28 | 28 | 0 |
| Topping Strawberry | 1 serv (1.2 oz) | 38 | 10 | 9 | 1 |
| Topping Strawberry | 1 serv (1 oz) | 101 | 16 | 15 | 0 |
| **BEVERAGES** | | | | | |
| Barqs Root Beer | 1 sm | 160 | 43 | 43 | 0 |
| Barqs Root Beer | 1 lg | 333 | 90 | 90 | 0 |
| Coca-Cola | 1 lg | 291 | 81 | 81 | 0 |
| Coca-Cola | 1 sm | 139 | 39 | 39 | 0 |
| Diet Coca-Cola | 1 sm | 1 | 0 | 0 | 0 |
| Diet Coca-Cola | 1 lg | 3 | 0 | 0 | 0 |
| Diet Sprite | 1 lg | 8 | 0 | 0 | 0 |
| Diet Sprite | 1 sm | 4 | 0 | 0 | 0 |
| Dr Pepper | 1 sm | 144 | 39 | 39 | 0 |
| Dr Pepper | 1 lg | 300 | 81 | 81 | 0 |
| Float Or Flurry Blue Coconut Slush | 1 reg | 424 | 57 | 52 | 0 |
| Limeade | 1 sm | 143 | 39 | 37 | 1 |
| Limeade | 1 lg | 303 | 83 | 78 | 2 |

| FOOD | PORTION | CALS | CARB | SUGAR | FIBER |
|---|---|---|---|---|---|
| Limeade Cherry | 1 sm | 169 | 46 | 44 | 1 |
| Limeade Cherry | 1 lg | 361 | 98 | 93 | 2 |
| Limeade Strawberry | 1 sm | 172 | 47 | 45 | 1 |
| Limeade Strawberry | 1 lg | 341 | 93 | 88 | 2 |
| Slush Blue Coconut | 1 lg | 521 | 134 | 132 | 0 |
| Slush Watermelon | 1 lg | 526 | 136 | 130 | 0 |
| Sprite | 1 sm | 138 | 37 | 37 | 0 |
| Sprite | 1 lg | 288 | 78 | 78 | 0 |
| **BREAKFAST SELECTIONS** | | | | | |
| Breakfast Burrito | 1 | 731 | 47 | 2 | 3 |
| Fruit Taquitos | 1 serv | 302 | 51 | 12 | 3 |
| Sunrise | 1 reg | 224 | 60 | 56 | 1 |
| Sunrise | 1 lg | 368 | 100 | 94 | 2 |
| Toaster Bacon Egg & Cheese | 1 | 500 | 40 | 3 | 2 |
| Toaster Ham Egg & Cheese | 1 | 436 | 41 | 4 | 2 |
| Toaster Sausage Egg & Cheese | 1 | 570 | 44 | 3 | 2 |
| **DESSERTS** | | | | | |
| Banana Split | 1 serv | 467 | 75 | 72 | 3 |
| Chocolate Covered Shake Banana | 1 reg | 625 | 66 | 60 | 2 |
| Chocolate Covered Shake Cherry | 1 reg | 587 | 59 | 51 | 1 |
| Chocolate Covered Shake Peanut Butter | 1 reg | 678 | 57 | 50 | 1 |
| Chocolate Covered Shake Strawberry | 1 reg | 608 | 64 | 56 | 1 |
| Cream Pie Shake Banana | 1 reg | 775 | 92 | 82 | 2 |
| Cream Pie Shake Chocolate | 1 reg | 795 | 96 | 86 | 1 |
| Cream Pie Shake Coconut | 1 reg | 721 | 79 | 71 | 1 |
| Dish Of Vanilla | 1 serv | 265 | 24 | 19 | 0 |
| Float Or Flurry Cherry Slush | 1 reg | 421 | 57 | 52 | 0 |
| Float Or Flurry Coca-Cola | 1 reg | 379 | 47 | 41 | 0 |
| Float Or Flurry Dr. Pepper | 1 reg | 377 | 47 | 41 | 0 |
| Float Or Flurry Grape Slush | 1 reg | 423 | 57 | 52 | 0 |
| Float Or Flurry Orange Slush | 1 reg | 422 | 56 | 52 | 0 |
| Float Or Flurry Rootbeer | 1 reg | 386 | 50 | 44 | 0 |
| Float Or Flurry Watermelon Slush | 1 reg | 427 | 56 | 53 | 0 |
| Ice Cream Cone | 1 | 285 | 24 | 23 | 0 |
| Shake Banana | 1 reg | 508 | 52 | 46 | 1 |

| FOOD | PORTION | CALS | CARB | SUGAR | FIBER |
|---|---|---|---|---|---|
| Shake Chocolate | 1 reg | 564 | 64 | 58 | 0 |
| Shake Pineapple | 1 reg | 615 | 83 | 74 | 1 |
| Shake Strawberry | 1 reg | 510 | 54 | 46 | 1 |
| Shake Vanilla | 1 reg | 454 | 41 | 32 | 0 |
| Sonic Blast Butterfinger | 1 reg | 636 | 59 | 56 | 1 |
| Sonic Blast M&M | 1 reg | 641 | 64 | 58 | 1 |
| Sonic Blast Oreo | 1 reg | 638 | 57 | 56 | 1 |
| Sonic Blast Reese's | 1 reg | 658 | 56 | 52 | 1 |
| Sundae Chocolate | 1 serv | 362 | 45 | 41 | 0 |
| Sundae Hot Fudge | 1 serv | 392 | 44 | 40 | 0 |
| Sundae Pineapple | 1 serv | 399 | 58 | 53 | 0 |
| Sundae Strawberry | 1 serv | 322 | 37 | 32 | 1 |
| **MAIN MENU SELECTIONS** | | | | | |
| Ched'R'Peppers | 1 serv | 256 | 29 | 5 | 4 |
| Cheese Fries | 1 reg | 265 | 23 | 1 | 4 |
| Cheese Fries | 1 lg | 322 | 31 | 2 | 5 |
| Cheese Tots | 1 lg | 435 | 41 | 2 | 4 |
| Chicken Strip Dinner | 1 serv | 749 | 86 | 5 | 5 |
| Chicken Strip Snack | 1 serv | 272 | 22 | – | 0 |
| Chicken Strips | 2 | 184 | 15 | – | 0 |
| Chili Cheese Fries | 1 reg | 299 | 24 | 2 | 4 |
| Chili Cheese Fries | 1 lg | 357 | 32 | 2 | 5 |
| Chili Cheese Tater Tots | 1 reg | 363 | 28 | 2 | 3 |
| Chili Cheese Tots | 1 lg | 547 | 43 | 3 | 5 |
| Corn Dog | 1 | 262 | 23 | 5 | 1 |
| Extra Long Coney Plain | 1 | 483 | 44 | 9 | 1 |
| French Fries | 1 lg | 252 | 30 | 2 | 5 |
| French Fries | 1 reg | 195 | 22 | 1 | 4 |
| Fritos Chili Pie | 1 serv | 611 | [illegible] | 3 | 36 |
| Hot Dog Plain | 1 | 262 | 22 | 5 | 1 |
| Jr. Burger | 1 | 353 | 27 | 7 | 1 |
| Mozzarella Sticks | 1 serv | 382 | 35 | 5 | 0 |
| No.1 Hamburger | 1 | 577 | 43 | 7 | 2 |
| No.1 Sonic Cheeseburger | 1 | 647 | 44 | 7 | 2 |
| No.2 Hamburger | 1 | 481 | 43 | 7 | 2 |
| No.2 Sonic Cheeseburger | 1 | 551 | 44 | 7 | 2 |
| Onion Rings | 1 reg | 331 | 66 | 23 | 7 |
| Sandwich Breaded Chicken | 1 | 582 | 66 | 6 | 2 |
| Sandwich Country Fried Steak | 1 | 748 | 56 | 7 | 2 |
| Sandwich Grilled Chicken | 1 | 343 | 31 | 6 | 2 |

| FOOD | PORTION | CALS | CARB | SUGAR | FIBER |
|---|---|---|---|---|---|
| Super Sonic No.1 | 1 | 929 | 45 | 7 | 2 |
| Super Sonic No.2 | 1 | 839 | 46 | 7 | 3 |
| SuperSonic Onion Rings | 1 serv | 706 | 141 | 39 | 11 |
| SuperSonic Tots | 1 serv | 485 | 53 | 3 | 5 |
| SuperSonic Fries | 1 serv | 358 | 44 | 2 | 7 |
| Tater Tots | 1 lg | 365 | 40 | 2 | 4 |
| Tater Tots | 1 reg | 259 | 27 | 1 | 3 |
| Toaster Sandwich BLT | 1 | 581 | 42 | 4 | 3 |
| Toaster Sandwich Bacon Cheddar Burger | 1 | 675 | 60 | 6 | 4 |
| Toaster Sandwich Chicken Club | 1 | 675 | 75 | 10 | 3 |
| Toaster Sandwich Country Fried Steak | 1 | 708 | 55 | 4 | 3 |
| Toaster Sandwich Grilled Cheese | 1 | 282 | 39 | 2 | 2 |
| Wrap Chicken Strip | 1 | 574 | 55 | 2 | 2 |
| Wrap Grilled Chicken | 1 | 539 | 40 | 2 | 2 |
| Wrap w/o Ranch Chicken Strip | 1 | 428 | 53 | 1 | 2 |
| Wrap w/o Ranch Grilled Chicken | 1 | 393 | 38 | 1 | 2 |
| **STARBUCKS** | | | | | |
| **BAKED SELECTIONS** | | | | | |
| Baby Bundt Cake Chocolate | 1 | 330 | 45 | 29 | 4 |
| Bagel | 1 | 430 | 92 | 5 | 3 |
| Bagel Cinnamon Raisin | 1 | 440 | 96 | 14 | 3 |
| Bagel Sesame | 1 | 440 | 92 | 5 | 6 |
| Bar Caramel Apple | 1 | 310 | 38 | 21 | 2 |
| Bar Carrot Cake | 1 | 420 | 46 | 35 | tr |
| Bar Lemon | 1 | 310 | 44 | 32 | 0 |
| Bar Oreo Dream | 1 | 420 | 33 | 22 | 2 |
| Bar Toffee Crunch | 1 | 430 | 56 | 37 | 1 |
| Biscotti Chocolate Hazelnut | 1 | 110 | 15 | 8 | 1 |
| Biscotti Vanilla Almond | 1 | 110 | 15 | 8 | 1 |
| Brownie Caramel | 1 | 580 | 60 | 44 | 2 |
| Brownie Enrobed Espresso | 1 | 430 | 48 | 32 | 3 |
| Brownie Espresso | 1 | 370 | 43 | 30 | 2 |
| Brownie Milk Chocolate Peanut Butter | 1 | 460 | 45 | 34 | 2 |
| Bundt Cake Lemon Yogurt | 1 serv | 350 | 56 | 34 | tr |

| FOOD | PORTION | CALS | CARB | SUGAR | FIBER |
|---|---|---|---|---|---|
| Caramel Pecan Sticky Roll | 1 | 730 | 75 | 39 | 7 |
| Cinnamon Roll | 1 | 620 | 80 | 41 | 3 |
| Cinnamon Twist | 1 | 320 | 37 | 13 | 1 |
| Coffee Cake | 1 serv | 570 | 75 | 45 | 2 |
| Coffee Cake Apple Walnut | 1 serv | 320 | 41 | 28 | 1 |
| Coffee Cake Blueberry Walnut | 1 serv | 340 | 43 | 30 | 1 |
| Coffee Cake Cinnamon Walnut | 1 serv | 360 | 46 | 31 | 1 |
| Coffee Cake Crumble Berry | 1 serv | 520 | 69 | 40 | 2 |
| Coffee Cake Hazelnut | 1 serv | 630 | 74 | 43 | 2 |
| Coffee Cake Sour Cream | 1 serv | 420 | 43 | 29 | 1 |
| Cookie Black And White | 1 | 430 | 68 | 53 | 2 |
| Cookie Double Chocolate Chunk | 1 serv | 430 | 58 | 37 | 3 |
| Cookie Oatmean Raisin | 1 | 390 | 65 | 34 | 3 |
| Cookie White Chocolate Macadamia Nut | 1 | 470 | 54 | 34 | 2 |
| Crisp Cinnamon Twist | 1 | 60 | 9 | 4 | 0 |
| Croissant Almond | 1 | 330 | 39 | 16 | 2 |
| Croissant Butter w/ Apricot Glaze | 1 | 320 | 37 | 13 | 1 |
| Croissant Raspberry & Cream Cheese | 1 | 260 | 34 | 11 | 1 |
| Crumb Cake | 1 serv | 670 | 89 | 44 | 1 |
| Danish Apple w/ Mocha Swirls | 1 | 370 | 44 | 18 | 2 |
| Danish Cheese w/ Mocha Swirls | 1 | 460 | 44 | 18 | 1 |
| Danish Raspberry w/ Mocho Swirls | 1 | 370 | 45 | 17 | 1 |
| Graham Dark Chocolate | 1 | 140 | 17 | 12 | tr |
| Graham Milk Chocolate | 1 | 140 | 17 | 12 | tr |
| Madeline | 1 | 80 | 11 | 6 | 0 |
| Muffin Blueberry | 1 | 380 | 49 | 28 | 1 |
| Muffin Cranberry Orange | 1 | 410 | 53 | 31 | 2 |
| Muffin Morning Sunrise | 1 | 330 | 54 | 32 | 2 |
| Muffin Chocolate Cream Cheese | 1 | 450 | 53 | 31 | 1 |
| Pound Cake Banana | 1 serv | 360 | 47 | 24 | 1 |
| Pound Cake Cranberry Walnut | 1 serv | 390 | 45 | 26 | 1 |
| Pound Cake Iced Carrot | 1 serv | 540 | 101 | 64 | 3 |

| FOOD | PORTION | CALS | CARB | SUGAR | FIBER |
|---|---|---|---|---|---|
| Pound Cake Marble | 1 serv | 400 | 49 | 29 | tr |
| Pound Cake Orange Poppy | 1 serv | 490 | 55 | 32 | 2 |
| Pound Cake Pumpkin | 1 serv | 310 | 47 | 27 | 2 |
| Pound Cake Zucchini | 1 serv | 370 | 47 | 27 | 2 |
| Pullman Banana | 1 serv | 400 | 57 | 31 | 2 |
| Pullman Chocolate | 1 | 380 | 54 | 33 | 2 |
| Pullman Cranberry Walnut | 1 | 360 | 53 | 28 | 2 |
| Pullman Lemon Glazed | 1 | 370 | 55 | 31 | tr |
| Pullman Marble Chocolate Chip | 1 | 440 | 61 | 37 | 1 |
| Pullman Orange Poppy Cheese | 1 | 450 | 55 | 34 | 1 |
| Pullman Pumpkin | 1 | 370 | 51 | 22 | 2 |
| Scone Blueberry | 1 | 460 | 68 | 24 | 3 |
| Scone Butterscotch Pecan | 1 | 520 | 64 | 22 | 2 |
| Scone Cinnamon Chip w/ Icing | 1 | 510 | 71 | 29 | 2 |
| Scone Maple Oat w/ Icing | 1 | 490 | 69 | 28 | 2 |
| Scone Apricot Currant | 1 | 450 | 67 | 17 | 3 |
| Scone Raspberry | 1 | 440 | 65 | 20 | 2 |
| Shortbread | 1 | 100 | 12 | 4 | 0 |
| **BEVERAGES** | | | | | |
| Apple Juice | 1 grande | 230 | 57 | 52 | 0 |
| Blended Coffee Of The Week | 1 grande | 10 | 2 | 0 | 0 |
| Caffe Americano | 1 grande | 150 | 3 | 0 | 0 |
| Caffe Au Lait Nonfat Milk | 1 grande | 90 | 13 | 11 | 0 |
| Caffe Au Lait Soy Milk | 1 grande | 110 | 15 | 12 | tr |
| Caffe Latte Whole Milk | 1 grande | 260 | 21 | 19 | 0 |
| Caffe Mocha Whip Whole Milk | 1 grande | 400 | 42 | 33 | 2 |
| Caffe Latte Soy Milk | 1 grande | 210 | 28 | 21 | 2 |
| Caffe Mocha No Whip Nonfat Milk | 1 grande | 230 | 43 | 32 | 2 |
| Caffe Mocha No Whip Soy Milk | 1 grande | 260 | 46 | 33 | 3 |
| Caffe Mocha Whip Nonfat Milk | 1 grande | 330 | 44 | 34 | 2 |
| Caffe Mocha Whip Soy Milk | 1 grande | 360 | 48 | 35 | 3 |
| Caffe Latte Nonfat Milk | 1 grande | 160 | 24 | 20 | 0 |
| Cappuccino Nonfat Milk | 1 grande | 100 | 14 | 11 | 0 |
| Cappucino Soy Milk | 1 grande | 120 | 17 | 12 | tr |
| Caramel Mocha No Whip Soy Milk | 1 grande | 340 | 66 | 52 | 3 |
| Caramel Macchiato Nonfat Milk | 1 grande | 230 | 40 | 35 | 0 |
| Caramel Macchiato Soy Milk | 1 grande | 300 | 49 | 36 | 1 |

| FOOD | PORTION | CALS | CARB | SUGAR | FIBER |
|---|---|---|---|---|---|
| Caramel Macchiato Whole Milk | 1 grande | 320 | 37 | 34 | 0 |
| Caramel Mocha Whip Soy Milk | 1 grande | 440 | 68 | 54 | 3 |
| Caramel Apple Cider No Whip | 1 grande | 300 | 72 | 64 | 0 |
| Caramel Apple Cider Whip | 1 grande | 410 | 76 | 68 | 0 |
| Caramel Mocha No Whip Whole Milk | 1 grande | 370 | 61 | 50 | 2 |
| Caramel Mocha Whip Nonfat Milk | 1 grande | 410 | 65 | 52 | 2 |
| Caramel Mocha Whip Whole Milk | 1 grande | 470 | 63 | 52 | 2 |
| Caramel Mocha No Whip Nonfat Milk | 1 grande | 300 | 63 | 51 | 2 |
| Chocolate Nonfat Milk | 1 grande | 240 | 45 | 36 | 2 |
| Chocolate Whole Milk | 1 grande | 340 | 42 | 35 | 2 |
| Cinnamon Spice Mocha No Whip Nonfat Milk | 1 grande | 250 | 47 | 40 | tr |
| Cinnamon Spice Mocha No Whip Whole Milk | 1 grande | 330 | 45 | 45 | tr |
| Cinnamon Spice Mocha Whip Nonfat Milk | 1 grande | 350 | 49 | 41 | tr |
| Cinnamon Spice No Whip Soy Milk | 1 grande | 290 | 51 | 41 | 2 |
| Cinnamon Spice Whip Soy Milk | 1 grande | 390 | 53 | 42 | 2 |
| Espresso Decaf Coffee Of The Week | 1 grande | 10 | 2 | 0 | 0 |
| Frappuccino Blended Coffee | 1 grande | 230 | 46 | 38 | 0 |
| Frappuccino Blended Coffee Mocha Coconut No Whip Whole Milk | 1 grande | 400 | 75 | 60 | 2 |
| Frappuccino Caramel Blended Coffee No Whip | 1 grande | 280 | 57 | 48 | 0 |
| Frappuccino Caramel Blended Coffee Whip | 1 grande | 430 | 61 | 52 | 0 |
| Frappuccino Chocolate Blended Creme No Whip | 1 grande | 400 | 73 | 63 | 1 |
| Frappuccino Chocolate Brownie Blended Coffee No Whip | 1 grande | 370 | 69 | 56 | 2 |
| Frappuccino Chocolate Brownie Blended Coffee Whip | 1 grande | 510 | 72 | 59 | 2 |

| FOOD | PORTION | CALS | CARB | SUGAR | FIBER |
|---|---|---|---|---|---|
| Frappuccino Chocolate Malt Blended Creme Whip | 1 grande | 610 | 90 | 72 | 2 |
| Frappuccino Mocha Blended Coffee No Whip | 1 grande | 290 | 58 | 48 | 0 |
| Frappuccino Mocha Blended Coffee Whip | 1 grande | 420 | 61 | 51 | 0 |
| Frappuccino Mocha Coconut Blended Coffee Whip | 1 grande | 550 | 80 | 64 | 2 |
| Frappuccino Mocha Malt Blended Coffee No Whip | 1 grande | 430 | 91 | 65 | 1 |
| Frappuccino Mocha Malt Blended Coffee Whip | 1 grande | 570 | 95 | 68 | 1 |
| Frappuccino Tazo Chai Creme Blended Tea No Whip | 1 grande | 370 | 69 | 64 | 0 |
| Frappuccino Tazo Chai Creme Blended Tea Whip | 1 grande | 500 | 72 | 66 | 0 |
| Frappuccino Tazoberry Blended Tea | 1 grande | 190 | 49 | 46 | tr |
| Frappuccino Tazoberry Creme Blended Tea No Whip | 1 grande | 330 | 74 | 60 | tr |
| Frappuccino Tazoberry Creme Blended Tea Whip | 1 grande | 460 | 76 | 71 | tr |
| Frappuccino Vanilla Blended Creme No Whip | 1 grande | 350 | 64 | 60 | 0 |
| Frappuccino Vanilla Blended Creme Whip | 1 grande | 480 | 66 | 62 | 0 |
| Frappuccino White Chocolate Mocha Blended Coffee No Whip | 1 grande | 320 | 62 | 54 | 0 |
| Frappuccino White Chocolate Mocha Blended Coffee Whip | 1 grande | 450 | 65 | 56 | 0 |
| Hot Chocolate No Whip Whole Milk | 1 grande | 340 | 42 | 35 | 2 |
| Hot Chocolate No Whip Nonfat Milk | 1 grande | 240 | 45 | 36 | 2 |
| Hot Chocolate Whip Nonfat Milk | 1 grande | 340 | 47 | 37 | 2 |
| Hot Chocolate Whip Whole Milk | 1 grande | 440 | 44 | 37 | 2 |
| Ice Caffe Mocha Whip Whole Milk | 1 grande | 350 | 37 | 27 | 2 |

| FOOD | PORTION | CALS | CARB | SUGAR | FIBER |
|---|---|---|---|---|---|
| Iced Cafe Latte Whole Milk | 1 grande | 160 | 13 | 11 | 0 |
| Iced Cafe Mocha Whip Nonfat Milk | 1 grande | 310 | 38 | 28 | 2 |
| Iced Cafe Mocha Whip Soy Milk | 1 grande | 330 | 40 | 28 | 3 |
| Iced Caffe Americano | 1 grande | 20 | 3 | 0 | 0 |
| Iced Caffe Mocha No Whip Whole Milk | 1 grande | 220 | 35 | 25 | 2 |
| Iced Caffe Latte Nonfat Milk | 1 grande | 100 | 14 | 11 | 0 |
| Iced Caffe Latte Soy Milk | 1 grande | 120 | 17 | 12 | tr |
| Iced Caffe Mocha No Whip Nonfat Milk | 1 grande | 180 | 36 | 26 | 2 |
| Iced Caffe Mocha No Whip Soy Milk | 1 grande | 200 | 38 | 26 | 3 |
| Iced Caramel Macchiato Nonfat Milk | 1 grande | 100 | 36 | 32 | 0 |
| Iced Caramel Macchiato Soy Milk | 1 grande | 230 | 39 | 33 | 1 |
| Iced Caramel Macchiato Whole Milk | 1 grande | 270 | 34 | 31 | 0 |
| Iced Shaken Coffee | 1 grande | 80 | 20 | 19 | 0 |
| Iced Tazo Chai Nonfat Milk | 1 grande | 230 | 50 | 45 | 0 |
| Iced Tazo Chai Whole Milk | 1 grande | 270 | 48 | 45 | 0 |
| Iced White Chocolate Mocha No Whip Soy Milk | 1 grande | 340 | 59 | 53 | tr |
| Iced White Chocolate Mocha No Whip Whole Milk | 1 grande | 360 | 56 | 52 | 0 |
| Iced White Chocolate Mocha Whip Nonfat Milk | 1 grande | 450 | 59 | 55 | 0 |
| Iced White Chocolate Mocha Whip Soy Milk | 1 grande | 470 | 61 | 55 | tr |
| Iced White Chocolate Mocha Whip Whole Milk | 1 grande | 490 | 58 | 54 | 0 |
| Iced White Chocolate No Whip Nonfat Milk | 1 grande | 320 | 57 | 53 | 0 |
| Milk Nonfat | 1 grande | 160 | 23 | 22 | 0 |
| Steamed Apple Cider | 1 grande | 230 | 57 | 52 | 0 |
| Steamed Nonfat Milk | 1 grande | 160 | 23 | 22 | 0 |
| Steamed Whole Milk | 1 grande | 270 | 21 | 21 | 0 |

| FOOD | PORTION | CALS | CARB | SUGAR | FIBER |
|---|---|---|---|---|---|
| Tazo Chai Whole Milk | 1 grande | 290 | 50 | 46 | 0 |
| Tazo Chai Nonfat Milk | 1 grande | 230 | 51 | 47 | 0 |
| Tazo Iced Tea | 1 grande | 80 | 20 | 19 | 0 |
| Tazo Tea Lemonade | 1 grande | 120 | 31 | 29 | 0 |
| Vanilla Creme Whip Nonfat Milk | 1 grande | 340 | 44 | 42 | 0 |
| Vanilla Creme Whip Whole Milk | 1 grande | 440 | 42 | 41 | 0 |
| Vanilla Creme No Whip Nonfat Milk | 1 grande | 240 | 43 | 40 | 0 |
| Vanille Creme No Whip Whole Milk | 1 grande | 340 | 40 | 39 | 0 |
| White Chocolate Mocha No Whip Nonfat Milk | 1 grande | 340 | 58 | 54 | 0 |
| White Chocolate Mocha No Whip Whole Milk | 1 grande | 410 | 56 | 53 | 0 |
| White Chocolate Mocha Whip Nonfat Milk | 1 grande | 440 | 60 | 56 | 0 |
| White Chocolate Mocha Whip Whole Milk | 1 grande | 510 | 58 | 55 | 0 |
| White Chocolate No Whip Soy Milk | 1 grande | 370 | 62 | 55 | 1 |
| White Chocolate Whip Soy Milk | 1 grande | 440 | 65 | 58 | 1 |
| White Hot Chocolate No Whip Nonfat Milk | 1 grande | 390 | 66 | 63 | 0 |
| White Hot Chocolate No Whip Whole Milk | 1 grande | 480 | 63 | 62 | 0 |
| White Hot Chocolate Whip Nonfat Milk | 1 grande | 490 | 68 | 65 | 0 |
| White Hot Chocolate Whip Whole Milk | 1 grande | 580 | 65 | 64 | 0 |
| Whole Milk | 1 grande | 270 | 21 | 21 | 0 |
| **TOPPINGS** | | | | | |
| Caramel | 1 tbsp | 15 | 2 | 2 | 0 |
| Chocolate | 1 tsp | 5 | 1 | 1 | 0 |
| Flavored Sugar Free Syrup | 1 pump | 0 | 0 | 0 | 0 |
| Flavored Syrup | 1 pump | 20 | 5 | 5 | 0 |
| Mocha Syrup | 1 pump | 25 | 6 | 4 | 0 |
| Sprinkles | 1 serv | 0 | tr | tr | 0 |

| FOOD | PORTION | CALS | CARB | SUGAR | FIBER |
|---|---|---|---|---|---|
| **SUBWAY** | | | | | |
| **BEVERAGES** | | | | | |
| Fruizle Smoothie Berry Lishus | 1 sm (13 oz) | 113 | 28 | 27 | 1 |
| Fruizle Smoothie Berry Lishus w/ Banana | 1 sm (17 oz) | 221 | 56 | 27 | 4 |
| Fruizle Smoothie Peach Pizazz | 1 sm (12 oz) | 103 | 26 | 26 | 0 |
| Fruizle Smoothie Pineapple Delight w/ Banana | 1 sm (17 oz) | 241 | 61 | 33 | 4 |
| Fruizle Smoothie Pineapple Delite | 1 sm (13 oz) | 133 | 33 | 33 | 1 |
| Fruizle Smoothie Sunrise Refresher | 1 sm (12 oz) | 119 | 29 | 28 | 1 |
| **COOKIES** | | | | | |
| Chocolate Chip | 1 | 215 | 30 | 18 | 1 |
| Chocolate Chunk | 1 | 217 | 30 | 17 | 1 |
| Double Chocolate | 1 | 209 | 30 | 20 | 1 |
| M&M | 1 | 215 | 30 | 17 | 1 |
| Oatmeal Raisin | 1 | 210 | 30 | 16 | 2 |
| Peanut Butter | 1 | 221 | 26 | 16 | 1 |
| Sugar | 1 | 227 | 28 | 14 | 0 |
| White Macadamia Nut | 1 | 221 | 28 | 17 | 1 |
| **SALAD DRESSINGS** | | | | | |
| Fat Free French | 1 serv (2 oz) | 70 | 17 | 12 | 0 |
| Fat Free Italian | 1 serv (2 oz) | 20 | 4 | 3 | 0 |
| Fat Free Ranch | 1 serv (2 oz) | 60 | 14 | 6 | 0 |
| **SALADS AND SALAD BARS** | | | | | |
| BMT | 1 serv | 275 | 11 | 1 | 3 |
| Cold Cut Trio | 1 serv | 234 | 11 | 1 | 3 |
| Ham | 1 serv | 112 | 11 | 1 | 3 |
| Meatball | 1 serv | 320 | 17 | 2 | 4 |
| Roast Beef | 1 serv | 117 | 10 | 1 | 3 |
| Roasted Chicken Breast | 1 serv | 130 | 9 | 0 | 3 |
| Seafood & Crab | 1 serv | 197 | 17 | 1 | 4 |
| Steak & Cheese | 1 serv | 181 | 12 | 2 | 4 |
| Subway Club | 1 serv | 146 | 12 | 2 | 3 |
| Subway Melt | 1 serv | 203 | 11 | 1 | 3 |
| Tuna | 1 serv | 238 | 10 | 0 | 3 |
| Turkey Breast | 1 serv | 105 | 11 | 1 | 3 |
| Turkey Breast & Ham | 1 serv | 117 | 11 | 1 | 3 |
| Veggie Delight | 1 serv | 50 | 9 | 0 | 3 |

| FOOD | PORTION | CALS | CARB | SUGAR | FIBER |
|---|---|---|---|---|---|
| **SANDWICHES** | | | | | |
| 6 Inch Steak & Cheese | 1 | 362 | 41 | 7 | 4 |
| 6 Inch Subway Melt | 1 | 384 | 40 | 6 | 3 |
| 6 Inch Sub BMT | 1 | 456 | 40 | 6 | 3 |
| 6 Inch Sub Cold Cut Trio | 1 | 415 | 40 | 5 | 3 |
| 6 Inch Sub Ham | 1 | 261 | 39 | 6 | 3 |
| 6 Inch Sub Meatball | 1 | 501 | 46 | 7 | 4 |
| 6 Inch Sub Roast Beef | 1 | 267 | 39 | 6 | 3 |
| 6 Inch Sub Roasted Chicken Breast | 1 | 291 | 40 | 6 | 3 |
| 6 Inch Sub Seafood & Crab | 1 | 378 | 46 | 6 | 3 |
| 6 Inch Sub Subway Club | 1 | 296 | 40 | 6 | 3 |
| 6 Inch Sub Tuna | 1 | 419 | 39 | 5 | 3 |
| 6 Inch Sub Turkey Breast | 1 | 254 | 39 | 5 | 3 |
| 6 Inch Sub Turkey Breast & Ham | 1 | 267 | 40 | 5 | 3 |
| 6 Inch Sub Veggie Delight | 1 | 200 | 37 | 4 | 3 |
| American Cheese Triangles | 2 | 41 | 0 | 0 | 0 |
| Asiago Caesar Sauce | 1.5 tbsp | 110 | 2 | 1 | 0 |
| Bacon Strips | 2 | 45 | 0 | 0 | 0 |
| Breakfast Bacon & Egg | 1 | 321 | 34 | 3 | 3 |
| Breakfast Cheese & Egg | 1 | 317 | 34 | 3 | 3 |
| Breakfast Ham & Egg | 1 | 338 | 34 | 4 | 3 |
| Breakfast Western Egg | 1 | 300 | 36 | 3 | 3 |
| Cheddar Triangles | 2 | 59 | 0 | 0 | 0 |
| Cucumber Slices | 3 | 2 | 0 | 0 | 0 |
| Deli Ham | 1 | 210 | 35 | 3 | 3 |
| Deli Roast Beef | 1 | 223 | 35 | 3 | 3 |
| Deli Tuna | 1 | 325 | 36 | 2 | 3 |
| Deli Turkey Breast | 1 | 215 | 36 | 3 | 3 |
| Deli Style Roll | 1 | 165 | 32 | 2 | 3 |
| Dijon Horseradish | 1.5 tbsp | 91 | 1 | 0 | 0 |
| Dijon Horseradish Melt | 6 inch | 465 | 47 | 67 | 4 |
| Fat Free Red Wine Vinaigrette | 1.5 tbsp | 29 | 6 | 3 | 0 |
| Fat Free Sweet Onion | 1.5 tbsp | 38 | 9 | 8 | 0 |
| Green Pepper Strips | 3 (0.2 oz) | 2 | 0 | 0 | 0 |
| Hearty Italian Bread | 6 inch | 207 | 41 | 5 | 3 |
| Honey Mustard | 1.5 tbsp | 28 | 7 | 6 | 0 |
| Honey Mustard Ham | 6 inch | 311 | 52 | 12 | 4 |
| Honey Oat Bread | 6 inch | 249 | 48 | 9 | 4 |

| FOOD | PORTION | CALS | CARB | SUGAR | FIBER |
|---|---|---|---|---|---|
| Italian Bread | 6 inch | 178 | 33 | 4 | 2 |
| Lettuce | 1 serv (0.7 oz) | 3 | 0 | 0 | 0 |
| Mayonnaise | 1 tbsp | 111 | 0 | 0 | 0 |
| Mayonnaise Light | 1 tbsp | 46 | 1 | 0 | 0 |
| Monterey Cheddar Bread | 6 inch | 235 | 39 | 5 | 3 |
| Mustard | 2 tsp | 7 | 1 | 0 | 0 |
| Olive Oil Blend | 1 tsp | 45 | 0 | 0 | 0 |
| Olive Rings | 3 (3 g) | 3 | 0 | 0 | 0 |
| Onions | 1 serv (0.5oz) | 5 | 1 | 0 | 0 |
| Parmesan Oregano Bread | 6 inch | 211 | 40 | 5 | 3 |
| Pepperjack Cheese Triangles | 2 | 40 | 0 | 0 | 0 |
| Pickle Chips | 3 pieces (0.3 oz) | 1 | 0 | 0 | 0 |
| Provolone Circles | 2 havles | 51 | 0 | 0 | 0 |
| Red Wine Vinaigrette Club | 6 inch | 350 | 53 | 9 | 4 |
| Roasted Garlic Bread | 6 inch | 225 | 45 | 7 | 4 |
| Sourdough Bread | 6 inch | 208 | 41 | 2 | 3 |
| Southwest Sauce | 1.5 tbsp | 86 | 2 | 1 | 0 |
| Southwest Turkey Bacon | 6 inch | 407 | 48 | 7 | 4 |
| Sweet Onion Chicken Teriyaki | 6 inch | 374 | 59 | 17 | 4 |
| Swiss Triangles | 2 | 53 | 0 | 0 | 0 |
| Tomato Slices | 3 (1.2 oz) | 7 | 2 | 0 | 0 |
| Vinegar | 1 tsp | 1 | 0 | 0 | 0 |
| Wheat Sub | 6 inch | 186 | 36 | 5 | 3 |
| Wrap Chicken Bacon Ranch w/ Swiss | 1 | 480 | 19 | – | – |
| Wrap Turkey Bacon Melt | 1 | 430 | 22 | – | – |
| **SOUPS** | | | | | |
| Black Bean | 1 cup | 180 | 27 | 4 | 15 |
| Brown & Wild Rice w/ Chicken | 1 cup | 190 | 17 | 3 | 2 |
| Cheese w/ Ham & Bacon | 1 cup | 230 | 13 | 4 | 2 |
| Chicken & Dumplings | 1 cup | 130 | 16 | 2 | 1 |
| Cream Of Broccoli | 1 cup | 130 | 12 | 5 | 1 |
| Cream Of Potato w/ Bacon | 1 cup | 210 | 20 | 3 | 4 |
| Golden Broccoli Cheese | 1 cup | 180 | 12 | 4 | 9 |
| Hearty Chili Beef | 1 cup | 250 | 31 | 9 | 9 |
| Minestrone | 1 cup | 70 | 11 | 2 | 0 |
| New England Clam Chowder | 1 cup | 140 | 19 | 2 | 1 |
| Potato Cheese Chowder | 1 cup | 210 | 22 | 3 | 2 |
| Roasted Chicken Noodle | 1 cup | 90 | 7 | 1 | 1 |

| FOOD | PORTION | CALS | CARB | SUGAR | FIBER |
|---|---|---|---|---|---|
| Tomato Bisque | 1 cup | 90 | 15 | 7 | 3 |
| Vegetable Beef | 1 cup | 90 | 14 | 4 | 2 |

## TACO CABANA

| FOOD | PORTION | CALS | CARB | SUGAR | FIBER |
|---|---|---|---|---|---|
| Black Beans | 1 serv (4 oz) | 111 | 21 | – | – |
| Borracho Beans | 1 serv (4 oz) | 108 | 17 | – | – |
| Breakfast Taco Bacon & Egg | 1 | 246 | 22 | – | – |
| Breakfast Taco Barbacoa | 1 | 307 | 2 | – | – |
| Breakfast Taco Chorizo & Egg | 1 | 248 | 22 | – | – |
| Breakfast Taco Potato & Egg | 1 | 234 | 27 | – | – |
| Burrito Bean & Cheese | 1 | 710 | 85 | – | – |
| Burrito Beef | 1 | 653 | 76 | – | – |
| Burrito Black Bean | 1 | 559 | 95 | – | – |
| Burrito Chicken | 1 | 665 | 74 | – | – |
| Calabacita | 1 serv (4 oz) | 78 | 6 | – | – |
| Chips | 1 serv (2 oz) | 285 | 36 | – | – |
| Elotes | 1 | 220 | 26 | – | – |
| Fajitas Beef | 1 serv (4 oz) | 245 | 3 | – | – |
| Fajitas Chicken Dark | 1 serv (4 oz) | 236 | 2 | – | – |
| Fajitas Chicken White | 1 serv (4 oz) | 191 | 3 | – | – |
| Grilled Chicken Dark | 1 serv (4.5 oz) | 298 | 1 | – | – |
| Grilled Chicken Dark No Skin | 1 serv (3.4 oz) | 170 | 1 | – | – |
| Grilled Chicken White | 1 serv (5 oz) | 295 | 1 | – | – |
| Grilled Chicken White No Skin | 1 serv (3.8 oz) | 167 | tr | – | – |
| Guacamole | 1 serv (1 oz) | 48 | 2 | – | – |
| Queso | 1 serv (3 oz) | 184 | 7 | – | – |
| Refried Beans | 1 serv (4 oz) | 171 | 21 | – | – |
| Sour Cream | 1 serv (1 oz) | 57 | 1 | – | – |
| Spanish Rice | 1 serv (4 oz) | 181 | 30 | – | – |
| Taco Bean & Cheese | 1 | 292 | 35 | – | – |
| Taco Black Bean | 1 | 216 | 37 | – | – |
| Taco Carne Guisada | 1 | 202 | 20 | – | – |
| Taco Crispy Beef | 1 | 148 | 13 | – | – |
| Taco Soft Chicken | 1 | 217 | 21 | – | – |
| Tortilla Corn | 1 6-inch | 70 | 11 | – | – |
| Tortilla Flour | 1 6-inch | 129 | 22 | – | – |
| Tortilla Soup | 1 lg | 371 | 32 | – | – |
| Tortilla Soup | 1 sm | 249 | 26 | – | – |

| FOOD | PORTION | CALS | CARB | SUGAR | FIBER |
|---|---|---|---|---|---|
| **TGI FRIDAY'S** | | | | | |
| Sizzling Chicken & Broccoli | 1 serv | 700 | 15 | – | – |
| Sizzling NY Strip Steak w/ Blue Cheese & Broccoli | 1 serv | 684 | 15 | – | – |
| **TIM HORTONS** | | | | | |
| **BAGELS AND CREAM CHEESE** | | | | | |
| Blueberry | 1 | 200 | 59 | 10 | 3 |
| Cinnamon Raisin | 1 | 300 | 58 | 12 | 4 |
| Cream Cheese | 1.5 oz | 150 | 7 | 7 | 0 |
| Cream Cheese | 1.5 oz | 150 | 3 | 1 | 0 |
| Cream Cheese Light | 1.5 oz | 90 | 3 | 3 | 0 |
| Cream Cheese Plain | 1.5 oz | 140 | 1 | 1 | 0 |
| Everything | 1 | 300 | 57 | 8 | 3 |
| Multigrain | 1 | 300 | 58 | 8 | 6 |
| Onion | 1 | 295 | 58 | 8 | 3 |
| Plain | 1 | 290 | 57 | 8 | 3 |
| Poppy Seed | 1 | 300 | 58 | 8 | 4 |
| Sesame Seed | 1 | 300 | 57 | 7 | 4 |
| Whole Wheat & Honey | 1 | 300 | 59 | 11 | 6 |
| **BAKED SELECTIONS** | | | | | |
| Biscuit Southern Country Cranberry | 1 | 470 | 68 | 21 | 2 |
| Biscuit Southern Country Raspberry | 1 | 470 | 68 | 19 | 2 |
| Cake Black Forest | 1 serv | 500 | 75 | 44 | 3 |
| Cake Celebration | 1 serv | 500 | 85 | 56 | 1 |
| Cake Chocolot Fantasy | 1 serv | 420 | 72 | 51 | 3 |
| Cake Shadow | 1 serv | 430 | 63 | 43 | 2 |
| Cookie Macaroon | 1 | 140 | 14 | 11 | 3 |
| Cookie Oatcakes | 1 | 190 | 22 | 10 | 1 |
| Cookie Oatmeal Raisin | 1 | 150 | 22 | 13 | 1 |
| Cookie Peanut Butter Chocolate Chunk | 1 | 170 | 18 | 11 | 1 |
| Croissant Butter | 1 | 210 | 25 | 3 | 1 |
| Croissant Cheese | 1 | 240 | 27 | 3 | 1 |
| Danish Cherry Cheese | 1 | 380 | 33 | 11 | 1 |
| Donut Apple Fritter | 1 | 300 | 40 | 14 | 2 |
| Donut Chocolate Dip | 1 | 230 | 33 | 11 | 0 |
| Donut Chocolate Glazed | 1 | 360 | 36 | 19 | 1 |

| FOOD | PORTION | CALS | CARB | SUGAR | FIBER |
|---|---|---|---|---|---|
| Donut Dutchie | 1 | 280 | 39 | 18 | 1 |
| Donut Honey Dip | 1 | 230 | 32 | 10 | 0 |
| Donut Maple Dip | 1 | 250 | 36 | 15 | 0 |
| Donut Old Fashion Glazed | 1 | 270 | 39 | 22 | 0 |
| Donut Old Fashion Plain | 1 | 220 | 24 | 8 | 0 |
| Donut Sour Cream Plain | 1 | 280 | 25 | 11 | 0 |
| Donut Sugar Twist | 1 | 230 | 32 | 9 | 0 |
| Donut Walnut Crunch | 1 | 320 | 36 | 17 | 2 |
| Donut Filled Angel Cream | 1 | 280 | 36 | 15 | 0 |
| Donut Filled Blueberry | 1 | 220 | 33 | 11 | 0 |
| Donut Filled Boston Cream | 1 | 230 | 36 | 13 | 0 |
| Donut Filled Canadian Maple | 1 | 230 | 36 | 13 | 0 |
| Donut Filled Strawberry | 1 | 220 | 33 | 10 | 0 |
| Donuts Honey Stick | 1 | 280 | 34 | 13 | 0 |
| Muffin Blueberry Bran | 1 | 300 | 51 | 21 | 5 |
| Muffin Carrot Whole Wheat | 1 | 410 | 52 | 24 | 4 |
| Muffin Chocolate Chip | 1 | 390 | 62 | 32 | 2 |
| Muffin Oatbran 'n Apple | 1 | 350 | 58 | 24 | 4 |
| Muffin Oatbran Carrot 'n Raisin | 1 | 340 | 57 | 26 | 4 |
| Muffin Oatmeal Raisin | 1 | 430 | 80 | 48 | 3 |
| Muffin Raisin Bran | 1 | 380 | 66 | 36 | 6 |
| Muffin Wild Blueberry | 1 | 330 | 54 | 27 | 2 |
| Muffin Low Fat Carrot | 1 | 260 | 60 | 30 | 6 |
| Muffin Low Fat Cranberry | 1 | 260 | 60 | 30 | 6 |
| Muffin Low Fat Honey | 1 | 290 | 66 | 33 | 6 |
| Pie Apple | 1 serv | 540 | 62 | 26 | 3 |
| Pie Banana Cream | 1 serv | 440 | 50 | 21 | 1 |
| Pie Cherry | 1 serv | 570 | 70 | 35 | 2 |
| Pie Chocolate Cream | 1 serv | 490 | 52 | 23 | 1 |
| Tart Fresh Strawberry | 1 serv | 220 | 36 | 10 | 2 |
| Tart Raisin Butter | 1 serv | 330 | 54 | 25 | 1 |
| Tea Biscuit Plain | 1 | 220 | 36 | 3 | 1 |
| Tea Biscuit Raisin | 1 | 250 | 47 | 15 | 2 |
| Timbits Chocolate Glazed | 1 | 70 | 9 | 5 | 0 |
| Timbits Dutchie | 1 | 60 | 10 | 5 | 0 |
| Timbits Honey Dip | 1 | 50 | 10 | 3 | 0 |
| Timbits Old Fashion Plain | 1 | 45 | 7 | 2 | 0 |
| Timbits Filled Banana Cream | 1 | 45 | 8 | 2 | 0 |
| Timbits Filled Lemon | 1 | 50 | 9 | 3 | 0 |

| FOOD | PORTION | CALS | CARB | SUGAR | FIBER |
|---|---|---|---|---|---|
| Timbits Filled Spiced Apple | 1 | 80 | 9 | 3 | 0 |
| Timbits Filled Strawberry | 1 | 50 | 9 | 3 | 0 |
| **BEVERAGES** | | | | | |
| Apple Juice | 1 (9 oz) | 140 | 36 | 34 | 0 |
| Cafe Mocha | 1 (10 oz) | 250 | 34 | 3 | 0 |
| Cappuccino English Toffee | 1 (10 oz) | 130 | 20 | 16 | 0 |
| Cappuccino French Vanilla | 1 (10 oz) | 130 | 20 | 16 | 0 |
| Cappuccino Iced | 1 (16 oz) | 430 | 54 | 52 | 0 |
| Chocolate Milk | 1 (14 oz) | 280 | 46 | 39 | 0 |
| Coffee Decaffeinated + Sugar & Cream | 1 (10 oz) | 80 | 10 | 10 | 0 |
| Coffee + Sugar & Cream | 1 (10 oz) | 80 | 10 | 10 | 0 |
| Coke | 1 (14 oz) | 170 | 44 | 44 | 0 |
| Diet Coke | 1 (14 oz) | 1 | 0 | 0 | 0 |
| Fruit Punch | 1 (10 oz) | 150 | 38 | 36 | 0 |
| Hot Chocolate | 1 (10 oz) | 200 | 44 | 43 | 0 |
| Iced Tea | 1 (14 oz) | 130 | 34 | 34 | 0 |
| Milk 2% | 1 (14 oz) | 210 | 20 | 20 | 0 |
| Orange Juice | 1 (10 oz) | 140 | 36 | 33 | 0 |
| Sprite | 1 (14 oz) | 160 | 41 | 41 | 0 |
| Tea + Sugar & Milk | 1 (10 oz) | 45 | 9 | 9 | 0 |
| **SANDWICHES** | | | | | |
| Albacore Tuna Salad | 1 serv | 350 | 49 | 50 | 3 |
| Black Forest Ham & Swiss | 1 serv | 640 | 53 | 4 | 2 |
| Chunky Chicken Salad | 1 serv | 380 | 50 | 6 | 3 |
| Fireside Roast Beef | 1 serv | 470 | 48 | 4 | 2 |
| Garden Vegetable | 1 serv | 460 | 50 | 6 | 3 |
| Harvest Turkey Breast | 1 serv | 470 | 53 | 4 | 2 |
| **SOUPS** | | | | | |
| Barley & Wild Rice | 1 serv | 120 | 22 | 1 | 1 |
| Chicken Noodle | 1 serv | 100 | 15 | 4 | 1 |
| Chili | 1 serv | 320 | 32 | 10 | 8 |
| Cream Of Broccoli | 1 serv | 190 | 27 | 9 | 1 |
| Cream of Mushroom | 1 serv | 195 | 21 | 4 | 1 |
| Hearty Vegetable | 1 serv | 130 | 27 | 4 | 2 |
| Minestrone | 1 serv | 125 | 25 | 4 | 2 |
| Potato Bacon | 1 serv | 195 | 29 | 3 | 1 |
| Vegetable Beef Barley | 1 serv | 110 | 14 | 5 | 2 |

| FOOD | PORTION | CALS | CARB | SUGAR | FIBER |
|---|---|---|---|---|---|
| **TOGO'S** | | | | | |
| **SALAD DRESSINGS** | | | | | |
| 1000 Island | 1 serv (2.3 oz) | 231 | 9 | – | 0 |
| Caesar | 1 serv (2.3 oz) | 241 | 8 | – | 0 |
| Oriental | 1 serv (2.3 oz) | 221 | 24 | – | 0 |
| Ranch | 1 serv (2.3 oz) | 321 | 5 | – | 0 |
| Reduced Calorie Italian | 1 serv (2.3 oz) | 60 | 4 | – | 0 |
| Reduced Calorie Ranch | 1 serv (2.3 oz) | 191 | 10 | – | 0 |
| **SALADS AND SALAD BARS** | | | | | |
| Caesar Salad | 1 serv | 471 | 23 | – | 2 |
| Garden Salad | 1 serv | 256 | 31 | – | 2 |
| Oriental Salad | 1 serv | 499 | 49 | – | 3 |
| Taco Salad | 1 serv | 943 | 76 | – | 11 |
| **SANDWICHES** | | | | | |
| Albacore Tuna | 1 sm | 701 | 78 | – | 3 |
| Avocado & Turkey | 1 sm | 675 | 80 | – | 6 |
| Avocado Cucumber & Alfalfa Sprouts | 1 sm | 637 | 85 | – | 7 |
| Bar-B-Q Beef | 1 sm | 724 | 94 | – | 3 |
| California Roasted Chicken | 1 sm | 510 | 73 | – | 3 |
| Cheese Swiss American Provolone | 1 sm | 859 | 77 | – | 3 |
| Chunky Chicken Salad | 1 sm | 636 | 72 | – | 3 |
| Egg Salad w/ Cheese | 1 sm | 728 | 76 | – | 3 |
| Ham & Cheese | 1 sm | 661 | 76 | – | 3 |
| Hot Pastrami | 1 sm | 705 | 85 | – | 3 |
| Hummus | 1 sm | 668 | 102 | – | 4 |
| Italian Salami & Cheese | 1 sm | 770 | 78 | – | 3 |
| Italian Salami Capicolla Mortadella Cotto & Provolone | 1 sm | 736 | 74 | – | 3 |
| Meatballs w/ Pizza Sauce & Parmesan | 1 sm | 707 | 78 | – | 4 |
| Pastrami Reuben | 1 sm | 875 | 85 | – | 2 |
| Roast Beef Hot & Cold | 1 sm | 552 | 73 | – | 3 |
| Turkey & Cranberry | 1 sm | 623 | 96 | – | 4 |
| Turkey & Bacon Club | 1 sm | 667 | 73 | – | 3 |
| Turkey & Cheese | 1 sm | 638 | 75 | – | 3 |
| Turkey & Ham w/ Cheese | 1 sm | 670 | 76 | – | 3 |

| FOOD | PORTION | CALS | CARB | SUGAR | FIBER |
|---|---|---|---|---|---|
| **WENDY'S** | | | | | |
| **BEVERAGES** | | | | | |
| Cola | 11 oz | 130 | 36 | 36 | 0 |
| Diet Cola | 11 oz | 0 | 0 | 0 | 0 |
| Frosty Junior | 6 oz | 170 | 26 | 21 | 0 |
| Frosty Medium | 16 oz | 440 | 73 | 56 | 0 |
| Frosty Small | 12 oz | 330 | 56 | 43 | 0 |
| Lemon-Lime Soda | 11 oz | 130 | 34 | 34 | 0 |
| **CHILDREN'S MENU SELECTIONS** | | | | | |
| French Fries Kid's Meal | 1 serv (3.2 oz) | 270 | 35 | 0 | 3 |
| Kid's Meal Cheeseburger | 1 (4.2 oz) | 310 | 33 | 6 | 2 |
| Kid's Meal Hamburger | 1 (3.9 oz) | 270 | 33 | 6 | 1 |
| Kids'Meal Chicken Nuggets | 4 pieces (2.1 oz) | 190 | 9 | 0 | 0 |
| **MAIN MENU SELECTIONS** | | | | | |
| ¼ lb Hamburger Patty | 1 (2.6 oz) | 200 | 0 | 0 | 0 |
| 2 Oz Hamburger Patty | 1 (1.3 oz) | 100 | 0 | 0 | 0 |
| American Cheese | 1 slice (0.6 oz) | 70 | 0 | 0 | 0 |
| American Cheese Jr. | 1 slice (0.4 oz) | 45 | 0 | 0 | 0 |
| Bacon | 1 strip (4 g) | 20 | 0 | 0 | 0 |
| Big Bacon Classic | 1 (9.9 oz) | 580 | 46 | 10 | 3 |
| Breaded Chicken Fillet | 1 (3.5 oz) | 230 | 13 | 0 | 0 |
| Cheddar Shredded | 2 tbsp (0.6 oz) | 70 | 1 | 0 | 0 |
| Chicken Breast Filet Sandwich | 1 (7.3 oz) | 430 | 46 | 6 | 2 |
| Chicken Club Sandwich | 1 (7.6 oz) | 470 | 47 | 6 | 2 |
| Chicken Nuggets | 5 pieces (2.6 oz) | 230 | 11 | 0 | 0 |
| Chili | 1 sm (8 oz) | 210 | 21 | 5 | 5 |
| Chili | 1 lg (12 oz) | 310 | 32 | 8 | 7 |
| Classic Single w/ Everything | 1 (7.6 oz) | 410 | 37 | 6 | 2 |
| French Fries | 1 Great Biggie (6.7 oz) | 570 | 73 | 1 | 7 |
| French Fries | 1 Biggie (5.6 oz) | 470 | 61 | 0 | 6 |
| French Fries | 1 med (5 oz) | 420 | 50 | 0 | 5 |
| Grilled Chicken Fillet | 1 (2.9 oz) | 110 | 1 | 0 | 0 |
| Grilled Chicken Sandwich | 1 (6.6 oz) | 300 | 36 | 8 | 2 |
| Honey Mustard Reduced Calorie | 1 tsp (7 g) | 25 | 2 | 2 | 0 |
| Hot Stuffed Baked Potato Plain | 1 (10 oz) | 310 | 72 | 5 | 6 |

| FOOD | PORTION | CALS | CARB | SUGAR | FIBER |
|---|---|---|---|---|---|
| Hot Stuffed Baked Potato Bacon & Cheese | 1 (12.6 oz) | 530 | 78 | 5 | 7 |
| Hot Stuffed Baked Potato Broccoli & Cheese | 1 (14.4 oz) | 470 | 80 | 6 | 9 |
| Jr. Bacon Cheeseburger | 1 (5.8 oz) | 380 | 34 | 5 | 2 |
| Jr. Cheeseburger | 1 (4.5 oz) | 310 | 34 | 6 | 2 |
| Jr. Cheeseburger Deluxe | 1 (6.3 oz) | 360 | 36 | 7 | 2 |
| Kaiser Bun | 1 (2.5 oz) | 200 | 38 | 6 | 2 |
| Ketchup | 1 tsp (7 g) | 10 | 2 | 1 | 0 |
| Lettuce | 1 leaf (0.5 oz) | 0 | 0 | 0 | 0 |
| Mayonnaise | 1½ tsp (9 g) | 30 | 1 | 0 | 0 |
| Mustard | ½ tsp (5 g) | 5 | 0 | 0 | 0 |
| Nuggets Sauce Barbeque | 1 pkg (1 oz) | 45 | 10 | 7 | 0 |
| Nuggets Sauce Honey Mustard | 1 pkg (1 oz) | 130 | 6 | 5 | 0 |
| Nuggets Sauce Sweet & Sour | 1 pkg (1 oz) | 50 | 12 | 10 | 0 |
| Onion | 4 rings (0.5 oz) | 5 | 1 | 1 | 0 |
| Pickles | 4 slices (0.4 oz) | 0 | 0 | 0 | 0 |
| Saltines | 2 (0.2 oz) | 25 | 4 | 0 | 0 |
| Sandwich Bun | 1 (2 oz) | 160 | 31 | 4 | 1 |
| Spicy Chicken Fillet | 1 (3.6 oz) | 210 | 10 | 0 | 0 |
| Spicy Chicken Sandwich | 1 (7.5 oz) | 410 | 43 | 5 | 2 |
| Tomatoes | 1 slice (0.9 oz) | 5 | 1 | 1 | 1 |
| Whipped Margarine | 1 pkg (0.5 oz) | 70 | 0 | 0 | 0 |
| **SALAD DRESSINGS** | | | | | |
| Blue Cheese | 1 pkg (2 oz) | 360 | 1 | 0 | 0 |
| French | 1 pkg (2 oz) | 250 | 13 | 11 | 0 |
| Hidden Valley Ranch | 1 pkg (2 oz) | 200 | 3 | 1 | 0 |
| Hidden Valley Ranch Reduced Fat Reduced Calorie | 1 pkg (2 oz) | 120 | 4 | 1 | 0 |
| Italian Reduced Fat Reduced Calorie | 1 pkg (2 oz) | 80 | 6 | 4 | 0 |
| Italian Caesar | 1 pkg (1.5 oz) | 230 | 1 | 0 | 0 |
| Thousand Island | 1 pkg (2 oz) | 260 | 7 | 6 | 0 |
| **SALADS AND SALAD BARS** | | | | | |
| Ceasar Side Salad w/o Dressing | 1 (3.2 oz) | 110 | 6 | 1 | 1 |
| Deluxe Garden Salad w/o Dressing | 1 (9.5 oz) | 110 | 10 | 5 | 4 |

| FOOD | PORTION | CALS | CARB | SUGAR | FIBER |
|---|---|---|---|---|---|
| Grilled Chicken Salad w/o Dressing | 1 (11.9 oz) | 200 | 10 | 5 | 4 |
| Side Salad w/o Dressing | 1 (5.4 oz) | 60 | 5 | 2 | 2 |
| Soft Breadstick | 1 (1.5 oz) | 130 | 23 | – | 1 |
| Taco Chips | 15 (1.5 oz) | 210 | 28 | 0 | 2 |
| Taco Salad w/o Dressing | 1 (16.4 oz) | 380 | 28 | 8 | 8 |